MACLEOD'S
CLINICAL EXAMINATION

EDITED BY

Graham Douglas BSc(Hons) MB ChB FRCPE

Consultant Physician
Aberdeen Royal Infirmary
Honorary Reader in Medicine
University of Aberdeen

Fiona Nicol BSc(Hons) MB BS FRCGP FRCPE

GP Principal and Trainer
Stockbridge Health Centre, Edinburgh
Assistant Director (General Practice Education)
Lister Postgraduate Institute, Edinburgh
Honorary Senior Lecturer
University of Edinburgh

Colin Robertson BA(Hons) MB ChB FRCPE FRCS(Ed) FFAEM

Consultant and Honorary Professor in Emergency Medicine
Royal Infirmary of Edinburgh

ILLUSTRATED BY ROBERT BRITTON

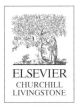

ELSEVIER
CHURCHILL
LIVINGSTONE

EDINBURGH LONDON NEW YORK OXFORD PHILADELPHIA ST LOUIS
SYDNEY TORONTO 2005

MACLEOD'S
CLINICAL EXAMINATION

EXAMINATION

ELEVENTH EDITION

ELSEVIER
CHURCHILL
LIVINGSTONE

First edition 1964
Second edition 1967
Third edition 1973
Fourth edition 1976
Fifth edition 1979
Sixth edition 1983
Seventh edition 1986
Eighth edition 1990
Ninth edition 1995
Tenth edition 2000
Eleventh edition 2005

ISBN 0443074046
International Student Edition 0443074054

British Library Cataloguing in Publication Data
A catalogue record for this book is available from the British Library

Library of Congress Cataloging in Publication Data
A catalog record for this book is available from the Library of Congress

Note
Medical knowledge is constantly changing. Standard safety precautions must be followed, but as new research and clinical experience broaden our knowledge, changes in treatment and drug therapy may become necessary or appropriate. Readers are advised to check the most current product information provided by the manufacturer of each drug to be administered to verify the recommended dose, the method and duration of administration, and contraindications. It is the responsibility of the practitioner, relying on experience and knowledge of the patient, to determine dosages and the best treatment for each individual patient. Neither the publisher nor the editors assumes any liability for any injury and/or damage to persons or property arising from this publication.
The Publisher

The publisher's policy is to use **paper manufactured from sustainable forests**

Printed in Spain

Commissioning Editor: Laurence Hunter
Project Development Manager: Helen Leng
Project Manager: Nancy Arnott
Designer: Erik Bigland

Preface

The skills involved in history taking and physical examination are central to the practice of clinical medicine despite diagnostic and therapeutic advances. This book describes these and is intended primarily for medical undergraduates who often have patient contact from their first days of study. It should also be of value to primary care and postgraduate hospital doctors, particularly those studying for higher clinical examinations or returning to a clinical environment after a period of research or specialized study. Nurse practitioners and other paramedical staff are involved increasingly in medical assessment and we hope that the book will provide a reference for them.

Medical education is changing. Much clinical teaching now occurs in general practice as well as in hospital and this is reflected in the new editorial team and contributors. Because English has no epicene third person pronoun, we have used the male pronoun in the book to aid clarity. Please be assured that this does not reflect any prejudice on our part.

The book has three sections: the first details the principles of history taking, general examination and the external features of disease. Chapters 3 to 10 are systems based. Chapters 11 and 12 are entirely new and cover specialized areas. Objective Structured Clinical Examination (OSCE) panels will assist with revision and the key points at the end of each chapter distil clinical experience.

We have made significant changes to the structure and content of the systems chapters. The gastrointestinal, renal and reproductive systems are now separate chapters reflecting trends in current teaching. The examination of the eye is incorporated into the nervous system as it is an integral part of that examination. Examination of the ear, nose and throat is a new chapter.

The two new chapters in Section 3 relate to the patient as a whole. The first outlines the examination of babies and children, while the second covers the approach to the critically ill patient. Both chapters emphasize an integrated and structured approach to these patients.

This edition contains more figures, diagrams and photographs than its predecessors. This is partly in response to feedback from readers. It is clear that many students find reading text laborious and information is often more easily assimilated pictorially. Clinical acumen is also, at least in part, based on pattern recognition. We have used line drawings to illustrate surface anatomy and techniques of examination, and photographs to show normal and abnormal clinical appearances.

Evidence-based medicine has become a mantra. This approach has yielded significant dividends for investigative techniques and therapeutics. The evidence-base for much of clinical examination is, however, scanty. We have tried to exclude techniques of little clinical value and excessively rare features. While recognizing the merits of anecdote and individual clinical experience, we are surprised at the lack of a rigorous evaluation of many clinical symptoms and signs. This offers challenges and opportunities. It is possible to open this book at almost any page and find a topic which is crying out for evidence-based analysis. We hope that one function of the book will be to stimulate this enquiry and we would be delighted to receive these results and incorporate them in future editions.

We are delighted that this edition of *Macleod's Clinical Examination* – full text and illustrations – will, for the first time, be available in an online version, as part of Elsevier's 'Student Consult' electronic library. This major development in the book's history will put it at the forefront of electronic initiatives in clinical practice.

This 11th edition of *Macleod's Clinical Examination* continues to be closely integrated with *Davidson's Principles and Practice of Medicine*, and is best read in conjunction with that text.

The Editors

v

Picture and table credits

We are grateful to the following individuals and organizations for permission to reproduce the figures and tables listed below:

Chapter 2
Fig. 2.28A–D Forbes CD, Jackson WF. Color Atlas of Clinical Medicine, 3rd edn. Edinburgh: Mosby; 2003.

Chapter 3
Figs 3.6 and **3.9** Haslett C, Chilvers ER, Boon NA, Colledge NR, eds. Davidson's Principles and Practice of Medicine. 19th edn. Edinburgh: Churchill Livingstone; 2002. **Figs 3.8, 3.16A–D** and **3.40** Forbes CD, Jackson WF. Color Atlas of Clinical Medicine. 3rd edn. Edinburgh: Mosby; 2003.

Chapter 6
Fig. 6.8 Pitkin J, Peattie AB, Magowan BA. Obstetrics and Gynaecology An Illustrated Colour Text. Edinburgh: Churchill Livingstone; 2003. **Figs 6.9A&B** Haslett C, Chilvers ER, Boon NA, Colledge NR, eds. Davidson's Principles and Practice of Medicine. 19th edn. Edinburgh: Churchill Livingstone; 2002.

Chapter 8
Figs 8.16A&B Forbes CD, Jackson WF. Color Atlas of Clinical Medicine. 3rd edn. Edinburgh: Mosby; 2003. **Fig. 8.19** Nicholl D, ed. Clinical Neurology. Edinburgh: Churchill Livingstone; 2003. **Figs 8.23A–D** and **8.40** Epstein O, Perkin GD, de Bono DP, Cookson J. Clinical Examination. 2nd edn. London: Mosby; 1997.

Chapter 9
Figs 9.4 and **9.6A** Dhillon RS, East CA. Ear, Nose and Throat and Head and Neck Surgery An Illustrated Colour Text. Edinburgh: Churchill Livingstone; 1994. **Figs 9.5, 9.6B, 9.6C, 9.11, 9.16, 9.17** and **9.25** Bull TR Color Atlas of ENT Diagnosis. 3rd edn. London: Mosby-Wolfe; 1995.

Chapter 10
Figs 10.3 and **10.9** Haslett C, Chilvers ER, Boon NA, Colledge NR, eds. Davidson's Principles and Practice of Medicine. 19th edn. Edinburgh: Churchill Livingstone; 2002. **Figs 10.8A** and **10.11B** Forbes CD, Jackson WF. Color Atlas of Clinical Medicine. 3rd edn. Edinburgh: Mosby; 2003. **Fig. 10.12** J Gibson.

Chapter 11
Figs 11.7, 11.8, 11.10A&B, 11.12 and **11.24** Lissauer T, Clayden G. Illustrated Textbook of Paediatrics. 2nd edn. Edinburgh: Mosby; 2001. **Fig. 11.18** Child Growth Foundation. **Fig. 11.19** Dr Jack Beattie, Royal Hospital for Sick Children, Glasgow. **Table 11.13** Dr Barry McCormick, Children's Hearing Assessment Centre, Nottingham.

Chapter 12
Figs 12.9 and **12.10** European Resuscitation Council. **Table 12.1** Adapted from Hillman K, Parr M, Flabouris A *et al* 2001 Redefining in-hospital resuscitation: the concept of the medical emergency team. Resuscitation 48(2): 105–110.

Acknowledgements

The editors are very grateful to all of the past contributors and editors of previous editions, and in particular owe an immeasurable debt to Dr John Munro and Dr Mike Ford for their teaching, support and wisdom both in the past and in relation to this project.

We greatly appreciate the constructive suggestions and help that we have received from past and present students and colleagues in the design and content of the book. We wish to thank the many individuals who have provided advice and support including: Carol Sinclair and Pauline Fraser for secretarial help; Jackie Fiddes for designing the manikins and her computer skills; Robin Mitchell, Jacques Kerr and Lindsay Robertson for reviewing and commenting on sections of the manuscript; Mark Dunn, Meghan Perry and Martin McKechnie for photographs which formed the basis for line drawings; and Jamie Douglas, Tom Ford and Laura Robertson for their helpful suggestions.

We particularly wish to thank Keith Duguid of the Department of Medical Illustration, University of Aberdeen and Dr Charles Swainson and the Lothian University Hospitals Trust for help in providing clinical photographic material.

Finally we wish to thank Helen Leng, project development manager, and Laurence Hunter, commissioning editor at Elsevier for their tolerance, support and encouragement.

J.G.D., F.N.,
C.E.R.

How to get the most out of this book

The purpose of this book is to document and explain how to:

- talk with a patient
- take the history from the patient
- examine a patient
- formulate your findings into differential diagnoses
- rank these in order of probability
- use investigations to support or refute your differential diagnosis.

Initially when you approach a section we suggest that you glance through it quickly looking at the headings and how it is laid out. This will help you to see in your mind's eye the framework you will be using.

Learn to speed-read. It is invaluable in medicine and life generally. Most probably the last lesson you had on reading was at primary school. Most people can dramatically improve their speed of reading *and* increase their comprehension by using and practising simple techniques.

Try making mind maps of the details to help you recall and retain the information as you progress through the chapter. Each of the systems chapters is laid out in the same order:

- Introduction and anatomy
- Common symptoms and definition
- The History, what questions to ask and how to follow them up
- The Clinical Examination, what and how to examine
- Investigations:
  - those done at the patient's side (near-patient tests)
  - laboratory investigations
  - invasive investigations including X-rays
- Key Points including some clinical points that will help you see how an experienced clinician thinks about problems.

Your purchase of this book entitles you to access the complete text online and search using key words or using the index. You can also view all the illustrations and use the hypertext linked page cross references to navigate quickly through the book. There are also integrated links which provide bonus content from other textbooks including *Davidson's Principles and Practice of Medicine*.

Return to this book to refresh your technique if you have been away from a particular field for some time. It is surprising how quickly your technique will deteriorate if you do not use it regularly. Practise at every available opportunity so that you become proficient at examination techniques and gain a full understanding of the range of normality.

Ask a senior colleague to review your examination technique regularly; there is no substitute for this and regular practice. Listen also to what patients say, not only about themselves but also about other health professionals, and learn from these comments. You will pick up good and bad points that you will want to emulate or avoid.

Finally, enjoy your skills. After all, you are learning to be able to understand, diagnose and help people. For most of us this is the reason we became doctors.

Objective Structured Clinical Examination panels

Most undergraduate and postgraduate clinical examinations, including PACES for MRCP(UK), have an Objective Structured Clinical Examination (OSCE) format. This edition contains a new feature of 27 OSCE revision panels, listed below, summarising common clinical examples which may arise in examinations.

⊙ Examine this patient with …	
Tiredness and pallor p. 44	Acute pelvic pain p. 211
Weight loss and a good appetite p. 56	Postmenopausal bleeding p. 211
Tiredness and low blood pressure p. 62	Rectal bleeding p. 225
A hand eruption p. 68	Sudden onset headache p. 241
A pigmented skin lesion on his back p. 76	Sudden loss of vision in one eye p. 255
Sudden onset central chest pain p. 106	Acute redness and pain in one eye p. 255
Sudden loss of consciousness p. 106	Suspected brain stem death p. 263
Acute pain and discoloration in his right foot p. 117	A sore ear p. 288
Pleuritic chest pain p. 142	A blocked nose p. 292
Acute breathlessness p. 144	A sore throat p. 295
Haemoptysis p. 145	Acute lumbar back pain p. 325
Jaundice p. 173	Acute hip pain felt in the groin p. 337
Haematuria p. 191	Pain in the knee aggravated by walking p. 341
Loin pain p. 191	

Contributors

Kim Ah-See FRCS FRCS(ORL-HNS) MD
Consultant Otolaryngologist – Head and Neck Surgeon;
Honorary Senior Lecturer, Aberdeen Royal Infirmary

Elaine D C Anderson MD FRCS(Ed)
Consultant Breast Surgeon, Western General Hospital;
Clinical Director, South-East Scotland Breast Screening
Programme, Edinburgh

Peter Berrey BSc MBChB DRCOG
General Practitioner, Stockbridge Health Centre,
Edinburgh; Project Doctor, Steve Retson Project, Glasgow;
GP Appraisals Adviser, Lothian & Borders

John S Bevan MD FRCPE
Consultant Endocrinologist, Aberdeen Royal Infirmary;
Honorary Senior Lecturer, University of Aberdeen

Andrew W Bradbury BSc MD FRCS(Ed)
Professor of Vascular Surgery, Head of Surgery, University
of Birmingham; Consultant Vascular Surgeon and Director
of Research and Development, Birmingham Heartlands
and Solihull NHS Trust (Teaching)

Sineaid Bradshaw MBChB BSc DRCOG MRCGP
Paediatric GP Fellow; Senior House Officer, Family
Planning Well Woman Service, Lothian NHS Trust,
Edinburgh

Nicki R Colledge BSc(Hons) FRCPE
Consultant Geriatrician, Liberton Hospital and Royal
Infirmary of Edinburgh; Honorary Senior Lecturer,
University of Edinburgh

Allan Cumming MD FRCPE
Professor and Director of Undergraduate Learning and
Teaching, College of Medicine and Veterinary Medicine,
University of Edinburgh; Honorary Consultant Physician,
Renal Medicine, Lothian University Hospitals Division

Graham Devereux MA MD PhD FRCPE
Consultant in Respiratory and General Medicine, Aberdeen
Royal Infirmary

Graham Douglas BSc(Hons) MB ChB FRCPE
Consultant Physician, Aberdeen Royal Infirmary; Honorary
Reader in Medicine, University of Aberdeen

David J Gawkrodger MD FRCP FRCPE
Consultant Dermatologist, Royal Hallamshire Hospital,
Sheffield; Honorary Professor of Dermatology, University
of Sheffield

Ailsa E Gebbie FRCOG MFFP
Consultant Gynaecologist, Family Planning Services,
Lothian Primary Care Division, NHS Lothian, Edinburgh

Alasdair J Gray MBChB FRCS(Ed)(A&E) FFAEM
Consultant and Honorary Senior Lecturer in Emergency
Medicine, Royal Infirmary of Edinburgh

Neil R Grubb BSc(Hons) MBChB MRCP MD
Consultant Cardiologist and Honorary Senior Lecturer,
Royal Infirmary of Edinburgh

**James S Huntley MA DPhil(Oxon) MBBChir(Cantab)
MRCS(Ed)**
Lecturer and Honorary Specialist Registrar in Orthopaedic
and Trauma Surgery, University of Edinburgh

Ian Laing MA MD FRCPE FRCPCH
Consultant Neonatologist, Royal Infirmary of Edinburgh

Robert B S Laing MD FRCPE
Consultant Physician in Infectious Diseases, Aberdeen
Royal Infirmary

Alastair MacGilchrist MD FRCPE
Consultant Gastroenterologist/Hepatologist, Royal
Infirmary of Edinburgh

George Masterton BSc MD FRCPsych FRCPE
Consultant Psychiatrist, Royal Infirmary of Edinburgh

Fiona Nicol BSc(Hons) MB BS FRCGP FRCPE
GP Principal and Trainer, Stockbridge Health Centre, Edinburgh; Assistant Director (General Practice Education), Lister Postgraduate Institute, Edinburgh; Honorary Senior Lecturer, University of Edinburgh

David B Northridge MB FRCPE
Consultant Cardiologist and Honorary Senior Lecturer, Western General Hospital, Edinburgh

John Olson MD FRCPE
Consultant in Medical Ophthalmology, Aberdeen Royal Infirmary; Honorary Clinical Senior Lecturer, University of Aberdeen

Rowan W Parks MD FRCSI FRCS(Ed)
Senior Lecturer in Surgery and Honorary Consultant Surgeon, Royal Infirmary of Edinburgh

James Y Paton MD FRCPCH
Reader in Paediatric Respiratory Medicine, University of Glasgow; Honorary Consultant in Paediatric Respiratory Medicine, Royal Hospital for Sick Children, Glasgow

Brian Pentland FRCPE
Consultant Neurologist, Lothian Primary & Community Division, Astley Ainslie Hospital, Edinburgh

David M Reid MD FRCPE
Professor of Rheumatology, University of Aberdeen; Honorary Consultant Rheumatologist, Aberdeen Royal Infirmary

Colin Robertson BA(Hons) MB ChB FRCPE FRCS(Ed) FFAEM
Consultant and Honorary Professor in Emergency Medicine, Royal Infirmary of Edinburgh

Hamish Simpson DM(Oxon) FRCS(Ed & England)
Professor of Orthopaedics and Trauma, University of Edinburgh

Norman C Smith MD FRCOG
Consultant Obstetrician and Honorary Senior Lecturer, Aberdeen Maternity Hospital

David Snadden MCISc MD FRCGP FRCP
Associate Vice President Medicine and Professor Northern Medical Program, University of Northern British Columbia; Associate Dean, Northern Medical Program and Affiliate Professor, Department of Family Practice, University of British Columbia, Canada

Patrick F X Statham MBBS FRCS(SN)
Consultant Neurosurgeon, Western General Hospital, Edinburgh

Contents

Section 1
HISTORY TAKING AND GENERAL EXAMINATION

History taking

DAVID SNADDEN • ROBERT LAING • GEORGE MASTERTON • NICKI COLLEDGE

TALKING WITH PATIENTS

People visit doctors for many reasons. Sometimes it is because something unexpected and catastrophic has happened to them, but usually it is because of an ongoing problem, a relatively minor complaint or because something 'isn't right'. Before coming to the doctor they may have spoken to family or friends, tried remedies suggested by them, spoken to other health professionals, e.g. pharmacists, or complementary practitioners, or may have found information on the internet and brought this with them. Their decision to go to a doctor may only have been made after these attempts to explain or heal their illness or problem have been unsuccessful. By the time they have reached a doctor most patients have formed some idea of what might be wrong with them and will have worries or concerns that they need to talk about.

The general practitioner (GP) or family doctor is usually the first point of contact. Even a straightforward visit can be a big event for patients. They have to decide to go, usually make an appointment, work out what they are going to say and may have to arrange time off work or for child care. They then have to sit in a waiting room. This is an almost universal human experience; think about how it affected you the last time you had to do this. Things can become even more perplexing if the visit is to a hospital outpatient department or part of a hospital admission when their anxiety and apprehension can get worse as this is where 'serious' things happen. Whatever the cause, patients are seeking explanation and meaning for their symptoms. Whatever the setting, the doctor needs to try to work out why patients are there, what they are most concerned about and to agree with them the best course of action. The first and major part of that is talking with the patient (Table 1.1). If you listen carefully they will probably tell you what is wrong with them, will certainly tell you what is concerning them, and the physical examination will help you to confirm this or not. Communication is integral to the clinical examination and is most important at the beginning to gather information, and at the end to share information and engage your patients in their management.

Patient participation

Good communication is essential in good patient care; it supports the building of trust between doctor and patient and helps you provide clear and simple information that improves health. This allows you and the patient to understand each other and agree goals together which suit each individual patient. Communication is much more than 'taking a history', it is an integral and important part of looking after patients and is the only way they can be involved effectively in their health care. Poor communication leads to misunderstanding, conflicting messages and patient dissatisfaction and is the root cause of many subsequent complaints and litigation.

Beginning

That all sounds very well but how do you do it? (Table 1.2) Our personal experience of illness is unique and often difficult or embarrassing to explain. To make this easier for your patient consider the following.

Where will you see your patient?

Ideally in a quiet, private space. This is usually easy in a GP surgery, but often difficult in hospital. In hospital outpatient departments nurses or students are often present, and in hospital wards privacy is often only afforded by curtains – which means no privacy at all. You must be sensitive to your patients' privacy and dignity in all circumstances. If you are seeing the patient in a room and have others with you, for example junior colleagues, introduce them and ask permission for them to be there. If your patient is in a

1.1 Effective communication skills positively influence health outcomes
• Active listening helps the doctor recognize what is wrong
• Patient satisfaction is improved if patients understand what is wrong and what they can do to help
• When a doctor and patient agree on mutual goals health outcomes are improved
• Positive support and empathy improve health outcomes and enhance the relationship between the doctor and the patient
• Medicine taking is improved by clear information about what a medicine is meant to do

1.2 BLISS: the stages of the consultation	
Beginning	Preparation Setting Introductions
Listening	Problems Ideas Concerns Expectations Clarify, summarize, context
Information gathering	Systematic enquiry Clinical examination
Sharing information	Chunk it Check it Share decisions
Setting goals	Ending Follow-up

hospital bed but can get up, a side room or interview room may be used. Often there is no alternative to speaking to patients at their bedside, so let them know that you understand that your conversation may be overheard and give them permission not to answer sensitive things if they feel too uncomfortable about it.

How long will you have?

Consultation length varies. In general practice in the UK the average length is 10 minutes. This is usually adequate as the doctor may have seen the patient on several occasions and know the family and social background. In hospital 5–10 minutes may be adequate for return outpatients, but for new and complex problems much longer – 20–30 minutes – may be needed. If you are a student learning to talk with and examine patients allow 30 minutes at least. Plan your time around how long you expect your patients to take so that others are not kept waiting, and be prepared to be flexible.

How will you sit?

Arrange the seating in a non-confrontational way. If you use a desk, arrange the seats at the corner of the desk. This is less formal and helps communication (Fig. 1.1A, B). If you use a computer make sure the screen and keyboard do not get in the way or provide a distraction. Turn away from the screen to talk to your patient. If you are in a ward, pull up a chair and sit level with your patient (Fig. 1.1C). It is important that you can see your patient easily and gain eye contact.

Non-verbal communication

First impressions are important. Your demeanour, attitude and dress influence your patient from the outset. At all times you need to be professional in dress and behaviour. This does not mean you need to be formal, but you must be neat, clean and polite. Showing concern for your patient's situation is important.

Pick up non-verbal cues from your patients. Are they distressed? What is their mood like and how do their demeanour and body language change during the consultation? This gives clues to difficulties they are having that they cannot express verbally. If people are getting uncomfortable during a line of questioning their body language may become 'closed', i.e. they may cross their arms and legs and fail to keep eye contact.

Starting the consultation

Before starting, make sure you are talking to the correct patient. Introduce yourself, as your patients should know who you are and what you do. If you are in training, tell

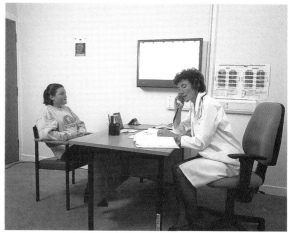

A

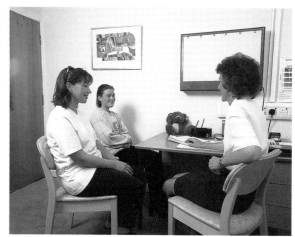

B

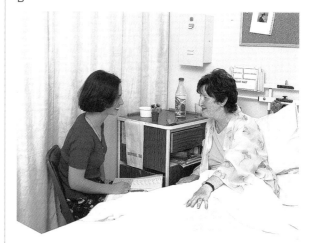

C

Fig. 1.1 Seating arrangements. (A) The desk as a defence mechanism. (B) A more appropriate arrangement of doctor and patient designed to put the patient at ease. (C) Appropriate arrangement of doctor and patient for a bedside interview.

them, as patients are usually eager to help. It helps to create a good impression if you appear to have prepared to see them. Look at the patient records and at any transfer or admission letters *before* the consultation. It is easier to give your patient your attention if you do not write notes during the consultation, but you may have to write some things, e.g. blood pressure readings or family trees, which are easily forgotten. If you are going to take notes let your patient know.

Throughout this part of the chapter there are examples of a doctor and a patient talking with each other. These are only illustrations, not hard and fast rules. Remember that it is the principles of communication that are important. If you get the principles right, then the words you use will change depending on the situation. To begin with, here are a few ideas on how to get an interview going.

> *Good morning Mrs Jones, I have got the right person haven't I? I am Mr Brown. I am a fourth year medical student. I've been asked if I could come and talk to you and examine you as you have just come into the ward today. Is that OK?*
>
> *It might take me 20–30 minutes if that is alright with you.*
>
> *I would like you to tell me what has been happening and then I'll want to ask a few questions and examine you.*
>
> *I see that you can't really get out of bed so I am afraid we'll need to talk here. I'll pull the screens round, but I'm sorry it is not that private, so if I ask you anything that you don't want to tell me in case others hear then just say so.*
>
> *Because I'll have to get quite a bit of information from you, I'll need to make a few notes. I hope that is alright because I'll forget otherwise. Now if I am writing things down it doesn't mean I'm not listening to you, I still will be.*
>
> *Are you happy with all that?*

Listening

The patient's own story is vital. Ask patients to tell you what has happened to bring them into the hospital, or, if in the community, try 'How can I help you today?' or 'What has brought you along to see me today?' Patients know doctors are busy and most will tell you their problem within 1–2 minutes so do not interrupt.

This first stage is '*active listening*'. This means encouraging patients to talk by looking interested, making encouraging comments or noises, e.g. 'tell me a bit more' or 'uhuh', and giving them the impression that you have time for them. Active listening is used to *gather information*. Also, it allows them to tell their story in their own words. This might not make complete sense to you, so you may have to ask for '*clarification*'. To do this ask them to explain a bit more about their symptoms. You can also tell them what you think they have said and ask if your interpretation is correct.

Can we start with you telling me what has happened to bring you into hospital? (Opening)

Well doctor, I have been getting this funny feeling in my chest over the last few months. It's been getting worse and worse till it got to the point today I had to call my GP and he sent me in. It was really awful this morning, I got really breathless and felt someone was standing on me.

Tell me a bit more about the feeling in your chest. (Open questioning)

Well it was here, across my chest, it was sort of tight and I was sweaty.

And did it go anywhere else? (Clarifying)

No, well maybe up here in my neck a bit.

So what you are saying is that you had this pain in your chest this morning that went on a long time – how long do you think? (Summarizing and clarifying)

Oh, a couple of hours.

And the pain was tight and up into your neck. How is it now? (Open questioning)

Oh it is not bad, the injections I had seem to have put it away.

OK, now you said that you had had the pain for the last few months. Can you tell me more about that? (Open questioning)

Well it was the same but not that bad, though it has been getting worse recently.

OK, can you remember when it first started? (Clarifying)

Oh 3 or 4 months ago.

And how often has it been coming? (Open questioning)

To start with just now and again, but in the last 2 to 3 weeks, probably every day anyway.

Does anything makes it worse? (Open questioning)

Well if I go up steps or up hills that can bring it on.

What do you do?

Stop and sometimes take my puffer.

Your what? (Clarifying)

This spray the doctor gave me to put in my mouth.

Can you show me it please?

OK.

And what does it do? (Clarifying)

Well it takes the pain away, but I get an awful headache with it.

OK, so for a few months you have had this tightness in your chest, which gets worse on going up hills and upstairs and which goes away if you use your spray. But today it came on and lasted a couple of hours but felt the same. Have I got that right? (Summarizing)

No, it was much worse this morning.

Once you have established what has happened, find out the patient's 'ideas', 'concerns' and 'expectations'.

I Ideas

C Concerns

E Expectations.

Patients will have thoughts and feelings about what has happened to them which may or may not be accurate, but which can help you. For instance, a patient with chest pain might think he has indigestion while you are considering angina. This can cause confusion so ask 'Do you have any thoughts about what might be happening to you?' A young mother bringing her child to the doctor with a sore throat may only want reassurance, not medicine. A simple question like 'What were you thinking I might do today?' can get surprising answers and avoid unnecessary prescriptions or investigations.

The way you ask a question is important. Open questions encourage the patient to talk. Closed questions seek specific information as part of a systematic inquiry. Both have their place. Open questions usually start with a word like '*where*' or '*what*', or a phrase like '*tell me more about …*', and are more useful at the beginning when you are trying to find out what is going on and to encourage the patient to talk. Closed questions, e.g. 'Have you been sick today?' invite yes or no answers.

Exploring your patient's context

Illness never happens in isolation. The context of our lives has a major influence on how we deal with illness. This can be complex, and finding out the context is a crucial part of gathering information about your patient. Many people call it the 'social history', but it is more than this. It allows you to understand the personal constraints and supports available to your patient. Your patient's context is a mixture of where they live, who they live with, where they work, who they work with, what they actually do, their cultural and religious beliefs and their relationships and past experience.

These are sensitive areas to explore. It may not be appropriate to explore all of them with everyone, but they are important in any long-term doctor–patient relationship. Understanding context modifies the information you give and the way you give it, the treatment you advise and the drugs you use.

Establish your patient's job, and explore in some depth what this job entails as it may have a bearing on the illness. This means you need to find out in detail not only what the job is, but what the patient actually does, whether there are any stresses in the job and whether there are any relationships at work that might affect the patient, e.g. a bullying boss or a harassing colleague.

Clearly, one job description can cover many tasks and you need to understand what your patient actually does. Patient A is under stress and patient B may be suffering the consequences of exposure to fungal spores which can cause farmer's lung. However, their initial answer to the first question was the same. Just as your patients' illness can have an influence on their ability to do their job, their job (past or present) may be an influence on their illness. A full

---

Doctor: *So tell me what your job is.*

Patient: I work on a farm.

Doctor: *Yes – but what do you actually do?*

Patient A: Well I own the farm and mostly do the bookwork and buying and selling of animals.

Patient B: I am a labourer on the farm.

Doctor: *So what are you doing at the moment?*

Patient A: It has been a terrible year with the drought, the yields are down and I am trying to get another loan from the bank manager.

Patient B: Well just now we are working in the barn first thing in the mornings cleaning up and then laying feed for the cattle. After that we are in the fields doing the early ploughing.

Doctor: *So when you are laying the feed, what are you doing?*

Patient B: We are unrolling last summer's hay bales.

Doctor: *So what does that mean?*

Patient B: Well we roll them out with the tractor and then spread it out for the cattle a bit with a fork.

Doctor: *Is there much dust?*

Patient B: Oh yes, it creates a real dust and it is very mouldy this year.

---

occupational history means your patients should tell you what jobs they have done in their working life. Try to find out if any of those could have had an influence on their symptoms (see Occupational history, p. 16).

Find out about their home circumstances. Relationships in modern society are complex, so choose your words carefully; for example 'Is there anyone at home with you?' or 'Is there anyone that can help?' are useful ways of finding out diplomatically.

You need to be equally tactful in enquiring about relationships and the home environment. For example, if a 15-year-old newly diagnosed diabetic is about to go home you need to know the home circumstances, who is there and whether the relationships are supportive. Different arrangements are made for a patient whose mother is a health worker in a stable home, compared to one from a deprived background, with one parent and poor relationships. The decision to return to work depends on the content of the job, the sympathy and support of the employer and the patient's financial situation.

Patients' beliefs influence health care. Religious beliefs affect how a family copes with a disability, a dying relative, or whether some people accept certain treatments, and you need to be sensitive to and tolerant of these issues. Other moral beliefs need to be explored in some situations, e.g. requests for termination of pregnancy.

Now gather information in a more systematic way to clarify any issues and focus on the actual problems. Do this through a detailed systematic inquiry and clinical examination of your patient. Once you have gathered that information you reach the most important part of the consultation, which is when you share your findings with your patient.

Sharing information

Clarifying and summarizing

Use the same techniques as at the beginning of your consultation, except now your patient needs to understand *your* use of words. Clarify and summarize what you say. Set realistic goals to achieve together. Your use of language is vital and you should use words that your patient understands. Tailor your explanation to your patient; you would use very different terms when dealing with a lawyer compared to dealing with a farm labourer.

First explain what you have found and what you think this means. Give important information first and check what has been understood. Put the information into small chunks and warn the patient how many important things are coming. For example 'There are two important things I want to discuss with you, the first is …'.

Use simple language, if you have to use a term like 'cancer', spend time ensuring your patient understands the treatment options and likely prognosis. If the news is bad, ensure you have time for patients to let the news sink in. Suggest they have a friend or relative with them if they wish. Go at your patients' pace and do not give more information than they want or can handle at any one time. Hearing bad news often blocks patients' ability to retain any further information so you should arrange follow-up to discuss all their further questions.

Some doctors try to avoid using emotive terms, e.g. cancer, but if you need to give bad news it should be accurate, unambiguous, and given sensitively. There is no place for being abrupt or for brutal honesty. Most people understand the word 'cancer', but 'tumour' can be interpreted in many ways.

Enabling

Make sure that your patients are involved in any decisions; this is called enabling. Share your own ideas with them,

make suggestions and encourage them to contribute their thoughts. Help their decision making by giving written information to take home or suggest other sources of information, e.g. self-help groups or the internet. Check they have understood you and discuss any investigations or treatment you think might be needed, including any risks or side-effects.

In this way negotiate a mutually agreeable plan. For example a patient with cancer may have the choice of surgery or radiotherapy, each of which has different risks and side-effects. It may not be easy to decide, but by involving your patients and discussing with them the pros and cons of treatments you will reach a decision that they understand and agree with. They have to live with the consequences of the treatment, and it is much easier for them to accept if they have had a hand in choosing.

Setting goals

Setting goals allows you and your patient to agree on what you are trying to achieve. These might be areas that your patient needs to work on. For example if patients are trying to stop smoking then you may set goals with them about when they are going to stop, what help they will use, e.g. support groups or nicotine replacement therapy or both, how they will identify risky situations, e.g. socializing, and how to handle these in an effort to avoid being tempted to have a cigarette.

Goals should follow the SMART principle:

S Specific
M Measurable
A Achievable
R Relevant
T Time related.

Outcomes that might be agreed are that you provide discussion of the problem, advice, or reassurance, or that you may advise referral, investigation, or drug treatment.

Finally, you need to arrange for follow-up if necessary, or give patients some idea as to when they might want to return. This depends on how they are feeling and the effects of any treatment you have suggested. End a complex discussion by very briefly summarizing what you have agreed, or ask your patient to summarize for you.

Situations which influence communication

Transference/countertransference

Transference is the process where your patient unconsciously projects on to you thoughts, behaviours and emotional reactions that originate with other significant relationships from childhood onwards. For example, people who are very ill or have just been given some news about a specific diagnosis, the implications of which are overwhelming, may behave in uncharacteristic ways. They might return to a

1.3	Talking with patients

- Speak clearly and audibly
- Do not use jargon
- Do not use unnecessarily emotive words
- Give the important information first in small amounts
  - *'Chunk it'*
  - *Check* what has been understood
- Negotiate a shared decision
- Set goals
- Summarize

position of dependency and may seek care and comfort that was absent in their past. If you do not provide this, patients may get very angry. These are difficult concepts, but have a major part to play in any doctor–patient relationship. You cannot avoid transference because it is an unconscious process, but be aware that it is happening.

Recognizing transference helps you to understand unexpected behaviour and to continue to provide care for your patient. Transference can be used positively, to enhance your communication with your patient. Many medical students have had a patient say 'Oh you are just like my son/daughter'.

Countertransference is where the doctor responds to patients in a way similar to significant past relationships. For example the repeated failure to listen to a patient's stories of failed relationships may echo experiences in a doctor's own life. The signs of countertransference are not listening, misjudging your patient's feelings, repeatedly going over the same story and always running late with the same patient. Self-awareness is the most important way to deal with these issues, which arise at some stage for all doctors.

Empathy

If your patients see you as an empathic doctor it will help your relationship with them, and improve their health outcomes. What is empathy and how do you express it? Empathy is not sympathy, the expression of sorrow; it is much more. It is helping your patients feel that you understand what they are going through. Try to see the problem from their point of view and relate that to them. For example, consider a young teacher who has recently had disfiguring facial surgery to remove a benign tumour from her upper jaw. She has recovered in terms of wound healing, but now has a drooping lower eyelid, and significant facial swelling. She returns to work. Think how you would feel and imagine yourself in this situation. You can express empathy by sensitive questions which show you can relate to your patient's experience.

> *... So you have all healed up from your operation now?*
> Yes – but I still have to put drops in my eye.
> *And what about the swelling under your eye?*
> That gets worse during the day, and sometimes by afternoon I can't see that well.
> *And how does that feel at work?*
> Well it is really difficult, you know the kids and everything, it is all a bit awkward.
> *I can understand that that must make you feel pretty uncomfortable and awkward – that must be very difficult. How do you cope? Thinking about that makes me wonder if there are any other areas that are awkward for you, maybe in the other bits of your life, like the social side ....*

Sensitive situations

Doctors have to explore questions of a personal or sensitive nature, or have to examine intimate parts. These need time and care.

If you are talking to a patient who you think may have a sexually transmitted disease, you need to be very sensitive in broaching this subject. First give some indication that you are going to ask questions in this area, and make sure the conversation is entirely private. Here are some examples of questions that might work.

> *Because of what you are telling me I need to ask you some rather personal questions, is that OK?*
> *Can you tell me if you have had any casual relationships recently?*
> *Are you worried that you might have picked anything up, I mean in a sexual way?*
> *Having told me that you think you are at risk of something, can I ask if you have a regular sexual partner?*
> *Follow this up with 'Is your partner male or female?' If there is no regular partner ask how many sexual partners there have been in the past year and how many have been male and how many female.*

Use the same sensitivity to seek permission to examine intimate areas. First warn your patients, then seek their permission to examine them and explain what you need to do. Offer a chaperone, and record in the notes if they do not wish this (see Ch. 7).

> *So I need to examine you down below since that seems to be where the problem is. I will need to examine you with my hands, I'll have gloves on. I will also need to look at you down below through a small instrument. Is that OK? It would be helpful if we had a chaperone who can help us. Would that be OK? So while I fetch her could you get undressed behind the screens and I'll examine you once you are ready?*

You also need to give your patients clear instructions about what clothes they need to remove.

There may be times when it is appropriate to delay an intimate examination until sufficient time, appropriate facilities or a chaperone is available.

Difficult situations

Breaking bad news is one of the most difficult communication tasks you will face. Always speak to the patient in a quiet and private environment, ideally, if the patient agrees, in the presence of a relative or partner and if possible with a nurse or counsellor. Be honest. Do not tell your patients anything that is not true; the truth always emerges over time. Your patients may only wish to know some things, and they may appear not to hear or retain what you tell them. This is called *denial* and is a normal defence mechanism. Go at your patients' pace; find out how much more they want to know and continually check their understanding. They will need time to reflect on what you have said and may need to return to see you at another time. They might ask for a prognosis: 'How long have I got?' is a common question. Take care with this and never give a specific time – you will usually be wrong. Even in the most difficult circumstances do not take away hope. There is always something that can be done for a patient.

Dealing with emotions

At some point you will encounter angry or distressed patients and relatives who may be crying inconsolably. You may also encounter talkative or over-familiar patients. Illness can bring anger and frustration. Getting angry yourself or ignoring their anger does not help. If you feel angry with your patients, it is likely that they feel angry themselves. Exploring the reasons for this often defuses the situation. Do this by recognizing that your patients are angry and asking them to explain why.

If an apology is needed, give it; it may defuse the situation. Use such phrases as, 'you seem angry about something' or 'is there something that is upsetting you?' Similarly with other emotions follow the same basic guidance. Recognize the emotion, show empathy and understanding, encourage your patient to talk and offer what explanations you can.

If your patients are too talkative, or where they want to deal with too many things, you have to sometimes lead with statements: 'Now I only have a short time left with you, so what is the most important thing we need to deal with now.' If they have a long list of complaints suggest: 'Well of the six things you have brought today I can only deal with two, so which are the most important to you and we will deal with the rest next time.' It is important to set professional boundaries if your patient becomes over-familiar: 'Well it would be inappropriate for me to discuss personal issues with you. I am here to help you so let's focus on your problem.'

Patients who are too ill to talk or who are confused

If your patient is very ill, confused or mentally ill, or impaired for whatever reason, obtain what information you can from third parties. Rapidly assess the situation, treat your patient, and review everything when your patient is fit enough (see Ch. 12).

1.4   Transcultural awareness
• Appropriateness of eye contact
• Appropriateness of hand gestures
• Personal space
• Physical contact between sexes (e.g. shaking hands)
• Cultures and beliefs surrounding illness
• What should happen as death approaches?
• What should happen after death?

Communication difficulties

When you see patients who cannot speak your language, are deaf or who have expressive problems, e.g. dysphasia, dysarthria or stammering, try to establish some method of communication. This may need an interpreter. Writing things down, lip reading, sign language or someone who is used to communicating with your patient often helps.

Transcultural issues

Be sensitive when dealing with someone from a culture different from your own (Table 1.4). The use of eye contact, touching and personal space is different in different cultures. In western, and North American cultures, holding eye contact for long periods is normal; in most of the rest of the world this is seen as confrontational or rude. In some cultures it is normal to shake hands between opposite sexes, but this is strictly forbidden in others. Understand and accept differences in your patients' cultures and beliefs and be aware of them. When in doubt ask the patients, this lets them know that you are aware of and sensitive to these issues.

Third party information

You may need to obtain information about your patient from someone else, usually a relative and sometimes a friend or carer. Ideally obtain your patient's permission and have the patient present. In this way confidentiality is not breached. You may be approached by third parties without your patient's knowledge. Find out who they are, their relationship to your patient, and whether your patient knows they are talking to you. Ensure that third parties understand that you can only listen to what they have to say and cannot divulge any of your clinical information about your patient. They may tell you about sensitive matters, e.g. mental illness, sexual abuse, drug or alcohol addiction. This information needs to be explored with your patients sensitively, as only they will be able to confirm the truth and agree to treatment. In all circumstances confidentiality of your patients' information is your first priority.

Read *Good Medical Practice* published by the General Medical Council, which describes the standards of competence, care and conduct expected of you in all aspects of your professional work.

THE PRESENTING COMPLAINT

1.5	Elements in a clinical history

- Presenting complaint
- Past medical history
- Drug history
- Family history
- Social history
- Occupational history
- Systemic or general symptom inquiry
- Further information from a third party

After introducing yourself and confirming your patient's name continue by asking for details of their background including age, date of birth, marital status and current occupation. Then establish your patient's presenting complaint. This is often described in a phrase, and helps to identify the principal problem. Start with open questions but then gradually focus down on symptoms by using closed questions. Choose your words carefully since patients may misinterpret questions such as 'What are you complaining of?' as implying that you regard them as complainers. Try:

- 'What would you say your main problem is?'
- 'When do you think you were last well?'
- 'When were you last your usual self?'

Follow up with 'What has happened to you since then?' If another doctor has referred your patient use the referral letter, e.g. 'Your own doctor has told me that you have been having some chest pain. Can you tell me about the pain please?'

Examples of presenting complaints are listed in Table 1.6. The list is not comprehensive but includes the most common

1.6	Systematic inquiry – cardinal symptoms			
General health	Well-being Appetite Weight change	Energy Sleep Mood		poor stream or flow terminal dribbling incontinence urethral discharge libido erectile difficulties

Cardiovascular system	Chest pain on exertion (angina)
	Breathlessness:
	    lying flat (orthopnoea)
	    at night (paroxysmal nocturnal dyspnoea)
	    on minimal exertion – record how much
	Palpitation
	Pain in legs on walking (claudication)
	Ankle swelling
			Women	Last menstrual period (consider pregnancy)
				Timing and regularity of periods
				Length of periods
				Abnormal bleeding
				Vaginal discharge
				Contraception
				If appropriate:
				    libido
				    pain during intercourse (dyspareunia)
				    incontinence (stress and urge)

Respiratory system	Shortness of breath (exercise tolerance) Cough Wheeze Sputum production (colour, amount) Blood in sputum (haemoptysis) Chest pain (due to inspiration or coughing)		**Nervous system**	Headaches Dizziness (vertigo or light-headed) Faints Fits Altered sensation (numbness or tingling (paraesthesiae)) Weakness Visual disturbance Hearing problems (deafness, tinnitus) Memory and concentration changes

Gastrointestinal system	Mouth (oral ulcers, dental problems)
	Difficulty swallowing (dysphagia – distinguish
	    from pain on swallowing, odynophagia)
	Nausea and vomiting
	Vomiting blood (haematemesis)
	Indigestion
	Heartburn
	Abdominal pain
	Change in bowel habit
	Change in colour of stools (pale, dark, tarry
	    black, fresh blood)
			Musculoskeletal	Joint pain, stiffness or swelling
				Mobility
				Falls

Genitourinary system	Pain passing urine (dysuria) Frequency passing urine (at night, nocturia) Blood in the urine (haematuria) Sexual partners – unprotected intercourse		**Endocrine**	Heat or cold intolerance Change in sweating Excessive thirst (polydipsia)

Men	If appropriate:
	    prostatic symptoms including difficulty starting –
	    hesitancy
			Other	Bleeding or bruising
				Skin rash

symptoms for each system. Follow up any positive finding by asking closed questions to clarify if the symptom is significant.

Diagnosis

The aim of talking with the patient is to make a diagnosis. To do this you need to know what symptoms are caused by each disease or problem. Each disease process or problem has specific characteristics that help you in this task. You will need to become expert in pattern recognition. Work out which organ is affected and what process is going on by identifying these characteristics and patterns in the patient's story. Diagnosis is based on recognizing the pattern of symptoms which each disease or problem commonly produces. You need to know these characteristics and then you will be able to ask useful questions. Initially you will not know enough to focus your questions and will have to use blanket questioning, but as you gain experience you can refine your questions according to the complaint. Build up your knowledge all the time by reading, seeing patients and listening to and observing colleagues. You should have a good idea of the diagnosis before you examine the patient and you should use your examination to support or refute it.

Make sure that patients tell you what they feel the principal problem is in their own words without pressure or interruption. Prompt to keep the history flowing, and use your knowledge of disease to direct your questioning. When finished their initial description of the presenting complaint, start with the symptom that seems to concern them most. Make sure that you understand exactly what they mean by any term that they use. For example, does 'weakness' mean true muscle weakness or are they simply tired? Explore each symptom offered by the patient. For each symptom work out its cardinal features.

The patient in the dialogue is a 65-year-old male smoker.

Each answer weights the probability of a particular diagnosis being more likely, while helping to exclude others. This is conditional probability as described in Bayes' theorem. In this example the age of the man and the fact he is a long-term smoker increase the probability of certain diagnoses related to smoking. A persistent cough for 2 months increases the likelihood of lung cancer and chronic obstructive pulmonary disease (COPD). The chest pain does not exclude COPD since the man could have pulled a muscle by coughing but it is less likely than pleuritic pain from infection due to obstruction of an airway caused by lung cancer. This is confirmed by his increasing shortness of breath. Haemoptysis lasting 2 months dramatically increases the chance of lung cancer. When the patient confirms his weight loss the positive predictive value of all these answers is very high for lung cancer and you will carry out your examination and plan investigations accordingly.

What would you say is the main problem? (Open question)

I've had a cough which I just can't seem to get rid of. I think it started after I had been ill with the flu about 2 months ago. I thought it would get better but it hasn't and it's driving me mad.

Can you tell me a bit more about the cough? (Open question)

Well, it is bad all the time. I cough and cough, and bring up some phlegm. I can't sleep at night sometimes and waken up feeling rough because I have slept so poorly and sometimes I get pains in my chest because I have been coughing so much. (Follow up by asking key questions to clarify the cough – see Table 4.1, p. 126.)

Tell me about the pains. (Open question)

Well they are here on my side when I cough.

Does anything else bring on the pains? (Open and prompting question)

No. (Follow this up by asking the key questions about pain – see Table 1.7.)

What colour is the phlegm? (Closed question, focusing on the symptom offered)

Clear.

Have you ever coughed up any blood? (Closed question)

Yes, sometimes.

How often? (Closed question, clarifying the symptom)

Oh most days.

How much? (Closed question, clarifying the symptom)

Oh just streaks, but sometimes a bit more.

Do you ever get wheezy or feel short of breath with your cough?

A bit (see Table 4.1, p. 126.)

How has your weight been? (Closed question, seeking additional confirmation of serious pathology)

I have lost about 6 kilos.

Pain

Pain is a very common symptom. Later chapters describe characteristic features of specific presentations, and by knowing these and asking appropriate questions to clarify the patient's symptoms you will be able to make a differential diagnosis.

Characteristics of pain are summarized in Table 1.7.

Associated symptoms

Ask about associated symptoms to help you work out the significance of any presenting complaint. Any severe pain can be associated with nausea, sweating and faintness as part of the vagal and sympathetic response. Particular associated symptoms may suggest an underlying cause, e.g. visual disturbance preceding a migraine headache or palpitation (suggesting an arrhythmia) in association with angina pain. If the pain is sufficiently severe to disturb sleep, this suggests a physical cause but also, because

1.7 Characteristics of pain	
Site	Somatic pain often well localized, e.g. sprained ankle Visceral pain more diffuse, e.g. angina pectoris
Onset	Speed of onset and any associated circumstances
Character	Described by adjectives, e.g. sharp/dull, burning/tingling, boring/stabbing, crushing/tugging, preferably using the patient's own description rather than offering suggestions
Severity	Difficult to assess as so subjective. Sometimes helpful to compare with other common pains, e.g. toothache
Radiation	Through local extension, or referred by a shared neuronal pathway to a distant, unaffected site, e.g. diaphragmatic pain at the shoulder tip via the phrenic nerve (C_3, C_4)
Associated symptoms	Visual aura accompanying classical migraine Numbness in the leg with back pain suggesting nerve root irritation
Timing (duration, course, pattern)	Since onset Episodic or continuous. If episodic, duration and frequency of attacks; if continuous, any changes in the severity Variation by day or night, during the week or month, e.g. relating to the menstrual cycle
Exacerbating and relieving factors	Circumstances in which pain is provoked or exacerbated e.g. food Specific activities or postures, and any avoidance measures that have been taken to prevent the onset Effects of specific activities or postures. Includes effects of medication and alternative medical approaches

patients are exhausted, this changes their perception of and ability to cope with the pain.

Effects on lifestyle

Ask 'How do you cope with the pain?' This helps you to gain insight into the patient's coping strategies and shows your empathy. Areas to be considered in relation to chronic pain are illustrated in Figure 1.2.

Attitudes to illness

This is a difficult area to evaluate objectively. Many symptoms, e.g. pain and fatigue, are subjective and two patients with identical conditions can present dramatically different histories. The following attitudes to illness should always be considered.

Pain threshold and tolerance. This varies considerably not only between patients but in the same person in different circumstances (Table 1.8). Patients also vary in their willingness to speak about their discomfort.

Past experience. Both personal and family experience of pain influence the response to symptoms. A family history of sudden death from heart disease may well affect how a person interprets and reacts to chest pain.

Somatization. When physical symptoms exist without signs of organic disease this is called somatization or functional disorder. It is an expression of emotional illness or distress. To the patient the symptoms are real. Do not sound dismissive of these symptoms. Phrases such as 'I realize these headaches are very disabling' or 'Your chest pain is clearly very distressing' help to reassure your patients that you take them seriously, while you explore the

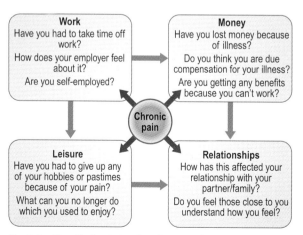

Fig. 1.2 The effects of chronic pain – questions you may ask. Note that pain affects several areas of a patient's life but that these are interlinked.

1.8 Pain threshold
Pain threshold can be *increased* by: • exercise • analgesia • positive mental attitude • up-beat personality Pain threshold can be *decreased* by: • sleep deprivation • depression • financial and personal worries • anxiety and fear about the cause • past experience

possibility of a non-physical cause. For example, a person may concentrate on the tension headache rather than the source of stress that is exacerbating it. Recognizing somatization helps to avoid inappropriate investigations which may ultimately reinforce illness behaviour.

Gains. Most illness brings some gains to the patient. These may simply be more attention from family and friends through to considerable financial benefits and being able to avoid unpleasant work or stress. Patients may not be conscious of these as demotivating factors in their illness but sometimes they deliberately exaggerate symptoms.

PAST HISTORY

Ask about relevant past medical history as part of the history of the presenting complaint, e.g. previous angina in the patient with chest pain. There is often a relationship between the past medical history and the presenting problem. For example, a patient presenting with dyspepsia may have had a past history of multiple attendances for minor injuries. This should raise the possibility of an alcohol problem which could also account for the current symptoms.

Strike a balance between asking open questions about the past history and obtaining relevant, meaningful information (Table 1.9). Asking if your patients have ever had an illness may invite a description of every cold, cough and headache that has troubled them, while asking only about serious illness is to unfairly ask them to decide about the nature of any previous ill health.

DRUG HISTORY

Ask about prescribed drugs and any other medications your patient is taking (Table 1.10). Include over-the-counter remedies and alternative medicine treatments, particularly herbal or homeopathic remedies, laxatives, analgesics and vitamin/mineral supplements. Note the name of each drug, the dose, dosage regimen and duration of treatment along with significant side-effects. In hospital contact the patient's general practitioner for a record of the current prescription, although many patients will have a computer counterfoil from their GP with details of medicines. If patients claim

---

1.9 Past history
• Have you had any illness that you saw your doctor about?
• Have you had to take time off work because of ill health?
• Have you had any operations?
• Have you attended any hospital clinics?
• Have you been a patient in hospital? If so, why was that?

---

to be taking unlikely combinations or amounts of drugs, confirm this with the last doctor to look after them. A drug addict may claim to be receiving a prescription for benzodiazepines and opioids in the hope of receiving the same from the admitting doctor. Always verify the patient's claims with their GP and inform the addict's dispensing pharmacy of the admission. This allows the prescription to be halted for the duration of admission and prevents it being collected by someone else on the patient's behalf.

Compliance/concordance

Compliance is the traditional model of medical care where patients take their medication as prescribed by the doctor. The modern term, concordance, means a shared decision between doctor and patient where they arrive at an agreement that respects the wishes and beliefs of the patient.

Half of all patients do not take medicines as directed. Ask them to describe how and when they take their medication. Give permission for them to admit that they do not take all their medicines by saying 'That must be difficult to remember'. Many GPs can use their computerized databases to confirm whether patients have picked up their prescriptions on time. However, this does not provide evidence that the patient has obtained the drugs from the pharmacist or taken them at the correct time.

Drug allergies/reactions

Always ask if your patient has ever had an allergic reaction to medication. In particular enquire about previous reactions before prescribing an antibiotic, particularly penicillin. Clarify exactly what patients mean by allergy, as this term is used loosely.

Ask about other allergies, e.g. foodstuffs, animal hair, pollen or metal. Record true allergies prominently in the

---

1.10 Example of a drug history				
Drug	**Dose**	**Duration**	**Indication**	**Notes**
Aspirin	75 mg daily	5 years	Started after myocardial infarction	
Amitriptyline	25 mg at night	6 months	Takes for poor sleep	Feels drowsy in morning
Atenolol	50 mg daily	5 years	Started after myocardial infarction	Causes cold hands (? compliance)
Codydramol (paracetamol+dihydrocodeine)	Up to 8 tabs daily	4 weeks	Back pain	Causes constipation

patient's case records and drug chart. Otherwise the patient may receive a substance which precipitates a life-threatening adverse reaction.

FAMILY HISTORY

Obtain the family history by asking open-ended questions, e.g. 'Are there any illnesses that run in your family?' It is possible that the presenting complaint directs you to a particular line of inquiry, e.g. 'Is there any history of heart disease in your family?' Many illnesses, e.g. thyroid disease, coronary artery disease, may be associated with a positive family history but are not due to a single gene disorder (Table 1.11), and so family history is just one risk factor.

Some patients require prompting with suggestions about common familial diseases, e.g. diabetes mellitus, thyroid disease or coeliac disease. Document illness in parents, any siblings and children. If there is a suspicion of an inherited disorder, e.g. Huntington's disease or haemophilia, family history should go back at least three generations with details of racial origins and consanguinity (Fig. 1.3). In these circumstances ask if your patient or any close relative has been adopted.

In addition to blood relatives, ask about the health of other household members since this gives clues about

1.11	Examples of single gene inherited disorders		
Autosomal dominant	**Autosomal recessive**	**X-linked**
Adult polycystic renal disease	Cystic fibrosis	Duchenne muscular dystrophy
Huntington's disease	Sickle cell anaemia	Haemophilia A
Myotonic dystrophy	Alpha thalassaemia	Fragile X syndrome
Neurofibromatosis	Alpha-1-antitrypsin deficiency	

environmental risks to the patient's health. For example, if a woman's husband died of lung cancer she may have been exposed to passive smoking.

SOCIAL HISTORY

The social history places a disease in the context of the patient's life and reveals factors relevant to the presenting illness (Table 1.12). A social history can be expansive, incorporating everything from childhood experiences to coffee intake. With experience you will focus on the relevant issues. It is rarely appropriate to ask an elderly woman with

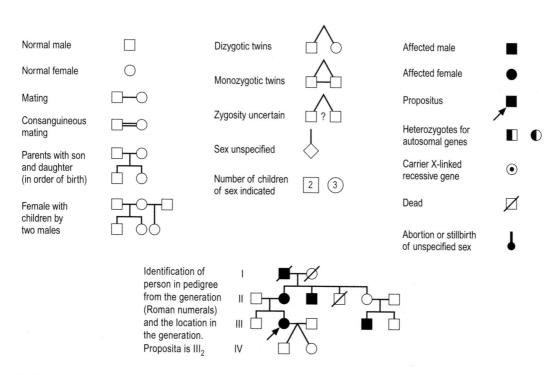

Fig. 1.3 Symbols used in, and example of a pedigree chart.

1.12 The social history

Upbringing

- Birth injury or complications
- Early parental attachments and disruptions
- Schooling, academic achievements or difficulties
- Further or higher education and training
- Behaviour problems

Home life

- Emotional, physical or sexual abuse[a]
- Experiences of death and illness
- Interest and attitude of parents

Occupation

- Current and previous (clarify exactly what a job entails)
- Exposure to hazards, e.g. chemicals, asbestos, foreign travel, accidents and compensation claims
- Unemployment, reason and duration
- Attitude to job

Finance

- Circumstances including debts
- Benefits from social security

Relationships and domestic circumstances

- Married or long-term partner
- Quality of relationship
- Problems
- Partner's health, occupation and attitude to patient's illness
- Who else is at home, any problems, e.g. health, violence, and bereavement?
- In trouble with the law

House

- Type of home, size, owned or rented
- Details of home including stairs, toilets, heating, cooking facilities, neighbours

Community support

- Social services involvement, e.g. home help, meals on wheels
- Attitude to needing help

Sexual history[a]

Leisure activities

- Exercise, hobbies and pastimes, pets

Substance misuse[a]

[a]Ask only if it is relevant to the history

a hip fracture whether she is injecting drugs but it is always necessary to know if she lives alone, has any friends or relatives nearby, what support services she receives and how well suited her house is for someone with poor mobility.

Remember that your patient's illness affects others. There may be an infirm relative at home for whom the patient cares or there may be no one at home to look after the patient because, although she is married, her husband works abroad for 3 weeks out of 4. GPs usually know the

social circumstances, so ask them if there is any doubt about the accuracy of the social history. If the GP referred the patient to hospital because of a crisis at home, your patient's discharge from hospital is likely to prove short-lived unless these problems, e.g. lack of downstairs toilet, no carer, a patient's inability to cook for himself, have been addressed along with the medical problems.

Ask about any dietary restrictions. These may be self-imposed or have been recommended by a health practitioner.

Occupational history

The work people do may have a profound influence on their health. Some occupations are known to be associated with certain illnesses (Table 1.13). You should take a full occupational history from all patients. An appropriate question to ask might be 'Please tell me about all the jobs you have done in your working life.' Follow this up by asking what the patient actually does when at work; in particular, any chemical or dust exposure, the use of protective devices and whether other workers have become ill. Symptoms which improve over the weekend or during holidays should always suggest an occupational disorder. Remember that hobbies may also be associated with certain illnesses, e.g. psittacosis pneumonia and extrinsic allergic alveolitis in those who keep birds.

Travel history

Travel is common for holidays, business and study purposes. One person in eight of those who travel outwith Europe or North America attend their GP on returning with possible travel-related illness. Travellers to hot climates are at risk of contracting tropical infections, and air travel itself may increase the risk of certain conditions e.g. middle ear problems and deep venous thrombosis. The incubation period is useful in deciding on the likelihood of an illness (Table 1.14). As well as the country your patient visited you should ask about the type of accommodation, e.g. a five-star hotel or a tent, and the activities undertaken, e.g. water sports, sexual contacts while abroad.

Sexual history

It is not always appropriate to take a full sexual history (see Ch. 7). If it is relevant, ask questions in an objective fashion. Precede the questions with a statement, e.g. 'As part of your medical history, I need to ask you some questions about your relationships. I hope that you don't mind this.'

Examples of some objective questions are

- Do you have a regular sexual partner at the moment?
- Is your partner male or female?
- Can I ask if you have had any (other) sexual partners in the last 12 months?
- How many were male? How many female?

1.13	Examples of occupational disorders		
Occupation	**Factor**	**Disorder**	**Presents**
Shipyard workers, boilermen	Asbestos	Pleural plaques Asbestosis Mesothelioma	Over 20 years later
Dairy farmers	*Leptospira hadjo* Fungus spores on mouldy hay	Lymphocytic meningitis Farmer's lung (extrinsic allergic alveolitis)	Within 1 week Within 4–18 hours
Divers	Surfacing from depth too quickly	Decompression sickness Central nervous system, skin, bone and joint symptoms	Immediately and up to 1 week
Industrial workers	Chemical exposure, e.g. chromium	Dermatitis on hands	Variable
Bakery workers	Flour mites	Occupational asthma	Variable
Healthcare workers	Cuts, needlestick injuries	Hepatitis B and C	Incubation period > 3 months
Disc jockeys Using noisy machinery	Excessive noise	Sensorineural hearing loss	Develops over months

1.14	Examples of incubation periods of travel-related infections		
Disease	**Incubation period**	**Travel to presentation**	**Usual symptoms**
Falciparum malaria	8–25 days	Up to 6 weeks	Fever
Vivax malaria	8–27 days	Up to 1 year	Fever
Typhoid fever	10–14 days	Up to 3 weeks	Fever, headache
Paratyphoid fever	8–12 days	Up to 3 weeks	Fever, diarrhoea
Dengue fever	3–15 days	Up to 3 weeks	Fever, headache
Schistosomiasis	2–63 days	Up to 10 weeks	Itch, fever, haematuria, abdominal discomfort
Hepatitis A	28–42 days	Up to 6 weeks	Jaundice
HIV infection	12–26 weeks	Up to ?12 years	Weight loss, pneumonia

- Do you use barrier contraception – sometimes, always or never?
- Have you ever had a sexually transmitted infection?

Tobacco

Ask if your patients have ever smoked; if so, for how long and how much. Record when they started and stopped. If they smoke ask what (cigarettes, cigars or pipe); the quantity (number of cigarettes/cigars or amount of pipe tobacco per day) and the duration. Use 'pack years' (Table 1.15) to estimate the risk of tobacco-related health problems in your patients (Fig. 1.4) (see Ch. 4).

Alcohol

Patients may be upset if you ask bluntly 'How much alcohol do you drink?' Try 'Do you ever drink any alcohol?' Sensitively work out with them how much and when. Do this

1.15	Calculating pack years of smoking

20 cigarettes = 1 packet

$$\frac{\text{No. of cigarettes smoked per day}}{20} \times \text{No. of years smoking}$$

For example, a smoker of 10 cigarettes a day who has smoked for 15 years would have smoked:

$$\frac{10}{20} \times 15 = 7.5 \text{ pack years}$$

by asking open questions giving permission for them to tell you, and do not appear to judge them. Then follow up with closed questions covering:

- What?
- When?
- How much?

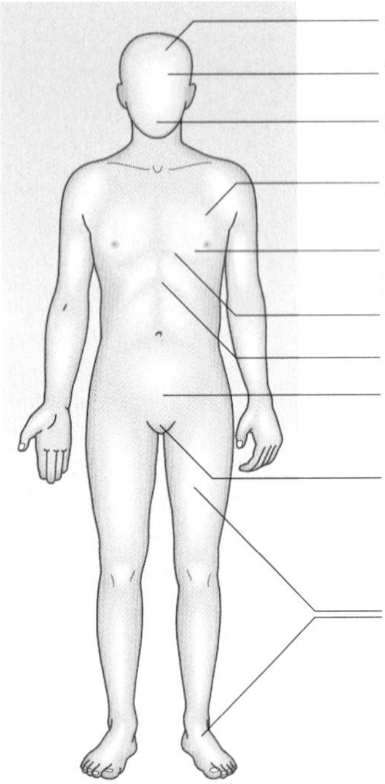
Cerebrovascular disease
Tobacco amblyopia
Oral cancer
Lung cancer
Chronic obstructive pulmonary disease
Ischaemic heart disease
Peptic ulceration
Small babies, and other obstetric problems
Erectile dysfunction
Peripheral vascular disease

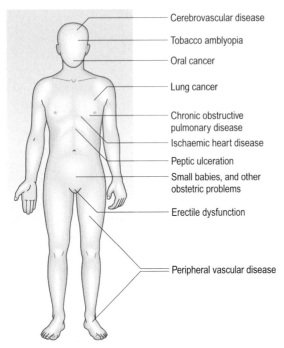

Fig. 1.4 Tobacco-related disorders.

If they still have difficulty answering, ask them:

- When did you last have a drink?
- What's the most you ever drink?

From this calculate the number of units of alcohol consumed each week. This can be calculated in one of two ways (Table 1.16).

1.16 Calculating units of alcohol

Method one	
Standard measure (1 unit) =	One small glass of wine One half pint of beer One short of spirits
Method two	
Standard measure (1 unit) =	25 ml of 40% alcohol 10 ml ethanol
x% proof – *x* units of alcohol per litre	
Examples 1 litre of 40% proof spirits contains 400 ml ethanol or 40 units 750 ml (standard bottle) contains 30 units alcohol 1 litre of 4% beer contains 40 ml ethanol or 4 units 500 ml can contains 2 units of alcohol	
Alternatively, use an online calculator, e.g. The Portman Group calculator: http://www.portmangroup.org.uk	

1.17 The content of a detailed alcohol history

- Quantity and type of drink
- Amount of money spent on alcohol
- Daily/weekly pattern (especially binge drinking and morning drinking)
- Usual place of drinking
- Alone or accompanied
- Purpose
- Attitudes to alcohol

The first uses standard measures but is inaccurate and often underestimates intake. The second method is based on direct calculation of the alcohol content of drinks. This is more accurate given the range of alcohol strengths in beers, cider and wine, but it is less convenient.

If a person drinks one glass of wine per night, the first method would estimate the intake to be 7 units per week. However, if the pure alcohol content of each glass was 17.5 ml (1.75 units in 175 ml) then the patient's intake by method two is 12.25 units per week. Many bottles of alcohol are now labelled with the number of units per bottle or per standard glass. Record alcohol consumption in the notes as units of alcohol consumed per week.

Table 1.17 lists the content of a detailed alcohol history.

Alcohol problems

Terms, e.g. problem drinking and alcohol dependence, are sometimes used interchangeably. It is more accurate to use the following terms.

Hazardous drinking. This is 'at-risk' drinking and is the regular consumption of:

- 24 g of pure ethanol (3 units) per day for men
- 14 g of pure ethanol (2 units) per day for women.

Drinking at this level doubles a man's risk of liver disease, raised blood pressure and violent death and increases a women's risk of developing breast cancer and liver disease. In anyone it increases the chance of depression and obesity, and impairs cognitive function.

The pattern of drinking is important because binge drinking of a large amount of alcohol causes *acute intoxication*. This is more likely to result in trauma, e.g. a head injury, than consuming the same amount over 4 or 5 days. Everyone should have at least 2 days per week when they drink no alcohol.

Harmful drinking. This is when the pattern of drinking has caused physical or mental health damage.

Alcohol dependence. This is where a person's use of alcohol takes a higher priority than other behaviours that previously had greater value. The features are:

- A strong, often overpowering, desire to take alcohol.
- Difficulty in controlling starting or stopping drinking and in the amount that is drunk.

- Tolerance, so that increased doses are needed to achieve the effects originally produced by lower doses.
- A withdrawal state when drinking is stopped or reduced. This produces tremor, sweating, rapid heart rate, anxiety, insomnia, and occasionally seizures, disorientation or hallucinations (delirium tremens). It is relieved by more alcohol.
- Progressive neglect of other pleasures and interests.
- Continuing to drink in spite of being aware of the harmful consequences.

Early detection of alcohol problems is important because of the health risks to patients and their families (Fig. 1.5). Screening tests help increase the detection of problem drinking. The CAGE questionnaire (Table 1.18) is still used by many clinicians but is not sensitive unless combined with two additional questions about the maximum daily intake and total weekly consumption. A more sensitive questionnaire is FAST but this has a more complex scoring system (Table 1.19).

Illicit drug use

You do not need to ask all patients about use of illicit drugs. But remember that about 30% of the adult population in Britain have used illicit drugs (mainly cannabis) at some time. Symptoms associated with drug use should prompt

1.18	The CAGE Questionnaire

Have you ever felt you should **C**UT down on your drinking?
Have people **A**NNOYED you by criticizing your drinking?
Have you ever felt bad or **G**UILTY about your drinking?
Do you ever have a drink first thing in the morning to steady you or help a hangover? (an **E**YE opener)

Positive answers to two or more questions suggest problem drinking; confirm this by asking about the maximum taken

you to ask further questions (Table 1.20). These questions are to confirm the patient is taking or has taken drugs and the amounts involved; to assess the degree of dependence and other coexistent problems and the patient's motivation to tackle the problem. Complications of drug misuse are listed in Table 1.21.

SYSTEMATIC INQUIRY

The purpose of the systematic inquiry is to uncover symptoms that the patient may have felt uncomfortable about disclosing earlier or has forgotten to mention. The patient's response to an open question is likely to be more important than that to the closed questions of systematic inquiry. A suitable open-ended question, often asked after the history of the presenting complaint, might be: 'Is there anything else you would like to tell me about?

Start by running through the symptoms in Table 1.6 (p. 11) as part of your routine history with every patient. You will eventually be able to focus on those symptoms that are most relevant. Experienced clinicians often carry out the systematic inquiry as they talk about the presenting complaint, but this takes practice and knowledge of the conditions you are trying to exclude or diagnose.

Follow up any positive response by asking questions to increase or decrease the probability of certain diseases.

Some examples of targeted systematic inquiry are:

- The smoker with weight loss: are there any respiratory symptoms, e.g. unresolving chest infection or haemoptysis, to suggest lung cancer? Are there any symptoms that suggest another organ being affected, e.g. bowel changes?
- The patient with recurrent mouth ulcers: do any alimentary symptoms suggest Crohn's disease or coeliac disease or do any locomotor symptoms suggest Behçet's disease?
- The patient with palpitation: are there any endocrine symptoms to suggest thyrotoxicosis, or a family history of thyroid disease?
- When you observe something that raises your suspicion, e.g. smell of alcohol, or an obvious goitre, ask questions about symptoms related to those conditions.

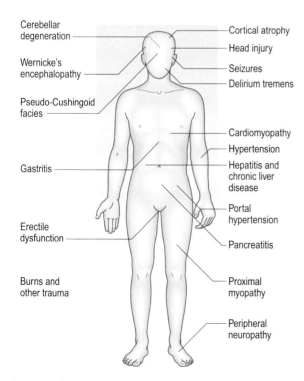

Cerebellar degeneration
Wernicke's encephalopathy
Pseudo-Cushingoid facies
Gastritis
Erectile dysfunction
Burns and other trauma

Cortical atrophy
Head injury
Seizures
Delirium tremens
Cardiomyopathy
Hypertension
Hepatitis and chronic liver disease
Portal hypertension
Pancreatitis
Proximal myopathy
Peripheral neuropathy

Fig. 1.5 Alcohol-related disorders.

1.19 The FAST Questionnaire

For the following questions please circle the answer that best applies

1 drink = ¹/₂ pint of beer or 1 glass of wine or 1 single measure of spirits

1. MEN: How often do you have EIGHT or more drinks on one occasion?
   WOMEN: How often do you have SIX or more drinks on one occasion?
   Never   Less than monthly   Monthly   Weekly   Daily or almost daily

2. How often during the last year have you been unable to remember what happened the night before because you had been drinking?
   Never   Less than monthly   Monthly   Weekly   Daily or almost daily

3. How often during the last year have you failed to do what was normally expected of you because of drinking?
   Never   Less than monthly   Monthly   Weekly   Daily or almost daily

4. In the last year has a relative or friend, or a doctor or other health worker been concerned about your drinking or suggested you cut down?
   Never   Yes, on one occasion   Yes, on more than one occasion

Scoring FAST

First stage
If the answer to question 1 is *Never* then the patient is probably not misusing alcohol
If the answer is *Weekly* or *Daily or almost daily* then the patient is a hazardous, harmful or dependent drinker
50% of people are classified using this one question

Second stage
Only use these questions if the answer is *Less than monthly* or *Monthly*
Score questions 1–3: 0, 1, 2, 3, 4
Score question 4: 0, 2, 4
Minimum score is 0
Maximum score is 16
Score for hazardous drinking is 3 or more

1.20 Illicit drug history

- What drugs are being taken?
- How often, how much?
- How long have they been taking drugs?
- Any periods of abstinence? If yes when and why did they relapse?
- What symptoms do they have if they cannot get drugs?
- Do they ever inject? If yes, where do they get their needles and syringes?
- Do they ever share needles and syringes?
- Do they see drug use as a problem?
- Do they want to make changes in their life or change the way they use drugs?

COMPLETING THE HISTORY TAKING

When you think you have got all the relevant information from the patient you should have an idea of the likely diagnosis, or at least differential diagnoses. Your examination should elicit signs that will confirm or refute this. Before you examine the patient:

- Briefly summarize what the patient has told you.
- Reflect this back to the patient. This allows the patient to:
  – correct anything you have misunderstood
  – add anything that may have been forgotten.
- Tell the patient what you are going to do next.

1.21 Complications of illicit drug misuse

Infections

- Hepatitis B and C
- HIV
- Abscesses, cellulitis and necrotizing fasciitis
- Septic pulmonary thromboembolism or lung abscesses
- Aspiration pneumonia
- Endocarditis
- Tetanus
- Wound botulism
- Sexually transmitted disease: many work in the sex industry to finance their habit

Injury

- Thrombophlebitis and deep vein thrombosis
- Arterial injury and occlusion
- Skin ulceration

Overdose

- Respiratory failure
- Rhabdomyolysis and renal failure

Chaotic life style leading to

- Poor nutrition
- Poor dental hygiene
- Failure to care for dependents
- Debt
- Prison

Key points

- Encourage patients to tell the story in their own words.
- Facilitate this by using open questions.
- Ask closed questions later to clarify symptoms.
- Clarify any medical or other terms the patient uses so that you both understand what is meant.
- Ask sensitive questions in an objective and non-judgemental way.
- Check drug history and other facts with the patient's GP or previous doctor.

- Quantify the use of tobacco, alcohol and illicit drugs.
- Summarize your understanding of the problems and reflect it back to the patient.
- Patients' previous experience and attitude influence their symptoms and presentation.
- You should have a good idea of the diagnosis after obtaining the history. If not, you are unlikely to make one during the examination.

THE PSYCHIATRIC HISTORY

Psychiatry is the medical specialty that deals with those disorders in which mental or behavioural abnormalities are the presenting complaint, or are most prominent. These conditions are classified by their clinical presentation rather than aetiology or pathology, and diagnoses are made by satisfying the inclusion and exclusion criteria according to either the World Health Organization's International Classification of Diseases (ICD 10) or the American Psychiatric Association's Diagnostic and Statistical Manual (DSM IV).

Mental and behavioural disorders are very common, with a prevalence of about 20% in the adult general population: they account for about 40% of consultations in primary care. Most conditions are mild, and are managed without specialist input. However, severe mental disorders pose serious threats to the health and safety of the patient, and sometimes to the well-being of others.

Physical and mental disorders often coexist – sometimes coincidentally but more often as cause and effect. For example, a severe infection may precipitate delirium (an acute confusional state), while intravenous drug abuse may result in the patient acquiring infections, e.g. hepatitis C and HIV. Consequently the prevalence of mental disorders (particularly organic brain disorders, mood illnesses and substance misuse disorders) is even greater among the physically ill, and affects mortality and morbidity. Because of these considerations all clinicians should be competent at basic psychiatric assessment of a patient.

HISTORY

Psychiatric interviewing has three core purposes:

- to obtain a history
- to assess the mental state of the patient
- to establish rapport that will facilitate further management.

Sometimes it is assumed that a psychiatric interview is invariably a lengthy procedure in which a detailed history of the patient's entire life is necessary: this is not so! Assessment interviews usually do have to cover background personal and social factors to establish an understanding of how the illness evolved and to guide management, but the focus, as in all history taking, is the presenting problem and its solution for the patient.

Before meeting the patient it is important to obtain as much background psychiatric, medical and social information as possible – from the source of referral and from ward staff if the patient is in hospital. It is particularly important to establish the nature of the problem and whether it is the patient's complaint or somebody else's concern. Additionally, it is helpful to establish whether:

- the patient knows about and accepts the referral
- the patient is able to understand and communicate
- the patient wishes to be seen alone or with somebody else
- there is an element of danger
- behavioural disturbance or other impediments to interview are likely.

Plainly, there are circumstances when a standard 'one-to-one interview' is not feasible, notably when the patient:

- is a child (when family or parental interviewing is the norm)
- has a severe learning disability
- has a mental disorder that prevents normal communication
- is too disturbed
- refuses to be assessed.

Otherwise, the interview follows conventional procedures:

- Put the patient at ease.
- Listen attentively and react to the patient's verbal and non-verbal cues – be empathic verbally and non-verbally.
- Allow patients to tell their story in their own words.
- Allow breaks and digressions (within reason) if the patient requires these – notably with sensitive topics or when distress emerges.

- Concentrate on the presenting complaint, using a technique of nested, open questions to explore the key elements.
- Switch to choice questions if the patient struggles with open questions.
- Clarify, echo, reflect, emphasize, summarize.
- Once the presenting situation is clear, the patient is settled and rapport permits, take greater control of the interview content through focused questioning and greater use of closed questions. Closed questions then enable the crucial background facts to be established.

Content

The content of a psychiatric history is as follows:

- Reason for referral
- Presenting complaint(s)
- History of presenting complaint(s)
- Family history (including psychiatric disorders specifically)
- Personal history – childhood; education; occupational history; sexual and marital history; children; current social circumstances
- Past medical/psychiatric history
- Prescribed medication; other remedies
- Psychoactive substance use, including alcohol, tobacco and caffeine
- Forensic history
- Premorbid personality.

Some aspects of psychiatric history taking differ from standard medical interviewing, and merit further consideration.

Risk assessment

Mental disorders can be associated with danger: classically depression with harm to self, and paranoid states with harm to others. Whenever the presentation suggests such hazards may be a possibility, then inquiries about thoughts, impulses and actions concerning suicide or violence must be made. How and when this is broached during the interview depends on cues: generally it is best left until rapport is firmly established, as patients often find these matters difficult to reveal. Many patients are relieved to be able to confide what is frightening to them and unacceptable to share with their family.

Sensitive issues

There are other themes that can be tricky for the patient and doctor during an interview, notably sexual matters and criminal activities. The sexual history is a component in a standard psychiatric history, the forensic history is another,

while illicit drug-taking is part of the history of psychoactive substance use. It is far more important to build an effective relationship than to obtain a complete account at the expense of alienating the patient. Enquiring about sensitive matters can and sometimes should be omitted from initial psychiatric history taking unless the presenting problem is such that there is an obvious relevance which the patient can understand, or it is essential for establishing management. Such topics can be returned to if necessary at later interviews when rapport will enable the patient to divulge such material more comfortably (and probably more accurately too).

Premorbid personality

Assessment of premorbid personality is, by convention, the last section in the psychiatric history. It is also the most difficult for students and non-psychiatrists. Personality influences vulnerability to mental illnesses, colours the clinical presentation, determines the patient's attitudes and coping strategies, and has to be taken into account in the management plan. Assessing premorbid personality involves evaluating what kind of person the patient was before the illness emerged – and because of this, it is the one section of history for which an informant who knew the patient well is essential. It is helpful to summarize premorbid personality under these subheadings:

- interests and hobbies
- social activities, friendships and other relationships
- moral/religious beliefs
- predominant mood
- coping strategies and reactions to stress and setback
- strengths, weaknesses, basic character.

One useful approach is to start by asking patients how they might have spent an average week in their life before they became ill.

Other sources of information

In psychiatric assessment, information obtained from other sources is usually necessary, sometimes vital and occasionally the only available history.

- Background medical information will be available in the case records of known patients and from the general practitioner.
- Speaking to a relative or carer will provide useful collateral history that may confirm, refute or supplement the patient's history.
- Contacting the patient's social worker, community nurse, counsellor or support worker is often helpful.
- With inpatients, speaking to ward nurses informs about aspects such as sleep pattern, hallucinatory activity and cooperation.

PHYSICAL EXAMINATION

Psychiatric assessment concentrates on mental functioning, but physical examination is often required too. The content and extent of the physical examination depend on the history and likely diagnosis; usually general observation, coupled with basic cardiovascular and neurological examination will suffice.

MENTAL STATE EXAMINATION

The mental state examination is a vital part of psychiatric assessment. Like a physical examination, it is systematic with the aim being to elicit signs of disorder. The main areas are:

- appearance
- behaviour
- speech
- mood
- thought content
- perception
- cognitive functioning
- insight.

Mental state examination involves:

- observation of the patient
- assimilation and analysis of the history
- consideration of the form as well as the content of the patient's mental life
- specific questions exploring various mental phenomena
- short tests of cognitive function.

This will be channelled by the history and potential diagnoses so, for example, when an organic brain disorder is suspected, more thorough assessment of cognitive functioning is required, while for depression the assessment of mood is central.

Appearance

- General, e.g. attire and cleanliness, especially evidence of self-neglect
- Facial appearance
- Posture and gait.

Behaviour

- Cooperation/reaction to the interview/eye contact/rapport
- Level of consciousness
- Social behaviour
- Motor overactivity – includes hyperkinesis (a disorder of children), restlessness, agitation, compulsions and rituals

- Motor underactivity – includes stupor, slowing (retardation) and poverty of movement (akinesis)
- Motor abnormality – includes involuntary movements and mannerisms.

Speech

- Rate – includes pressure of speech and slowing
- Quantity – includes mutism, poverty of speech and pressure of speech
- Articulation – includes stammering, stuttering and dysarthria
- Form – covers the way in which a patient speaks rather than the content:
  - flights of ideas: where ideas flow rapidly but remain connected although sometimes by unusual associations, e.g. clang words (associated with mania)
  - loosening of association/formal thought disorder (found in schizophrenia): when the logical sequence of ideas is lost; specific abnormalities include thought blocking when thinking suddenly ceases and there is a pause before a different thought emerges, and word salad which is the extreme case when words emerge as a jumble
  - perseveration: an inability to change theme, resulting in inappropriate repetition of a response
  - circumstantiality: slowed thinking, loaded down with unnecessary detail and digression, but maintaining the goal of the thought
  - neologisms: invented words, or established words with a novel meaning.

Mood

Mood is defined in DSM IV as 'a pervasive and sustained emotion that in the extreme colours the patient's perception of the world'. Examining mood involves consideration of the patient's subjective emotional state and your objective evaluation.

Subjective mood

Subjective mood is established by inquiry, introduced by an open question, e.g. 'How have you been feeling recently?' or 'How do you feel in your spirits?' This leads on to further exploration in the usual way.

Objective mood

Objective mood is picked up during the interview. It requires a degree of experience as well as empathy to assess accurately. It takes into account the patient's demeanour, facial expression and behaviour as well as observed emotional expression. Not infrequently you can sense the patient's emotional state, be it sadness, anger, irritability, anxiety, bewilderment or elation, by considering your own response during the interview.

Dysphoric (abnormal) mood states take two forms:

- abnormal pervasive mood
- abnormal expression of mood.

Abnormal pervasive mood states occur in many types of mental disorder, but are the central feature of:

- depression, when there is sustained low mood which may include sadness, tearfulness, hopelessness, despair and, in severe illness, loss of emotion such that the patient feels nothing
- mania, when the patient feels elated or euphoric
- anxiety, when worry, apprehension and tension feature.

Abnormal expression of mood includes:

- labile mood, when emotions are superficial, rapidly changing and poorly controlled; extreme lability is sometimes emotional incontinence (associated with multi-infarct dementia)
- incongruous mood, when the emotional expression is inappropriate for the thought
- blunting, when normal expression of mood is diminished or lost (sometimes termed flattening of affect).

Incidentally, the terms mood and affect are often used interchangeably, but they are subtly different. Mood refers to the pervasive emotional state, whereas affect is the observable expression of emotions, which is variable over time. A useful analogy is to think of a patient's mood as a climate, in which case the patient's affect is the current weather.

Thought content

This is a central part of the mental state examination, and is primarily based on the history the patient has provided. Thought content is subdivided into preoccupations and abnormal beliefs.

Preoccupations

Preoccupations include:

- Ruminations: repetitive ideas or themes on which the patient broods. Ruminations often reflect the mood state, e.g. incessant worrying in anxiety states and morbid thinking in depression (Table 1.22). Morbid ideation includes ideas of guilt, unworthiness, burden and blame as well as dwelling on past losses, failures and disappointments. Suicidal or homicidal ruminations are particularly important to establish and evaluate (Table 1.23).
- Hypochondriasis: a specific, unjustified preoccupation with having a serious disease.

1.22 Typical preoccupations associated with mood disorder	
Anxiety state	Anxiousness, worry, fear, apprehension, doubt, uncertainty
Depressive disorder	Loss of self-worth, confidence, ability Guilt, burden, failure, catastrophe, hopelessness Death, suicide Unlovable, unlikeable, self-denigration

1.23 Questions to ask to determine the possibility of suicidal thoughts in a patient
• How have you been feeling recently? • Do you feel brighter in the morning or in the evening? • Have you any difficulties with sleeping/night waking? • Do you feel worried, irritable or depressed? • Has life seemed less worthwhile? • Have you ever seriously considered taking your own life?

- Obsessional thoughts: a form of rumination that involves senseless preoccupation with a topic from which the patient cannot desist in spite of realizing it is irrational. Compulsions are the behavioural expression and have the same characteristics.
- Phobias: the opposite of obsessions. Instead of feeling compelled to think or do something, the phobic patient feels compelled to avoid a situation, object or activity because of an irrational fear.

Abnormal beliefs

Abnormal beliefs are subdivided into overvalued ideas and delusions.

Overvalued ideas. These are not pathognomonic of mental illness. They are beliefs that are held, expressed and acted on by the patient about matters which are of particular importance to them – but to a degree that others from the same culture would regard as unreasonable. Eccentrics and unconventional people, e.g. members of unusual sects or cults, exemplify this phenomenon: while some may be mentally ill, many are not.

Delusions. Delusions are invariably of clinical significance. A delusion is a false belief which is held with total conviction, which is not shared by others from the same culture and which is maintained in spite of proof or logical argument to the contrary. Together with hallucinations, delusions are regarded as 'psychotic symptoms': psychosis is a collective term that encompasses mental illnesses in which the patient's experience and reasoning do not reflect reality.

Delusions are subdivided into primary and secondary. Primary delusions, which are characteristic of schizophrenia, are fully formed de novo. Secondary delusions, which can occur in various mental illnesses, can be understood to have arisen in a context of another mental process – usually an abnormal mood state or abnormal perceptions. In this setting, they provide an explanation for patients as to why they are having these feelings or experiences.

The content of delusions can give a clue to the nature of the mental illness – for instance, grandiose delusions are associated with mania, nihilistic delusions with depression, and paranoid delusions with delirium and schizophrenia. When delusions are bizarre their recognition is easy, but delusions may seem quite ordinary ideas, e.g. being followed, victimized or impoverished, when establishing their psychotic nature can be much harder.

When conducting a psychiatric interview it is inappropriate to ask routinely about delusions: such inquiries will upset many patients and damage rapport, while deluded patients are unlikely to give a straight answer anyway. Exploring delusions requires tact and timing. Questions usually have to be focused on information the patient has provided, or sometimes other information brought to your attention. Technique generally involves greater use of closed questions to pin down the beliefs, e.g. 'Do you really believe that you are the Messiah?' If the patient answers 'yes' then explore this as a nest for further inquiry; for example, lead on with 'What proof can you give me?'

Perception

Alterations in normal perception consist of changes to our normal, familiar awareness of ordinary experiences. Abnormal experiences may be referred to:

- the environment, which includes illusions, hallucinations and derealization
- the patient, which includes somatic hallucinations and depersonalization.

An *illusion* is a false perception of a real, external stimulus. Such misinterpretations may affect any sensory modality but auditory and visual illusions are commonest. Frequently, illusions arise from a sensory impairment, e.g. partial sightedness or deafness, or because of clouding of consciousness (common in delirium), and the illusion is an understandable attempt to fill in the gap. For example, a coat hanging behind a door may give the illusion of a person standing there.

An *hallucination* is a false perception which is not based on a real stimulus, so a person is seen at the door where there is no stimulus to prompt this sighting. Hallucinations are located in external space and are authentic to the patient. Hallucinations can affect any of the sensory modalities although visual and auditory are commonest. Visual hallucinations are particularly associated with delirium and auditory hallucinations with schizophrenia, but almost any form of hallucination is possible in any of the mental illness in which psychotic features can occur.

Some hallucinatory experiences are normal, for example on going to sleep (hypnagogic) and on wakening (hypnopompic), while people in mourning may experience visual, auditory or tactile hallucinations that involve contact with the deceased. Similarly, *depersonalization* (a feeling of having become unreal or that the body has altered in some way) and *derealization* (when the same changes have occurred in the patient's surroundings) often occur as a normal experience, especially when tired or stressed.

Hallucinations need to be distinguished from pseudo-hallucinations which are common, and often lead to a misdiagnosis of psychotic illness. Pseudohallucinations are identified by patients as arising from within their own mind, and are experienced as an internal phenomenon, sometimes described as an inner voice or eye. They tend to lack the reality for the patient of true hallucinations, i.e. they have an 'as if' quality, and so do not have knock-on effects on other mental functions.

As with assessment of delusions, it is necessary to explore this aspect of the mental state tactfully and timeously in order to avoid damage to rapport ('You must think I'm mad').

Cognitive functions

Assessing attention and concentration is routine in mental state examination. Other aspects can be tested more selectively, but this becomes essential and wide-ranging when an organic brain disorder is suspected. This phase of the examination must be carefully explained before starting so that the patient does not get upset or annoyed by questions that could justifiably be regarded as insulting or silly.

Cognitive assessment comprises:

- attention and concentration
- orientation
- memory
- general knowledge and intelligence.

Attention and concentration

Attention and concentration can be impaired in many mental disorders. It is important to establish the presence of impairment because this will affect the patient's ability to retain and comply with information given and treatment requirements, and hence has a major bearing on how the management plan is formulated. When testing indicates significant impairment, it is unnecessary to proceed to test registration, immediate recall and short-term memory as these will inevitably be affected as a consequence.

Impaired attention is usually evident at interview as increased distractibility, with the patient responding to extraneous cues – both real that would normally be ignored (e.g. a muffled conversation outside the room), and unreal (e.g. auditory hallucinations).

Testing involves examining patients' ability to follow sequences that should be familiar to them (i.e. do not involve new learning). The traditional method is the serial sevens test. The patient is asked to count back aloud in sevens from 100 as quickly as possible and as far as possible. Mistakes are noted and the patient is asked to try again. Time taken, number of errors and the finishing point should be noted. This test requires some mathematical ability and hence is influenced by intelligence and educational attainment. When these attributes are dubious, serial threes, counting back from 20 in the same manner, is an alternative. However, sequencing months in reverse from December is a better method.

Orientation

Disorientation is the best sign of an organic mental disorder. Orientation should be checked for time, date (including day of the week), place and person. Minor anomalies can occur normally in hospital when the patient's routine is broken and the passage of time is lost through severe illness or an operation. Other evidence should be incorporated, for instance a relative's information that the patient wanders from home at night, thinking it is daytime, and then cannot find the way home.

Memory

Memory function is subdivided into registration and immediate recall, short-term memory, recent memory and long-term memory. It is unnecessary to test all of these in all patients, the extent of examination being determined by the history and likely diagnosis. The following summarizes simple tests that can be used:

- Registration and immediate recall: immediate repetition of a series of digits. Normal forward digit span is seven or more; five or fewer indicates impairment.
- Short-term memory: name and address test. Give the patient a six-item fictitious name and address to remember (not your own!) after explaining what you are doing. Registration and immediate recall is tested by getting the patient to repeat this information back immediately. This should be scored, e.g. 4/6 items correct, and then repeated until 6/6 is obtained; count the number of attempts required and abandon the test after five attempts if the patient cannot assimilate all the information. Ask for the information again after 5 minutes during which other inquiries have been made. Note the score, the nature of errors and the patient's attempts at correction/awareness of mistakes. Normal scores are 5 or 6; 4 is borderline; fewer than 4 indicates significant memory impairment.
- Recent memory: ask the patient about current events reported in the news over the past week, bearing in mind the patient's access to information and interests.

Alternatively ask about visitors or events in the patient's own life over the past week, making sure that the answers can be verified.
- Long-term memory: problems are evident from the history, for example failing to remember key events, dates and people in the patient's life. In dementing illnesses, long-term memory is often spared until later stages of the disorder, sometimes to a remarkable degree when compared with other memory functions.

General knowledge/intelligence

General knowledge is an expression of both intelligence and long-term memory, and as such it is not particularly useful to assess. Impaired intelligence, notably learning disability, is usually evident:

- in the history – schooling and educational attainment in particular, but also occupational history
- in the presentation – use of language, understanding of language and concepts, abilities to plan, organize, anticipate.

Formal standard tests include closed questions on subjects like history (e.g. the dates of major wars), geography (e.g. capitals of countries) and important people (e.g. names of prime ministers, monarchs or American presidents). Another technique is to check breadth of knowledge by asking the patient to name different kinds of items in a collection, e.g. 10 kinds of fruit, vegetable, flower or colour. Finally basic numeracy and literacy should be checked by asking the patient to do simple calculations and to read newspaper headlines.

Insight

Insight refers to how patients understand or explain their condition. Insight is almost invariably present to some extent but rarely completely; it also fluctuates during the course of the illness and may appear to vary depending on the nature of the inquiry – for example, patients not infrequently deny they are mentally ill yet accept psychiatric admission. Hence commenting that insight is present or absent is unhelpful. In assessing insight, three elements are important:

- recognition of illness
- acceptance of illness
- willingness to accept treatment and agree to a management plan.

PSYCHIATRIC RATING SCALES

The use of psychiatric rating scales as clinical tools in psychiatric assessment is increasingly widespread. Most of

1.24	Abbreviated mental test

1. Time (nearest hour)?
2. Day of week?
3. Month?
4. Year?
5. Age?
6. Place?
7. Names of three objects at 2 minutes, e.g. apple, table, coin (score 1 if only one item is remembered)
8. Dates of Second World War?
9. Name of Prime Minister?
10. Count backwards from 20 to 1 (0 for any uncorrected error)

Each item scores 1 point
Normal scores 8–10
Mild–moderate dementia 4–7
Moderate–severe dementia 0–3

THERAPEUTIC ROLE OF THE PSYCHIATRIC INTERVIEW

When conducting a psychiatric assessment interview, you must bear in mind the third purpose mentioned at the start of this chapter. This is establishing rapport that will facilitate further management. Patients need to feel that they have derived something from the encounter and not simply answered a lot of questions, some of which seem irrelevant or are frankly embarrassing, for no apparent reason other than to satisfy your need to complete the records. Active listening, sensitive questioning, tolerating difficult thoughts, experiences and emotions, empathizing, supporting and reassuring when appropriate are all therapeutic activities that facilitate further management and ensure that the patient leaves the interview, it is hoped, feeling better and certainly not feeling worse.

◆ Key points

- ◆ Get as much background information and history from other sources as you can (with the patient's permission if indicated).
- ◆ Concentrate initially on establishing rapport by helping your patient feel at ease and enabling him to tell his story as he wishes.
- ◆ Be willing to modify the extent, order and content of the assessment to take account of your patient's background and presentation.
- ◆ Observe your patient closely to gain objective evidence of his mental state, especially nonverbal information.
- ◆ Your patient's speech gives you access to his thought form and content, mood and cognitive functioning.
- ◆ Consider your own response to your patient: you can often sense his mood. Do you feel sad, angry, irritated or confused, for example?
- ◆ Use brief formal tests to assess cognitive function.
- ◆ Consider standardized rating scales as a screening tool (and sometimes to monitor progress).
- ◆ Do not forget the importance of selective physical examination.
- ◆ Remember to assess these key issues – potential risks to self or others, degree of distress and disability, capacity to take decisions, insight into illness.

these scales were developed for research purposes, either to identify potential cases or to provide a numerical measure of change in a condition. Some scales require special training; all require to be used sensibly and appropriately. Rating scales should never replace standard psychiatric interviewing, but they can be useful adjuncts, either to screen for a disorder or to provide a reliable indication of change in an illness.

Screening tools should be brief, easy to use, valid and reliable: widely used examples are the CAGE and FAST (alcohol problems), Hospital Anxiety and Depression Scale (HADS) (mood disorders) and the Abbreviated Mental Test (AMT) (organic brain disorders) (Table 1.24). Progress measures have to be used repeatedly, so they tend to be longer to reduce practice learning and to enable finer discrimination of change. Although screening measures, e.g. HADS and AMT, can be used, good examples are the Beck Depression Inventory (BDI) (depression) and the Mini Mental State Examination (MMSE) (organic brain disorders).

DOCUMENTING THE FINDINGS – THE CASE NOTES

The case notes, sometimes called case records, are the written record of a patient's medical condition (Table 1.25). The notes include your initial findings, proposed investigations and the plan of management for your patient's condition, together with information about the patient's progress.

They allow information to be recorded and shared by all the staff caring for the patient, not simply during one episode of illness, but over time. When a patient presents in the future, the new findings can be compared with those found at any earlier presentation. Notes must therefore be accurate,

1.25 Information in the case record
• History and examination findings
• Investigations and results
• The management plan
• Assessments of other health professionals, e.g. dieticians, health visitors
• Information and education provided to patients and their relatives
• Correspondence about the patient
• The patient's progress
• Advance directives or 'living will'
• Contact details about next of kin.

1.26 Describing wounds
Position
• Where on the body, including which aspect of a limb
Size and orientation
• e.g. 5 cm by 3 mm vertical scratch
Appearance
• e.g. colour, shape
Type of lesion
• *Abrasion:* loss of the outer skin due to impact with a rough surface
• *Scratch:* linear abrasion due to drawing of a sharp point over the skin
• *Bruise:* bleeding within the tissues beneath the skin
• *Laceration:* tearing of the skin due to blunt trauma; ragged edges
• *Incised wound:* cut or gash; sharp edges
• *Penetrating wound:* depth is greater than length; breaches full skin thickness

legible and clearly signed. In primary care, case records may span the whole of a person's life and record the development of a condition over several consultations.

You may write notes while talking to the patient and taking the history but do not let this interrupt the flow of your discussion, and maintain as much eye contact as possible. Active listening is difficult if you are writing, so practice making brief notes at the time so that you do not forget important points. Write up the full history after you have left the patient. If the consultation is short, you can write up the notes afterwards because it is easier to remember all the details. Write up the physical findings when you have completed the examination and not as you proceed. Only record objective findings and never make judgemental, flippant or pejorative comments. This is unprofessional, and remember that patients or their lawyer may subsequently read their notes.

Although structured proformas for recording the initial history and examination findings are used as an aide-memoire in many hospitals, it is not possible to record every detail of the history and examination in every patient. Only record negative findings if they are relevant; for instance, in a patient presenting with breathlessness, the negative details of the respiratory inquiry are important but you can condense the negative responses to the gastrointestinal inquiry to one entry of 'none' or 'nil'. You may use abbreviations but they should not be obscure or ambiguous. Widely recognized ones are included in the case example (Fig. 1.6). The prefix '°' is often used to signify 'no', for example °tenderness, or °headache. Use diagrams to show the site and size of superficial injuries or ulcers, and for the abdomen to illustrate the position of tenderness, masses or scars (see Fig. 5.9, p. 168). Describe injuries accurately, because if the patient has been the victim of assault you may be asked to give legal evidence from the notes months or years after the event (Table 1.26).

Unitary notes

Unitary or 'multidisciplinary' notes allow the whole team to record their findings in one document, rather than each health professional keeping separate case records. Although a bulky unitary record can be cumbersome, it encourages a shared approach to care, avoids duplication and makes it easy for different professionals to access information.

Primary care

Primary care records follow the patient between practices and contain the whole story of a patient's health, rather than discrete episodes of hospital care. Diagnoses in primary care may emerge over a series of consultations so the entries are often short, but include a description of the problem, any working diagnosis, advice given, investigations or treatment arranged, follow-up and the doctor's initials or signature.

Computer records

Most records are still held on paper but comprehensive computer records are increasingly used in primary care and hospital settings. Computer records allow easy access to medical and prescribing information during the consultation, and paper summary sheets are an easy way of transferring legible, relevant information. Many general practices, however, still use a mixture of paper and electronic records, although in the future smart cards carried by patients will hold their entire medical record. Paperless practices have all patient information held on computer. It is arranged to highlight important medical events unobscured by routine information. This can be downloaded onto portable palmtops for domiciliary use.

Clinical coding

When computers are used, conditions and diagnoses are documented systematically so that information can be

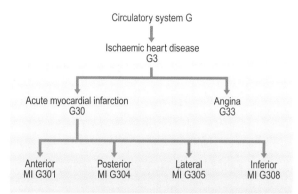

Circulatory system G

↓

Ischaemic heart disease
G3

Acute myocardial infarction
G30

Angina
G33

Anterior
MI G301

Posterior
MI G304

Lateral
MI G305

Inferior
MI G308

Fig. 1.6 An example from the Read Code of Clinical Terms system.

retrieved in a way that makes clinical sense. In the UK, Read Codes are used. These are a comprehensive list of clinical terms that describe the diagnoses, care and treatment of patients in a hierarchical way (Fig. 1.6). Each clinical term has a unique Read Code and, once coded, the data can be used for audit and statistical analysis.

The College of American Pathologists has developed a different clinical classification called SNOMED®. This system is now being combined with the Read Code system to produce SNOMED CT which will bring together the two leading international clinical terms systems to provide one unified system for worldwide use. These clinical terms systems are not classifications of diseases but systems of coding clinical terms in everyday use.

Confidentiality

The case record is confidential and must be stored securely. It is also a legal document that may be used in a court of law.

Details cannot be shared with anyone who is not involved in a patient's care, unless the patient gives full, informed, written consent. This includes insurance companies, lawyers, the police and research workers. You may only break confidence if a patient is a risk to him/herself or other members of the public. For example in the UK, if your patient with active epilepsy continues to drive against medical advice, you must inform the Driving and Vehicle Licensing Centre, advise the patient you are doing so and record this clearly in the notes.

In the UK the Health Records Act of 1990 gives patients the right to see and receive a copy of their paper case record. Some patients already hold their own paper records, usually when care is shared between hospital and community, for example in antenatal care and diabetic care. The Data Protection Act 1998 gives patients the right to see anything held on computer about them. You can stop patients seeing a part of their case record if you think this would cause serious harm to their physical or mental health or to any other individual. Remember this when you record information about third parties, for example in cases of sexual abuse.

◆ Key points

◆ Always record, date and sign your findings, investigations and management plan for the patient.
◆ Record only objective findings.
◆ Record all abnormal findings but only record the negative findings if they are relevant.
◆ The notes are confidential and details must be shared only with professionals directly involved in the patient's care.
◆ Patients have the right to see their case notes, should they wish.

Date : 03.08.04
Time : 14.00

MARY BROWN aged 76
32 Tartan Cresc.
Edinburgh
DOB 17.09.22

Emergency admission to CCU via GP: Dr Wells, High St., Edinburgh

History from patient   **PC** Chest pain   2 hours
                              Breathlessness   1 hour
                              Dizziness   30 mins

HPC
Severe pain 'like a band around chest' while watching TV which has now lasted 2 hours despite using GTN.
Radiates to jaw and inner aspect of L arm.
Has gradually become breathless over the last hour and dizzy in last 30 minutes.

First began six months ago: episode of lower retrosternal chest pain after walking about ¹/2 mile uphill.
     • relieved by rest after 5 minutes
     • no associated palpitation or SOB
Two further episodes over the next 3 months

3 months ago: increasing frequency of pain
     • now brought on by walking 200 yards on the flat or climbing 1 flight of stairs
     • worse after heavy meals
     • other features of pain as before

2 months ago: visited GP who diagnosed angina. Prescribed GTN which gave effective relief.

1 week ago: 3 episodes of chest pain at rest, all immediately relieved by GTN.

Smokes 20/day since aged 19
°blackouts °pain in calves on exertion.

PH   Tonsillectomy   1952   Hospital X
         Perforated peptic ulcer   1977   Hospital Y
         COPD   Since 1990   General practitioner

         °MI, °DM, ° J, °HBP, °Stroke, °RF, °TB

DH   DOSE   FREQUENCY   DURATION

         Salbutamol inhaler   2 puffs   4 times daily   3 years
         Temazepam   10mg   At night   6 months
         Senokot (self medication) 2 tabs   2–3 times per week   10 years
         GTN spray   1 puff   As required   2 months
         NKA.

FH
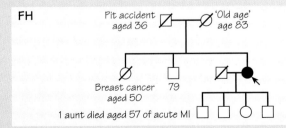

                    1

Fig. 1.7   Case notes example.

Demographic Details
Always record
• The patient's name and address, date of birth and age
• Any national health identification number such as CHI in the UK
• Source of referral e.g. from Accident and Emergency
  or General Practitioner
• GP's name and address
• Source of history e.g. patient, relative, carer
• Date and time of examination

Presenting Complaint (PC)
State the major problem in one or two of the patient's own
words (or give a brief list), followed by the duration of each.
Do not use medical terminology.

History of Presenting Complaint (HPC)
Describe the onset, nature and course of each symptom.
Paraphrase the patient's account and condense it if necessary.
Omit irrelevant details.
Put particularly telling comments in inverted commas.
Include other parts of the history if relevant, such as the smoking
history in patients with cardiac or respiratory presentations,
or family history in disorders with a possible genetic trait such
as hypercholesterolaemia or diabetes.
Correct grammar is not necessary.
GTN – glyceryl trinitrate
SOB – short of breath

Past History (PH)
Tabulate in chronological order.
Include important negatives, e.g. in a patient with chest pain ask
about previous myocardial infarction, angina, hypertension or
diabetes mellitus and record whether these are present or absent.
Jaundice is important because it may pose a risk to health care
workers if due to hepatitis B or C.

COPD – Chronic obstructive pulmonary disease
   MI – Myocardial infarction
   DM – Diabetes mellitus
    J – Jaundice
  HBP – Hypertension
   RF – Rheumatic fever

Drug History (DH)
Tabulate these and include any allergies particularly to drugs.
Record any previous adverse drug reactions prominently on
the front of the notes as well as inside.

NKA – No known allergies

Family History (FH)
Record the age and current health or the causes of or the
ages at death of the patient's parents, siblings and children.
Use the symbols shown in Chapter 1 (p. 15) to construct
a pedigree chart.

SH
Retired cleaner.
Widow for 3 years. Lives alone in sheltered housing.
Smoked 20/day from age 19.
Teetotal.
HH once a week for cleaning and shopping. Daughter nearby visits regularly

SE
CVS: See above

RS: Long-standing cough most days with white sputum on rising in morning only. °haemoptysis
Wheezy in cold weather.

GI: Weight steady
Nil else of note

GUS: PARA 1 + 0. °PMB °urinary symptoms

CNS: Nil of note

MSS: Occasional pain and stiffness in right knee on exertion for 5 years

ES: Nil of note

O/E
Anxious, frail, cachectic lady.
Weight 45 kg. Height 1.25 m
2 cm craggy mass in upper, outer quadrant L breast. Fixed to underlying tissues.
<u>Patient unaware of this</u>
1 cm node in apex of left axilla.
°pallor, °cyanosis, °jaundice, °clubbing

CVS
P90 reg, small volume, normal character,
BP 140/80 JVP + 3 cms normal character °oedema AB 5ICS MCL °thrills
HS I + II + 2/6 ESM at LLSE °radiation
°bruits
PP:

	Radial	Brachial	Carotid	Femoral	Popliteal	Post. Tibial	Dorsalis pedis
R	+	+	+	+	+/-	+/-	+/-
L	+	+	+	+	+	+	+

(Normal +, Reduced +/-, Absent -)

RS
Trachea central. Reduced cricosternal distance and intercostal indrawing on inspiration.
Expansion reduced but symmetrical.
PN resonant
BS vesicular and quiet
VR normal and symmetrical

Social History (SH)
Occupation
Marital status
Living circumstances; type of housing and with whom
Smoking
Alcohol
Illicit drug use (if appropriate)
Social support in the frail or disabled

HH – home help

Systematic Enquiry (SE)
Document positive responses that do not feature in the HPC.

CVS – Cardiovascular system
RS – Respiratory system
GI – Gastrointestinal system
GUS – Genito-urinary system
PMB – Postmenopausal bleeding
CNS – Central nervous system
MSS – Musculoskeletal system
ES – Endocrine system

General / On examination (OE)
Physical appearance e.g. frail, drowsy, breathless
Mental state e.g. anxious, distressed, confused
Undernourished, cachectic, obese
Abnormal smells e.g. ketones, alcohol, uraemia, foetor hepaticus
Record height, weight and waist circumference
Skin e.g. cyanosis, pallor, jaundice, any specific lesions or rashes
Breasts, normal or describe any mass
Hands; finger clubbing, or abnormalities of skin and nails
Lymph nodes; characteristics and site

Cardiovascular system (CVS)
Pulse (P) rate, rhythm, character and volume
Blood pressure (BP)
Jugular venous pressure (JVP) height and character
Presence or absence of ankle oedema
Apex beat (AB) position, character, presence of thrills
Heart sounds (HS) any added sounds, murmurs and grade
Peripheral pulses (PP) and bruits

5ICS – 5th intercostal space
MCL – Mid clavicular line
ESM – Ejection systolic murmur
LLSE – Lower left sternal edge

Respiratory System (RS)
Any chest wall deformity
Trachea central or deviated
Signs of hyperinflation
Expansion and its symmetry
Percussion note (PN) and site of any abnormality
Breath sounds (BS), any added sounds and site of abnormality
Vocal resonance (VR) and site of abnormality

Abdo.
Normal oral mucosa
Upper midline scar
Hernial orifices intact
°tenderness or guarding
°masses
°LKKS or ascites
BS normal
PR faecal loading. No mucosal abnormality
FOB negative
PV not performed

Scar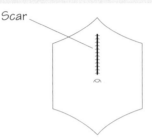

CNS

AMT 9
Cranial nerves II–XII: PERLA, NAD
Speech normal

	RIGHT		LEFT	
	UL	LL	UL	LL
Power	5	5	5	5
Tone	normal (n)	n	n	n
Light touch	n	n	n	n
Position	n	n	n	n
Coordination	n	n	n	n

Reflexes	K	A	B	T	S	Pl
R	++	+	++	+	+	flexor
L	++	+	++	+	+	flexor

(increased +++, normal ++, diminished +, absent -)

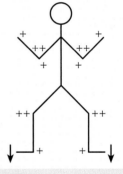

MSS
Heberden's nodes on index and middle fingers bilaterally.
Full ROM in all joints.
Crepitus in right knee. No other bony abnormality

IMPRESSION △

Active problems
1 Chest pain suggestive of angina or acute myocardial infarction (MI)
2 Left breast lump and axillary node suspicious of cancer
3 Smoker

Inactive problems
1 Stable COPD
2 Perforated duodenal ulcer 1977
3 Possible osteoarthritis of right knee

3

Abdominal System (AS)
Mouth
  Any abnormality–own teeth or dentures
Abdo
  Scars and site
  Shape, distended or scaphoid
  Hernial orifices
  Tenderness and guarding and site of this
  Masses and description of these
  Enlargement of liver, kidneys or spleen (shorten to LKKS)
  Ascites if present
  Bowel sounds (BS); presence and character
  Rectal examination (PR) record whether or not it was
  performed and your findings
  In women; vaginal examination (VE) is only carried
  out if relevant
  In men; external genitalia

FOB–Faecal occult blood testing

Central Nervous System (CNS)
In older patients record the abbreviated mental test (AMT) score
In impaired consciousness, head injury or possible raised
intracranial pressure record the Glasgow Coma Scale (GCS)
(pp. 239–240)

Abnormal speech
Cranial nerves; record abnormalities only
Fundoscopy
Tabulate the remaining examination
If it is relevant record the presence or absence of tremor, gait,
abnormality, fasciculation, dyspraxia, two point discrimination,
stereognosis or sensory neglect.

PERLA–Pupils equal and react to light and accommodation
    NAD–No abnormality detected
      UL–Upper limb
      LL–Lower limb
       K–Knee
       A–Ankle
       B–Biceps
       T–Triceps
       S–Supinator
      Pl–Plantar

Musculoskeletal System (MSS)
Gait if abnormal
Muscle or soft tissue changes
Swelling, colour, heat, tenderness
Deformities in the bones of joints
Limitations of ranges of movements (ROM) in any affected joint

Clinical Diagnosis or Impression
Record your conclusions and the most likely diagnoses in order
of probability.
In patients with multiple pathology make a problem list so the key
issues are seen immediately

△ Diagnosis

Plan

ECG performed on admission shows sinus rhythm and deep ST depression in leads II, III and aVF

Troponin at 12 hours
Repeat ECG in 1 hour
Chest X-ray
Full blood count
Urea and electrolytes, glucose

Oxygen and cardiac monitor
Aspirin and clopidogrel
Buccal nitrate
Low molecular weight heparin
Diltiazem as beta-blocker contraindicated due to COPD
Advice to stop smoking

When stable
1 Review anti-anginal management
2 Referral for mammography and fine needle aspiration of breast lump
3 Spirometry and assessment of inhaler technique

Information given

Diagnosis and treatment explained to patient and family
N.B. Breast lump not mentioned at this stage until discussed with senior staff

A. Doctor

A. DOCTOR   (House Officer)

Progress notes

3.8.04
1800 Ward Round—Dr Consultant

No further chest pain

O/E
P70 BP 100/70
JVP not elevated °oedema
HS I + II and ESM as above
Chest clear
Breast lump noted

ECG at 4 hours—resolution of inferior ST changes

Impression

Probable unstable angina—now settling
Await troponin

Plan

Continue LMW heparin until pain-free for 48 hours
Check cholesterol
For echocardiography in view of murmur
Spirometry and assessment of inhaler technique

Consultant to discuss finding of breast lump
with patient and daughter

A. Doctor

A. DOCTOR   (House Officer)

4

Plan
• List the investigations required. When a result is already available, for example of an electrocardiograph, record it.
• Record any immediate management instigated
• If uncertain about an investigation or treatment, precede with a '?' and discuss with a more senior member of staff

Information given
Document what you have told the patient and any other family member. It is also important to document any diagnosis that you have not discussed.
If the patient voices any concerns or fears, document these too.

Progress Notes
Follow the same structure with these additions
• Changes in the patient's symptoms
• Examination findings
• Results of new investigations
• Clinical impression of the patient's progress
• Plans for further management, particularly drug changes
Make progress notes regularly depending on the speed of change in the patient's condition; in an intensive therapy setting, this may be several times a day but, in a stable situation, daily or alternate days.
Date and sign all entries.
Record any unexpected change in the patient's condition as well as routine progress notes.

General examination

JOHN S. BEVAN • DAVID J. GAWKRODGER

THE GENERAL EXAMINATION

The setting for a physical examination

Patients attending a general practitioner are seen in the surgery or at home, whereas hospital examinations take place in outpatient clinic rooms or on the wards. Privacy is essential but may be difficult in a ward setting. Pulling the curtains around the bed obscures vision but not sound, it is therefore important to talk with the patient quietly but at a level sufficient for good communication. This may be difficult with deaf, elderly patients.

Perform the physical examination in a warm and well-lit environment. Subtle abnormalities of complexion, such as mild jaundice, are easier to detect in natural rather than artificial light. The examination couch or bed should be of adjustable height, with a step or stool to allow patients to get up easily. An adjustable backrest is essential, particularly for breathless patients who cannot lie flat.

Sensitively, but adequately, expose the areas of the body to be examined and cover the rest of the patient with a blanket or sheet. Take care to avoid unnecessary exposure and embarrassment. A female patient will appreciate the opportunity to replace her brassière after you have completed the chest examination and before you examine her abdomen. Make sure your patient does not become cold during the examination.

Tactfully ask relatives to leave the room before the physical examination. Sometimes it is appropriate for one to remain if the patient is very apprehensive, or if you need a translator or if the patient requests it. Parents should always be present when you examine small children (see Ch. 11). For any intimate examination you should have a chaperone to prevent misunderstandings and provide support and encouragement for the patient. Some patients do not wish this; respect their wishes and record it in the notes (see Ch. 1).

The equipment you will need to carry out a full examination is listed in Table 2.1.

Sequence for performing a physical examination

With experience, you will develop your own style and sequence of physical examination. A regular routine helps to reduce the chance of you missing things out.

The sequence of examination is:

- **Inspection**
- **Palpation**
- **Percussion**
- **Auscultation.**

You will learn to integrate these smoothly into each component of the physical examination, sometimes combining two

2.1   Equipment required for a full examination
• Stethoscope
• Pen-torch
• Measuring tape
• Ophthalmoscope
• Sphygmomanometer
• Tendon hammer
• Tuning fork
• Cotton wool
• Disposable Neurotips
• Wooden spatula
• Magnifying glass
• Disposable gloves, lubricant jelly and a proctoscope may also be required
• Facilities for obtaining blood samples, urinalysis and faecal occult blood testing should be available
• Accurate weighing scales and a height-measuring device (preferably a Harpenden stadiometer)

or more. There is no single correct way of performing a physical examination; Table 2.2 provides a suggested sequence.

The physical examination starts as soon as you see the patient. Assess patients' general demeanour, external appearance and watch how they rise from their chair and walk into the room. Often your general observations point

2.2   A personal system for performing a physical examination
• Handshake and introduction
• Note general appearances while talking:
– does the patient look well?
– any immediate and obvious clues, e.g. obesity, plethora, breathlessness
– complexion
• Hands and radial pulse
• Face
• Mouth
• Neck
• Thorax:
– breasts
– heart
– lungs
• Abdomen
• Lower limbs:
– oedema
– circulation
– locomotor function and neurology
• Upper limbs:
– movement and neurology
• Cranial nerves, including fundoscopy
• Blood pressure
• Height and weight
• Urinalysis

to a specific diagnosis or to the system causing problems. For example, if you notice that a tired patient is abnormally pigmented, this should suggest a possible diagnosis of adrenal insufficiency (Addison's disease).

After taking a detailed history you should have a differential diagnosis in mind. Carry out your examination specifically trying to elicit the signs that will confirm or refute your diagnoses.

First impressions

The handshake

Greet your patient in a friendly but professional manner. Introduce yourself and shake hands. This may provide diagnostic clues (Table 2.3). Note if the right hand is functional; in patients with a right hemiparesis you may need to shake their left hand. Avoid too firm a grip in a patient with signs of arthritis; a painful handshake is not a good start to a consultation.

Facial expression and general demeanour

Ask yourself 'Does this patient look well?' As you talk to the person, ask yourself 'How does this patient make *me* feel?' If *you* are aware of feeling tense, your patient may be anxious or, rarely, have hyperthyroidism.

Facial expression and eye-to-eye contact may be useful indicators of physical and psychological well-being (Table 2.4). Note that in some cultures direct eye-to-eye contact is not considered polite. A patient admitted to hospital with deliberate self-harm often covers his face with the bedclothes and is reluctant to communicate. Actively recognize the features of anxiety, fear, anger or grief, and explore the reasons for these. Some patients conceal their anxieties with a demeanour of inappropriate cheerfulness; watch out for this and do not be deflected by it.

2.3	Information from a handshake
Features	**Diagnosis**
Cold, sweaty hands	Anxiety
Cold, dry hands	Raynaud's phenomenon
Hot, sweaty hands	Hyperthyroidism
Large, fleshy, sweaty hands	Acromegaly
Dry, coarse skin	Regular water exposure Manual occupation Hypothyroidism
Delayed relaxation of grip	Myotonic dystrophy
Deformed hands/fingers	Dupuytren's contracture Rheumatoid arthritis

2.4	Abnormal facial expressions
Features	**Diagnosis**
Poverty of expression	Parkinsonism
Startled expression	Hyperthyroidism
Apathy, with poverty of expression and poor eye contact	Depression
Apathy, with pale and puffy skin	Hypothyroidism
Lugubrious expression with bilateral ptosis	Myotonic dystrophy
Agitated expression	Anxiety Hyperthyroidism Hypomania

Clothing

Obtain information about patients' personality, state of mind and social circumstances by taking note of their clothing. Young people wearing dirty clothes in a poor state of repair may have problems with alcohol or drug addiction or may simply be making a statement about themselves. Elderly patients with similar clothing and faecal or urinary soiling are unable to look after themselves. This may be because of physical disease, immobility, dementia or other mental illness. Anorectic patients may wear baggy clothing to cover weight loss. Completely inappropriate dress suggests psychiatric illness. Skin piercing is fashionable and local infection may occur at these sites. Skin tattoos may prompt consideration of blood-borne viral infections, e.g. hepatitis B. A MedicAlert bracelet (Fig. 2.1) or necklace highlights important medical conditions and treatments, and may be life-saving if the patient is too ill to give a history.

Complexion

Patients, their friends or family may notice abnormalities of their complexion. The colour of the face depends upon the combination of, and variations in, levels of

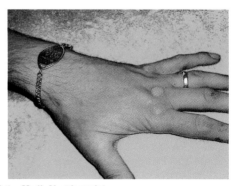

Fig. 2.1 MedicAlert bracelet.

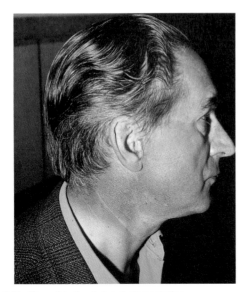

Fig. 2.2 Phenothiazine-induced pigmentation.

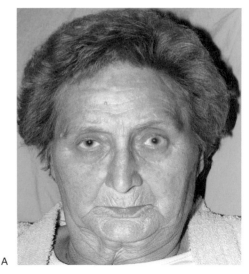

A

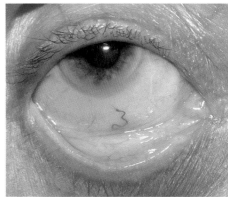

B

Fig. 2.3 Anaemia. (A) Facial and (B) conjunctival pallor.

oxyhaemoglobin, reduced haemoglobin, melanin and, to a lesser extent, carotene. Unusual skin colours, excluding those applied externally, are due to abnormal pigments, such as the sallow yellow-brownish tinge seen in uraemia. A bluish tinge is produced by abnormal haemoglobins, e.g. sulphaemoglobin and methaemoglobin, and may be caused by drugs, e.g. dapsone. Excessive pink colour is seen rarely in severe carbon monoxide poisoning due to high carboxyhaemoglobin levels. Metabolites of some drugs cause striking abnormal coloration of the skin, particularly in exposed areas, e.g. mepacrine (yellow), clofazamine (brownish-black), amiodarone (bluish-grey) and pheno-thiazines (slate-grey) (Fig. 2.2).

Haemoglobin. Untanned Caucasian skin is pink due to the red pigment oxyhaemoglobin in the superficial capillary–venous plexuses. The contribution of haemoglobin to the complexion is influenced by the proportion that is oxygenated or reduced.

Pallor from vasoconstriction occurs in patients who faint or are frightened. If relatives or friends have noticed increasing pallor it may be a feature of progressive anaemia. Examine the mucous membranes of the conjunctivae and mouth to recognize the pallor of anaemia (Fig. 2.3).

Vasodilatation may produce a deceptively pink com-plexion even in the presence of anaemia. Perimenopausal women and patients with carcinoid syndrome commonly have transient, pink flushing, particularly of the face, due to vasodilatation. Chronic flushing may result in permanent telangiectasia.

An unduly plethoric complexion is seen in polycythaemia in which the haematocrit is raised, some alcohol abusers with pseudo-Cushing's syndrome and in Cushing's syn-drome itself (Fig. 2.4). The plethora of Cushing's syndrome is due to thinning of the skin with enhanced visibility of superficial blood vessels.

Cyanosis. Cyanosis is an abnormal blue discoloration of the skin and mucous membranes and requires an absolute concentration of deoxygenated haemoglobin of > 50 g/l. It can be difficult to detect, particularly in black and Asian patients. *Central cyanosis* is seen at the lips and tongue and requires good lighting conditions (Fig. 2.5). Central cyanosis is usually due to arterial hypoxaemia and always indicates underlying disease – usually cardiac or pulmonary (see p. 134). In patients with a normal haemoglobin concentration central cyanosis can be detected when the arterial oxygen saturation falls below 90%, corresponding to an arterial oxygen tension of approximately 8 kPa (60 mmHg). Anaemic or hypovolaemic patients rarely have central cyanosis because severe hypoxia is required to produce the necessary concentration of deoxygenated haemoglobin. In contrast, patients with polycythaemia can become cyanosed at higher arterial oxygen tensions.

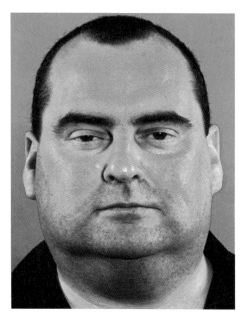

Fig. 2.4 Cushingoid facies.

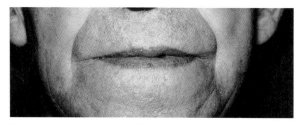

Fig. 2.5 Central cyanosis of lips.

Peripheral cyanosis is seen in the hands or feet. Peripheral cyanosis occurs when central cyanosis is present, but is more commonly seen with poor peripheral circulation. This may have an arterial, e.g. atheromatous peripheral arterial disease and Raynaud's phenomenon, or venous cause, e.g. venous obstruction. Peripheral cyanosis is most commonly seen in normal patients when the hands are exposed to cold.

Melanin. The amount and distribution of melanin is modified in a number of conditions (Table 2.5). *Vitiligo* is a condition which can occur at any age, where irregular depigmentation causes white patches of skin to develop (Fig. 2.6). *Albinism* is a group of inherited conditions that may affect any race. These patients have little or no melanin in their skin, or hair. The amount of pigment in the eyes varies and while some individuals have reddish eyes, most have blue eyes. The characteristic pallor of *hypopituitarism* is apparent only in white races (Fig. 2.7).

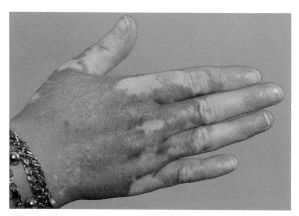

Fig. 2.6 Vitiligo.

2.5 Causes of abnormal melanin production	
Underproduction	**Mechanism**
Vitiligo (patchy depigmentation)	Autoimmune destruction of melanocytes
Albinism	Genetic deficiency of tyrosinase
Hypopituitarism	Reduced pituitary secretion of melanotrophic peptides, growth hormone and sex steroids
Overproduction	
Adrenal insufficiency (Addison's disease)	Increased pituitary secretion of melanotrophic peptides
Nelson's syndrome (may occur after bilateral adrenalectomy for Cushing's disease)	Increased pituitary secretion of melanotrophic peptides
Cushing's syndrome due to ectopic ACTH secretion by tumours (e.g. small cell lung cancer)	Ectopic release of melanotrophic peptides by dysregulated tumour cells
Pregnancy and oral contraceptives	Increased levels of sex hormones
Haemochromatosis	Iron deposition and stimulation of melanocytes

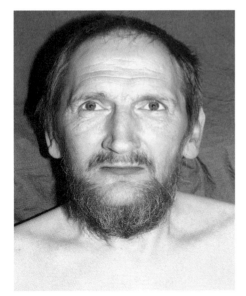

Fig. 2.7 Pallor of hypopituitarism.

In adrenal insufficiency overproduction of melanin results in brown pigmentation of the skin (Fig. 2.8A), particularly in skin creases, recent scars, overlying bony prominences and areas exposed to pressure such as belts and bra straps. Melanin may also be deposited in the mucous membranes of the lips and of the mouth, where it results in muddy brown patches (Fig. 2.8B).

Pregnancy and oral contraceptives may be associated with blotchy pigmentation of the face (chloasma). Pregnancy also causes increased pigmentation of areas that were darker before pregnancy, e.g. the areolae, armpits and genital skin. Sometimes a dark line develops in the midline of the lower abdomen (linea nigra). In Addison's disease and hypopituitarism, vasoconstriction occurs in the skin, so that pigmentation and pallor are accentuated. In hypopituitarism, growth hormone and sex steroid deficiencies also contribute to skin thinning.

⊙ Examine this patient with tiredness and pallor

1. Look for signs of chronic blood loss or *iron deficiency* – pallor, angular stomatitis, koilonychia.
2. Look at face for puffiness about the eyes (*hypothyroidism*) and in men poor beard growth (*hypopituitarism*).
3. Listen to voice – slow, deliberate, croaky (*hypothyroidism*).
4. Measure blood pressure – hypotension in hypovolaemia, and *hypopituitarism*.
5. Feel the neck for goitre (*hypothyroidism*).
6. Palpate abdomen for tenderness, masses and hepatosplenomegaly.
7. Examine for absence of axillary and pubic hair (*hypopituitarism*).
8. Examine external genitalia – small testes in men (*hypopituitarism*).
9. Examine visual fields – bitemporal hemianopia (*pituitary tumour*).
10. Percuss tendon reflexes – delayed relaxation in *hypothyroidism*.

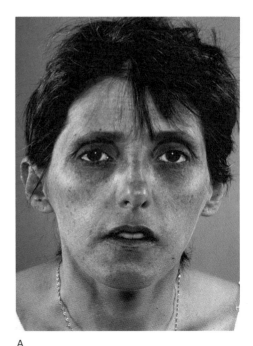

A

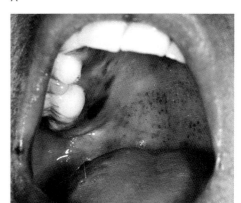

B

Fig. 2.8 Addison's disease. (A) Facial and (B) buccal pigmentation.

Carotene. Hypercarotenaemia occurs occasionally in people who eat excessive amounts of raw carrots and tomatoes. A yellowish discoloration is seen particularly on the face, palms and soles but is distinguished from jaundice as it does not affect the sclerae. Hypercarotenaemia may affect the face in hypothyroidism because of impaired hepatic metabolism of carotene.

Bilirubin. In jaundice, the sclerae, mucous membranes and skin are yellow. Jaundice is usually clinically detectable when the serum bilirubin concentration is $> 50\ \mu mol/l$. It is useful to look for jaundice in the sublingual mucosa.

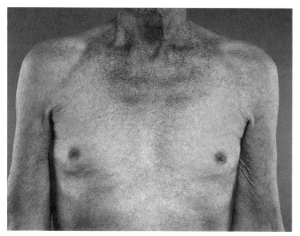

Fig. 2.9   Haemochromatosis with increased skin pigmentation.

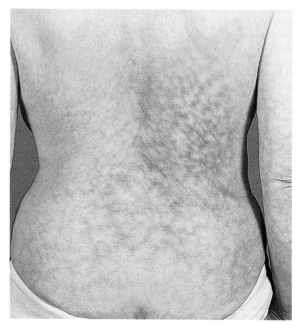

Fig. 2.10   Erythema ab igne.

Patients with pernicious anaemia may have a characteristic lemon-yellow complexion due to a combination of mild jaundice and anaemia. If jaundice is deep and longstanding, a greenish colour develops in the sclerae and skin due to the presence of biliverdin.

Iron.   In haemochromatosis, increased skin pigmentation is due to a combination of iron deposition and increased melanin production (Fig. 2.9). In combination with diabetes mellitus the clinical syndrome is known as 'bronzed diabetes'.

Haemosiderin, a haemoglobin breakdown product, may be deposited locally in the lower legs because of extravasation of blood into the subcutaneous tissues as a result of venous insufficiency. Local deposition of haemosiderin (erythema ab igne or 'granny's tartan') may occur with heat-damage to the skin. This may occur when a person (most often elderly) sits too close to a fire, or in patients who apply local heat, e.g. a hot water bottle, to the site of pain (Fig. 2.10).

Sounds

Normal speech depends upon the tongue, lips, palate and nose, the integrity of the mucosa, muscles and nerve supply of the larynx and the ability to expel sufficient air from the lungs. The neurological abnormalities causing disturbances of voice and speech are described on page 238. Other causes such as a cleft palate, nasal obstruction, loose dentures or a dry mouth can be found on inspection. Hoarseness of the voice may be due to infective laryngitis, heavy smoking or a neurological cause.

In severe hypothyroidism the voice may be characteristic, even allowing the diagnosis to be made over the telephone. The speech is low-pitched, slow and deliberate, and laboured. This is due to myxoedematous infiltration of the tissues concerned in voice production.

Other types of abnormal sound may help in the differentiation of breathlessness, e.g. musical wheezing, the rattling of bronchial secretions or the crowing noise of stridor (see p. 134).

Odours

The body normally produces an odour. This largely arises from apocrine sweat contaminated by skin bacteria and may be reduced by antiperspirants and deodorants or concealed with perfume. Excessive sweating causes an increase in body odour. Poor personal hygiene increases this and the smell may be compounded by dirty or soiled clothing and stale urine. Excessive body odour occurs in:

- the very elderly, infirm or demented
- alcohol or drug misuse
- physical disability preventing normal hygiene
- severe learning difficulties.

Some odours are diagnostic:

- Stale 'mousy' smell of the volatile amine, methyl mercaptan, on the breath of patients with liver failure (*fetor hepaticus*).
- Sweetness of the breath in diabetic or starvation ketoacidosis due to acetone. Note that this smell is obvious to some observers but not others.

- Fetid smell of chronic suppuration, necrotic tumours or some skin disorders.
- Fishy smell of anaerobic bacterial vaginosis.

Bad breath (*halitosis*) is often unrecognized by the patient. It is caused by decomposing food wedged between the teeth, gingivitis, stomatitis, atrophic rhinitis and tumours of the nasal passages. Bronchiectasis may be associated with offensive breath. In patients with gastric outlet obstruction, foul-smelling belching may occur. The most offensive odour of this type is associated with a gastrocolic fistula. Sometimes, halitosis occurs without any obvious explanation.

Tobacco has a characteristic lingering smell which pervades skin, hair and clothing. Marijuana can also be identified by smell. The smell of alcohol on a patient's breath in the morning suggests an alcohol problem.

Movements

Tremor may be present in anxiety, hyperthyroidism and alcohol dependence. It also occurs after administration of a β_2 agonist, e.g. salbutamol. Involuntary movements may be due to disease of the central nervous system, particularly when the extrapyramidal system is involved (see p. 264). Twitching and myoclonic jerks may be observed in patients with uraemia. The 'flapping tremor' (*asterixis*) of hepatic failure or carbon dioxide retention may be apparent only when the patient's arms are outstretched with the hands dorsiflexed (Fig. 2.11).

Posture and gait

Gait may range from brisk, erect and confident to shuffling, slouched and hesitant. Many abnormal gaits are caused by neurological or musculoskeletal disorders. Look carefully at the patient's posture in bed. If the patient looks uncomfortable and never changes posture there may be a generalized weakness or neurological disability. 'Cot sides', a ripple mattress or a urinary catheter are further indicators of poor mobility.

'Spot diagnoses'

Many conditions can be diagnosed at first glance, e.g. morbid obesity. Others are more subtle. Endocrine conditions with an insidious onset, e.g. hypothyroidism or acromegaly, may be diagnosed instantly by a doctor who has never seen the patient before, yet have been overlooked by a relative in daily contact with the patient (Fig. 2.12).

THE HANDS

Looking at the hands is a gentle, non-threatening way to begin the examination, which can yield a wealth of diagnostic clues.

Examination sequence

→ Inspect the dorsal and then palmar aspects of both hands.
→ Note changes in the:
  → skin
  → nails
  → soft tissues
  → tendons
  → joints.
→ Look for evidence of muscle wasting.
→ Assess the temperature and circulation.

Common abnormalities

Posture. This may be diagnostic. Common examples include the flexed hand and arm of hemiplegia or radial nerve palsy, and ulnar deviation of the hands in longstanding rheumatoid arthritis.

Shape. Trauma is the commonest cause of deformity of the hand. Long thin fingers (arachnodactyly) are typical of Marfan's syndrome. Short metacarpals, especially of the ring and little fingers, are found in pseudohypoparathyroidism and are best seen when the patient is asked to make a fist (Fig. 2.13).

Size. In acromegaly the hands are large, broad and fleshy (Fig. 2.14). The soft tissues of the hands are also thickened in myxoedema. Localized oedema of an arm and hand may arise from venous obstruction, lymphatic blockage or disuse due to muscle paresis.

Colour. The colour of the hands is usually similar to that of the rest of the skin. Note any tobacco staining of the fingers. Look at the skin creases for pigmentation but remember that pigmentation is normal in many non-Caucasian races (Fig. 2.15).

Temperature. In a cold or cool climate the temperature of the patient's hand is a good guide to peripheral perfusion.

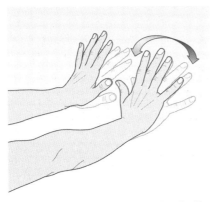

Fig. 2.11 Hand and arm position for observing the 'flapping tremor' of hepatic encephalopathy.

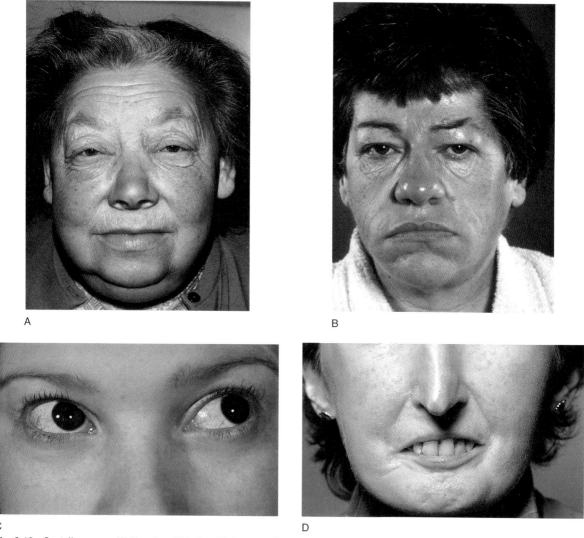

A

B

C

D

Fig. 2.12 Spot diagnoses. (A) Hypothyroid facies. (B) Acromegalic facies. (C) Blue sclera of osteogenesis imperfecta. (D) Scleroderma facies with 'beaking' of nose and taut skin around the mouth.

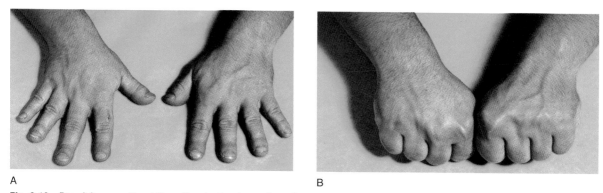

A

B

Fig. 2.13 Pseudohypoparathyroidism. The short metacarpals are best seen when the patient makes a fist.

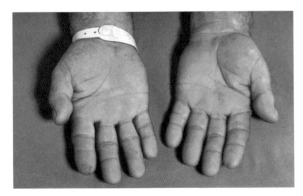

Fig. 2.14 Acromegaly.

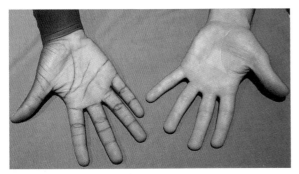

Fig. 2.15 Normal palms: African (left) Caucasian (right).

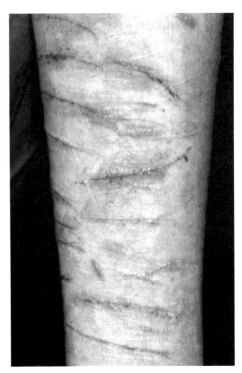

Fig. 2.16 Self-cutting.

In chronic obstructive pulmonary disease, the hands may be cyanosed due to reduced arterial oxygen saturation and warm due to elevated arterial carbon dioxide levels. In some patients with heart failure the hands are cold and cyanosed due to vasoconstriction in response to a low cardiac output. If they are warm, heart failure may be due to a high-output state, e.g. hyperthyroidism.

Skin

Children have smooth hairless hands, but in an adult male this suggests hypogonadism. Manual work may produce specific callosities due to pressure at characteristic sites. In contrast, disuse results in a soft, smooth palmar skin. This is also seen on the soles of the feet in patients who are bedbound.

While examining the hands, look at the flexor surfaces of the wrists and forearms. Note any linear (usually transverse), multiple wounds or scars which suggest deliberate self-harm (Fig. 2.16). There is an association between repeated 'self-cutting' in adolescents and past, or on-going, child sexual abuse.

Nails (Fig. 2.17)

In chronic iron deficiency the nails become brittle, flat and eventually spoon-shaped (*koilonychia*). White nails (*leukonychia*) are a sign of hypoalbuminaemia and occur in chronic liver disease, nephrotic syndrome, protein-losing enteropathy and protein malnutrition (kwashiorkor). Beau's lines, due to temporary arrest of nail growth, are transverse white grooves which appear at the same time on all nails shortly after a severe illness and which move out to the free margins as the nails grow. Although one or two splinter haemorrhages are commonly seen under the nails of manual workers, multiple lesions raise the possibility of infective endocarditis.

Subcutaneous tissues

Dupuytren's contracture causes thickening and shortening of the palmar fascia, resulting in flexion deformities of the little and ring fingers.

Finger clubbing is discussed on page 135. Autoimmune hyperthyroidism may be associated with a specific type of finger clubbing known as thyroid acropachy, more pronounced in the digits on the radial side of the hand, and pretibial myxoedema may occur on the lower limbs in such patients (Fig. 2.18).

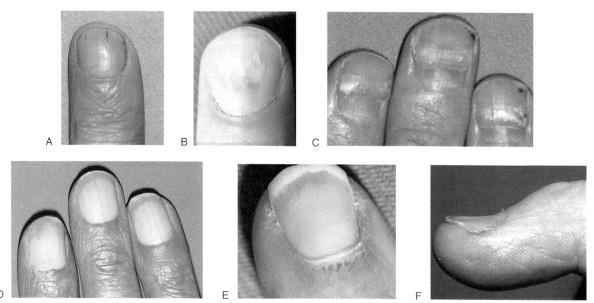

Fig. 2.17 **The nail as a diagnostic aid.** (A) Splinter haemorrhages. (B) Onycholysis with pitting in psoriasis. (C) Beau's lines. (D) Leukonychia. (E) Dilated capillaries in the proximal nail fold in systemic lupus erythematosus. (F) Koilonychia.

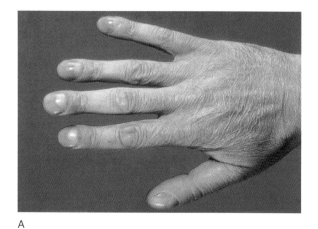

Fig. 2.18 **Autoimmune hyperthyroidism.** (A) Thyroid acropachy. (B) Pretibial myxoedema.

Joints

Arthritis frequently involves the small joints of the hands. Common conditions include rheumatoid arthritis (meta-carpophalangeal and proximal interphalangeal joints), and osteoarthritis and psoriatic arthropathy (distal interphalangeal joints) (see Ch. 10).

Muscles

Muscle wasting is common in rheumatoid arthritis producing 'dorsal guttering' of the hands. In carpal tunnel syndrome, median nerve compression may result in wasting of the thenar muscles – this may occur in rheumatoid arthritis, hypothyroidism and acromegaly, or be associated with pregnancy. Cervical spondylosis with radiculopathy may cause small muscle wasting.

Blood vessels

Palmar erythema is a bright-red cutaneous vasodilatation seen mainly over the thenar and hypothenar eminences. Although found in normal individuals, it is common in hyperthyroidism and chronic liver disease.

Characteristic haemangiomata with central bright-red feeding arterioles and radiating capillaries, known as *spider naevi*, are a feature of chronic liver disease. They may occur on the hands or in any other site on the upper half of the body (Fig. 2.19). They are oestrogen-dependent and up to five may be present in normal women during the reproductive years; this number often increases during pregnancy.

Arteritis may occur in connective tissue disorders and cause small necrotic lesions around the base of the nail and on the pulps, most commonly in systemic lupus erythematosus (see Fig. 2.17E).

The linear marks of thrombosed veins caused by intra-venous drug injection in addicts ('mainliners') are characteristic (Fig. 2.20).

THE LYMPH GLANDS

Lymph glands are often palpable in normal people, especially in the submandibular, axilla and groin regions (Fig. 2.21). Distinguish between normal and pathological glands. Pathological lymphadenopathy may be local or generalized. It is of diagnostic and prognostic significance in the staging of lymphoproliferative and other malignancies.

Size. Normal glands in adults are seldom greater than 0.5 cm diameter.

Consistency. Normal glands feel soft, rubbery or 'shotty'. In contrast, in Hodgkin's disease they are characteristically 'rubbery', in tuberculosis they may be 'matted' and in metastatic cancer they feel 'craggy'. Calcified glands feel stony hard.

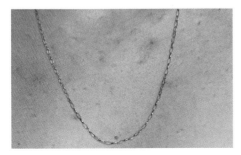

Fig. 2.19   Spider naevi.

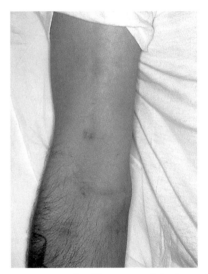

Fig. 2.20   The linear marks of intravenous injection at the right elbow.

Tenderness. Tenderness is usually a feature of acute viral or bacterial infection. With tender cervical lymphadenopathy, common sources include infectious mononucleosis, dental sepsis and tonsillitis.

Fixation. Fixation of glands to deep structures or skin usually indicates malignancy.

⤷ Examination sequence

General principles
→ Inspect for any visible lymphadenopathy.
→ Palpate one side at a time using the fingers of one hand.
→ Compare with the glands on the contralateral side.
→ Assess:
  → site
  → size
  → consistency.
→ Record the measurements of the main glands.
→ Note any tenderness.
→ Determine if the gland is fixed to:
  → surrounding and deep structures
  → skin.
→ Examine the cervical and axillary glands with the patient sitting.
→ Examine for the inguinal and popliteal glands with the patient lying down.

Cervical glands
→ From behind, examine the submental, submandibular, preauricular, tonsillar, supraclavicular and deep cervical glands in the anterior triangle of the neck (Fig. 2.22A).
→ Palpate deeply for the scalene nodes (Fig. 2.22B).
→ From the front of the patient, examine the posterior triangles, up the back of the neck and the posterior auricular and occipital nodes (Fig. 2.22C).

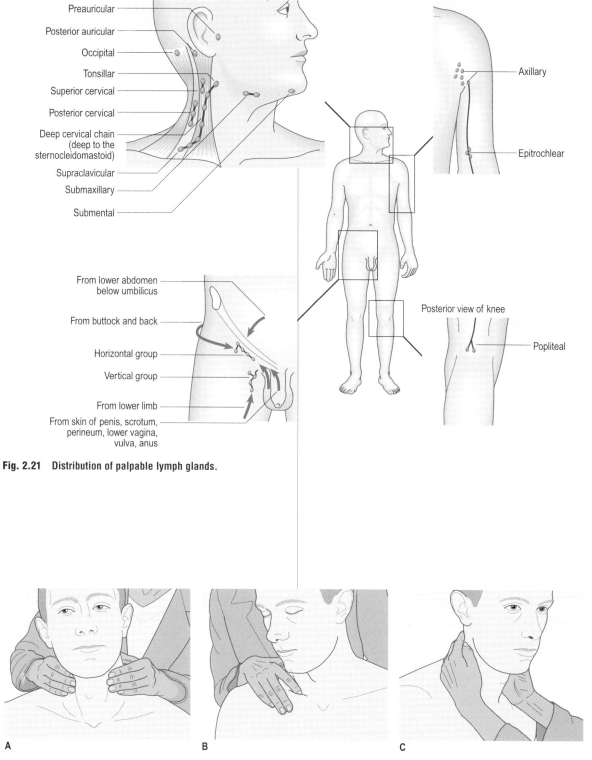

Preauricular

Posterior auricular

Occipital

Tonsillar

Superior cervical

Posterior cervical

Deep cervical chain
(deep to the
sternocleidomastoid)

Supraclavicular

Submaxillary

Submental

Axillary

Epitrochlear

From lower abdomen
below umbilicus

From buttock and back

Horizontal group

Vertical group

From lower limb

From skin of penis, scrotum,
perineum, lower vagina,
vulva, anus

Posterior view of knee

Popliteal

Fig. 2.21   Distribution of palpable lymph glands.

A   B   C

Fig. 2.22   Palpation of the cervical glands. (A) Examine the glands of the anterior triangle from behind using both hands, (B) examine for the scalene nodes from behind with your index finger in the angle between the sternocleidomastoid muscle and the clavicle, (C) examine glands in the posterior triangle from the front.

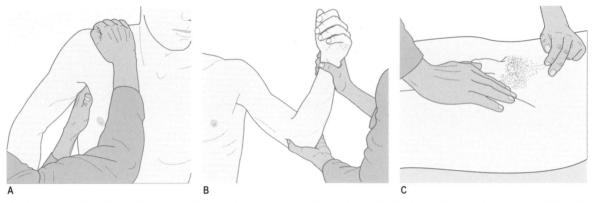

Fig. 2.23 **Palpation of the axillary, epitrochlear and inguinal glands.** (A) Examination for the right axillary lymphadenopathy, (B) for left epitrochlear glands and (C) left inguinal glands.

Axillary glands
→ From in front of the patient, support the arm on the side under examination. Palpate the right axilla with your left hand and vice versa (Fig. 2.23A). Gently place your finger tips into the vault of the axilla and then draw them downwards feeling the medial, anterior and posterior axillary walls in turn. Make sure your nails are short to avoid causing your patient discomfort.

Epitrochlear glands
→ Support the patient's right wrist with your left hand, grasp the patient's partially flexed elbow with your right hand and use your thumb to feel for the epitrochlear gland. Examine the left epitrochlear gland with your left thumb (Fig. 2.23B).

Inguinal glands
→ Palpate over the horizontal chain, which lies just below the inguinal ligament, and then over the vertical chain along the line of the saphenous vein (Fig. 2.23C).

Popliteal glands
→ Use both hands to examine the popliteal fossa with the knee flexed and limb muscles relaxed.

Common abnormalities

If you find localized lymphadenopathy, examine the areas which drain to that site. Most often infection causes localized tender lymphadenopathy (*lymphadenitis*), e.g. in acute tonsillitis the submandibular lymph glands are involved. If the lymphadenopathy is non-tender, look for a malignant cause, tuberculosis or features of HIV infection. Generalized lymphadenopathy occurs in a number of conditions (Table 2.6). Look for enlargement of the liver and spleen and for other haematological features, e.g. purpura or petechiae.

2.6	Important common causes of lymphadenopathy
Generalized	
Viral	Epstein–Barr virus (glandular fever or Burkitt's lymphoma), cytomegalovirus, HIV
Bacterial	Brucellosis, syphilis
Protozoal	Toxoplasmosis
Malignancy	Lymphoma, acute or chronic lymphocytic leukaemia
Inflammatory	Rheumatoid arthritis, systemic lupus erythematosus, sarcoidosis
Localized	
Infective	Acute or chronic, bacterial or viral
Malignancy	Secondary metastases, lymphoma (Hodgkin's or non-Hodgkin's lymphoma)

THE THYROID GLAND

Anatomy

The thyroid is a butterfly-shaped gland, comprising two symmetrical lobes joined by a central isthmus that normally covers the second and third tracheal rings (Fig. 2.24A). The gland may extend into the superior mediastinum, or may occasionally be entirely retrosternal. Rarely, the gland may be located higher in the neck along the line of the thyroglossal duct. When situated at the back of the tongue, it is known as a lingual goitre and may be visible through the open mouth.

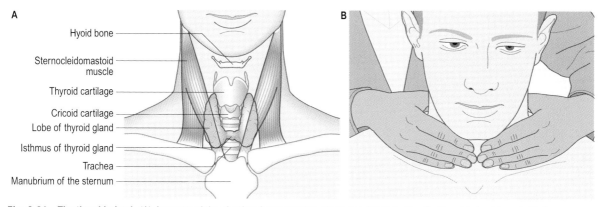

Fig. 2.24   The thyroid gland. (A) Anatomy of the gland and surrounding structures. (B) Palpating the thyroid gland from behind.

The normal thyroid gland is palpable in about 50% of females and 25% of males. A *goitre* is enlargement of the thyroid gland and is commonly discovered during examination of the neck.

⊡ Examination sequence

→ Inspect the neck from the front.
→ Look for a thyroid swelling while the patient swallows a sip of water. The thyroid (or a thyroglossal cyst) moves upwards on swallowing since it is enveloped in the pretracheal fascia, which is attached to the cricoid cartilage.
→ Ask the patient to sit with the neck muscles relaxed and stand behind the patient.
→ Place your hands gently on the front of the patient's neck with your index fingers just touching (Fig. 2.24B). Ask the patient to swallow a sip of water while you feel over the gland. Some patients find this unpleasant so be alert for any signs of distress.
→ Note the size, shape and consistency of any goitre, and the presence or absence of a thrill. Measure any discrete nodules with calipers.
→ Listen with the diaphragm of your stethoscope for a thyroid bruit.

Abnormal findings

Shape and surface. Simple goitres are relatively symmetrical in their earlier stages but often become nodular with time. The surface of the thyroid gland is usually smooth and diffuse in Graves' disease, whereas it is irregular in uninodular or multinodular goitre (Fig. 2.25).

Mobility. Most goitres move upwards with swallowing. However, invasive thyroid cancer may fix the gland to surrounding structures. Very large goitres may also be immobile.

Consistency. The consistency, texture and smoothness of the surface of the gland may vary. Nodules in the substance of the gland may be large or small, single or multiple. A very hard consistency suggests malignant change in the gland. Large, firm lymph nodes near a goitre also suggest thyroid cancer.

Tenderness. Diffuse tenderness is typical of viral thyroiditis, whereas localized tenderness may follow bleeding into a cyst.

Thyroid bruit. This indicates abnormally high blood flow and can be associated with a palpable thrill. It occurs in hyperthyroidism. A thyroid bruit may be confused with other sounds. A bruit arising from the carotid artery or transmitted from the aorta will be louder along the line of the artery. Transient gentle pressure over the root of the neck will interrupt a venous hum from the internal jugular vein.

SWELLINGS

Patients often present with a lump that they have suddenly found. This does not necessarily mean that it has only recently developed. Ask if they have noted any change in size or other characteristics since it was first detected and whether there are any associated features, e.g. pain, tenderness or colour change. Sometimes on physical examination you will find a lump of which the patient was unaware.

Table 2.7 lists features to note in any lump or swelling.

⊡ Examination sequence

→ Inspect the swelling, noting any change in colour or texture of the overlying skin.
→ Gently palpate for tenderness or change in skin temperature.

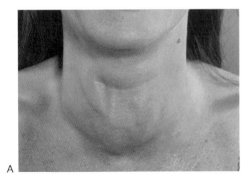

A

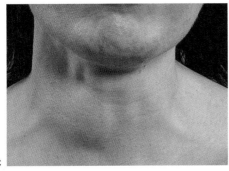

B

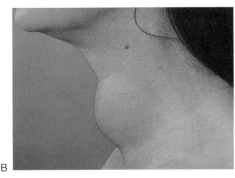

C

Fig. 2.25 Goitres. (A and B) Diffuse. (C) Uninodular.

→ Define the site and shape of the swelling.
→ Measure its size and record the findings diagrammatically.
→ Feel the swelling for a few moments to determine if it is *pulsatile* (moves in time with the arterial pulse).
→ Assess the consistency, surface texture and margins of the swelling.
→ Attempt to pick up an overlying fold of skin to assess whether it is fixed to the skin.
→ Determine if it is fixed to deeper structures by attempting to move the swelling in different planes relative to the surrounding tissues.
→ Look for fluctuation by compressing the swelling on one side and seeing and feeling if a bulge is created on the opposite side. Confirm the presence of fluctuation in two planes.
→ Auscultate for bruits and other sounds.
→ Transilluminate.

Size. Accurately measure the size of any swelling so with time you can detect significant change.

Position. The origin of some swellings may be obvious, e.g. in the breast, thyroid or parotid gland. In other sites, e.g. the abdomen, this is less clear. Multiple swellings may occur in neurofibromatosis (Fig. 2.26), skin metastases, lipomatosis and lymphomas.

Attachments. Lymphatic obstruction causes fixation of the skin with fine dimpling at the opening of the hair follicles resembling orange skin (*peau d'orange*) (see Fig. 7.5, p. 200). This is commonly due to malignant disease. Fixation to deeper structures may occur in a breast

2.7 Features to note in any lump or swelling
• Size
• Position
• Attachments
• Surface
• Edge
• Consistency
• Transillumination
• Inflammation:
– redness
– tenderness
– heat
• Thrills, bruits and noises

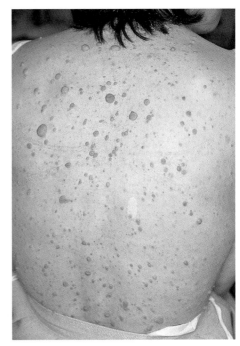

Fig. 2.26 Neurofibromatosis.

cancer which is fixed to underlying muscle. Arterial swellings (*aneurysms*) and highly vascular tumours are pulsatile. Other swellings may be pulsatile if they lie over a major blood vessel.

Surface. The surface and shape of a swelling may be characteristic. Examples in the abdomen include an enlarged spleen or liver, a distended bladder or the fundus of the uterus in pregnancy. The surface may be smooth or irregular and may provide a clue to the pathological process. For example, the surface of liver is smooth in acute hepatitis but is often nodular in metastatic disease.

Edge. The edge or margin may be well delineated or ill defined, regular or irregular, sharp or rounded. The margins of enlarged organs, e.g. thyroid gland, liver, spleen or kidney, can usually be defined more clearly than those of inflammatory or malignant masses. An indefinite margin may suggest an infiltrating malignancy in contrast to the clearly defined edge of a benign tumour.

Consistency. The consistency of a swelling may vary from soft to 'stony' hard. Very hard swellings are usually malignant or calcified, or consist of dense fibrous tissue.

Fluctuation indicates a swelling containing fluid, e.g. abscess or cyst. Soft encapsulated tumours such as lipomas may also show some degree of fluctuation.

Transillumination. In a darkened room, press the lighted end of a pen-torch onto one side of the swelling. A cystic swelling will light up if the fluid is translucent, provided that the covering tissues are not too thick.

Inflammation. Redness, warmth and tenderness suggests inflammation.

Redness (erythema). The skin over acute inflammatory lesions is usually red due to vasodilatation. In haematomas the pigment from extravasated blood may produce the range of colours familiar in a bruise (*ecchymosis*).

Tenderness. Inflammatory swellings are usually tender or painful. Some swellings, e.g. lipomas, skin metastases, neurofibromas, are characteristically painless. Severe and intractable pain may result from malignancy or nerve involvement.

Temperature. Inflammatory swellings and some tumours, especially if rapidly growing, may feel warm.

Thrills, bruits and noises. If the blood flow through a swelling is increased, a systolic murmur (bruit) may be audible on auscultation and, if sufficiently marked, a thrill may be palpable. Bruits may also be heard over arterial aneurysms and arteriovenous malformations. Bowel sounds may be heard over a hernia which contains intestine.

MEASUREMENT OF HEIGHT AND WEIGHT

Clinical examination should include the measurement of weight and height, both for their immediate value and for future reference. Serial weight measurements are useful in monitoring acutely ill patients and those with chronic disease.

Women have a smaller percentage of total body water than men. However, women of reproductive age often have cyclical fluctuations in weight due to perimenstrual fluid retention.

Measure the body mass index, rather than weight alone, as it is independent of the patient's height. Body mass index is derived from the formula Weight/Height^2 (using metric units, kg/m^2). It can be calculated from this formula or derived from a nomogram (Fig. 2.27).

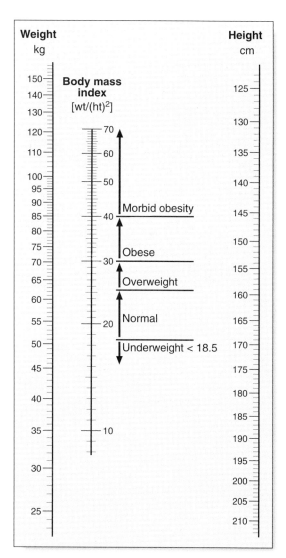

Fig. 2.27 Desirable weights of adults according to body mass index.

The relationship between body mass index and nutritional status is as follows:

	Body mass index
Underweight	< 18.5
Normal	18.5–24.9
Overweight	25–29.9
Obese	30–39.9
Morbid obesity	≥40

Body mass index does not, however, describe the distribution of body fat. This is important because excess intra-abdominal fat is an independent predictor of health risk. To assess this measure waist circumference, which correlates with visceral fat and indirectly measures central adiposity. There is an increased risk to health when *waist circumference* exceeds 94 cm (37 inches) for men and 80 cm (32 inches) for women.

➡ Examination sequence

→ Note any abnormalities in stature or body proportions.
→ Measure height using a vertical scale with a rigid, adjustable arm-piece, with the patient standing erect and without shoes. In the serial assessment of growth in children and teenagers, measure height to the nearest millimetre using a calibrated stadiometer (p. 365).
→ Weigh patients wearing indoor clothing without shoes. In hospital, patients should wear their night clothes.
→ Calculate and record the body mass index.
→ Look for abnormal fat distribution.
→ Measure the waist with the patient standing. This is the girth at the level equidistant between the costal margin and iliac crest. It should be the maximum diameter so measure over any abdominal fat and not under it.
→ Look for any evidence of malnutrition or specific vitamin deficiencies.

Common abnormalities

Tall stature

Most individuals with heights above the 95th centile are not abnormal and you should ask about the height of close relatives. Abnormal causes of increased height are:

- Marfan's syndrome
- hypogonadism
- pituitary gigantism.

In Marfan's syndrome, the limbs are long in relation to the length of the trunk, and the arm-span exceeds the height (Fig. 2.28A). Additional features include long slender fingers (*arachnodactyly*) (Fig. 2.28B), narrow feet, a high-arched palate (Fig. 2.28C), upward dislocation of the lenses of the eyes (Fig. 2.28D) and cardiovascular abnormalities including mitral valve prolapse, and dilatation of the aortic root with aortic regurgitation.

Around puberty, the epiphyses close in response to stimulation from the sex hormones. Consequently, in some patients with hypogonadism, the limbs continue to grow for longer than usual. Their sitting height is considerably less than half their total standing height. The arm-span may exceed the standing height or, more significantly, twice the sitting height.

Pituitary gigantism is a rare cause of tall stature due to excessive growth hormone secretion before epiphyseal fusion has occurred. *Acromegaly* occurs when growth hormone excess develops after epiphyseal closure. It is characterized by coarsening of the soft tissues, a large tongue, prognathism with separation of the teeth and enlarged hands and feet. The enlarging pituitary tumour may cause visual field defects, e.g. bitemporal hemianopia.

Short stature

Short stature is usually familial. However, any significant childhood illness will reduce the rate of growth and may limit final height. Some pathological conditions causing short stature can be identified from their associated features (see Table 11.8); other disorders, e.g. renal tubular acidosis, intestinal malabsorption, and hypothyroidism, may be less obvious in young people, with delay in diagnosis. Loss of height is part of normal ageing but is accentuated by compression fractures of the spine due to osteoporosis, particularly in women.

Obesity

Obesity is a major heath problem in many countries. It is associated with sleep apnoea, hypertension, hyperlipidaemia, type 2 diabetes mellitus, and certain cancers, and shortens life expectancy (Fig. 2.29).

Obesity occurs in most patients when dietary intake exceeds energy expenditure. Genetic, social and psychological factors are important. Rarely, obesity is secondary to

---

⊙ Examine this patient with weight loss and a good appetite

1. Observe patient's demeanour – hyperactive, 'staring eyes' (*hyperthyroidism*).
2. Examine eyes for lid lag and proptosis (*thyroid eye disease*).
3. Look for signs of dehydration – dry tongue, lack of skin turgor (e.g. *diabetes mellitus, coeliac disease*).
4. Examine hands for finger clubbing (*coeliac disease*), warmth, sweating, fine tremor (*hyperthyroidism*).
5. Examine nails for any onycholysis or thyroid acropachy (*hyperthyroidism*).
6. Feel pulse – tachycardia in *hyperthyroidism* bradycardia in *hypothyroidism*.
7. Palpate neck for goitre (diffuse or nodular).
8. Look at legs for *pretibial myxoedema*.
9. Look at optic fundi for *diabetic retinopathy*.
10. Perform urinalysis for glycosuria (*diabetes mellitus*).

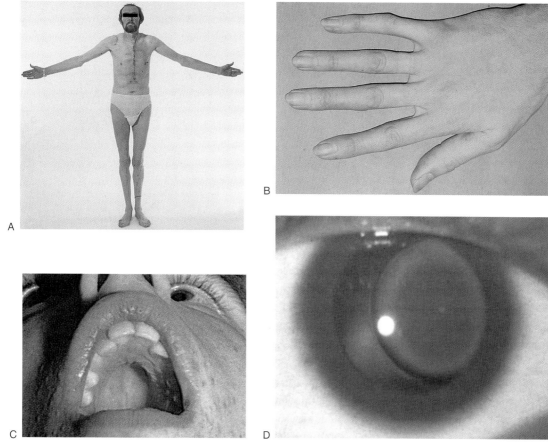

Fig. 2.28 Marfan's syndrome. This is an autosomal dominant condition, with (A) tall stature, and reduced upper segment to lower segment ratio (note surgery for aortic dissection); (B) long fingers and toes; (C) a high arched palate; (D) dislocation of the lens in the eye.

conditions such as hypothyroidism, Cushing's syndrome, Prader–Willi syndrome or drugs, e.g. glucocorticoids.

Abnormalities of fat distribution

Regional distribution of fat is of greater prognostic significance than the absolute degree of obesity. The waist–hip ratio provides a simple assessment of visceral adipose fat. Subjects with a 'pear-shaped' configuration and a waist–hip ratio of 0.8 or less in females or < 0.9 in males have a good prognosis, whereas 'apple-shaped' subjects with a greater waist–hip ratio have an increased risk of cardiovascular disease (Fig. 2.30).

  Specific abnormalities of fat distribution.

- *Localized deposits*. Lipomas are commonly found around the trunk and are benign soft, fluctuant, circumscribed, lobulated swellings.
- *Progressive lipodystrophy* is a rare condition in which subcutaneous fat is reduced in the face, neck, arms and lower legs but may be deposited in excess on the lower trunk and thighs. Associated diabetes mellitus due to severe insulin resistance is common. Lipodystrophy is common in patients with HIV infection receiving highly active antiretroviral therapy.
- *Localized atrophy of subcutaneous fat* may develop in diabetic patients at the sites of insulin injection. This was common with animal-derived insulins but is rarely seen with highly purified human insulin.
- In *Cushing's syndrome* the distribution of fat is abnormal. The syndrome is usually due to prolonged systemic glucocorticoid administration. Rarely, these features are caused by excessive endogenous secretion of adrenocorticotrophic hormone by the pituitary (*Cushing's disease*). Fat deposition tends to be centrally distributed, on the neck and trunk (Fig. 2.31). The face is plethoric and rounded (so-called 'moon' face; see Fig. 2.4, p. 43). The limbs are often noticeably thin, due to muscle wasting.

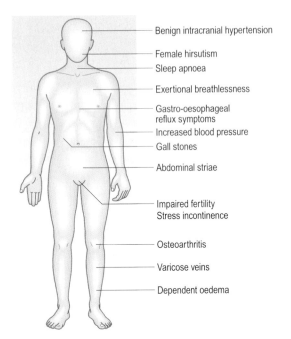

Benign intracranial hypertension
Female hirsutism
Sleep apnoea
Exertional breathlessness
Gastro-oesophageal reflux symptoms
Increased blood pressure
Gall stones
Abdominal striae
Impaired fertility
Stress incontinence
Osteoarthritis
Varicose veins
Dependent oedema

Fig. 2.29 Complications of obesity.

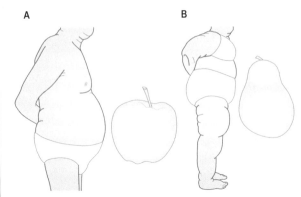

Fig. 2.30 Abdominal obesity and generalized obesity.
(A) Abdominal obesity (apple shape). (B) Generalized obesity where fat deposition is mainly on the hips and thighs (pear shape).

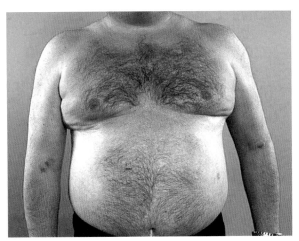

Fig. 2.31 Cushing's syndrome showing central fat deposition and muscle wasting of limbs.

ASSESSMENT OF NUTRITIONAL STATUS

Malnutrition and starvation remain major problems in many parts of the world. Recent estimates have suggested that malnutrition affects 15–40% of UK hospital admissions. Malnutrition may be due to poverty or the result of illness. Malnutrition occurs in anorexia nervosa and in abuse of alcohol or other addictive drugs. It is a prominent feature of untreated, advanced HIV infection.

Illness may produce profound changes in an individual's nutritional requirements, and alter the appetite and the ability to eat and communicate needs. Malnutrition delays recovery from illness and surgery and increases the risk of complications. Measure height, weight, and body mass index as part of the initial nutritional assessment. Repeat measurements at least weekly in an acute setting, and at least monthly in outpatients or in the community.

Vitamin C deficiency (scurvy) (Fig. 2.32) occurs particularly in elderly people living alone or younger people with dietary fads. Consider in patients with extensive bruising.

Vitamin D deficiency is common and usually results from reduced dietary intake and decreased formation in the skin.

MEASUREMENT OF TEMPERATURE

The 'normal' oral or ear temperature is 37°C but may range between 35.8 and 37.2°C. There is a circadian variation with the lowest readings occurring in the early morning. Rectal temperature is usually about 0.5°C higher than in the mouth which, in turn, is 0.5°C higher than the axilla, but the axilla is not recommended as a site for reliable measurement. Body temperature may be taken beneath the tongue, or in the rectum or the external auditory meatus. Mercury thermometers are increasingly being replaced by electronic devices, which are safer and more accurate.

Skin warmth to the touch usually provides an indication of fever, but the skin of a patient with a normal temperature may feel cold, and an apparently normal skin temperature does not exclude hypothermia. Accordingly, temperature should always be measured.

Increase in body temperature is an important physical sign. It may be a response to raised ambient temperature (often in humid environments) – *heat illness*. *Fever* is an increase in body temperature caused by a cellular response

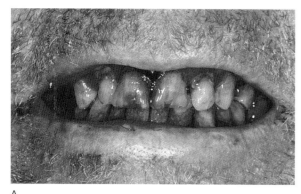

 A

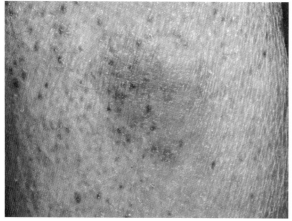

B

Fig. 2.32 Scurvy. (A) Bleeding gums and (B) bruising and perifollicular haemorrhages.

2.8 Clinical features of hypothermia	
Core temperature	**Clinical features**
36°C	Increased metabolic rate, vasoconstriction
35°C (hypothermia)	Shivering maximal, impaired judgement
34°C	Uncooperative
33°C	Depressed conscious level
28–32°C (severe hypothermia)	Progressive depression of conscious level, muscle stiffness Failure of vasoconstrictor response and shivering Bradycardia, hypotension, J waves present on ECG, risk of arrhythmias
< 28°C	Coma, patient may appear dead, absent pupillary and tendon reflexes Spontaneous ventricular fibrillation
20°C	Asystole/profound bradyarrhythmias

to infection, immunological disturbance or malignancy. A *rigor* is an episode of shivering or shaking followed by excessive sweating that follows a rapid increase in body temperature. The *pattern* of a fever is not usually specific or sensitive as an indicator of a particular disease, but patients with collections of pus commonly have a high swinging fever with rigors.

Hypothermia is a core temperature < 35°C. It is easily missed and may mimic clinical death. Use a low-reading mercury thermometer or an electronic device to measure the rectal temperature. The rectum is the most accessible site and rectal temperature the best approximation to core temperature.

As body temperature falls, conscious level is progressively impaired, and coma is common with core temperatures < 28°C (Table 2.8).

Hypothermia may occur in various situations:

- elderly immobile patients living alone, particularly during the winter
- water immersion and near-drowning
- prolonged unconsciousness in low ambient temperatures, especially in combination with alcohol intoxication (which causes peripheral vasodilatation), drug overdosage, stroke or head injury
- severe hypothyroidism.

ASSESSMENT OF HYDRATION

In adults, water comprises 60–65% of body mass. A person weighing 70 kg has about 45 l of body fluid. Two-thirds of this is intracellular (30 l). Of the remainder, interstitial fluid comprises two-thirds (10 l) and the circulating blood volume is approximately 5 l.

Examination sequence

→ Assess the state of hydration by testing skin turgor. Gently pinch a fold of skin on the neck or anterior chest wall, hold it for a few seconds, then release it. Well-hydrated skin springs back into position immediately, whereas dehydrated skin subsides abnormally slowly.

→ Record the pulse rate and supine/erect blood pressures. Look for postural hypotension (a fall > 15 mmHg) in systolic pressure.

→ Check for oedema in the ankles and legs. In patients in bed check for sacral oedema.

→ Examine the jugular venous pulse (JVP) (p. 94).

Dehydration

Unless you consider the possibility of dehydration, you may overlook or underestimate its severity. Assess hydration in all patients especially those with excessive fluid loss, e.g. vomiting, diarrhoea, sweating, burns and polyuria, and in conditions of raised ambient temperature. A detailed history of the nature and the quantity of fluid loss is important. If the usual weight is known, useful information is obtained by weighing the patient.

A dry tongue is a poor sign since it is often due to mouth breathing. Loss of skin turgor relates more to reduced collagen elasticity than to water loss and an adult can lose 4–6 l before the skin becomes dry and loose.

The blood pressure may be low, and postural hypotension may indicate intravascular volume depletion.

Oedema

Oedema means swelling of tissues due to an increase in interstitial fluid.

- *Generalized oedema* may be due to a disorder of the heart, kidneys, liver or gut or may be nutritional in origin.
- *Localized oedema* may arise from venous or lymphatic obstruction, allergy or inflammation.
- *Postural oedema* is relatively common in the lower limbs of inactive patients.

Clinical manifestations of oedema

When oedema is due to generalized fluid retention (Fig. 2.33), its distribution is determined by gravity. It is usually found in the legs, backs of the thighs and the lumbosacral area in the semirecumbent patient. If the patient lies flat, it may involve the face and hands, as in children with nephrotic syndrome.

The cardinal sign of subcutaneous oedema is pitting of the skin, made by applying firm pressure with your fingers or thumb for a few seconds (Fig. 2.34). The pitting may persist for several minutes until it is obliterated by the slow return of the displaced fluid. Pitting on pressure may not be demonstrable until body weight has increased by as much as 10–15%. Day-to-day alterations in body weight are usually the most reliable index of changes in body water.

Hypothyroidism is characterized by mucinous infiltration of the tissues (*myxoedema*). In contrast to oedema, myxoedema and chronic lymphoedema do not pit on pressure.

Generalized oedema

There are two principal causes of generalized oedema, hypoproteinaemia and fluid overload. These may be distinguished by the jugular venous pulse (JVP), which is usually elevated in fluid overload but not in hypoproteinaemia.

Hypoproteinaemia. Ions freely cross the vascular endothelium, so the osmotic pressure within capillaries is largely determined by the plasma proteins. Albumin is the

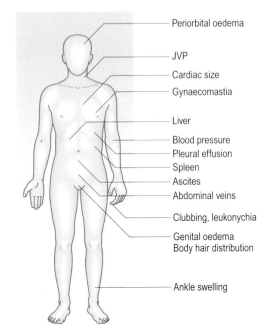

Periorbital oedema
JVP
Cardiac size
Gynaecomastia
Liver
Blood pressure
Pleural effusion
Spleen
Ascites
Abdominal veins
Clubbing, leukonychia
Genital oedema
Body hair distribution
Ankle swelling

Fig. 2.33 Features to look for in oedema.

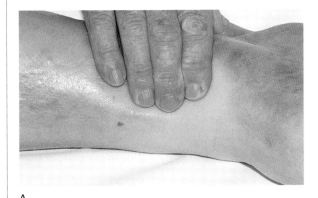

A

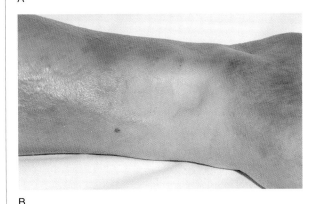

B

Fig. 2.34 Demonstration of pitting oedema.

principal protein in plasma, and the *colloid osmotic* (or *oncotic*) *pressure* of plasma is mostly due to albumin. Decreased plasma albumin concentration predisposes to oedema. Hypoproteinaemia may occur because of inadequate protein intake, absorption, production or excess protein loss.

Inadequate protein intake or absorption

- Kwashiorkor develops when there is inadequate intake of protein. This, and true famine, are the most important nutritional disorders in the world.
- Failure of digestion of dietary protein results from impairment of pancreatic exocrine function, as in chronic pancreatitis.
- Malabsorption of the products of digestion may occur in conditions such as Crohn's disease or coeliac disease, or after extensive small bowel resection.

Inadequate protein production

- Reduced synthesis of albumin is found in chronic liver disease including cirrhosis. When the portal venous pressure is high, ascites may be more prominent than dependent oedema.

Excessive loss of protein

- Heavy protein loss in the urine (> 5 g/day) results in the nephrotic syndrome.
- Repeated removal of body fluids, especially ascites, may cause protein depletion.
- Protein may be lost through the gut wall in protein-losing enteropathy, e.g. coeliac disease.

Several of these factors may be present in the same patient. In addition, a low intravascular volume may cause secondary hyperaldosteronism via the renin–angiotensin system, promoting sodium retention and causing a further increase in oedema.

The cause of hypoproteinaemia can usually be identified from the history. Nephrotic syndrome can be excluded in the absence of heavy proteinuria and most patients with a hepatic cause will have features of chronic liver disease.

Fluid overload.

Cardiac causes. Several factors are responsible for oedema in patients with heart failure:

- *Impairment of renal blood flow.* This promotes excessive reabsorption of salt and water.
- *Increased venous pressure.* A rise in venous pressure proximal to the failing heart promotes oedema.
- *Endocrine adaptations.* Secondary hyperaldosteronism and increased vasopressin encourage salt and water retention.
- *Reduced plasma oncotic pressure.* Chronic congestion of the liver due to right heart failure reduces albumin

synthesis. This may be aggravated by poor appetite and reduced protein intake.

Renal causes. In some renal disease, e.g. acute glomerulonephritis, there is an increased circulating and extracellular fluid volume with increased tubular reabsorption of sodium and reduction in urine volume.

Iatrogenic causes. Excessive fluid replacement, especially intravenously, may produce fluid overload – infants and young children are particularly vulnerable. Patients with diminished (*oliguria*) or absent (*anuria*) urine production due to renal failure are at particular risk of fluid overload.

Localized oedema

This may be caused by venous, lymphatic, inflammatory or allergic problems.

Venous causes. Any cause of increased venous pressure will increase capillary pressure, producing oedema in the area drained by that vein. This may be a problem with the vein itself, e.g. external pressure from a tumour, thrombosis, or valvular incompetence from previous thrombosis or surgery. Conditions which impair the normal pumping action of muscles, e.g. hemiparesis, forced immobility, also increase venous pressure by impairing venous return. Oedema may accordingly occur in immobile, bedridden patients, in a paralysed limb, or even in a healthy person sitting for long periods, e.g. during air travel.

Lymphatic causes. Normally oedema does not develop, because interstitial fluid returns to the central circulation via the lymphatic system. Any cause of impaired lymphatic flow, e.g. intraluminal or extraluminal obstruction may produce localized oedema (*lymphoedema*) (Fig. 2.35). If the condition persists, fibrous tissues proliferate in the interstitial space and the affected area becomes hard and no longer pits on pressure. Lymphoedema is common in some tropical countries because of lymphatic obstruction by filarial worms. The legs, external genitalia and the female breast are most frequently involved. Eventually the skin in affected areas becomes very thick and rough (*elephantiasis*). In the UK, lymphoedema is most often due to congenital hypoplasia of the lymph vessels of the legs (Milroy's disease), recurrent lymphangitis (resulting in lymphatic fibrosis), or may affect an arm after radical mastectomy and/or irradiation for breast cancer.

Inflammatory causes. Any cause of tissue inflammation including infection, injury or ischaemia, liberates mediators such as histamine, bradykinin and cytokines which cause vasodilatation and increase capillary permeability. Inflammatory oedema is accompanied by the other features of inflammation – redness, heat and pain – and you should avoid testing for pitting on pressure.

Allergic causes. Increased capillary permeability occurs in allergic conditions but, in contrast to inflammation, is not painful. The affected area may be red and itchy

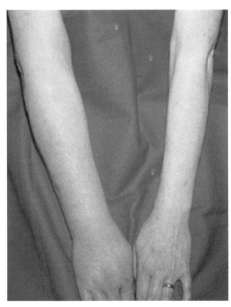

Fig. 2.35 Lymphoedema of the right arm. Following mastectomy and radiotherapy on the right side.

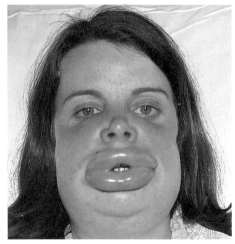

Fig. 2.36 Angio-oedema following a wasp sting.

(*pruritic*), because of local histamine and other inflammatory mediators. *Angio-oedema* is a specific form of allergic oedema which affects the face, lips and mouth (Fig. 2.36). Swelling may develop rapidly and may be life-threatening if the upper airway is affected.

◉ Examine this patient with tiredness and low blood pressure

1. Look for signs of dehydration, e.g. prolonged diarrhoea.
2. Look for pigmentation in skin creases, scars and buccal mucosa (*Addison's disease*).
3. Look for signs of blood loss – pallor and postural hypotension.
4. Look for signs of iron deficiency – angular stomatitis, koilonychia.
5. Look for vitiligo (*autoimmune disorders*).
6. Feel pulse for bradycardia (*heart block, Stokes–Adams attack*) or tachycardia (*supraventricular tachycardia, ventricular tachycardia*) and irregularity (*atrial fibrillation*).
7. Listen to heart – pansystolic murmur (*post-myocardial infarction ventricular septal defect* or *mitral incompetence*), pericardial friction rub (*pericarditis*).

◆ Key points

- The physical examination starts as soon as you meet the patient.
- Ask yourself: 'Does this patient look well?'
- Examine patients in a warm and well-lit environment.
- There is no *one* correct way of performing a physical examination, but you should develop a systematic routine to reduce the chance of missing things.
- Some important medical conditions are diagnosed from inspection only.
- The handshake may provide diagnostic clues.
- Abnormalities in the hands point to a wide variety of systemic disorders.
- Subtle abnormalities of complexion may not be apparent in artificial lighting.

ENDOCRINE EXAMINATION

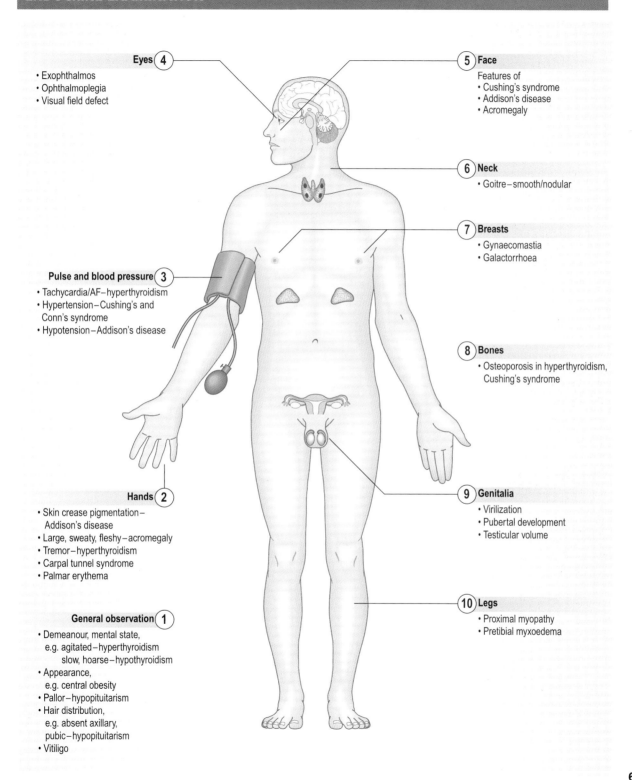

Eyes (4)
- Exophthalmos
- Ophthalmoplegia
- Visual field defect

(5) Face
Features of
- Cushing's syndrome
- Addison's disease
- Acromegaly

(6) Neck
- Goitre – smooth/nodular

(7) Breasts
- Gynaecomastia
- Galactorrhoea

Pulse and blood pressure (3)
- Tachycardia/AF – hyperthyroidism
- Hypertension – Cushing's and Conn's syndrome
- Hypotension – Addison's disease

(8) Bones
- Osteoporosis in hyperthyroidism, Cushing's syndrome

Hands (2)
- Skin crease pigmentation – Addison's disease
- Large, sweaty, fleshy – acromegaly
- Tremor – hyperthyroidism
- Carpal tunnel syndrome
- Palmar erythema

(9) Genitalia
- Virilization
- Pubertal development
- Testicular volume

General observation (1)
- Demeanour, mental state,
  e.g. agitated – hyperthyroidism
      slow, hoarse – hypothyroidism
- Appearance,
  e.g. central obesity
- Pallor – hypopituitarism
- Hair distribution,
  e.g. absent axillary,
  pubic – hypopituitarism
- Vitiligo

(10) Legs
- Proximal myopathy
- Pretibial myxoedema

SKIN EXAMINATION

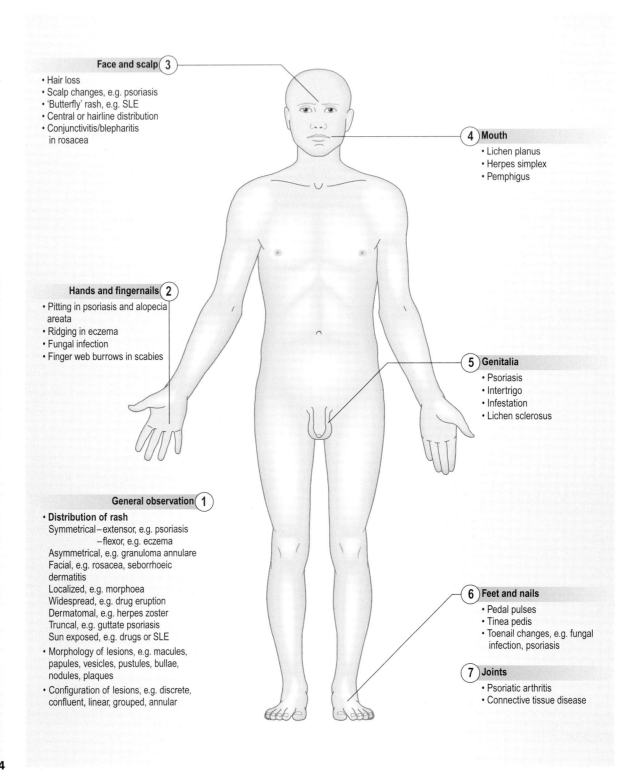

Face and scalp ③
- Hair loss
- Scalp changes, e.g. psoriasis
- 'Butterfly' rash, e.g. SLE
- Central or hairline distribution
- Conjunctivitis/blepharitis in rosacea

④ **Mouth**
- Lichen planus
- Herpes simplex
- Pemphigus

Hands and fingernails ②
- Pitting in psoriasis and alopecia areata
- Ridging in eczema
- Fungal infection
- Finger web burrows in scabies

⑤ **Genitalia**
- Psoriasis
- Intertrigo
- Infestation
- Lichen sclerosus

General observation ①
- **Distribution of rash**
  Symmetrical – extensor, e.g. psoriasis
  – flexor, e.g. eczema
  Asymmetrical, e.g. granuloma annulare
  Facial, e.g. rosacea, seborrhoeic dermatitis
  Localized, e.g. morphoea
  Widespread, e.g. drug eruption
  Dermatomal, e.g. herpes zoster
  Truncal, e.g. guttate psoriasis
  Sun exposed, e.g. drugs or SLE
- Morphology of lesions, e.g. macules, papules, vesicles, pustules, bullae, nodules, plaques
- Configuration of lesions, e.g. discrete, confluent, linear, grouped, annular

⑥ **Feet and nails**
- Pedal pulses
- Tinea pedis
- Toenail changes, e.g. fungal infection, psoriasis

⑦ **Joints**
- Psoriatic arthritis
- Connective tissue disease

Anatomy and function of the skin

The skin is the largest organ in the body, with a surface area of approximately 1.8 m^2 and comprises about 16% of body weight. Its most important function is as a barrier to protect the body from noxious external factors and to keep the internal organs intact (Table 2.9). Skin is composed of three layers: the epidermis, the dermis and the subcutis (Fig. 2.37).

Epidermis. The epidermis is a stratified squamous epithelium which acts as a protective barrier. It is normally ~0.1 mm thick, but is thicker (0.8–1.4 mm) on the palms of the hands and soles of the feet. It has four layers (basal, prickle, granular and horny) representing the stages of maturation of keratin. Cells lose their nuclei in the granular layer and, as flat plates, form the horny layer. The main cell is the keratinocyte, which produces the protein keratin. Melanocytes make up 5–10% of the basal cell population and synthesize melanin, transferring it to the keratinocytes via dendritic processes. Melanocytes are most numerous on the face and other exposed sites and originate from the neural crest. Langerhans cells are dendritic and immunologically active antigen-presenting cells that form a network throughout the epidermis.

Dermis. The dermis consists of a supportive connective tissue matrix containing specialized structures that is thin (0.6 mm) on the eyelids and thicker (3 mm or more) on the back, palms and soles. It contains fibroblasts, dendritic cells, mast cells, macrophages and lymphocytes. Collagen fibres make up 70% of the dermis and give strength and toughness. Elastin fibres provide elasticity to the skin. Glycosaminoglycans form a semisolid matrix that allows some movement of dermal structures, e.g. hair follicles, sweat glands, blood and lymphatic vessels and nerves.

Subcutis. This is a loose connective tissue and fat layer of variable thickness but may be up to 3 cm thick on the abdomen.

Anatomy and function of hair and nails

Hair and nails are specialized epidermal structures. Hair has a protective and sexual function. Hairs are found over the entire surface of the skin, with the exception of the glabrous skin of the palms and soles, the glans penis and vulval introitus. The follicle density is greatest on the face.

Hair

The hair shaft consists of an outer cuticle that encloses a cortex of packed keratinocytes with, in terminal hairs, an inner medulla. The germinative cells in the hair bulb are associated with melanocytes, which synthesize pigment. There are three types of hair:

- *Lanugo* hairs are formed in the fetus and are fine and long. They are normally shed before birth, but are seen in premature babies.
- *Vellus* hairs are short, fine, light-coloured hairs that cover most body surfaces.
- *Terminal* hairs are longer, thicker and darker, and are found on the scalp, eyebrows, eyelashes, pubic, axillary and beard areas.

Amounts and type of hair vary and are influenced by racial and genetic factors. Caucasians have straight hair, black Africans curly hair, Mongoloids have sparse facial and body hair, while Mediterranean people have more body hair than northern Europeans.

Hair cycle. Hairs pass through regular cycles: growth (*anagen*), resting (*telogen*) and shedding (*catagen*). The cycle may last up to 5 years for scalp hair, less for eyebrow, axillary and pubic hair. Usually, adjacent hairs are not in the same phase but illnesses or childbirth can synchronize the hair cycle and the loss of large amounts of hair (*telogen effluvium*) can give worrying results.

Puberty. Body hair develops throughout the years of sexual maturity, although there is wide variation in its pattern. At puberty, stimulation by androgens induces vellus hairs of the pubic region to develop into terminal hairs. This begins earlier in girls (average age 11.5 years) than in boys (average age 13.5 years). Gonadotrophins are not involved

2.9 Functions of skin
Barrier
• To chemicals, particles, microbes, UV radiation • Against mechanical injury • To loss of body fluids
Homeostasis
• Regulation of body temperature
Sensation
• Touch, temperature, pressure, pain
Mobility
• Provides a surface for grip
Metabolism
• Role in vitamin D production
Immunity
• Outpost for immune surveillance
Psychology
• Sexual attraction, self-image

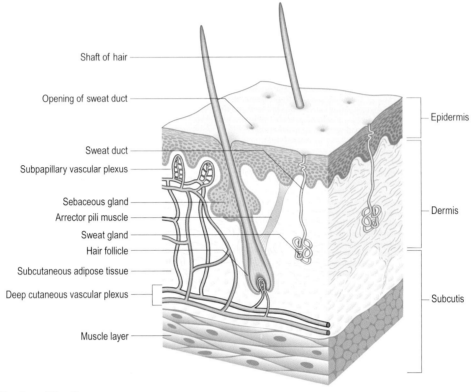

Fig. 2.37 Structure of the skin.

Labels (Fig. 2.37):
- Shaft of hair
- Opening of sweat duct
- Sweat duct
- Subpapillary vascular plexus
- Sebaceous gland
- Arrector pili muscle
- Sweat gland
- Hair follicle
- Subcutaneous adipose tissue
- Deep cutaneous vascular plexus
- Muscle layer
- Epidermis
- Dermis
- Subcutis

in this process, so patients with gonadotrophin deficiency have pubic hair but no other pubertal development. Axillary hair appears 2 years after pubic hair and coincides with onset of facial hair in boys (p. 366).

Nails

The nail (Fig. 2.38) is a plate of hardened densely packed keratin. Nails protect the finger tip and facilitate grasping and tactile sensitivity in the finger pulp. The *nail matrix* contains dividing cells that mature, keratinize and move forward to form the *nail plate*, which has a thickness of 0.3–0.5 mm and grows at a rate of 0.1 mm/24 h for the fingernail. Toenails grow more slowly. Adjacent dermal capillaries produce the pink colour of the nail; the white lunula is the visible distal part of the matrix.

COMMON SYMPTOMS

Patients with skin disease often complain of:

- itch and sleep disturbance (scabies and infestation with lice are characteristically itchy)
- physical presence of a growth or a rash

- discharge, crusting and odour
- dropping off of scales from skin or scalp
- disfigurement and psychological distress
- inability to work or pursue leisure activities (e.g. swimming).

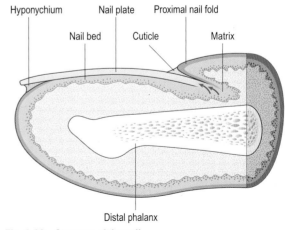

Labels (Fig. 2.38):
- Hyponychium
- Nail plate
- Proximal nail fold
- Nail bed
- Cuticle
- Matrix
- Distal phalanx

Fig. 2.38 Structure of the nail.

THE HISTORY

Presenting complaint

Ask about when, where and how the eruption or lesions began, their initial appearance and how it evolved. Note associated features such as itch and aggravating factors.

Past and drug histories

Ask about previous skin disease, atopic symptoms (hayfever, asthma, childhood eczema), medical disorders that may involve the skin e.g. Stevens–Johnson syndrome caused by mycoplasma pneumonia, herpes simplex or drugs (Fig. 2.39) or have cutaneous features, and prescribed or self-medicated drugs, including creams and cosmetics.

Social, family and genetic histories

Foreign travel may allow exposure to tropical infections or sunlight that could cause a photosensitive eruption. Psoriasis and atopic eczema have strongly inherited traits.

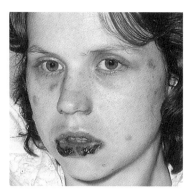

A

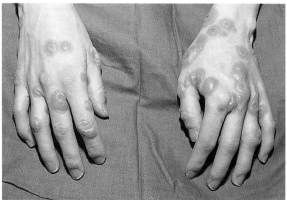

B

Fig. 2.39 Stevens–Johnson syndrome. (A) Facial and oral lesions. (B) 'Target lesions' on hands.

Occupational and environmental histories

Chemicals encountered at work or in leisure pursuits may be a cause of contact dermatitis. Suspect an industrial dermatitis if the eruption improves when the patient is away from work.

EXAMINATION

Conduct the skin examination in a warm well-lit place. A chaperone is desirable. Ask patients to undress to their underclothes if lesions are widespread to get a clear impression of the distribution and variation of the eruption, its composition in terms of the nature of individual lesions, and the patterns in which lesions are arranged (*configuration*). A hand-lens is useful to examine individual lesions. Wear examination gloves if the skin is broken.

Look for:

- Distribution
- Variation
- Composition in terms of the nature of individual lesions
- Patterns in which lesions are arranged ('configuration').

A synthesis of these variables in the light of the history allows you to make a diagnosis.

➡ Examination sequence

→ Stand back and look at the skin: is it abnormal?
→ Assess the distribution and colour of any lesions.
→ Observe the individual lesion in terms of size, shape, consistency, border changes and spatial interrelationships.
→ Palpate any lesions with your finger tips to find their consistency.
→ Look at the nails, hair and mucous membranes.
→ Examine local lymph nodes if indicated (see p. 51–52).
→ Take a skin scraping for culture if you suspect fungal infection.

Skin eruptions and lesions

Common distribution patterns

The distribution may be characteristic and indicate the diagnosis. Generally, symmetrical or universal eruptions suggest systemic or constitutional causes (Table 2.10). Asymmetrical rashes that spread from one focus are more likely to be due to fungal, bacterial or viral infection. Common patterns include:

- *Flexural.* Eruption in the antecubital and popliteal fossae indicates atopic eczema, an inflammatory dermatitis affecting 15% of children in Europe that typically involves the flexures of the popliteal fossa, antecubital fossa, neck and face (Fig. 2.40A).
- *Extensor.* Plaques on elbows and knees suggest psoriasis, which is seen in 1% of the population in westernized

2.10 Some examples of skin lesions and systemic disease		
Skin lesions	**Associations**	**Ask about**
Erythema nodosum	Sarcoidosis, tuberculosis, post-streptococcal infection, connective tissue diseases, drugs.	Cough and sputum, breathlessness, sore throat, drugs, etc.
Pyoderma gangrenosum	Ulcerative colitis, rheumatoid arthritis	Rectal bleeding, joint symptoms
Dermatitis herpetiformis	Gluten enteropathy	Family history, change in bowel habit
Generalized purpura	Idiopathic thrombocytopenic purpura and other haematological disorders	Family history, haematuria, fever and weight loss
Dermatitis artefacta	Personality disorders	Stresses or anxieties

countries and characteristically affects the extensor surfaces of the knees or elbows (Fig. 2.40B) in addition to the scalp and sacrum.

- *Facial.* Location on the forehead, nasolabial folds and scalp suggests seborrhoeic dermatitis (Fig. 2.41A), thought to represent an inflammatory reaction to yeasts on the skin. Facial involvement is a feature of acne (Fig. 2.41B), where comedones, pustules and cysts can also affect the chest and back, and rosacea, in which there is telangiectasia with pustules. The face is a prominent site for sun damage and for common malignant tumours, e.g. basal cell cancer (Fig. 2.41C).
- *Truncal.* An eruption on the trunk may suggest:
  – guttate psoriasis, which may follow a streptococcal throat infection
  – pityriasis rosea (Fig. 2.42A), which usually starts with one lesion, the 'herald patch'
  – tinea versicolor, an infection with pityrosporum yeast sometimes characterized by hypopigmentation

---

⊙ Examine this patient with a hand eruption

1. Enquire about the duration of the eruption; recent onset may indicate new environmental exposure.
2. Ask about previous skin disease, e.g. *atopic eczema*, and occupation, e.g. exposure to noxious chemicals, water, detergents, latex gloves, foodstuffs or industrial oils.
3. Ask about previous treatments, e.g. contact allergy to wood alcohols in a barrier cream applied at work.
4. Look at distribution:
   finger tips involved, e.g. *garlic allergy* in a chef
   small papules at the wrists extending up the forearm (*lichen planus*)
   nails involved, e.g. pitting in *psoriasis.*
5. Are there skin lesions elsewhere on the body, e.g. *atopic eczema* affecting the antecubital or popliteal fossae, or *psoriasis* on the elbows, knees or scalp?
6. Look for burrows on the sides of the fingers (*scabies*).
7. Are there small blisters (vesicles) with redness, fissuring and scaling (*eczema*) or are the changes those of plaques with nail pitting (*psoriasis*).
8. Consider referral for further investigations, for example:
   patch testing for cell-mediated allergy, e.g. to chemicals
   skin prick testing for immediate allergy, e.g. to latex.

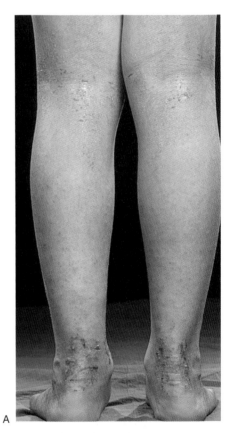

A

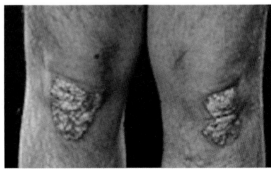

B

Fig. 2.40 Distribution: flexural and extensor aspects. (A) Atopic eczema in the popliteal fossae and ankles. (B) Psoriasis on the knees.

– urticaria (Fig. 2.42B), which is diagnosed by wheals that clear within 24 hours.

• *Peripheral.* A distribution around the wrists suggests lichen planus (Fig. 2.43); looking at the buccal mucosa might help. Some eruptions are typically found on the lower leg, e.g. necrobiosis lipoidica (Fig. 2.44A), erythema nodosum (associated with sarcoidosis or tuberculosis) or vasculitis (Fig. 2.44B), caused by circulating immune complexes damaging dermal blood vessels. The hands or feet are affected by fungal infection, typically 'athlete's foot' (Fig. 2.44C).

• *Sun-exposed.* An eruption caused by the sun typically involves the face (sparing areas beneath the eyes and lower lip), the V of the neck or the posterior neck, and exposed areas of the arms and legs. A rash on sun-exposed sites of face and arms suggests connective tissue diseases (e.g. systemic lupus erythematosus), use of photosensitizing drugs (e.g. thiazide diuretics or non-steroidals) or a primary sun sensitivity condition, e.g. polymorphic light eruption, or a photosensitive eczema.

• *Dermatomal.* A rash showing dermatomal distribution suggests herpes zoster (shingles) (Fig. 2.45).

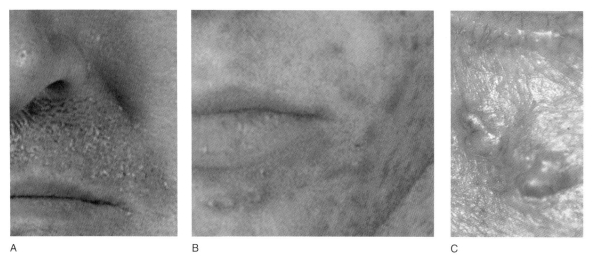

A   B   C

Fig. 2.41 **Distribution: facial.** (A) Seborrhoeic dermatitis. (B) Acne vulgaris. (C) Basal cell cancer showing pearly papules with telangiectasia.

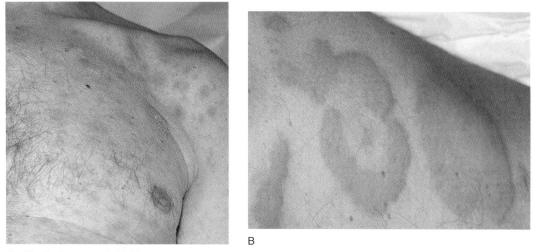

A   B

Fig. 2.42 **Distribution: truncal.** (A) Pityriasis rosea. (B) Urticaria.

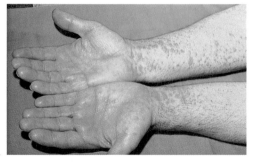

A

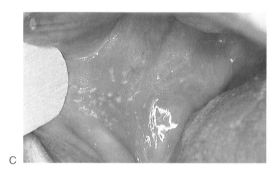

C

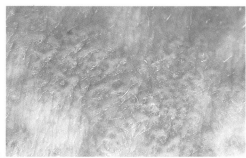

B

Fig. 2.43 Diagnostic sequence, lichen planus. (A) Discrete flat-topped papules on the wrist. (B) Wickham's striae visible on close inspection. (C) White lacy network of striae on buccal mucosa.

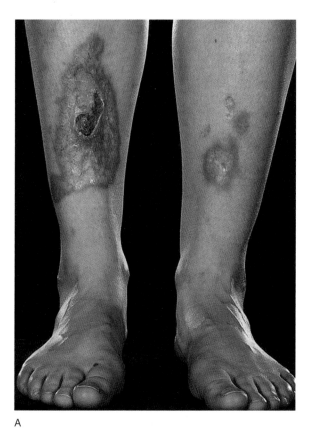

A

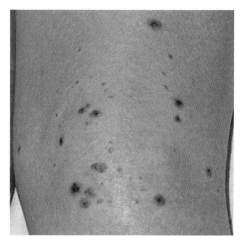

B

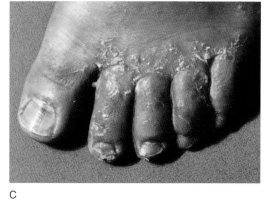

C

Fig. 2.44 Distribution: peripheral. (A) Necrobiosis lipoidica. (B) Vasculitis. (C) Fungal infection.

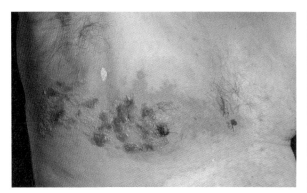

Fig. 2.45   Distribution. Dermatomal distribution suggests shingles.

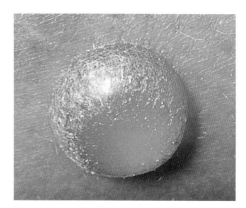

Fig. 2.47   Bulla from an insect bite.

Common morphological patterns

The ability to use terminology to define the nature of the primary lesions is difficult to grasp at first but comes with use and permits a meaningful description of an eruption (Figs 2.46–2.49, Table 2.11). Primary lesions are often complicated by secondary changes such as crusting, erosion and excoriation. Variability in morphology can be useful: for example, lesions are *monomorphic* (all of one appearance) in guttate psoriasis and *pleomorphic* (of differing appearance) in chickenpox. Common patterns of configuration include linear, grouped, annular and the Koebner phenomenon (Fig. 2.51).

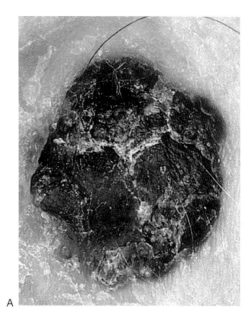

A

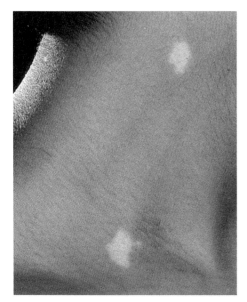

Fig. 2.46   Macule. Macules can be pigmented, as in a freckle, erythematous as in a haemangioma, or hypopigmented, as shown here in vitiligo, an autoimmune condition in which there is often symmetrical loss of pigment through destruction of melanocytes.

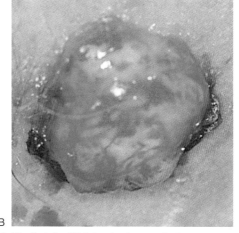

B

Fig. 2.48   Nodule. (A) Seborrhoeic wart. (B) Squamous cell cancer.

2.11	Definitions of skin lesion terminology
Term	**Definition**
Abscess	A localized collection of pus
Atrophy	Loss of epidermis, dermis or both, resulting in thin, translucent and wrinkled skin with visible blood vessels
Bulla	A fluid-filled blister > 5 mm diameter
Burrow	A tunnel in the skin caused by a parasite, e.g. acarus of scabies
Callus	Local hyperplasia of the horny layer, often on palm or sole, due to pressure
Comedo	A plug of sebum and keratin wedged in a dilated pilosebaceous orifice on the face
Crust	Dried exudate, e.g. serum, blood or pus, on the skin surface
Cyst	A nodule consisting of an epithelial-lined cavity filled with fluid or semisolid material
Ecchymosis	A macular red or purple haemorrhage, > 2 mm diameter, in skin or mucous membrane
Erosion	A superficial break in the epidermis, not extending into dermis, which heals without scarring
Erythema	Redness of the skin due to vascular dilatation
Excoriation	A superficial abrasion, often linear, due to scratching
Fissure	A linear split in epidermis, often just extending into dermis
Freckle	A macular area showing increased pigment formation by melanocytes
Lichenification	Chronic thickening of skin with increased skin markings, resulting from rubbing or scratching
Macule	A localized area of colour or textural change in the skin
Milium	A small white cyst that contains keratin
Nodule	A solid elevation of skin > 5 mm diameter
Papilloma	A nipple-like projection from the surface of the skin
Papule	A solid elevation of skin < 5 mm diameter
Petechia	A haemorrhagic punctate spot 1–2 mm diameter
Plaque	A palpable elevation of skin > 2 cm diameter and < 5 mm in height
Purpura	Extravasation of blood resulting in red discoloration of skin or mucous membranes
Pustule	A visible collection of pus in a blister
Scale	Accumulation of easily detached fragments of thickened keratin
Scar	Replacement of normal tissue by fibrous connective tissue at site of an injury
Stria	Atrophic linear band in skin, white, pink or purple in colour, the result of connective tissue changes
Telangiectasia	Dilated dermal blood vessels resulting in a visible lesion
Ulcer	A circumscribed area of skin loss extending into the dermis
Vesicle	A clear, fluid-filled blister
Wheal	A transitory, compressible papule or plaque of dermal oedema, red or white in colour, and usually indicating urticaria

Common patterns of hair disease

Hair loss (*alopecia*) or too little hair has several common patterns:

- *Diffuse alopecia.* In common male-pattern hair loss (Fig. 2.52A), terminal scalp hairs undergo miniaturization to vellus hairs. This is an ageing phenomenon that has a strong inherited component and is dependent on androgens. Women may show age-related hair loss that is more diffuse. Non-scarring diffuse hair loss is a feature of many conditions including hypothyroidism, hypopituitarism and iron deficiency and may be drug induced, e.g. cytotoxic agents.

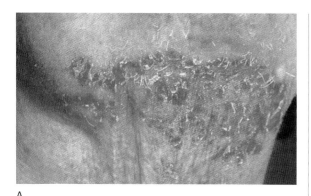

A

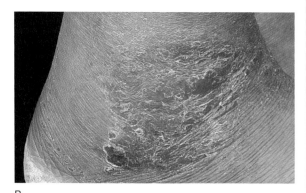

B

Fig. 2.49 Plaque. (A) Lupus vulgaris (tuberculosis of the skin). (B) Tuberculoid leprosy.

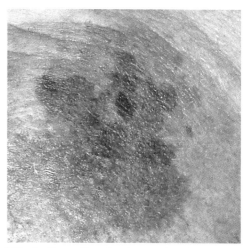

Fig. 2.50   Lentigo malignant melanoma. Irregular margin and pigmentation.

2.12 Causes of hirsutism	
Type	**Example**
Pituitary	Acromegaly
Adrenal	Cushing's syndrome, virilizing tumours, congenital adrenal hyperplasia
Ovarian	Polycystic ovary syndrome, virilizing tumours
Drugs	Androgens, progestogens
Idiopathic	End-organ hypersensitivity to androgens

- *Localized non-scarring alopecia.* In the autoimmune condition *alopecia areata* (Fig. 2.52B) there is circumscribed loss of scalp, beard or eyebrow hair. Hair loss in alopecia areata may extend to involve the whole scalp (*alopecia totalis*) or the entirety of body hair (*alopecia universalis*). Localized hair loss can also be caused by fungal infection (Fig. 2.52C), hair pulling, traction from braiding and secondary syphilis.
- *Scarring alopecia.* When the scalp is scarred the hair follicles are destroyed and hair loss is permanent. Causes include burns, severe infections, e.g. herpes zoster, lichen planus and systemic lupus erythematosus.
- *Loss of secondary sexual hair.* In old age, cirrhosis and hypopituitarism, axillary and pubic hair is lost. Axillary and pubic hair never develops in primary hypogonadism.

Excessive hair growth takes two forms:

- *Hirsutism* occurs in females. There is a male-pattern growth of terminal hair, including the facial and pubic hair. The pubic hair growth is no longer flat topped but extends up to the umbilicus ('the male escutcheon'). Most commonly it is a racial trait or idiopathic – representing increased end-organ sensitivity to androgens. A rare cause is an androgen-secreting tumour

(Table 2.12). In these cases there are usually other features of virilization, e.g. male-pattern hair loss, cliteromegaly or a deep voice.
- *Hypertrichosis* is excess terminal hair growth in a non-androgenic distribution and may occur in males or females. Hypertrichosis is less common than hirsutism and is usually due to a systemic disorder, e.g. porphyria cutanea tarda, malignancy, anorexia nervosa, malnutrition or drugs, e.g. ciclosporin, minoxidil, and phenytoin. Localized hypertrichosis is found with scarring, melanocytic naevi and over the lower back in spina bifida.

Common patterns of nail abnormality
(see Fig. 2.17, p. 49)

Nail disorders

Nail changes can be useful in diagnosing internal conditions and skin diseases (Table 2.13):

- Onycholysis (separation of the nail from the nail bed) and pitting are found in psoriasis.

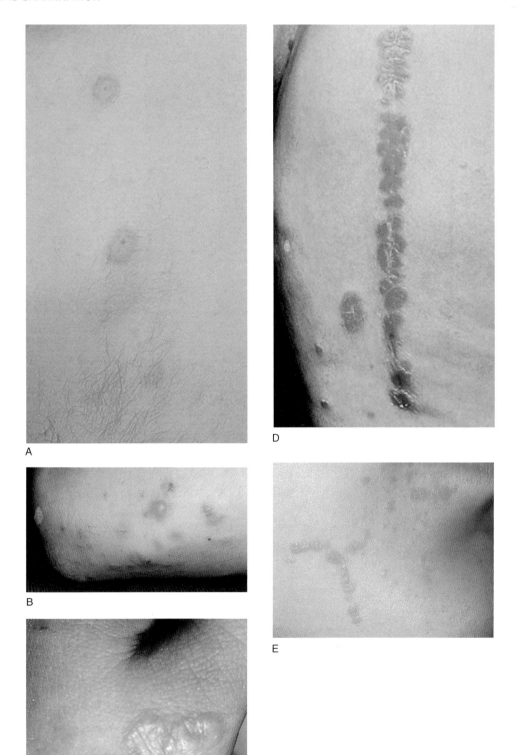

Fig. 2.51 Configuration. (A) Insect bites – linear. (B) Dermatitis herpetiformis – grouped. (C) Granuloma annulare – annular. (D) Psoriasis showing the Koebner phenomenon – the appearance of lesions in an area of trauma. (E) Viral warts – Koebner phenomenon.

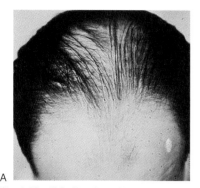
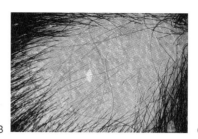
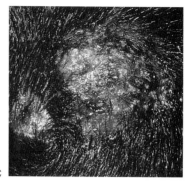

Fig. 2.52 Hair disorders. (A) Male-pattern baldness with hair loss from the temples and vertex of the scalp. (B) Alopecia areata with 'exclamation mark' hairs, which taper as they approach the skin. (C) Scalp ringworm with secondary bacterial infection and localized hair loss.

2.13 Nail changes in systemic disease and skin disorders

Change	Description of nail	Differential diagnosis
Beau's lines	Transverse grooves	Any severe systemic illness which affects growth of the nail matrix
Brittle nails	Nails break easily, usually at distal margin	Effect of water and detergent, iron deficiency, hypothyroidism, digital ischaemia
Colour change	Blue	Cyanosis, antimalarials, haematoma
	Blue-green	*Pseudomonas* infection
	Brown	Fungal infection, staining from cigarettes, chlorpromazine, gold, Addison's disease
	Brown longitudinal streak	Melanocytic naevus, malignant melanoma, Addison's disease, racial variant
	Red streaks (splinter haemorrhages)	Infective endocarditis, trauma
	White spots	Trauma to nail matrix (*not* calcium deficiency)
	White/brown 'half and half' nails	Chronic renal failure
	White (leuconychia)	Hypoalbuminaemia, e.g. associated with cirrhosis
	Yellow	Psoriasis, fungal infection, jaundice, tetracycline
	Yellow nail syndrome	Defective lymphatic drainage – pleural effusions may occur
Koilonychia	Spoon-shaped depression of nail plate	Iron deficiency anaemia; lichen planus, repeated exposure to detergents
Nail fold	Dilated capillaries and erythema at nail fold	Connective tissue disorders including systemic sclerosis, systemic lupus erythematosus, dermatomyositis
Onycholysis	Separation of nail from nail bed	Psoriasis, fungal infection, trauma, thyrotoxicosis, tetracyclines (*photo-onycholysis*)
Pitting	Fine or coarse pits may be seen in nail bed	Psoriasis, eczema, alopecia areata, lichen planus
Ridging	Transverse (across nail)	Beau's lines (see above), eczema, psoriasis, tic-dystrophy, chronic paronychia
	Longitudinal (up/down)	Lichen planus, Darier's disease

- Fungal infection (onychomycosis) causes thickening and sometimes whitening of the nail plate.
- Beau's lines are the result of disturbance to nail growth by a severe systemic illness.
- Clubbing can be congenital or signify serious cardiac or respiratory disease.
- Splinter haemorrhages may be seen with trauma but might signify infective endocarditis.
- Nail fold erythema and telangiectasia is a feature of systemic lupus erythematosus, other connective tissue diseases and vasculitis.
- Eczema, e.g. ridging and dystrophy.
- Alopecia areata, fine 'thimble' pitting.

- Darier's disease in which there are longitudinal ridges and triangular nicks at the distal nail edge.
- 'Spoon-shaped' nail (koilonychia) of iron deficiency.

Abnormal findings in mucous membranes and other sites

With any unusual or atypical eruption, look at the mucous membranes of the mouth and genitalia for changes such as oral involvement by Wickham's striae in lichen planus, oral lesions in Kaposi's sarcoma (Fig. 2.53) or vulval involvement with lichen sclerosus. Always examine the lymph nodes in patients with suspected skin cancer. In

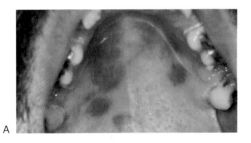

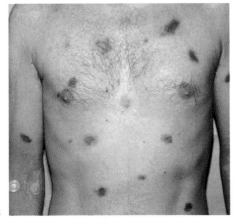

Fig. 2.53 Kaposi's sarcoma. (A) In the mouth and (B) on the skin.

---

skin lymphoma, a full examination is needed, looking particularly for lymphadenopathy and hepatosplenomegaly. In patients with leg ulcers, feel the leg and foot pulses to assess the arterial supply.

INVESTIGATIONS

Microscopy. View skin scrapings treated with potassium hydroxide solution under a light microscope to confirm the presence of fungal hyphae. In scabies, the acarus can be extracted using a needle and viewed under the microscope.

Wood's light. A hand-held ultraviolet lamp can show vitiligo that is not apparent in ordinary light or fluorescence in a fungal infection.

Surgical biopsy. A biopsy for histology or direct immunofluorescence can help make the diagnosis.

Doppler studies. An index of the dorsalis pedis blood pressure over brachial blood pressure of < 0.8 helps diagnose arterial disease in a patient with a leg ulcer (see p. 117).

Photography. Record the eruption or lesion for future comparison.

Patch tests. Application of prepared allergens on small aluminium discs to the upper back for 2 days with readings at 2 and 4 days after application permits a diagnosis of delayed-type contact allergy, e.g. to fragrances.

Prick tests. Pricking of prepared allergen solution into the dermis with reading at 15 minutes using histamine and saline as positive and negative controls allows diagnosis of immediate allergy, e.g. to latex.

> ○ **Examine this patient with a pigmented skin lesion on his back**
>
> 1. Does the patient have a fair skin type, i.e. does he/she burn easily and tan poorly or not at all? (*Skin cancers* are more common in those with a pale skin.)
> 2. Has the patient had a lot of sun exposure or used sun beds regularly? (*Skin cancers* are common with excessive sun exposure and sun bed use.)
> 3. Is there a family history of *malignant melanoma* or other forms of *skin cancer*? (A family history is found in 10% of patients with *malignant melanoma*.)
> 4. Has the mole appeared recently or has the change occurred in an existing lesion? (*Malignant melanoma* can occur in an existing melanocytic naevus or as a new lesion.)
> 5. Ask if this mole has got bigger, been itchy or bled (*malignant melanoma*).
> 6. Is this mole irregular in outline, variable in pigmentation, inflamed or ulcerated? (*Malignant melanoma* commonly shows variation in pigmentation or outline.)
> 7. Examine the patient's entire skin for any other suspicious moles or *skin cancers*. (Abnormal moles may be found in patients who have a *malignant melanoma*.)
> 8. Request urgent surgical excision biopsy for histological examination.

◆ Key points

- ◆ Ask about the time of onset and evolution of the eruption or lesion.
- ◆ Ask about atopic symptoms, general medical conditions and record use of drugs and topical therapies.
- ◆ Look at the entire skin surface, use a hand lens where necessary and ensure good lighting.
- ◆ Gently feel the skin to assess texture, wearing gloves if the skin is broken.
- ◆ Look for distribution, individual morphology and configuration of the lesions.
- ◆ Examine nails, hair, mouth and genitalia if indicated, and always be sensitive to the patient's modesty.

Section 2
SYSTEMIC EXAMINATION

The cardiovascular system

3

DAVID NORTHRIDGE • NEIL GRUBB • ANDREW BRADBURY

CARDIOVASCULAR EXAMINATION

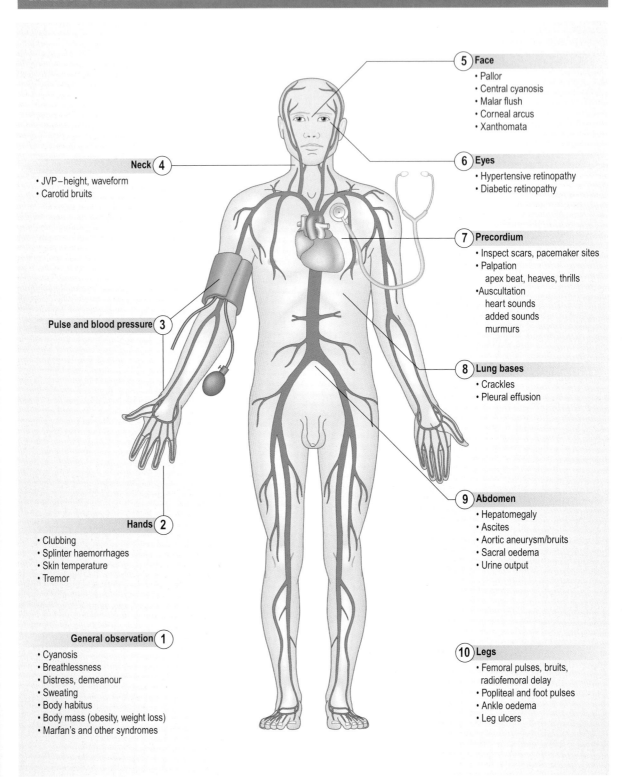

5 **Face**
- Pallor
- Central cyanosis
- Malar flush
- Corneal arcus
- Xanthomata

6 **Eyes**
- Hypertensive retinopathy
- Diabetic retinopathy

7 **Precordium**
- Inspect scars, pacemaker sites
- Palpation
  apex beat, heaves, thrills
- Auscultation
  heart sounds
  added sounds
  murmurs

8 **Lung bases**
- Crackles
- Pleural effusion

9 **Abdomen**
- Hepatomegaly
- Ascites
- Aortic aneurysm/bruits
- Sacral oedema
- Urine output

10 **Legs**
- Femoral pulses, bruits, radiofemoral delay
- Popliteal and foot pulses
- Ankle oedema
- Leg ulcers

Neck **4**
- JVP – height, waveform
- Carotid bruits

Pulse and blood pressure **3**

Hands **2**
- Clubbing
- Splinter haemorrhages
- Skin temperature
- Tremor

General observation **1**
- Cyanosis
- Breathlessness
- Distress, demeanour
- Sweating
- Body habitus
- Body mass (obesity, weight loss)
- Marfan's and other syndromes

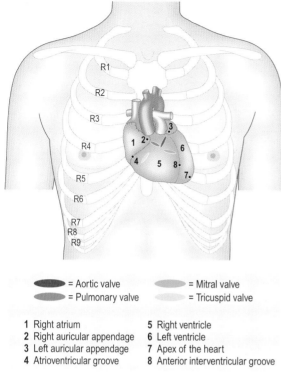

= Aortic valve   = Mitral valve
= Pulmonary valve   = Tricuspid valve

1 Right atrium   5 Right ventricle
2 Right auricular appendage   6 Left ventricle
3 Left auricular appendage   7 Apex of the heart
4 Atrioventricular groove   8 Anterior interventricular groove

Fig. 3.1   Surface anatomy of the chambers and valves of the heart.

INTRODUCTION

Most chronic cardiac diseases are initially asymptomatic and this *silent* phase may last for many years. Cardiac pathology may be diagnosed during 'routine' examination or because of the development of a complication (e.g. atrial fibrillation in mitral stenosis). The cardinal symptoms of heart disease are *chest discomfort, breathlessness, palpitation, syncope* and *peripheral oedema* (Table 3.1). The probability that a particular symptom is caused by heart disease depends upon many factors, including the patient's age, sex, family history, social history and the physical findings.

3.1 Common symptoms of heart disease		
Symptom	**Cardiovascular causes**	**Other causes**
Chest discomfort	Myocardial infarction Angina Pericarditis Aortic dissection	Oesophageal spasm Pneumothorax Musculoskeletal pain
Breathlessness	Heart failure Angina Pulmonary embolism Pulmonary hypertension	Respiratory disease Anaemia Obesity
Palpitation	Tachyarrhythmias Ectopic beats	Anxiety Hyperthyroidism Drugs
Syncope/dizziness	Arrhythmias Postural hypertension Aortic stenosis Hypertrophic obstructive cardiomyopathy Atrial myxoma	Simple faints Epilepsy
Oedema	Heart failure Constrictive pericarditis Venous stasis	Nephrotic syndrome Liver disease Drugs

COMMON SYMPTOMS

CHEST DISCOMFORT

Various types of chest discomfort caused by cardiovascular disorders are listed in Table 3.2. It is important to consider all degrees of discomfort, since patients will not necessarily find their condition *painful*.

Angina pectoris

Angina is the most important cause of recurrent chest discomfort. It is the symptomatic manifestation of myocardial ischaemia and usually has typical features with well-recognized precipitating, aggravating and relieving factors.

Site and radiation

Angina is characteristically felt in the centre of the chest. Pain at the cardiac apex is unlikely to be ischaemic. The patient's body language may be helpful – anginal discomfort is poorly localized and usually indicated using the open hand or a fist rather than the finger tip (Fig. 3.2). It may radiate to either or both arms, to the throat or jaw (occasionally it can be confused with toothache) and, less commonly, to the

3.2 Types of cardiac pain

Type	Cause	Characteristics
Angina	Coronary stenosis (rarely aortic stenosis, hypertrophic cardiomyopathy)	Precipitated by exertion, eased by rest and/or glyceryl trinitrate Characteristic distribution
Myocardial infarction	Coronary occlusion	Similar sites to angina, more severe, persists at rest
Pericarditic pain	Pericarditis	Sharp, raw or stabbing Varies with movement or breathing
Aortic pain	Dissection of the aorta	Severe, sudden onset, radiates to the back

3.4 Canadian Cardiovascular Society: functional classification of stable angina

Grade 1	Ordinary physical activity, such as walking and climbing stairs, does not cause angina. Angina with strenuous or rapid or prolonged exertion at work or recreation
Grade 2	Slight limitation of ordinary activity. Walking or climbing stairs rapidly, walking uphill, walking or stair climbing after meals, in cold, in wind, or when under emotional stress, or only during the few hours after awakening
Grade 3	Marked limitation of ordinary physical activity. Walking one to two blocks on the level and climbing less than one flight in normal conditions
Grade 4	Inability to carry on any physical activity without discomfort – angina may be present at rest

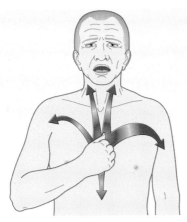

Fig. 3.2 Site and radiation of angina.

back or epigastrium. Discomfort at one of these sites may be the principal complaint with no associated chest pain.

Duration, precipitating and relieving factors

Angina is a short-lived discomfort, usually lasting less than 10 minutes, and is precipitated by conditions which temporarily increase myocardial oxygen demand, i.e. anything that increases heart rate, blood pressure or force of left ventricular contraction (Table 3.3). It usually occurs predictably, at a certain level of activity or excitement, but is provoked more readily by exercise after a meal, or in cold

3.3 Factors worsening or relieving angina

Aggravating	Relieving
Exertion	Rest
Emotional excitement	Glyceryl trinitrate
Cold weather	Warm up before exercise
Exercise after meal	

windy weather. Many patients find that after an attack of angina they can resume exercise without recurrent chest pain, the phenomenon of *second wind* (warm-up phenomenon).

The impact on functional capacity should be assessed as described below. The Canadian Cardiovascular Classification provides a more objective assessment (Table 3.4).

Patients quickly learn that their angina is rapidly relieved by rest or after taking sublingual glyceryl trinitrate.

Character

Patients describe angina as a tightness or heaviness and it is usually not severe, a 'discomfort' rather than a 'pain'. *Severity* of angina relates to the degree of functional limitation and the frequency of symptoms rather than the intensity of the pain. Initially patients may blame 'indigestion' for their symptoms and may not appreciate their significance.

Angina is commonly accompanied by a feeling of breathlessness. Occasionally this is the primary complaint. Autonomic symptoms such as profuse sweating, nausea and vomiting are not features of angina, but do occur in acute myocardial infarction.

Special types of angina

Unstable angina is angina of recent onset or increasing severity, duration or frequency. Pain may occur on minimal exertion or at rest. Unstable angina is a medical emergency because, untreated, it may culminate in myocardial infarction.

Crescendo angina is a specific type of unstable angina where attacks are progressively more frequent each day.

Nocturnal or *decubitus angina* may occur because of the increased venous return produced by lying down, or when antianginal preparations, which are commonly taken in the morning, lose their efficacy. It usually indicates severe coronary disease.

It may be difficult to distinguish between angina and other cardiac or non-cardiac causes of chest pain (Table 3.5).

3.5 Differential diagnosis: angina vs oesophageal pain	
Angina	**Oesophageal pain**
Usually precipitated by exertion	Can be worsened by exertion, but often present at other times
Rapidly relieved by rest	Not rapidly relieved by rest
Retrosternal and radiates to arm and jaw	Retrosternal or epigastric, sometimes radiates to arm or back
Seldom wakes patient from sleep	Often wakes patient from sleep
No relation to heartburn (but patients often have 'wind')	Sometimes related to heartburn
Rapidly relieved by nitrates	Often relieved by nitrates
Typical duration 2–10 minutes	Variable duration

3.7 Characteristics of pericarditic pain	
Site	Retrosternal, may radiate to left shoulder or back
Prodrome	May be preceded by a viral illness
Onset	No obvious initial precipitating factor; tends to fluctuate in intensity
Nature	May be stabbing or 'raw' – 'like sandpaper'. Often described as sharp, rarely as tight or heavy
Made worse by	Changes in posture, respiration
Helped by	Analgesics, especially non-steroidal anti-inflammatory drugs
Accompanied by	Pericardial rub

The diagnosis of angina involves an assessment of cardio-vascular risk: atypical symptoms in a 60-year-old male smoker with a history of diabetes are probably angina, whereas even a characteristic history is unlikely to represent angina if the patient is a non-smoking, young female.

Myocardial infarction

Myocardial infarction causes pain similar to angina in site, radiation and character but it is usually much more severe and prolonged and persists despite taking glyceryl trinitrate (Table 3.6). Autonomic symptoms such as sweating, nausea and vomiting are common, particularly in inferior wall infarcts, and can direct your attention away from the heart to the upper gastrointestinal tract. Patients may also be breathless, restless and distressed and may experience a sensation of impending death.

The symptoms of myocardial infarction are not always severe. Painless or 'silent' myocardial infarction is not uncommon, particularly in diabetic patients and the elderly. These patients may present later with complications from their infarct such as cardiac failure or an arrhythmia, or the diagnosis may be made retrospectively from a routine electrocardiogram (ECG).

Pericardial pain

Pericarditis causes chest pain which is usually more localized than ischaemic pain. Patients describe a sharp pain which is commonly accentuated by exertion, respiration and changes in posture, such as leaning forward (Table 3.7). Pericarditis may occur following myocardial infarction, viral infections and thoracic radiotherapy.

Aortic dissection

The sudden development of a linear tear in the wall of the aorta is called acute dissection. The length of aorta affected varies from a few centimetres to the whole vessel from root to bifurcation, and major branches may also be involved. Predisposing factors include hypertension, Marfan's syndrome, aortic dilatation and trauma.

Acute dissection causes very severe chest pain of sudden onset. It is often described as 'tearing' and frequently radiates to the back between the shoulder blades (Table 3.8). It is commonly associated with autonomic symptoms such as

3.6 Differential diagnosis: angina vs myocardial infarction	
Angina	**Myocardial infarction**
Site: retrosternal, radiates to arm, epigastrium, neck	As for angina
Precipitated by exercise or emotion	Often no obvious precipitant
Relieved by rest, nitrates	Not relieved by rest, nitrates
Mild/moderate severity	Usually severe (may be 'silent')
Anxiety absent or mild	Severe
No increased sympathetic activity	Increased sympathetic activity
No nausea or vomiting	Nausea and vomiting are common

3.8 Characteristics of pain caused by dissection of the thoracic aorta	
Site	Often first felt between shoulder blades, and/or behind the sternum
Onset	Usually sudden
Nature	Very severe pain, often described as 'tearing'
Relieved by	No, tends to persist. Patients often restless with pain
Accompanied by	Hypertension, asymmetric pulses, unexpected bradycardia, early diastolic murmur, syncope, focal neurological symptoms and signs

3.9 Some mechanisms and causes of heart failure	
Mechanism	**Cause**
Reduced ventricular contractility (systolic dysfunction)	Myocardial ischaemia Myocardial infarction Cardiomyopathy Myocarditis Drugs with negative inotropic actions, e.g. beta-blockers
Impaired ventricular filling (diastolic dysfunction)	Left ventricular hypertrophy Constrictive pericarditis
Increased metabolic and cardiac demand	Pregnancy Anaemia } aggravating factors which rarely cause heart failure alone Fever Thyrotoxicosis Arteriovenous fistulae Paget's disease
Arrhythmia	Tachycardia especially atrial fibrillation Bradycardia
Valvular or structural cardiac lesions	Mitral and/or aortic valve disease Tricuspid and/or pulmonary valve disease (rare) Ventricular septal defect Hypertrophic obstructive cardiomyopathy
Fluid overload	Excessive IV infusion. Drugs, e.g. non-steroidal anti-inflammatory drugs, steroids
Other	Intercurrent non-cardiac illness in patients with cardiac disease

sweating, and may cause syncope and/or focal neurological symptoms and signs.

BREATHLESSNESS

The sensation of breathlessness (dyspnoea) on effort may be normal. It becomes a symptom of disease if it occurs at exercise levels below those expected for the patient's age and degree of previous fitness. This chapter deals specifically with dyspnoea of cardiac origin, though respiratory disease (see Ch. 4) may coexist.

Dyspnoea on exertion is the usual presenting symptom of heart failure, the common causes of which are listed in Table 3.9. Patients may complain of associated fatigue 'I just know I have to stop', but symptoms of tiredness or a lack of energy are rarely cardiac in origin. To assess the degree of symptomatic limitation caused by exertional breathlessness objectively, use the New York Heart Association classification (Table 3.10).

Patients with severe or acute heart failure typically caused by acute myocardial infarction may develop dyspnoea at rest. Other cardiovascular causes of acute dyspnoea at rest include arrhythmias and pulmonary embolism. Patients with acute pulmonary oedema usually prefer to be upright, while those with pulmonary embolism are often more comfortable lying flat and may faint (syncope) if made to sit upright.

3.10 New York Heart Association classification of heart failure symptom severity	
Class I	No limitations. Ordinary physical activity does not cause undue fatigue, dyspnoea or palpitation (asymptomatic left ventricular dysfunction)
Class II	Slight limitation of physical activity. Such patients are comfortable at rest. Ordinary physical activity results in fatigue, palpitation, dyspnoea or angina pectoris (symptomatically 'mild' heart failure)
Class III	Marked limitation of physical activity. Less than ordinary physical activity will lead to symptoms (symptomatically 'moderate' heart failure)
Class IV	Symptoms of congestive cardiac failure are present even at rest. With any physical activity increased discomfort is experienced (symptomatically 'severe' heart failure)

Orthopnoea and paroxysmal nocturnal dyspnoea

Orthopnoea is dyspnoea on lying flat. Lying flat increases venous return to the heart and in patients with a failing left ventricle may precipitate pulmonary venous congestion and pulmonary oedema. To avoid this unpleasant symptom, the patient will typically try to lie propped up, e.g. using extra pillows or sleeping upright in a chair. Orthopnoea is usually

Mechanism

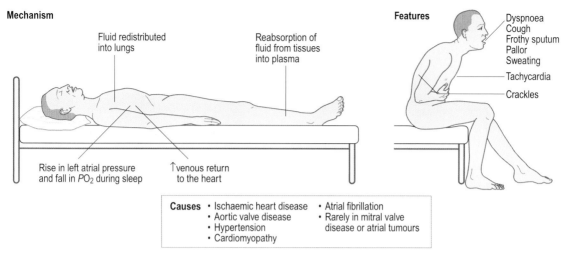

Features

Dyspnoea
Cough
Frothy sputum
Pallor
Sweating

Tachycardia

Crackles

Fluid redistributed
into lungs

Reabsorption of
fluid from tissues
into plasma

Rise in left atrial pressure
and fall in PO_2 during sleep

↑venous return
to the heart

Causes	• Ischaemic heart disease	• Atrial fibrillation
	• Aortic valve disease	• Rarely in mitral valve
	• Hypertension	disease or atrial tumours
	• Cardiomyopathy	

Fig. 3.3 Paroxysmal nocturnal dyspnoea.

found when heart failure is advanced and rarely occurs in the absence of dyspnoea on effort.

Paroxysmal nocturnal dyspnoea is a form of orthopnoea (Fig. 3.3). The patient is comfortable lying down to sleep, but is woken later with acute, severe, breathlessness which is relieved by sitting up. The intensity of the symptom is often described as like suffocation and patients may get out of bed, occasionally throwing open the windows to relieve their distress. Characteristically, they have an associated cough producing frothy sputum which may be streaked with blood. Distinguish paroxysmal nocturnal dyspnoea from nocturnal asthma (Ch. 4).

PALPITATION

Palpitation is the sensation of the heart beating in the chest. Patients often use terms such as thumping, pounding, fluttering, jumping, racing and skipping a beat. Ask patients to tap out, with their fingers, the pattern of palpitation they experience. This helps to clarify the rate and rhythm.

Palpitation may be due to heightened awareness of the heart beating in sinus rhythm, occasional irregularities of the heartbeat, e.g. ventricular extrasystoles, or awareness of the heart beating in an abnormal rhythm. Most patients complaining of palpitation do not have a sustained arrhythmia and not all patients with arrhythmia have palpitations, e.g. atrial fibrillation is commonly asymptomatic. Investigation is usually required to confirm the diagnosis, but the history can frequently distinguish between the different types of palpitation (Table 3.11). Ask about:

- the mode of onset and termination
- specific triggers of exercise, alcohol, caffeine

3.11	Descriptions of arrhythmias
Arrhythmia	**Patient's description**
Ventricular or atrial extrasystoles	'Heart misses a beat' Heart 'jumps' or 'flutters'
Atrial fibrillation	Heart 'jumping about' or 'racing' Associated breathlessness May be unnoticed
Supraventricular tachycardia	Heart racing or fluttering Associated polyuria
Ventricular tachycardia	Heart racing or fluttering Associated breathlessness May present as syncope rather than as palpitation

- frequency
- duration of attacks
- rhythm (ask patient to tap out).

Awareness of heart beating in normal sinus rhythm

Most healthy people experience this at some time, usually in relation to sympathetic nervous system overactivity, e.g. after strenuous exercise, when given a fright or waiting for an interview or examination. It may be most noticeable in bed at night when external visual and auditory inputs are minimal and visceral sensations more prominent. Similar palpitation occurs with excessive caffeine intake in coffee, tea, cola or other drinks and with nicotine from smoking.

Common irregularities of the heartbeat

Ventricular ectopic beats are a benign cause of palpitation and occur more often at rest and subside with physical activity. Patients with ectopic beats may take their own pulse and describe 'missed beats', followed by a particularly strong heartbeat. This occurs because the premature (ectopic) depolarization results in a low stroke volume producing an impalpable impulse following incomplete left ventricular filling. The subsequent compensatory pause leads to over-filling of the ventricle and a more forceful contraction and greater stroke volume with the next beat.

Palpitation due to sustained arrhythmias

Palpitation caused by a tachycardia is usually of sudden onset, lasts for minutes or longer and is unrelated to anxiety or stress. You need to identify the nature of the arrhythmia and its underlying pathology. The questions to ask depend upon the specific arrhythmia.

- Is there a family history of premature heart disease or sudden death?
- Is there a past history of rheumatic fever, previous heart attacks or other heart disease?
- What is the daily caffeine and weekly alcohol consumption (see p. 17)?
- Are any drugs being taken, whether prescribed, over the counter or recreational?
- Are there any non-specific symptoms of recent ill health (to consider unusual causes such as infective endocarditis or Lyme disease etc.)?
- If the attacks are paroxysmal:
  - are there any precipitating factors (e.g. exercise, anxiety or stress)?
  - what is the nature of the onset of the attacks and are there associated symptoms (such as presyncope or chest discomfort)?
  - are there any relieving factors (e.g. breath-holding, exercise)?

Patients with coronary heart disease or cardiomyopathy are at particular risk of ventricular arrhythmias. Consider such patients with palpitation or syncope to have a potentially life-threatening ventricular arrhythmia until proven otherwise.

SYNCOPE AND DIZZINESS

It is uncommon for dizziness to be caused by cardiac disease. However, loss of consciousness (syncope) or the feeling of impending loss of consciousness (presyncope) may be cardiac in origin. There are three groups of causes:

- postural hypotension
- arrhythmias
- left ventricular outflow obstruction.

3.12	Symptoms related to medication
Dyspnoea	Beta-blockers in patients with asthma Exacerbation of heart failure by beta-blockers, some calcium channel antagonists, non-steroidal anti-inflammatory drugs
Dizziness	Vasodilators, e.g. nitrates, alpha-blockers and angiotensin-converting enzyme inhibitors
Angina	Aggravated by thyroxine or drug-induced anaemia, e.g. aspirin or non-steroidal anti-inflammatory drugs
Oedema	Fluid retention from steroids, non-steroidal anti-inflammatory drugs Oedema from calcium channel antagonists (e.g. nifedipine, amlodipine)
Palpitation	Tachycardia and/or arrhythmia from thyroxine, beta-2 stimulants (e.g. salbutamol), digoxin toxicity, hypokalaemia from diuretics, tricyclic antidepressant drugs

Postural hypotension

Postural hypotension is a significant (> 20 mmHg) fall in systolic blood pressure on standing. It is commonly caused by antihypertensive drug therapy, especially diuretics and vasodilators (Table 3.12). It is also a symptom of autonomic neuropathy (see Ch. 8).

Arrhythmias

Supraventricular tachyarrhythmias such as atrial fibrillation rarely cause syncope. The commonest cause is bradyarrhythmia, related to sick sinus syndrome or atrio-ventricular block (i.e. Stokes–Adams attacks), which can be aggravated by drugs including digoxin, beta-blockers and verapamil. Ventricular tachyarrhythmias may also cause syncope or presyncope, especially in patients with impaired left ventricular function.

Left ventricular outflow obstruction

Severe aortic stenosis and hypertrophic cardiomyopathy are associated with obstruction of the left ventricular outflow tract. They may cause syncope or presyncope, especially on exertion when cardiac output fails to meet the increased metabolic demand. Clinical examination may reveal a systolic murmur.

Other cardiovascular causes

Recurrent syncope may occur because of an enhanced vagal response (malignant vasovagal syncope). Fainting results from sudden bradycardia in association with vasodilatation. Patients often give a previous history of fainting due to specific stimuli, e.g. at the sight of blood. A related cause, sharing a similar mechanism, is carotid sinus hypersensitivity. Gentle pressure on the carotid sinus may produce the patient's symptoms by causing a profound bradycardia. Atrial myxoma is a rare cause of syncope.

PERIPHERAL OEDEMA

Oedema can be both a symptom (ankle swelling) and a sign. It is usually found in the lower limbs, especially the

3.13 Causes of unilateral and bilateral leg oedema
Unilateral
• Deep vein thrombosis • Soft tissue infection • Trauma • Immobility, e.g. hemiplegia
Bilateral
• Heart failure • Chronic venous insufficiency • Hypoproteinaemia, e.g. nephrotic syndrome, kwashiorkor, cirrhosis • Lymphatic obstruction, e.g. pelvic tumour, filariasis • Drugs, e.g. non-steroidal anti-inflammatory drugs, nifedipine, amlodipine, fludrocortisone • Inferior vena caval obstruction • Thiamine deficiency (wet beri-beri) • Milroy's disease (more common in females, unexplained lymphoedema which appears at puberty) • Immobility

ankles, or over the sacrum in patients lying in bed. Although oedema may occur in heart failure, it is also seen in a number of other diseases, and is sometimes drug induced (Table 3.13).

OTHER SYMPTOMS

Non-cardiac symptoms may be the presenting complaint in patients with cardiac disease (Table 3.14). Infective endocarditis often presents with non-specific symptoms including weight loss, tiredness and night sweats.

3.14 Cardiovascular disease presenting with 'non-cardiac' symptoms		
System	**Symptom**	**Cause**
Central nervous system	Stroke	Cerebral embolism Endocarditis Hypertension
Gastrointestinal	Jaundice	Liver congestion secondary to heart failure
	Abdominal pain	Mesenteric embolism
Renal	Oliguria	Heart failure

THE HISTORY

The history is as important as clinical examination in the evaluation of the patient with cardiac disease. Indeed the most common cause of cardiac symptoms, coronary heart disease, commonly occurs without abnormal physical findings.

Presenting complaint

Establish the frequency, duration and severity of symptoms and causative and relieving factors. Episodes of chest pain or breathlessness of recent onset demand more urgent attention than symptoms that are stable. Many cardiac diseases are slowly progressive so determine the evolution of symptoms over time since this guides the timing of investigations and therapeutic intervention (e.g. valve surgery).

Functional impairment

Assess the impact of symptoms of exertional chest pain or breathlessness on the patient's *functional capacity*. Establish the intensity of exercise required to induce symptoms, e.g.

gentle walking or only more strenuous exercise like climbing hills or stairs, as well as the extent of domestic (e.g. cooking, cleaning, shopping), social (e.g. mobility, hobbies, sport) and occupational disability. Ask patients whether or not they are able to keep up when walking with their partners or friends of the same age.

Past history

Ask about rheumatic fever or heart murmurs during childhood. Specifically enquire about conditions associated with cardiac disease, including:

• diabetes mellitus
• glomerulonephritis and hypertensive heart disease
• thyrotoxicosis and atrial fibrillation
• amyloidosis and cardiomyopathy.

In cases of suspected infective endocarditis ask about recent dental work and other potential causes of bacteraemia. Other seemingly unrelated problems may also suggest an associated or underlying cardiovascular problem. For example, a patient with Marfan's syndrome may have aortic incompetence. In women, the obstetric history may help in assessing the haemodynamic significance of a valvular or congenital heart abnormality.

Drug history

Medication may be responsible for, or may aggravate, symptoms such as breathlessness, chest pain, oedema, palpitation or syncope (see Table 3.12). Starting thyroxine may precipitate or aggravate angina. Remember to ask about over-the-counter purchases such as non-steroidal anti-inflammatory drugs and alternative medicine and herbal remedies, as these may contain ingredients with cardiovascular actions.

Family history

Many cardiac disorders have a genetic component (Table 3.15). Ask if there is a family history of either premature coronary heart disease in a first-degree relative (< 55 years in a female or < 50 years in a male) or of sudden unexplained death at a young age, raising the possibility of a cardiomyopathy or inherited tendency to arrhythmia.

Social history

The aetiological role of smoking in coronary and peripheral vascular disease necessitates a detailed smoking history. Consumption of alcohol is also relevant since drinking to excess is associated with atrial fibrillation, hypertension and, occasionally, dilated cardiomyopathy. Caffeine consumption can cause palpitation, and some recreational drugs are associated with cardiac symptoms (e.g. cocaine and chest pain).

Occupational history

Cardiac disease may impair patients' physical activity and affect their employment. This may be a source of anxiety and an indication for therapeutic intervention. The diagnosis of cardiac disease may also have medicolegal consequences in certain occupations, e.g. commercial drivers, pilots (Table 3.16).

3.16 Occupational aspects of cardiovascular disease	
Occupational exposure associated with cardiovascular disease	
Organic solvents	Arrhythmias
	Cardiomyopathy
Vibrating machine tools	Raynaud's phenomenon
Publicans	Alcoholic cardiomyopathy
Occupational exposure exacerbating pre-existing cardiac conditions	
Cold exposure	Angina
	Raynaud's disease
Deep-sea diving	Embolism through foramen ovale
Occupational requirements for high standards of cardiovascular fitness	
Pilots	
Public transport/heavy goods vehicle drivers	
Armed forces	
Police	

3.15 Genetically determined cardiovascular disorders	
Single-gene defects	**Polygenic inheritance**
Hypertrophic cardiomyopathy	Ischaemic heart disease
Marfan's syndrome	Hypertension
Familial hypercholesterolaemia	Type 2 diabetes mellitus
Muscular dystrophies	Hyperlipidaemia
Long Q-T syndrome	

THE PHYSICAL EXAMINATION

The patient's condition determines how you perform the examination. In some situations it is not necessary to perform a comprehensive examination. There are three broad situations to consider:

- patients with cardiac or respiratory arrest requiring resuscitation
- severely ill patients that require immediate treatment
- stable patients.

The management of cardiac arrest is discussed in Chapter 12. Examining severely ill patients needs a focused examination

adapted to the specific situation. In haemodynamically stable patients you should have a set routine for physical examination.

GENERAL EXAMINATION

Consciously look at the patient's general appearance and ask yourself 'does the patient *look* unwell?'. This is the most important skill to learn in examination. Is the patient frightened or distressed? Note the patient's colour – pale, cyanosed, grey, or sweaty. The hands (Ch. 2) and the face (Fig. 3.4) can reveal important signs of cardiac disease. Look for the physical signs of alcohol abuse (see Fig. 1.5, p. 19) or tobacco consumption (see Fig. 1.4, p. 18).

Central cyanosis is an important sign (see Ch. 4). The most common cardiac cause is pulmonary oedema. Patients with congenital heart disease may have central cyanosis resulting from the development of a right-to-left shunt. They usually have finger clubbing and the cyanosis is not corrected by breathing high-flow oxygen.

Look for specific physical signs to support certain diagnoses. For example, hyperlipidaemia is an important risk factor in vascular disease and may cause:

- Palmar or tendon xanthomata (Fig. 3.5).
- Corneal arcus. This is a creamy yellow discoloration at the boundary of the iris and cornea caused by precipitation of cholesterol crystals. It can occur in those over 50 years in the absence of hyperlipidaemia (Fig. 3.6).

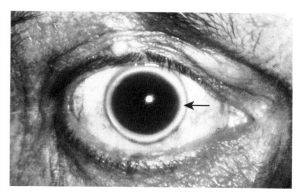

Fig. 3.6   Corneal arcus (arrow).

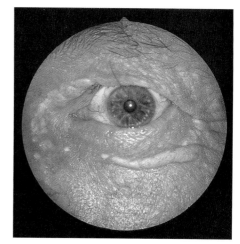

Fig. 3.7   Xanthelasma.

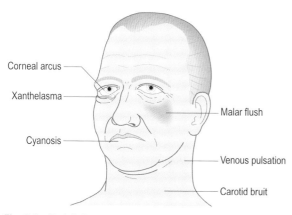

Fig. 3.4   Facial clues to heart disease.

Corneal arcus
Xanthelasma
Cyanosis
Malar flush
Venous pulsation
Carotid bruit

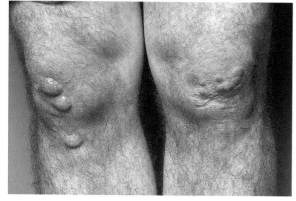

Fig. 3.5   Eruptive xanthomata.

- Xanthelasma. Yellowish cholesterol plaques are found around the eyelids and periorbital area (Fig. 3.7).

In patients with suspected infective endocarditis, look for:

- Splinter haemorrhages – multiple linear reddish-brown marks found along the axis of the finger- and toenails (see Ch. 2). Up to two isolated haemorrhages are a common finding in healthy individuals.
- Roth's spots – flame-shaped retinal haemorrhages with a 'cotton-wool' centre (Fig. 3.8). They are thought to result from septic emboli. Similar appearances may occur in patients with anaemia or leukaemia.
- A skin rash typically consisting of multiple petechiae, often on the legs and conjunctivae (Fig. 3.9), due to vasculitis. This can be confused with the rash of meningococcal disease.
- Finger clubbing is a rare feature of chronic endocarditis.
- Microscopic haematuria.

Clinical features are identified in Figure 3.10

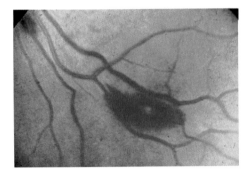

Fig. 3.8   A Roth spot.

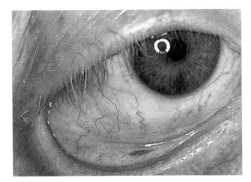

Fig. 3.9   Petechial haemorrhages.

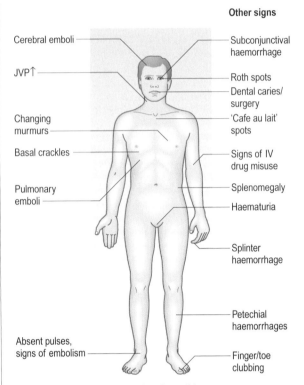

Fig. 3.10   Clinical features of endocarditis.

Other signs

Cerebral emboli
JVP↑
Changing murmurs
Basal crackles
Pulmonary emboli
Absent pulses, signs of embolism

Subconjunctival haemorrhage
Roth spots
Dental caries/ surgery
'Cafe au lait' spots
Signs of IV drug misuse
Splenomegaly
Haematuria
Splinter haemorrhage
Petechial haemorrhages
Finger/toe clubbing

ARTERIAL PULSES

Anatomy

The *radial pulse* is found at the wrist, lateral to the flexor carpi radialis tendon (Fig. 3.11A). Use this to assess pulse rate and rhythm. The *brachial pulse* is found in the antecubital fossa medial to the biceps tendon. The *carotid pulse* is most easily palpable at the angle of the jaw, anterior to the sternocleidomastoid muscle. Palpate the larger brachial and carotid arteries for a more reliable assessment of pulse volume and character than is given by the radial pulse.

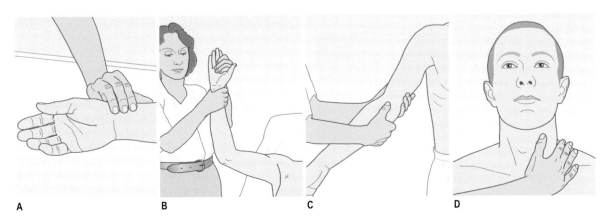

A   B   C   D

Fig. 3.11   The radial, brachial and carotid pulses. (A) Locating and palpating the radial pulse. (B) Feeling for a collapsing radial pulse. (C) Assessing the brachial pulse with a thumb. (D) Locating the carotid pulse with a thumb.

➡ Examination sequence

Radial pulses
➜ Place your three middle fingers over the right radial pulse.
➜ Use the pads of your fingers to assess the rate, rhythm and volume (Fig. 3.11A).
➜ Count the pulse for 15 seconds and multiply by four to obtain the pulse rate in beats per minute (b.p.m.).
➜ To detect a collapsing pulse, raise the patient's arm and feel across the pulse with your fingers (Fig. 3.11B).
➜ Now palpate the left radial pulse. If either pulse feels diminished in volume, confirm any difference by simultaneous palpation.

Brachial pulses
➜ Use your thumb (right thumb for right arm and vice versa) with your fingers cupped round the back of the elbow (Fig. 3.11C).
➜ Feel medial to the tendon of the biceps muscle to find the pulse and assess its character.

Carotid pulses
➜ Palpate the carotid pulse with the patient lying on a bed or couch in case you induce a reflex bradycardia.
➜ Never compress both carotid arteries simultaneously.
➜ Use your left thumb for the right carotid pulse and vice versa.
➜ Place the tip of your thumb between the larynx and the anterior border of the sternocleidomastoid muscle.
➜ Press your thumb gently backwards to feel the pulse (Fig. 3.11D).
➜ Listen for bruits over both carotid arteries using the diaphragm of your stethoscope while the patient holds his breath.

Normal findings

A normal adult resting pulse rate is between 60–100 b.p.m. Bradycardia is a pulse rate of < 60 b.p.m. and tachycardia > 100 b.p.m. These are arbitrary definitions and you should assess the heart rate in the context of the clinical situation. A pulse rate of 50 b.p.m. may be normal in a fit young person, whereas a pulse rate of 65 b.p.m. may be slow in acute heart failure.

A normal cardiac rhythm is called *sinus rhythm* because it arises from the sinoatrial node. Sinus rhythm seldom produces a completely regular pulse because the heart speeds up during inspiration and slows at the beginning of expiration in response to changes in vagus nerve activity. This *sinus arrhythmia* is most obvious in children, young adults and athletes.

Volume and character. Volume is the movement imparted to your fingers and reflects the pulse pressure – the difference between systolic and diastolic blood pressure. Character is the impression of the pulse waveform obtained. Pulse volume and character are best appreciated from a major pulse, such as the carotid. Recognizing characteristic waveforms is difficult and needs considerable experience.

3.17 Causes of fast or slow pulse	
Fast heart rate (tachycardia, > 100/min)	
Sinus tachycardia	**Arrhythmia**

Exercise
Pain
Excitement/anxiety
Fever
Hyperthyroidism
Medication:
  sympathomimetics
  vasodilators
	Atrial fibrillation
	Atrial flutter
	Supraventricular tachycardia
	Ventricular tachycardia

Slow heart rate (bradycardia, < 60/min)	
Sinus bradycardia	**Arrhythmia**

Sleep
Athletic training
Hypothyroidism
Medication:
  beta-blockers
  digoxin
  verapamil, diltiazem
	Carotid sinus hypersensitivity
	Sick sinus syndrome
	Second-degree heart block
	Complete heart block

Common abnormalities

Heart rate. Causes of tachycardia and bradycardia are shown in Table 3.17. Sinoatrial disease causes sinus bradycardia and sinus pauses. Atrioventricular nodal disease may produce complete heart block (third-degree atrioventricular block) in which the cardiac rhythm is regular, with a rate of 30–40 b.p.m. This rhythm can be intermittent and may cause the patient to lose consciousness (Stokes–Adams attacks).

The most common cause of tachycardia is sinus tachycardia due to exercise, pain, anxiety or fever. Tachyarrhythmias are abnormal rhythms caused by increased excitability, or by abnormal conducting pathways, in or between the atria and ventricles.

Pulse rhythm. It is important to identify any irregularity of the pulse rhythm, and whether this is permanent or intermittent. Common causes of an irregular pulse are listed in Table 3.18. A normal pulse rhythm may be interrupted by ectopic beats or extrasystoles originating from the atria or ventricles (Fig. 3.12). Often the pulse wave produced by the ectopic beat is too weak to be felt at the wrist. This produces a *pulse deficit*, a difference between the heart rate at the apex and the rate palpable at the radial pulse. Ventricular ectopic beats are followed by a compensatory diastolic pause which allows increased ventricular filling, and produces a larger stroke volume in the sinus beat following the ectopic beat. Sometimes ectopic beats occur regularly, e.g. after every normal beat. This is called *pulsus bigeminus* and may give the false impression of a very slow pulse.

Atrial fibrillation causes a chaotic ventricular rhythm leading to a pulse which is completely irregular in timing

3.18	Causes of irregular pulse

- Sinus arrhythmia
- Atrial extrasystoles
- Ventricular extrasystoles
- Atrial fibrillation
- Atrial flutter with variable response
- Second-degree heart block with variable response

3.19	Common causes of atrial fibrillation

- Hypertension
- Cardiac failure
- Myocardial infarction
- Thyrotoxicosis
- Alcohol-related heart disease
- Mitral valve disease
- Infection, e.g. respiratory, urinary tract
- Following surgery, especially cardiothoracic surgery

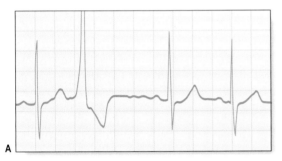

A

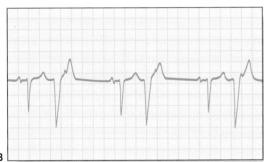

B

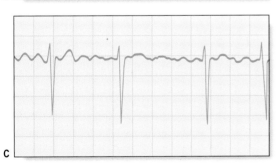

C

Fig. 3.12 ECG rhythm strip. (A) Ventricular ectopic beat. (B) Bigeminy. (C) Atrial fibrillation with 'controlled' ventricular response.

and of variable volume. Untreated atrial fibrillation usually produces a rapid ventricular rate during which the interval between successive ventricular contractions may be too short to allow proper filling. This can produce a considerable pulse deficit. When the ventricular response to atrial fibrillation is rapid, assess the heart rate by listening at the apex or from an ECG. Common causes of atrial fibrillation

are given in Table 3.19. Lone, or idiopathic, atrial fibrillation is unusual. If atrial fibrillation occurs in the absence of structural cardiac disease, it is important to check for thyrotoxicosis and alcohol as potential causes.

Pulse volume. A large volume pulse may be due to aortic regurgitation, or a high cardiac output state. Exercise, emotion, heat and pregnancy are physiological factors causing vasodilatation and increased cardiac output, which also occurs with fever, thyrotoxicosis, anaemia, peripheral arteriovenous shunts and Paget's disease of bone.

A low volume pulse is associated with reduced stroke volume due to heart failure, or peripheral vascular disease. The pulse may be thin and 'thready' in hypovolaemia due to haemorrhage or dehydration.

Coarctation is a congenital narrowing of the aorta, usually situated immediately distal to the left subclavian artery. In children with coarctation the upper limb pulses are normal, while all lower limb pulses are reduced or impalpable. In adults, coarctation usually presents with hypertension. Femoral pulses are usually palpable because of the development of collaterals but are of low volume and delayed with respect to the radial pulse (Fig. 3.13).

Pulsus alternans is rare and describes a beat-to-beat variation in pulse volume in the presence of a regular rhythm. It occurs in advanced heart failure and is often initially detected when measuring the blood pressure.

Pulsus paradoxus is a pulse that increases in volume on expiration and decreases in volume in inspiration. This variation occurs in health but is not normally easy to detect. This variation in pulse pressure is abnormal if it is exaggerated to the point that it is clinically detectable. It occurs with severe airways obstruction e.g. acute asthma, because of extreme changes in intrathoracic pressure, and in pericardial tamponade due to a large pericardial effusion. Pulsus paradoxus is best assessed by measuring the difference in systolic blood pressure during inspiration and expiration. A difference > 15 mmHg is pathological.

Pulse character. A *slow-rising pulse* has a gradual upstroke to the pulse waveform and a reduced peak that occurs late in systole. It is a feature of severe aortic stenosis. A *bisferiens pulse*, which occurs with mixed aortic stenosis and regurgitation, has two systolic peaks separated by a distinct midsystolic dip. A *collapsing pulse* occurs in severe

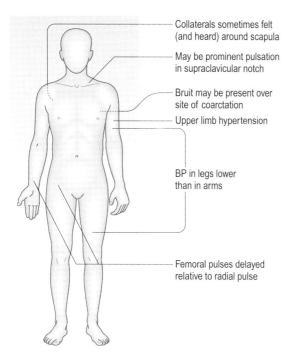

- Collaterals sometimes felt (and heard) around scapula
- May be prominent pulsation in supraclavicular notch
- Bruit may be present over site of coarctation
- Upper limb hypertension
- BP in legs lower than in arms
- Femoral pulses delayed relative to radial pulse

Fig. 3.13   Features of coarctation of the aorta.

aortic regurgitation when the peak of the pulse wave occurs early and is followed by a rapid descent. This rapid fall in pulse pressure imparts the 'collapsing' sensation. It is exaggerated by raising the patient's arm well above the level of the heart (see Fig. 3.11B).

BLOOD PRESSURE

It is essential to measure blood pressure (BP) as described. Pay attention to the details. Blood pressure is usually measured using a sphygmomanometer cuff wrapped round the upper arm (Fig. 3.14). Use the correct size of cuff; an undersized cuff leads to overestimation of blood pressure. A bladder length of 30–35 cm and width of 12 cm is suitable for most adults but if the Velcro fastening 'tears' while pumping up use a larger sized cuff.

Examination sequence

- Rest the patient for five minutes
- In ambulant patients, measurements are normally made with the patient seated. Either arm can be used.
- Support the patient's arm comfortably at about heart level.
- Apply the cuff to the upper arm with the centre of the bladder over the brachial artery.
- Palpate the brachial pulse.
- Inflate the cuff until the pulse is impalpable. Note the pressure on the manometer. This is a rough estimate of systolic pressure.

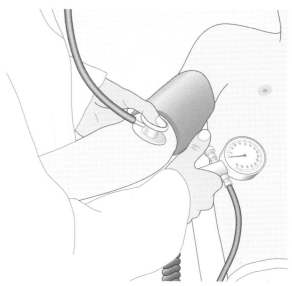

Fig. 3.14   Measuring the blood pressure.

- Now inflate the cuff another 10 mmHg and listen through the stethoscope over the brachial artery.
- Deflate the cuff slowly until regular sounds are first heard. Note the reading to the nearest 2 mmHg. This is the systolic pressure.
- Continue to deflate the cuff slowly until the sounds disappear.
- Record the pressure at which the sounds completely disappear as diastolic pressure. Occasionally muffled sounds persist and do not disappear, in which case the point of muffling is the best guide to the diastolic pressure

Normal findings

Blood pressure is written as systolic pressure/diastolic pressure, e.g. 146/92 mmHg.

Blood pressure varies with excitement, stress and environment. Repeated measurements, made on separate occasions, in a stress-free environment, are required to diagnose hypertension. In some patients simply measuring blood pressure can cause it to rise – so-called 'white coat' hypertension. Ambulatory blood pressure monitoring removes the stress of the clinic environment and helps identify this problem. Numerous devices are now available which can be set to make BP measurements, including systolic, diastolic and mean arterial pressures at set intervals for 24 hours. Many patients also use automatic machines which allow them to measure their own BP at home.

Common abnormalities

Hypertension is defined as a systolic blood pressure of > 140 mmHg and/or a diastolic pressure of > 90 mmHg. It is common and its prevalence increases with age. Hypertension has no specific symptoms but, untreated, can lead to death or morbidity from heart failure, cerebrovascular accident or renal failure. It is a major risk factor for coronary heart disease and atrial fibrillation. Clinical assessment of the hypertensive patient has four aims:

- to identify any underlying cause
- to assess the severity of the problem, as this dictates treatment
- to identify end-organ damage (cardiac, renal and retinal)
- to assess risk of cardiovascular disease in the context of other risk factors (Fig. 3.15).

Essential, or primary hypertension is a diagnosis of exclusion. Hypertension is often familial, and is commonly associated with obesity and alcohol misuse. A cause of hypertension (secondary hypertension) is identified in < 15% of patients, most of whom are < 40 years.

The commonest secondary cause is chronic renal disease or renal artery stenosis. A history of paroxysmal headaches, vomiting, sweating, pallor and weight loss, may suggest phaeochromocytoma, a tumour of the adrenal medulla that secretes high levels of catecholamines. Other secondary causes include Conn's syndrome (a tumour of the adrenal cortex that secretes aldosterone), Cushing's disease (caused by a microadenoma of the pituitary that secretes

adrenocorticotrophic hormone), and coarctation of the aorta. Conn's and Cushing's syndromes have no specific symptoms but should be suspected in patients with hypokalaemia. They are confirmed by specific endocrine tests.

The choice of treatment is influenced by the presence or absence of complications. Beta-adrenoceptor antagonists and calcium-channel antagonists are particularly useful in treating hypertensive patients with angina because of the dual action of these agents. Similarly angiotensin-converting enzyme inhibitors are especially helpful if there is associated left ventricular dysfunction.

➜ Examination sequence

➜ Check the pulse for atrial fibrillation (common association).
➜ Make several recordings of the blood pressure.
➜ Check for radiofemoral delay in patients < 40 years old.
➜ Examine the optic fundi for hypertensive retinopathy (Fig. 3.16).
➜ Look for features of Cushing's syndrome (see p. 57) or virilization.
➜ Palpate the abdomen for renal enlargement (see p. 189).
➜ Listen for bruits over the renal arteries.
➜ Examine the heart for features of left ventricular hypertrophy.
➜ Look for evidence of cardiac failure.
➜ Perform microscopic examination of the urine (see p. 194), looking for red cell casts.

JUGULAR VENOUS PRESSURE AND WAVEFORM

Anatomy

There are no valves between the right atrium and the internal jugular vein. The degree of distension of this vein is therefore dictated by the right atrial pressure, and the venous waveform provides information about cardiac function. The internal jugular vein enters the neck behind the mastoid process. It runs deep to the sternocleidomastoid muscle before entering the thorax between the sternal and clavicular heads and can only be examined when the neck muscles are relaxed. When the pressure in the internal jugular vein is elevated you can see a diffuse pulsation, although not the vein itself.

The external jugular vein is more superficial and prominent. Do not examine this routinely because it is prone to kinking and partial obstruction as it traverses the deep fascia of the neck.

Normal findings

Jugular venous pressure (JVP). Mean right atrial pressure is normally < 7 mmHg (9 cmH$_2$O). Since the sternal angle is approximately 5 cm above the right atrium the

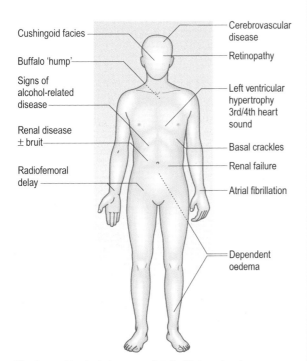

Cushingoid facies

Buffalo 'hump'

Signs of alcohol-related disease

Renal disease ± bruit

Radiofemoral delay

Cerebrovascular disease

Retinopathy

Left ventricular hypertrophy 3rd/4th heart sound

Basal crackles

Renal failure

Atrial fibrillation

Dependent oedema

Fig. 3.15   Physical signs associated with hypertension.

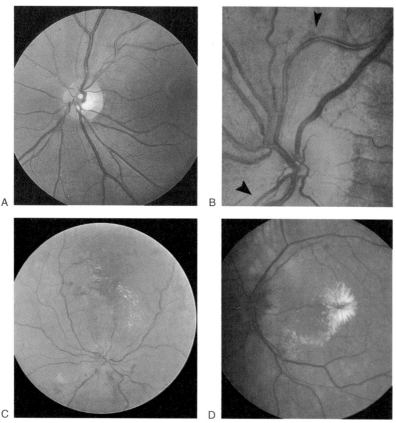

Fig. 3.16 Hypertensive retinopathy. (A) Grade 1: very early and minor changes – increased tortuosity of a retinal vessel and increased reflectiveness (silver wiring) of a retinal artery, are seen at 1 o'clock. (B) Grade 2: increased tortuosity and silver wiring (coarse arrow) with 'nipping' of the venules at arteriovenous crossings (fine arrow). (C) Grade 3: the same changes as in grade 2 plus flame-shaped retinal haemorrhages and soft 'cotton-wool' exudates. (D) Grade 4: swelling of the optic disc (papilloedema), retinal oedema, and hard exudates around the fovea, producing a 'macular star'.

normal jugular venous pulse should extend not more than 4 cm above the sternal angle (Fig. 3.17). When a healthy subject sits upright the pulse is hidden behind the clavicle and sternum. When the patient reclines at 45° the upper limit of the JVP is at the level of the clavicle. If you cannot see the JVP, press firmly over the centre of the abdomen for a few seconds after explaining to the patient what you are about to do. This increases venous return to the heart, transiently increasing right atrial pressure and the height of the jugular venous pulse by 2–3 cm (abdominojugular reflux).

JVP waveform. The normal waveform has two peaks per cardiac cycle, which helps distinguish it from the carotid arterial pulse (Table 3.20). The first peak ('a' wave) coincides with right atrial contraction and occurs just before the first heart sound. The second peak ('v' wave) is caused by atrial filling during ventricular systole when the tricuspid valve is closed (Fig. 3.18A). A third peak, the 'c' wave, is

3.20 Differences between carotid and jugular pulsation	
Carotid	**Jugular**
Rapid outward movement	Rapid inward movement
One peak per heartbeat	Two peaks per heartbeat (in sinus rhythm)
Palpable	Impalpable
Pulsation unaffected by pressure at the root of the neck	Pulsation diminished by pressure at the root of the neck
Independent of respiration	Height of pulsation varies with respiration
Independent of position	Varies with position of patient
Independent of abdominal pressure	Rises with abdominal pressure

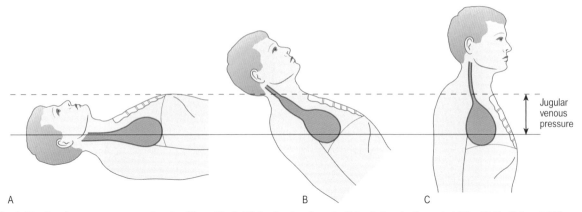

Fig. 3.17 Jugular venous pressure in a healthy subject. (A) Supine: jugular vein distended, pulsation not visible. (B) Reclining at 45°: point of transition between distended and collapsed vein can usually be seen to pulsate just above the clavicle. (C) Upright: upper part of vein collapsed and transition point obscured.

a transmitted pulsation from the carotid artery and is rarely visible.

Normally the JVP falls with inspiration because the fall in intrathoracic pressure is transmitted to the right atrium. Identification of the JVP waveform is difficult and requires experience.

⮕ Examination sequence

→ Position the patient reclining supine at 45° in good light.
→ Ensure that the neck muscles are relaxed by resting the back of the head on a pillow.
→ Look across the neck from the right side of the patient (Fig. 3.18A).
→ Identify the internal jugular pulsation (if necessary use the abdominojugular reflux).
→ Estimate the vertical height in centimetres between the top of the venous pulsation and the sternal angle to give the venous pressure (Fig. 3.18B).
→ If necessary, readjust the position of the patient until the waveform is clearly visible.
→ Identify the timing and form of the pulsation and note any abnormality.

Common abnormalities

The commonest cause of an elevated JVP is heart failure (Table 3.21). It is also elevated in other disorders characterized by fluid overload, e.g. renal failure, hepatic failure, IV fluid administration. Mechanical obstruction of the superior vena cava and massive pulmonary embolism can cause the JVP to be so high that it is not seen in the semirecumbent position. With superior vena caval obstruction the JVP is elevated and non-pulsatile. Pericardial constriction causes a specific respiratory pattern of elevation in which there is a paradoxical rise on inspiration (Küssmaul's sign).

Abnormalities of JVP waveform. In atrial fibrillation there is no atrial systole, which results in the loss of the 'a' wave.

Prominent 'a' waves are seen in any condition that restricts blood flow from the right atrium to the right ventricle, e.g. pulmonary hypertension and, rarely, tricuspid stenosis.

Cannon waves are giant 'a' waves that occur when the right atrium contracts against a closed tricuspid valve. They are seen as impulses shooting up the neck. Irregular cannon waves may be seen in complete heart block, and regular cannon waves occur during junctional bradycardias and some ventricular and supraventricular tachycardias.

A prominent 'v' wave is characteristic of severe tricuspid regurgitation. Liver pulsation is sometimes observed because of regurgitation of blood into the hepatic veins.

3.21 Abnormalities of the jugular venous pulse	
Condition	**Abnormalities**
Heart failure	Elevation, sustained abdominojugular reflux
Pulmonary embolism	Elevation
Pericardial effusion	Elevation, prominent 'y' descent
Pericardial constriction	Elevation. Küssmaul's sign
Superior vena caval obstruction	Elevation, loss of pulsation
Atrial fibrillation	Absent 'a' waves
Tricuspid stenosis	Giant 'a' waves
Tricuspid regurgitation	Giant 'v' waves
Complete heart block	'Cannon' waves

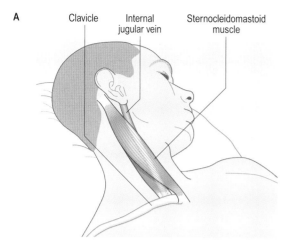

A

Clavicle / Internal jugular vein / Sternocleidomastoid muscle

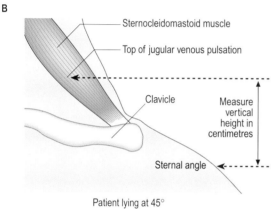

B

Sternocleidomastoid muscle

Top of jugular venous pulsation

Clavicle

Measure vertical height in centimetres

Sternal angle

Patient lying at 45°

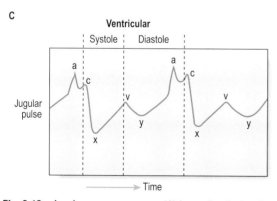

C

Ventricular

Systole | Diastole

Jugular pulse

a c v y x a c v y x

Time

Fig. 3.18 Jugular venous pressure. (A) Inspecting the jugular venous pressure from the side (the internal jugular vein lies deep to the sternocleidomastoid muscle). (B) Measuring the height of the JVP. (C) Form of the venous pulse wave tracing from the internal jugular vein: a = atrial systole; c = transmitted pulsation of carotid artery at onset of ventricular systole; v = peak pressure in right atrium immediately prior to opening of tricuspid valve; a – x = descent, due to atrial relaxation; v – y = descent at commencement of ventricular filling.

THE PRECORDIUM

Anatomy and function

Knowledge of the surface anatomy of the heart is important. The auscultatory areas (aortic, pulmonary area, etc.) do *not* correspond with the surface markings of the heart valves, but are the areas where transmitted sounds and murmurs are heard best. The *cardiac impulse* results from the heart rotating, moving forward and striking against the chest wall during systole. The apex beat is the most lateral and inferior position where the cardiac impulse can be felt.

Normal findings

The apex beat is normally found in the 5th left intercostal space (the space below the 5th rib) medial to the mid-clavicular line. Count the rib spaces down from the sternal angle – which is at the junction of the sternum and second rib. The midclavicular line is halfway between the supra-sternal notch and the acromioclavicular joint.

A normal apical impulse briefly lifts the palpating fingers and is localized. In overweight or muscular subjects the apex beat may be impalpable. It may also be impalpable in patients with asthma or emphysema because the chest is hyperinflated. Remember that, very occasionally, the heart may be on the right side (dextrocardia).

▶ Examination sequence

→ Inspect the precordium with the patient sitting at a 45° angle with shoulders horizontal. Look for surgical scars, visible pulsations and chest deformity.

→ Lay your whole hand flat over the precordium to obtain a general impression of cardiac activity (Fig. 3.19A).

→ Locate the apex beat by laying your fingers on the chest parallel to the rib spaces (Fig. 3.19B); if you cannot feel it, ask the patient to roll onto the left side (Fig. 3.19C).

→ Assess the character of the apex beat and its position.

→ Feel for the right ventricle using the heel of your hand applied firmly to the left parasternal position. Ask the patient to hold his breath in expiration (Fig. 3.19C).

→ Palpate for thrills at the apex and both sides of the sternum.

→ If you hear a murmur feel again for a thrill using the flat of your fingers while the patient is in the optimum position.

Common abnormalities

Chest deformities can affect the rest of the examination. Pectus excavatum (posterior displacement of the lower sternum) and pectus carinatum ('pigeon chest') may displace the heart and affect palpation and auscultation. A midline sternotomy scar usually indicates previous coronary bypass surgery or valve replacement. A left submammary scar is usually the result of a surgical mitral valvotomy. Infra-clavicular scars are seen after pacemaker implantation,

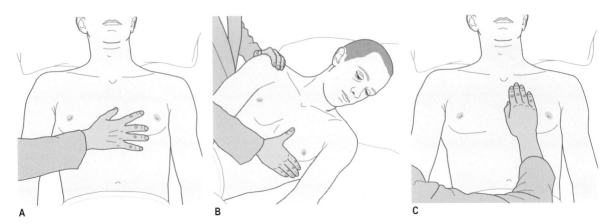

Fig. 3.19   Palpating the heart. (A) Use the hands to palpate the cardiac impulse. (B) Localize the apex beat with a finger (roll the patient, if necessary, into the left lateral position). (C) Palpate from apex to sternum for parasternal pulsations.

and the bulge of the pacemaker may be obvious in thin subjects.

Displacement of the apex beat.   The apex may be displaced laterally in subjects with chest deformity, or because of mediastinal shift secondary to a large pleural effusion, tension pneumothorax (away from the affected side) or pneumonectomy or lung collapse (towards the affected side). In these situations the trachea may also be deviated. Left ventricular dilatation causes the apex beat to be diffusely displaced inferiorly and laterally.

Character of the apical impulse.   A *heave* is a palpable impulse that feels as though it 'lifts' your hand from the patient's chest. Conditions that cause left ventricular hypertrophy, such as hypertension and aortic stenosis, produce a forceful apical impulse that is not significantly displaced. This thrusting apical 'heave' is quite different from the diffuse impulse of left ventricular dilatation. A pulsation over the left parasternal area (right ventricular heave) is usually abnormal in adults and indicative of right ventricular hypertrophy or dilatation, e.g. in pulmonary hypertension. The 'tapping' apex beat found in mitral stenosis represents a palpable first heart sound, and is not usually displaced.

A double apical impulse is characteristic of hypertrophic obstructive cardiomyopathy.

A *thrill* is a palpable murmur and feels rather like placing your hand on a purring cat. The most common thrill is that of aortic stenosis which may be palpable at the apex, the lower sternum, or in the neck. The thrill caused by a ventricular septal defect is best felt at the left sternal edge. Diastolic thrills are very rare.

LISTENING TO THE HEART

General considerations

Auscultation requires a stethoscope equipped with a bell and a diaphragm. The bell emphasizes low-pitched sounds such as the murmur of mitral stenosis. The diaphragm filters out these sounds and helps to identify high-pitched sounds such as normal heart sounds and most systolic murmurs. The earpieces of the stethoscope should fit comfortably. The tubing should be about 25 cm long and thick enough to reduce external sound. Make sure the room is quiet when auscultating.

Normal heart valves make a sound when they close (lub-dub) but not when they open. You must know the surface anatomy of the heart to understand how and where the sounds and murmurs radiate and basic cardiac physiology to appreciate their timings (Figs 3.1 and 3.20).

Use a regular routine for auscultation. Listen first at the apex and identify the two heart sounds. Simultaneously feel the carotid pulse with your thumb to time the sounds and murmurs. The first heart sound precedes the carotid pulsation, the second sound follows it.

Identify and describe the following:

- the first and second heart sounds
- extra heart sounds (third and fourth heard in diastole)
- additional sounds, e.g. clicks and snaps
- pericardial rubs
- murmurs in systole and/or diastole.

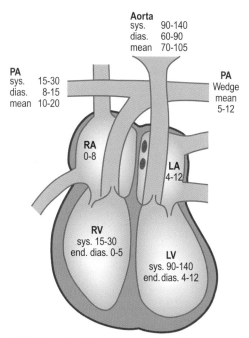

Fig. 3.20 Normal resting pressures (mmHg) in the heart and great vessels.

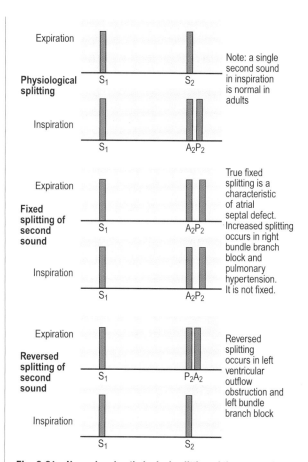

Fig. 3.21 Normal and pathological splitting of the second heart sound.

Heart sounds and added sounds

Normal findings

The first heart sound (S_1) is caused by the closure of the mitral and tricuspid valves at onset of ventricular systole. It is best heard at the apex.

The second heart sound (S_2) is caused by closure of the pulmonary and aortic valves at the end of ventricular systole and is best heard at the left sternal edge. It is louder and higher pitched than the first sound, and normally the aortic component is louder than the pulmonary one.

Physiological splitting of the second heart sound occurs because contraction of the left ventricle slightly precedes that of the right ventricle so that the pulmonary valve closes after the aortic valve. This splitting increases at end-inspiration because the increased venous filling of the right ventricle further delays pulmonary valve closure. This separation disappears on expiration (Fig. 3.21). Splitting of the second sound is best heard at the left sternal edge using the diaphragm. On auscultation, the clinician hears 'lub d/dub' (inspiration) 'lub-dub' (expiration).

A third heart sound (S_3) is a low-pitched early diastolic sound best heard with the bell at the apex. It coincides with rapid ventricular filling immediately after opening of the atrioventricular valves. A third heart sound is therefore heard after the second as 'lub-dub-dum'. A third heart sound

is a normal finding in children, young adults and during pregnancy.

➔ Examination sequence

➔ Explain that you wish to examine the chest and ask the patient to remove his clothing above the waist.

➔ With the patient lying at approximately 45° to the horizontal, listen over the precordium at the base of the heart, apex, and upper left and right sternal edges with both bell and diaphragm. Also listen over the carotid arteries and the axilla.

➔ At each site identify the first and second heart sounds and assess their character and intensity; note any splitting of the second heart sound.

➔ Concentrate in turn on systole (the interval between S_1 and S_2) and diastole (the interval between the S_2 and S_1). Listen for added sounds and then for murmurs.

➔ Roll the patient on to the left side. Listen at the apex using light pressure with the bell, to detect the mid-diastolic and presystolic murmur of mitral stenosis (Fig. 3.22A).

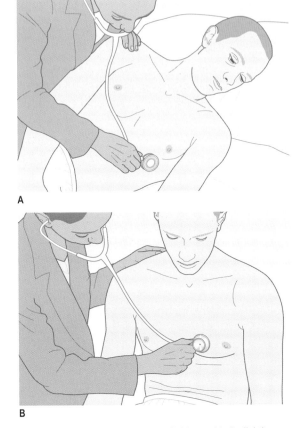

3.22	Abnormalities of intensity of the first heart sound
Quiet	Low cardiac output Poor left ventricular function Long P–R interval (first-degree heart block) Rheumatic mitral regurgitation
Loud	Increased cardiac output Large stroke volume Mitral stenosis Short P–R interval Atrial myxoma (rare)
Variable	Atrial fibrillation Extrasystoles Complete heart block

3.23	Abnormalities of the second heart sound
Quiet	Low cardiac output Calcific aortic stenosis Aortic incompetence
Loud	Systemic hypertension (aortic component) Pulmonary hypertension (pulmonary component)

Split	Widens in inspiration (enhanced physiological splitting):
	  right bundle branch block
	  pulmonary stenosis
	  pulmonary hypertension
	  ventricular septal defects
	Fixed splitting (unaffected by respiration):
	  atrial septal defect
	Widens in expiration (reverse splitting):
	  aortic stenosis
	  hypertrophic cardiomyopathy
	  left bundle branch block
	  ventricular pacemaker

Fig. 3.22 Auscultating the heart. (A) Listen with the lightly applied bell with the patient in the left lateral position for the murmur of mitral stenosis. (B) Listen with the diaphragm with the patient leaning forward for the murmur of aortic incompetence.

→ Sit the patient up and forwards, and ask the patient to breathe out fully and then hold his breath (Fig. 3.22B).
→ Listen over the right second intercostal space and over the left sternal edge with the diaphragm for the murmur of aortic incompetence.
→ Note the character and intensity of any murmur heard.

Common abnormalities

First heart sound. In mitral stenosis the intensity of the first heart sound is often increased due to the elevated left atrial pressure (Table 3.22).

Second heart sound. The aortic component of the second heart sound is sometimes quiet or absent in calcific aortic stenosis and may be reduced in aortic incompetence (Table 3.23). The aortic component is loud in systemic hypertension, and the pulmonary component is increased in pulmonary hypertension.

Wide splitting of the second heart sound with preservation of the normal respiratory variation occurs in conditions that delay right ventricular emptying, e.g. right bundle branch block. Fixed splitting of the second heart sound is a feature of atrial septal defect (Fig. 3.23). In this condition the right ventricular stroke volume is larger than the left, and the splitting is fixed because the defect equalizes the pressure between the two atria throughout the respiratory cycle.

In reversed splitting the two components of the second heart sound occur together on inspiration and separate on expiration. This occurs when left ventricular emptying is delayed so that the aortic valve closes after the pulmonary valve. Examples include left bundle branch block and right ventricular pacing.

Third heart sound. A third heart sound causes a 'triple rhythm' and is usually pathological after the age of 40 years (Table 3.24). The commonest causes are left ventricular failure and mitral regurgitation. In cardiac failure S_3 is usually accompanied by a tachycardia and S_1 and S_2 are quiet. The resulting 'triple rhythm' is called a 'gallop' rhythm.

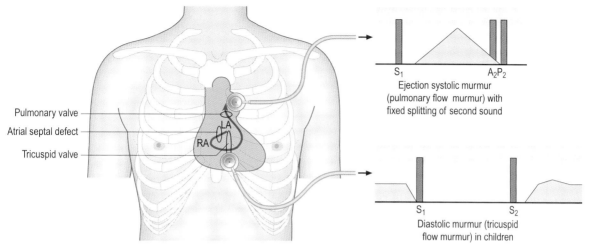

Fig. 3.23 Auscultatory features of atrial septal defect.

3.24	Causes of a third heart sound
Physiological	Healthy young adults Athletes Pregnancy Fever
Pathological	Large, poorly contracting left ventricle Mitral regurgitation

Fourth heart sound. A fourth heart sound (S_4) is less common. It is soft and low pitched, best heard with the bell of the stethoscope at the apex. It occurs just before the first sound (da-lub-dub). It is always pathological and is caused by forceful atrial contraction against a non-compliant or stiff ventricle. A fourth heart sound may be heard in left ventricular hypertrophy, hypertension and aortic stenosis.

Added sounds. An *opening snap* is commonly heard in mitral (rarely tricuspid) stenosis. It results from sudden opening of a stenosed valve and occurs early in diastole, just after the second heart sound (Fig. 3.24A). The opening snap of mitral stenosis is best heard at the apex.

Ejection clicks occur early in systole just after the first heart sound, in patients with congenital pulmonary or aortic stenosis (Fig. 3.24B). The mechanism is similar to that of an opening snap. Ejection clicks do not occur in calcific aortic stenosis because the cusps are rigid.

Midsystolic clicks occur in mitral valve prolapse (Fig. 3.24C) and may be associated with a late systolic murmur (see Fig. 3.25). They are high pitched and best heard at the apex.

Mechanical heart valves make a sound both when they close and open. The closure sound is normally louder. The

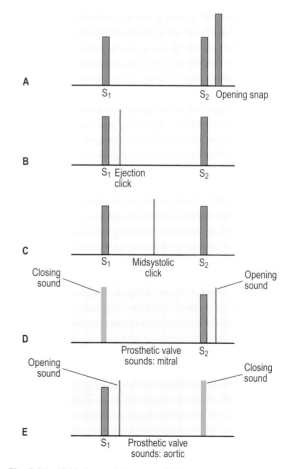

Fig. 3.24 'Added sounds' on auscultation.

sounds are high pitched, 'metallic', often palpable and may be heard without a stethoscope. A mechanical mitral valve replacement makes a metallic first heart sound and a sound like a loud opening snap (Fig. 3.24D). Mechanical aortic valves have loud, metallic second heart sounds and an opening sound like an ejection click (Fig. 3.24E). They invariably also cause a flow murmur.

Pericardial rub. A pericardial rub is usually best heard using the diaphragm of the stethoscope with the breath held in expiration. It is a superficial scratching sound which often has systolic and diastolic components. It may be audible over any part of the precordium and is often very localized. It is most often heard in acute viral pericarditis and sometimes 24–72 hours after myocardial infarction. Pericardial rubs vary in intensity over time, and with the position of the patient. A *pleuropericardial* rub is a similar sound that occurs in time with the cardiac cycle but is also influenced by respiration and is pleural in origin.

Murmurs

General considerations

Heart murmurs are produced by turbulent blood flow across an abnormal valve, septal defect or outflow obstruction, or by increased volume or velocity of blood flow through a normal valve. Murmurs may occur in a healthy heart. These 'innocent' murmurs occur when stroke volume is increased, e.g. during pregnancy, and in athletes with resting bradycardia or children with fever.

Timing

When you hear a murmur first determine whether it is systolic or diastolic.

Systole begins with the first heart sound (mitral and tricuspid valve closure). This occurs when left and right ventricular pressures exceed the corresponding atrial pressures. For a short period all four cardiac valves are closed (pre-ejection period). Ventricular pressures continue to rise until they exceed those of the aorta and pulmonary artery and then the aortic and pulmonary valves open. Systole ends with the closure of these valves, producing the second heart sound.

Diastole is the interval between the second and the first heart sound. Physiologically it is divided into three phases:

- *Early diastole (isovolumic relaxation)* – the time from the closure of the aortic and pulmonary valves until the opening of the mitral and tricuspid valves
- *Mid-diastole* – the period of passive ventricular filling
- *Presystole* which coincides with atrial systole.

Murmurs of aortic (and pulmonary) incompetence start in early diastole and extend into mid-diastole. The murmurs of mitral or tricuspid stenosis *cannot* start before mid-diastole.

Likewise third heart sounds occur in mid-diastole; fourth heart sounds in presystole.

Duration

The murmurs of mitral (and tricuspid) regurgitation start simultaneously with the first heart sound and continue throughout systole (pansystolic). The murmur produced by mitral valve prolapse does not begin until the mitral valve leaflet has prolapsed during systole, producing a late systolic murmur (Fig. 3.25). The ejection systolic murmur of aortic or pulmonary stenosis begins *after* the first heart sound, reaches maximal intensity in midsystole, then fades, stopping before the second heart sound (Fig. 3.26).

Character and pitch

The quality of murmurs is hard to define. Terms such as harsh, blowing, musical, rumbling, high or low pitched are used. High-pitched murmurs often correspond with high-pressure gradients, so the diastolic murmur of aortic incompetence is higher pitched than that of mitral stenosis.

Intensity

There are six grades of intensity (Table 3.25) used to describe murmurs. Diastolic murmurs are rarely louder than grade 4. The severity of valve dysfunction cannot be determined from the intensity of the murmur. For instance the murmur of critical aortic stenosis can be quiet and occasionally inaudible. Changes in intensity are important as they often denote *progression* of a valve lesion. Rapidly changing murmurs are sometimes heard with infective endocarditis because of valve destruction.

Location

Record the site(s) where you hear the murmur best. This helps to differentiate diastolic murmurs (mitral stenosis at the apex, aortic regurgitation at the left sternal edge), but is less helpful with systolic murmurs, which are often loud and audible all over the precordium.

Radiation

Murmurs radiate in the direction of the blood flow causing the murmur to specific sites outwith the precordium. Do not

3.25 Grades of intensity of murmur
1. Heard by an expert in optimum conditions
2. Heard by a non-expert in optimum conditions
3. Easily heard; no thrill
4. A loud murmur, with a thrill
5. Very loud, often heard over wide area, with thrill
6. Extremely loud, heard without stethoscope

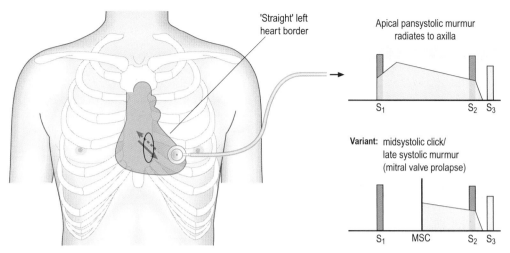

Fig. 3.25   Features of mitral regurgitation. The murmur begins at the moment of valve closure and may obscure the first heart sound. It varies little in intensity throughout systole. In mitral valve prolapse, the murmur begins in mid or late systole and there is often a midsystolic click.

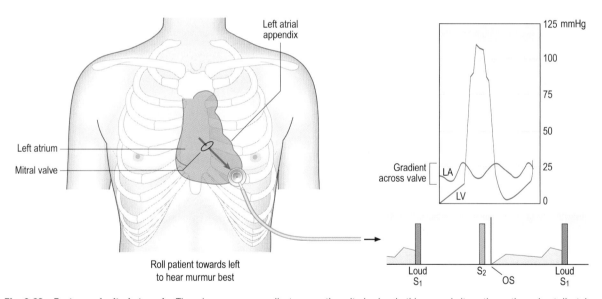

Fig. 3.26   Features of mitral stenosis. There is a pressure gradient across the mitral valve; in this example it continues throughout diastole. This causes a sharp movement of the tethered anterior cusp of the mitral valve at the time when the flow commences, and the opening snap results. The jet through the stenotic valve (arrow) strikes the endocardium at the cardiac apex.

confuse this with location. The pansystolic murmur of mitral regurgitation radiates towards the left axilla, the murmur of ventriculoseptal defect towards the right sternal edge, and that of aortic stenosis to the aortic area and the carotid arteries.

Common abnormalities

Systolic murmurs.   Ejection systolic murmurs are caused by increased stroke volume (flow murmur), or a stenosed aortic or pulmonary valve (Table 3.26). Aortic flow murmurs can be caused by pregnancy, fever, severe anaemia **103**

3.26 Causes of systolic murmurs
Ejection systolic murmur

Increased flow through normal valves
• 'Innocent systolic murmur':
  – fever
  – athletes (bradycardia → large stroke volume)
  – pregnancy (cardiac output maximum at 15 weeks)
• Atrial septal defect (pulmonary flow murmur)
• Severe anaemia

Normal or reduced flow though stenotic valve • Aortic stenosis • Pulmonary stenosis
Other causes of flow murmurs • Hypertrophic obstructive cardiomyopathy (obstruction at subvalvular level) • Aortic regurgitation (aortic flow murmur)
Pansystolic murmurs
All caused by a systolic leak from a high to a lower pressure chamber • Mitral regurgitation • Tricuspid regurgitation • Ventricular septal defect • Leaking mitral or tricuspid prosthesis

or bradycardia. Atrial septal defect is characterized by a pulmonary flow murmur.

The murmur of aortic stenosis is usually audible all over the precordium, including the apex (Fig. 3.27). It is harsh, high pitched and musical, and radiates to the upper right sternal edge and carotids. It is usually loud and there may be a thrill. In very severe aortic stenosis stroke volume may be so reduced that the intensity of the murmur is diminished.

Pansystolic murmurs are most often caused by mitral regurgitation. The murmur is often loud and blowing in character, best heard at the apex and radiating to the axilla. With mitral valve prolapse, regurgitation begins in early or midsystole producing a pan- or late systolic murmur (see Fig. 3.25). Tricuspid regurgitant murmurs are usually heard at the lower left sternal edge and if significant are associated with a 'v' wave in the JVP and a pulsatile liver.

A ventricular septal defect also causes a pansystolic murmur. Small congenital defects produce a loud murmur audible at the left sternal border, radiating to the right sternal border and often associated with a thrill. Rupture of the interventricular septum can complicate myocardial infarction and produces a harsh pansystolic murmur. Other causes of a murmur after myocardial infarction include acute mitral incompetence due to rupture of a papillary muscle or functional incompetence caused by left ventricular dilatation.

Diastolic murmurs.

Early diastolic murmur. The term early diastolic murmur is somewhat misleading because the murmur usually lasts throughout diastole, but it is *loudest* in early diastole. Early diastolic murmurs are usually caused by aortic regurgitation (Fig. 3.28). They are heard at the left sternal edge (occasionally louder at the right sternal edge) and are most obvious in expiration with the patient leaning forward. Since the regurgitant blood volume must be ejected during the subsequent systole, significant aortic regurgitation leads to

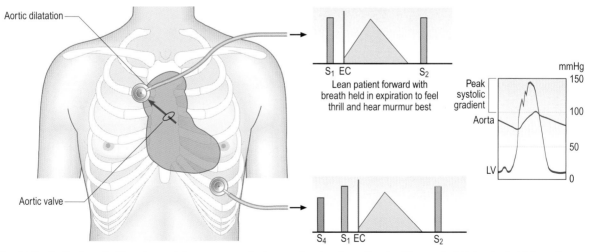

Fig. 3.27 Aortic stenosis. There is a systolic pressure gradient across the stenotic aortic valve. The resultant high-velocity jet (arrow) impinges on the wall of the aorta, and the diaphragm placed near to this on the chest detects the murmur best. Alternatively, the bell may be placed in the suprasternal notch. The diagrammatic representation of the phonocardiogram shows the ejection systolic murmur preceded by an ejection click (EC). A fourth heart sound may be heard at the apex.

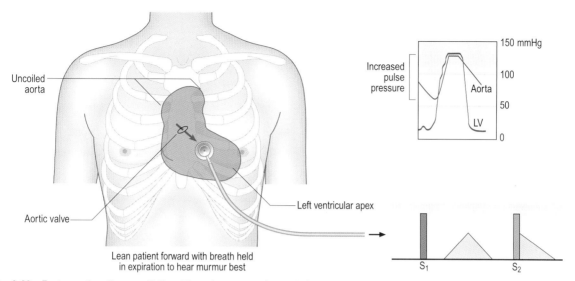

Fig. 3.28   Features of aortic regurgitation. The pulse pressure is usually increased; the jet from the aortic valve is directed inferiorly towards the left ventricular outflow tract (arrow) during diastole, producing a high-pitched murmur which is best heard with the diaphragm. The diagrammatic representation of the phonocardiogram also shows the associated systolic murmur, which is common because of the increased flow through the aortic valve in systole.

increased stroke volume and is almost always associated with a systolic flow murmur.

Pulmonary regurgitation is uncommon. It may be caused by pulmonary artery dilatation in pulmonary hypertension (Graham Steell murmur) or to a congenital defect of the pulmonary valve.

Mid-diastolic murmur. A mid-diastolic murmur is usually caused by mitral stenosis. This is a low-pitched, rumbling sound which may follow an opening snap (see Fig. 3.26). It is best heard with the bell of the stethoscope at the apex with the patient rolled to the left side. The murmur can be accentuated by listening after exercise. The whole cadence sounds like 'lup-ta-ta-roo' where 'lup' is the loud first heart sound, 'ta-ta' the second sound and opening snap and 'roo' the mid-diastolic murmur. If the patient is in sinus rhythm, left atrial contraction increases the blood flow across the

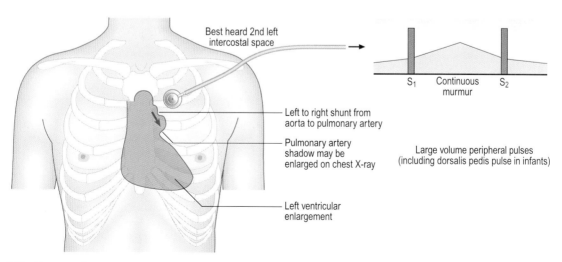

Fig. 3.29   Features of a persistent patent arterial duct. A continuous murmur is heard because aortic pressure always exceeds pulmonary arterial pressure resulting in continuous ductal flow. The pressure difference is greatest in systole producing a louder systolic component to the murmur.

stenosed valve leading to presystolic accentuation of the murmur. The murmur of tricuspid stenosis is similar but rare.

An *Austin Flint* murmur is a mid-diastolic murmur that accompanies aortic regurgitation. It is caused by the regurgitant jet striking the anterior leaflet of the mitral valve, restricting inflow to the left ventricle.

Continuous murmurs are rare in adults. The commonest cause is a patent arterial duct, which connects the upper descending aorta and pulmonary artery in the fetus and normally closes just after birth. The murmur is best heard at the upper left sternal border and radiates over the left scapula. Its continuous character is described as 'machinery-like' (Fig. 3.29).

Interpretation of findings

Auscultation remains an important clinical skill despite the ready availability of echocardiography. You must be able to detect abnormal signs to prompt appropriate investigation. Furthermore, certain auscultatory signs, such as the third or fourth heart sounds and pericardial friction, have no direct equivalent on echocardiography but are helpful prognostically.

Some patients, especially those with rheumatic heart disease, have multiple heart valve defects and the interpretation of physical signs is important. For example, a patient with mixed mitral stenosis and regurgitation will probably have dominant stenosis if the first heart sound is loud, but dominant regurgitation if there is a third heart sound.

● Examine this patient with sudden onset central chest pain

1. Feel the pulse for bradycardia (*heart block*, etc.), tachycardia (*supraventricular tachycardia, ventricular tachycardia*, etc.) and irregularity (*atrial fibrillation, multiple ventricular extrasystoles*).
2. Palpate carotid and femoral pulses (may be weak or absent in aortic dissection).
3. Measure the blood pressure.
4. Look for the JVP – raised in *heart failure*.
5. Examine the trachea and cardiac apex beat for mediastinal shift (*tension pneumothorax*).
6. Palpate the epigastrium for tenderness (*gastro-oesophageal reflux, peptic ulcer, oesophagitis*).
7. Listen to the heart for extra heart sounds or gallop **rhythm** (*heart failure*), pansystolic murmur radiating to the left axilla (*mitral incompetence* due to *papillary muscle rupture post-myocardial infarction*), pansystolic murmur at the left sternal edge (*ventricular septal defect post-myocardial infarction*) and pericardial friction rub (*pericarditis*).

● Examine this patient with sudden loss of consciousness

1. Feel the pulse for bradycardia (faint or *syncope; heart block* or *Stokes–Adams attack*), (*supraventricular tachycardia* or *ventricular tachycardia; sinus tachycardia* after seizure) and irregularity (e.g. sudden onset *atrial fibrillation*).
2. Measure the blood pressure for hypotension (e.g. septicaemia, acute *myocardial infarction*).
3. If possible measure the BP erect and supine (postural fall of > 20 mmHg systolic BP).
4. Check temperature – raised in *meningitis* and *subarachnoid haemorrhage*.
5. Listen for structural heart disease (e.g. *valvular heart disease, ventricular septal defect post-myocardial infarction, cardiac tamponade*).
6. Listen to the carotids for bruits (*embolic cerebrovascular accident*).
7. Examine for focal neurological signs (*post-epileptic seizure, cerebral haemorrhage*).
8. Inspect the tongue for lacerations and check for urinary incontinence (*post-epileptic seizure*).
9. Assess level of consciousness (*epileptic seizure, subarachnoid haemorrhage*, intracranial lesion).

COMMON CARDIAC INVESTIGATIONS

Indications for common cardiac investigations are given in Table 3.27.

Electrocardiography (ECG)

The standard 12-lead ECG (Fig. 3.30) uses recordings made from six precordial electrodes (V_1–V_6) and six different recordings from the limb electrodes (left arm, right arm and left leg). The right leg electrode is used as a reference.

Ambulatory ECG monitoring

Ambulatory recording can be made using cassette tape recorders or solid-state devices with digital memory. These make a continuous ECG recording that can be analysed by computer and checked by a cardiac technician. A typical recording lasts 24–48 hours. Patient-activated recorders are useful for capturing occasional arrhythmias and are activated only when symptoms occur (Fig. 3.31).

3.27 Common cardiac investigations		
Investigation	**Indications**	**Implications**
ECG	Numerous (medical and medico-legal)	Confirms the cardiac rhythm and reveals abnormalities in conditions such as left bundle branch block and Wolff–Parkinson–White syndrome. Diagnosis of myocardial infarction. Assessing for left ventricular hypertrophy. May reveal ischaemia; however, the resting ECG is usually normal in patients with angina
Exercise ECG	Chest pain	Ischaemic changes during exercise, especially when associated with symptoms, support a diagnosis of angina. However, exercise test can be normal in angina (false negative) and abnormal in healthy individuals (false positive)
	Post-myocardial infarction	Provides prognostic information
Ambulatory ECG monitoring	Palpitation	Confirms whether patients' symptoms are coincident with cardiac arrhythmia, e.g. ventricular ectopic beats or atrial fibrillation
	Syncope or presyncope	May show intermittent bradycardia or tachyarrhythmia if symptoms occur during monitoring
Chest X-ray	Numerous	Cardiothoracic ratio: maximum width of the cardiac silhouette/widest part of lung fields, usually the base. Increased in heart failure and valve disease. Pulmonary oedema in heart failure
Echocardiography	Cardiac murmur	Stenotic valve lesion readily diagnosed and accurately quantified. Regurgitation readily detected with semiquantitative assessment
	Breathlessness	Left ventricular function can be assessed. Impaired in heart failure
	Infective endocarditis	Valve vegetations confirm the diagnosis. Transoesophageal echocardiogram is more sensitive
Radionuclide studies	Breathlessness	Blood pool scanning provides an accurate assessment of left ventricular function, usually expressed as ejection fraction (end-diastolic volume – end-systolic volume/end-diastolic volume)
	Chest pain Pulmonary embolism	Myocardial perfusion scan reveals ischaemic deficits in ischaemic heart disease. Lung scan shows a perfusion deficit compared with simultaneous ventilation scan
Cardiac catheterization	Angina	Coronary angiography reveals the extent and severity of coronary stenoses. This determines the therapeutic approach
	Valve disease	Better evaluated non-invasively by echocardiography. Cardiac catheterization is only indicated to assess the coronary anatomy in patients who require heart valve surgery
	Heart failure	Right heart catheterization in patients with severe heart failure helps determine suitability for cardiac transplantation

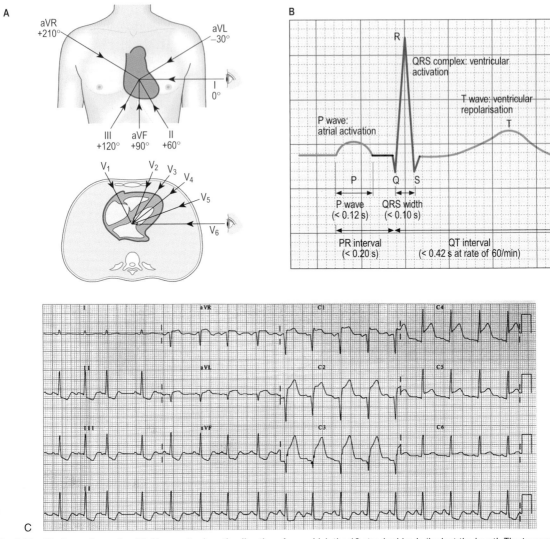

Fig. 3.30 Electrocardiography. (A) Diagram to show the directions from which the 12 standard leads 'look at the heart'. The transverse section is viewed from below like a CT scan. (B) Normal PQRST complex. (C) Acute anterior myocardial infarction. Note ST elevation in leads V1-6 and aVL and 'reciprocal' ST depression in leads II, III and aVF.

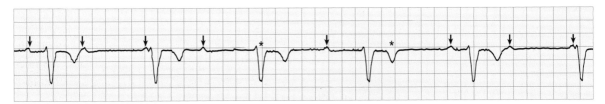

Fig. 3.31 Printout from 24-hour ambulatory ECG recording, showing complete heart block. Arrows indicate visible P waves; at times these are masked by the QRS complex or T wave (*).

Exercise ECG

Patients with stable angina often have a normal ECG at rest and an abnormal ECG during stress. An exercise ECG is a form of controlled physiological stress that may unmask evidence of coronary heart disease. Severe ECG abnormalities, or changes that occur during minor exertion, are of prognostic significance and may prompt invasive investigation with cardiac catheterization.

Chest X-ray

The chest X-ray is important in the investigation of heart disease. An enlarged heart, as judged by the cardiothoracic ratio (p. 148), is a common feature of valvular heart disease and heart failure. In heart failure this is often accompanied by distension of the upper lobe pulmonary veins, diffuse shadowing within the lungs due to pulmonary oedema and the finding of Kerley B lines (horizontal engorged lymphatics at the periphery of the lower lobes) (Fig. 3.32).

Echocardiography

Echocardiography was originally devised to evaluate valve abnormalities, but is now most commonly used to assess left ventricular function. In addition to imaging cardiac structure, blood flow can be displayed (Doppler echocardiography), and analysed to quantitate valve stenosis and regurgitation. Most scans are performed through the anterior wall of the chest (transthoracic) but when high-resolution images of posterior structures (e.g. left atrium or descending aorta) are required transoesophageal imaging is employed. This can be carried out safely in outpatients using topical anaesthesia and intravenous sedation (Fig. 3.33).

Radionuclide studies

Radionuclides are injected intravenously and detected using a gamma camera. Technetium-99 is used to label the circulating blood and provide an accurate assessment of left ventricular function. Thallium and sesta-MIBI are taken up by myocardial cells and provide an indication of myocardial perfusion, both at rest and during exercise.

Cardiac catheterization

This invasive procedure involves introducing fine catheters, approximately 2 mm in diameter, into the femoral (or radial) artery and/or vein, and advancing them to the left or right side of the heart respectively. Originally these techniques were developed to measure pressures in the different cardiac chambers in patients with valve disease. However, patients are now fully evaluated by echocardiography. Coronary angiography is performed using catheters designed to select the left and right coronary arteries and inject X-ray contrast medium into them. The findings are used to determine the need for, and mode of, revascularization in patients with coronary artery disease (Fig. 3.34).

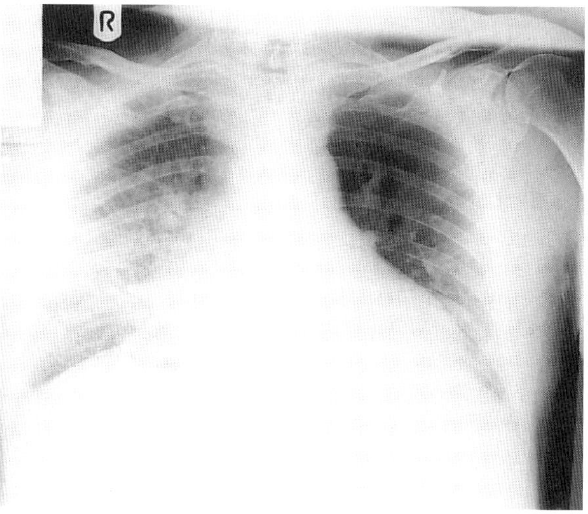

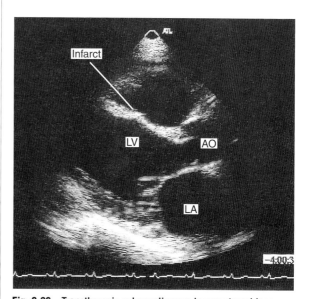

Fig. 3.33 Transthoracic echocardiogram in parasternal long axis view. This shows thinning of the interventricular septum, which has an irregular shape and bright echoes indicating fibrous scarring. This is the site of an old infarct. LA, left atrium; LV, left ventricle; AO, aortic root.

Fig. 3.32 Chest X-ray of heart failure.

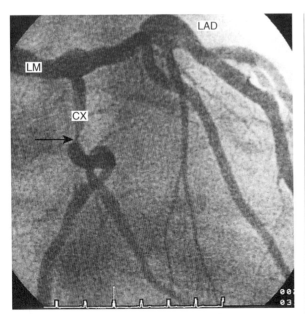

Fig. 3.34 Coronary angiography. The arrow indicates a severe discreet stenosis in the circumflex coronary artery. LM, left main; LAD, left anterior descending; CX, circumflex.

CT and MR scanning

Computerized tomography (CT) and magnetic resonance imaging can be used to identify structural defects of the heart and great vessels. MR imaging is helpful in congenital heart defects and infiltrative disorders, e.g. cardiac sarcoidosis. Recently *electron beam* CT has been used to screen for coronary arterial calcification, an early marker of coronary atherosclerosis.

◆ Key points

- ◆ Significant cardiac disease is often asymptomatic.
- ◆ The severity of cardiac symptoms is affected by the patient's daily activity level. Inactivity may mask symptoms.
- ◆ Look for disorders which can cause, or aggravate, cardiac symptoms, e.g. anaemia, hyperthyroidism, alcohol excess.
- ◆ An irregular pulse is usually caused by atrial fibrillation. Check the heart rate by auscultation and look for evidence of an underlying cause – thyrotoxicosis, hypertension, alcohol abuse, valve disease, and heart failure.
- ◆ Assess pulse character from a large artery, e.g. the carotid.
- ◆ Never palpate both carotid arteries simultaneously.
- ◆ Pulsatile elevation of the JVP indicates elevated right atrial pressure.
- ◆ Recurrent chest pain unresponsive to glyceryl trinitrate is very unlikely to be angina.
- ◆ Look for evidence of aortic outflow obstruction, e.g. aortic stenosis or hypertrophic obstructive cardiomyopathy, in any patient with unexplained syncope.

PERIPHERAL VASCULAR DISEASE

ARTERIAL DISEASE

25% of patients over the age of 60 in 'developed' countries have evidence of peripheral arterial disease but, of these, only a quarter are symptomatic. In the great majority of cases the underlying pathology is atherosclerosis affecting large and medium-sized vessels.

The identification of patients with peripheral arterial disease is important because:

- peripheral arterial disease is a marker for premature cardiovascular and cerebrovascular death
- if not recognized, the first manifestation of peripheral arterial disease may be a life- or limb-threatening complication such as stroke, acute limb ischaemia or ruptured abdominal aortic aneurysm

- modifying vascular risk factors improves outcomes
- peripheral arterial disease may affect medical and surgical treatment for a range of other conditions, e.g. the prescription of a beta-blocker may precipitate claudication.

Common symptoms

There are four major ways in which peripheral arterial disease patients may present:

- limb symptoms
- neurological symptoms
- abdominal symptoms
- vasospastic symptoms.

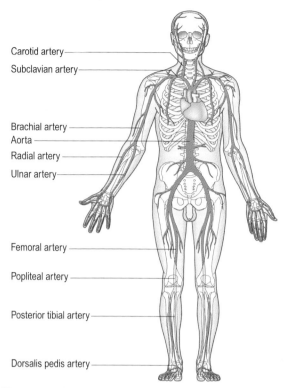

Carotid artery
Subclavian artery

Brachial artery
Aorta
Radial artery
Ulnar artery

Femoral artery

Popliteal artery

Posterior tibial artery

Dorsalis pedis artery

Fig. 3.35 The arterial system.

3.28	Classification of lower limb ischaemia
I	Asymptomatic
II	Intermittent claudication
III	Rest pain
IV	Tissue loss (ulceration/gangrene)

It is the commonest symptom of peripheral arterial disease. The pain typically occurs in the calf but may be felt in the thigh and/ or buttock if proximal obstruction to blood flow is present. Patients often describe a tightness or 'cramp-like' pain which develops after a relatively constant distance, which is shorter if walking uphill. The pain disappears completely within a few minutes of rest but recurs on walking. The *claudication distance* is how far patients say they can walk before pain starts. Patients often underestimate this.

Neurogenic claudication is leg pain on walking due to neurological and musculoskeletal disorders of the lumbar spine.

Venous claudication is pain due to venous outflow obstruction from the leg following extensive deep vein thrombosis. Neurogenic and venous claudication are much less common than arterial claudication and can be distinguished on history and examination (see Table 3.30).

Night/rest pain. This occurs typically when the patient goes to bed and falls asleep but is woken 1–2 hours later by severe pain in the foot, usually in the instep. This is because the beneficial effects of gravity on lower limb perfusion are lost on lying down. Sleep is also associated with a reduction in heart rate, blood pressure and cardiac output. Patients usually find relief by hanging the leg out of bed or by getting up and walking around. But when they return to bed, symptoms recur. The pain and sleep disturbance may be so debilitating that they sleep in a chair. This leads to dependent oedema, and the increased interstitial tissue pressure causes further reduction in tissue perfusion and more pain.

Rest pain usually indicates the presence of severe, multi-level arterial disease. In diabetic patients with rest pain it may be difficult to differentiate between an arterial cause and diabetic neuropathy. Both may be worse at night. However, unlike ischaemic pain, neuropathic pain is not usually confined to the foot, is often associated with burning and tingling, is not relieved by dependency and is often associated with dysaesthesia (many patients cannot even bear the pressure of bedclothes on their feet).

Tissue loss (ulceration and/or gangrene). In patients with rest pain caused by peripheral arterial disease with critical limb ischaemia, trivial injuries fail to heal and provide a portal of entry for bacteria, leading to gangrene and/or ulceration. Without revascularization the ischaemia

Limb symptoms

The legs are eight times more commonly affected than the arms because:

* arterial supply to the legs is less well developed in relation to the muscle mass
* the lower limb is more frequently affected by atherosclerosis.

There are four well-defined stages of lower limb ischaemia (lack of blood supply) (Table 3.28).

Asymptomatic ischaemia. Lower limb ischaemia is defined as an ankle : brachial pressure index of < 0.8 (see p. 117). Most patients are asymptomatic, either because they choose not to walk very far, or because their exercise tolerance is limited by other pathology. These patients have as high a risk from 'vascular' complications as those with symptoms and should be assessed and treated as if they have intermittent claudication.

Intermittent claudication. Intermittent claudication is pain felt in the legs on walking due to arterial insufficiency.

rapidly progresses and amputation and/or death is usually inevitable.

The history

General considerations

Ask about risk factors for atheroma (smoking, hypercholesterolaemia, hypertension, diabetes) and any family history of premature arterial disease. Enquire specifically about diabetes because it is associated with the early development of atheroma which progresses rapidly and is widespread. The clinical manifestations of diabetic arterial disease are frequently exacerbated by coexisting peripheral neuropathy.

The impact that claudication has on patients relates to their age and lifestyle. A postman who can walk only 400 m has a serious problem but an elderly man who simply wants to get across the road to the shops and the pub may cope well. Rather than focusing upon absolute distances, ask specific questions like:

- Can you walk to the clinic from the bus stop or car park without stopping?
- Can you do your own shopping?
- What are you prevented from doing because of the pain?

Ask about the patient's other medical conditions. There is little point in subjecting patients with intermittent claudication to the risks of vascular surgery, only to find that they are then equally limited by osteoarthritis of the hip, angina or severe breathlessness.

Male patients with buttock (gluteal) claudication due to internal iliac disease almost invariably cannot achieve or maintain an erection. Discretely enquire into sexual activity (p. 16) as many patients are extremely concerned by this symptom yet too embarrassed to mention it.

The physical examination

General considerations

Follow the routine described for the heart, looking for evidence of anaemia or cyanosis, signs of heart failure and direct or indirect evidence of vascular disease (Table 3.29). Then you should perform a detailed examination of the arterial pulses. Abnormally prominent pulsation in the neck of the elderly is rarely of clinical significance and is normally caused by tortuous arteries rather than a carotid aneurysm or carotid body tumour.

Anatomy

The anatomy of the radial, brachial and carotid pulses has been described (p. 90).

The *femoral artery* is situated just below the inguinal ligament, midway between the anterior superior iliac spine and the pubic symphysis (the mid-inguinal point). It is

3.29 Signs suggesting vascular disease	
Sign	**Implication**
Hands and arms	
Tobacco stains	Smoking
Purple discoloration of the finger tips	Atheroembolism from a proximal subclavian aneurysm
Pits and healed scars in the finger pulps	Secondary Raynaud's syndrome
Calcinosis and visible nail fold capillary loops	Scleroderma and the CREST (calcinosis, Raynaud's phenomenon, (o)esophageal dysfunction, sclerodactyly, telangiectasis) syndrome
Wasting of the small muscles of the hand	Thoracic outlet syndrome
Face and neck	
Corneal arcus and xanthelasma	Hypercholesterolaemia
Horner's syndrome	Carotid artery dissection or aneurysm
Hoarseness of the voice and 'bovine' cough	Recurrent laryngeal nerve palsy from a thoracic aortic aneurysm
Prominent veins in the neck, shoulder and anterior chest	Axillary/subclavian vein occlusion
Abdomen	
Epigastric/umbilical pulsation	Aortoiliac aneurysm
Mottling of the abdomen	Ruptured abdominal aortic aneurysm or saddle embolism occluding aortic bifurcation
Evidence of weight loss	Visceral ischaemia

immediately lateral to the femoral vein and medial to the femoral nerve (Fig. 3.36).

The *popliteal artery* lies posteriorly in relation to the knee joint, at the level of the knee crease, deep in the popliteal fossa.

The *posterior tibial artery* is located 2 cm below and posterior to the medial malleolus, where it passes beneath the flexor retinaculum between flexor digitorum longus and flexor hallucis longus.

The *dorsalis pedis artery* is the continuation of the anterior tibial artery on the dorsum of the foot. It passes lateral to the tendon of extensor hallucis longus and is best felt at the proximal extent of the groove between the first and second metatarsals. It may be absent or abnormally sited in 10% of normal subjects, sometimes being 'replaced' by a palpable perforating peroneal artery.

Record individual pulses as:

normal	+
reduced	±
absent	−
aneurysmal	++

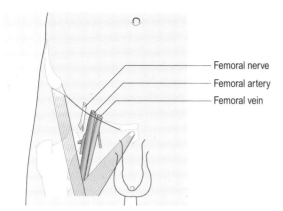

Fig. 3.36   Femoral triangle: vessels and nerves.

Femoral nerve
Femoral artery
Femoral vein

Examination of pulses

If you are in any doubt about which pulse is being felt, palpate your own pulse at the same time. If it is not synchronized with yours it is the patient's pulse.

➡ Examination sequence

→ Start at the head of the patient and work down the body using the sequence and principles of inspection, palpation and auscultation for each area.

The arms

→ Examine the radial, brachial and carotid pulses.
→ Measure the blood pressure in both arms. Many patients with peripheral arterial disease have asymptomatic subclavian artery disease. A difference of up to 10 mmHg in systolic pressure between the two arms is normal. If the discrepancy is greater than this, then the higher value is the true central pressure.

The abdomen

→ Look for obvious pulsation.
→ Palpate and listen over the abdominal aorta. If the aorta is easily palpable, consider the possibility of an abdominal aortic aneurysm, which is present in 5% of men > 65 years.

The legs

→ Inspect the legs and feet for changes of ischaemia including temperature and colour changes.
→ Note scars from previous vascular or non-vascular surgery and the position, margin, depth and colour of any ulceration.
→ Specifically look between the toes and at the heels for ischaemic changes.

Femoral pulse

→ With the patient supine, firmly press down and towards the patient's head in the groin crease (Fig. 3.37A) using two or three extended fingers. It can be difficult to feel in the obese.
→ Listen for bruits using the diaphragm of your stethoscope.
→ Check for radiofemoral delay.

Popliteal pulse

→ Patients should lie on a firm comfortable surface so they can relax their muscles.
→ Flex the patient's knee to 30°.
→ With your thumbs in front of the knee and your fingers behind, press firmly in the midline over the popliteal artery. It is sometimes difficult to feel.
→ By sliding your fingers 2–3 cm below the knee crease it may be possible to compress the artery against the back of the tibia as it passes under the soleal arch (Fig. 3.37B) making it easier to feel.
→ If the popliteal artery is especially easy to feel, consider the possibility of an aneurysm and request an ultrasound scan.

Posterior tibial pulse

→ Feel 2 cm below and 2 cm behind the medial malleolus, using the pads of your index and middle fingers (Fig. 3.37C).

Dorsalis pedis pulse

→ Feel in the middle of the dorsum of the foot just lateral to the tendon of extensor hallucis longus (Fig. 3.37D).

Common abnormalities

Chronic lower limb ischaemia.   Ischaemic changes may be present, e.g. absence of body hair on the legs, dorsum of the feet and toes. Other clinical features of arterial claudication are illustrated in Table 3.30.

In many patients the pedal pulses are absent or diminished. The presence of pedal pulses at rest does not exclude significant lower limb peripheral arterial disease. If the history is convincing ask the patient to walk until the onset of pain. Recheck the pulses because if the patient's symptoms are vascular in origin the pulses may disappear.

Patients with critical limb ischaemia typically have an ankle blood pressure < 50 mmHg and a positive Buerger's test.

Buerger's test

• With the patient lying supine, stand at the foot of the bed. Raise the feet and support the legs at 45° to the horizontal for 2–3 minutes
• Then ask the patient to sit up and hang the legs over the edge of the bed. Observe the patient's feet for another 2–3 minutes. Pallor on elevation (with emptying or 'guttering' of the superficial veins) followed by reactive hyperaemia (rubor) on dependency is a positive test and implies significant peripheral arterial disease.

Acute limb ischaemia.   The features of acute limb ischaemia are known as the 6 Ps (Table 3.31). Of these, loss of motor (ability to wiggle the toes/fingers) and/or sensory function (light touch over the forefoot/dorsum of the hand) are the most important and indicate nerve ischaemia. A limb with these features will become irreversibly damaged unless the circulation is restored within a few hours. Calf muscle tenderness is a grave sign indicating impending muscle

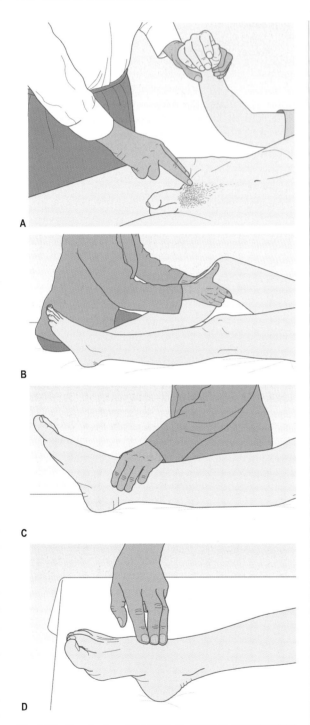

Fig. 3.37   Examination of the femoral, popliteal, posterior tibial and dorsalis pedis arteries. (A) Examine the femoral artery, while simultaneously checking for radiofemoral delay. (B) Feel the popliteal artery with the finger tips, having curled both hands into the popliteal fossa. (C) Examination of the posterior tibial artery. (D) Examination of the dorsalis pedis artery.

infarction. The common causes of acute limb ischaemia are embolus (usually cardiac in origin in association with atrial fibrillation), thrombotic occlusion of a narrowed atherosclerotic arterial segment and compartment syndrome (Table 3.32).

Acute arterial occlusion is associated with intense spasm in the arterial tree distal to the blockage and the limb appears 'marble white'. Over a few hours, the spasm relaxes and the skin microcirculation fills with deoxygenated blood leading to mottling which is light blue or purple, has a fine reticular pattern and blanches on pressure. As ischaemia progresses, blood coalescing in the skin produces a coarser pattern which is dark purple, almost black, and does not blanch. In the final stage large patches of fixed staining lead to blistering and liquefaction. Fixed mottling of an anaesthetic, paralysed limb, in association with muscle rigidity and turgor, indicates irreversible ischaemia and amputation is the only option.

Neurological presentations

A stroke is a focal central neurological deficit of vascular cause. Approximately 80% of strokes are ischaemic (as opposed to haemorrhagic). Of these, up to half are due to embolism from an atheromatous plaque at the common carotid bifurcation.

A bruit may arise from stenosis in the external or internal carotid arteries. Hearing a bruit in the neck is an unreliable sign of either the presence or the severity of internal carotid artery stenosis. There may be so little blood flow through a critical internal carotid artery stenosis that no bruit is audible. This applies to all other sites such as the femoral and subclavian arteries.

Vertebrobasilar artery territory. Transient ischaemic attacks and strokes in this territory cause different signs and symptoms. These may comprise giddiness, collapse, with or without loss of consciousness, transient occipital blindness or complete loss of vision in both eyes.

Patients with subclavian artery stenosis or occlusion proximal to the origin of the vertebral artery may experience vertebrobasilar symptoms as part of the 'subclavian steal' syndrome. This happens when the arm is exercised. The increased blood supply requirement in the arm is met by blood travelling up the carotid arteries and then, via the circle of Willis, down the vertebral artery into the arm, so 'stealing' blood from the posterior cerebral circulation. Signs of this include asymmetry of the pulses and blood pressure in the arms and sometimes a bruit over the subclavian artery in the supraclavicular fossa.

Abdominal presentations

Visceral ischaemia. Owing to the rich collateral circulation in the gut usually two of the three major visceral arteries (coeliac axis, superior and inferior mesenteric arteries) must

3.30 The clinical features of arterial, neurogenic and venous claudication

	Arterial	Neurogenic	Venous
Pathology	Stenosis or occlusion of major lower limb arteries	Lumbar nerve root or cauda equina compression (spinal stenosis)	Obstruction to the venous outflow of the leg due to iliofemoral venous occlusion
Site of pain	Muscles, usually the calf but may involve thigh and buttocks	Ill-defined. Whole leg. May be associated with numbness and tingling	Whole leg. 'Bursting' in nature
Laterality	Unilateral if femoropopliteal, and bilateral if aortoiliac disease	Often bilateral	Nearly always unilateral
Onset	Gradual after walking the 'claudication distance'	Often immediate upon walking or even standing up	Gradual, often from the moment walking commences
Relieving features	On the cessation of walking, the pain disappears completely in 1–2 minutes	Eased by bending forwards and stopping walking. May have to sit down to obtain full relief	Usually necessary to elevate leg to relieve discomfort
Colour	Normal or pale	Normal	Cyanosed. Often visible varicose veins
Temperature	Normal or cool	Normal	Normal or increased
Oedema	Absent	Absent	Always present
Pulses	Reduced or absent	Normal	Present but may be difficult to feel owing to oedema
Straight leg raising	Normal	May be limited	Normal

3.31 Signs of acute limb ischaemia

Soft signs	Hard signs (indicating a threatened limb)
Pulseless	**P**araesthesia
Pallor	**P**aralysis
Perishing cold	**P**ain on squeezing muscle

3.32 Acute limb ischaemia – embolus vs thrombosis in situ

	Embolus	Thrombosis
Onset and severity	Owing to lack of pre-existing collateral, the onset is acute (seconds or minutes) and the ischaemia profound	Owing to pre-existing collaterals, onset is more insidious (hours or days) and ischaemia less severe
Embolic source	Present (usually atrial fibrillation)	Absent
Previous claudication	Absent	Present
Pulses in contralateral leg	Present	Often absent
Diagnosis	Clinical	Angiography
Treatment	Embolectomy and anticoagulation	Medical, bypass surgery, thrombolysis

be critically stenosed or occluded before a patient develops symptoms and signs of chronic mesenteric arterial insufficiency. Typically, the patient develops severe central abdominal pain (*mesenteric angina*) 10–15 minutes after eating. This leads to fear of eating and significant weight loss. Diarrhoea may be a feature and visceral ischaemia may mimic a whole range of gastrointestinal pathologies. The patient may have had numerous investigations, even laparotomy, before the clinical diagnosis is made and confirmed by angiography.

Acute mesenteric ischaemia is a surgical emergency. The patient typically presents with severe abdominal pain, shock, bloody diarrhoea and profound metabolic acidosis. Rarely, renal angle pain occurs from renal infarction or ischaemia and is associated with micro- or macroscopic haematuria.

Abdominal aortic aneurysm. Abdominal aortic aneurysm is present in 5% of men aged > 65 years and is three times commoner in men than in women. Coexistent smoking habit and hypertension further increase these figures. Most patients are asymptomatic until the aneurysm ruptures, although they may present with abdominal and/or back pain or an awareness of abdominal pulsation.

The aortic bifurcation is at the level of the umbilicus, so feel in the epigastrium for a palpable abdominal aortic aneurysm. A pulsatile mass below the umbilicus suggests an iliac aneurysm. In thin patients a tortuous but normal-diameter aorta can feel aneurysmal. If the abdominal girth exceeds 38–40 inches (96–102 cm), even a large abdominal aortic aneurysm can be missed by experts. Ultrasound

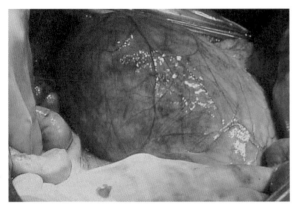

Fig. 3.38 Abdominal aortic aneurysm at laparotomy. The aorta is grossly and irregularly dilated.

studies clearly show that clinical examination is unreliable in establishing the presence of an abdominal aortic aneurysm, or estimating its size. Previous practice of determining whether an abdominal aortic aneurysm is present by assessing whether or not pulsation is expansile is also inaccurate. If you have *any* doubt or concern obtain an ultrasound scan (Figs 3.38 and 3.39).

A ruptured abdominal aortic aneurysm can be difficult to diagnose because many patients do not have the classical features of abdominal and/or back pain, pulsatile abdominal mass and hypotension. The commonest misdiagnosis is renal colic.

Embolism of atheromatous material (atheroembolism) and associated platelet debris and thrombotic material may arise from an abdominal aortic aneurysm and cause the

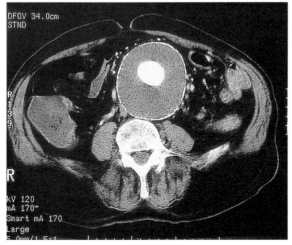

Fig. 3.39 CT scan of the abdomen showing abdominal aortic aneurysm.

'blue toe syndrome' characterized by purple discoloration of the toes and forefoot with a full set of pedal pulses.

Vasospastic presentations

Raynaud's phenomenon is digital ischaemia induced by cold and emotion and has three phases (Figs 3.40 and 3.41):

1. pallor due to digital artery spasm and/or obstruction
2. cyanosis due to deoxygenation of static venous blood (this phase may be absent)
3. redness due to reactive hyperaemia.

Raynaud's phenomenon may be primary (Raynaud's disease) due to idiopathic digital artery vasospasm, or secondary (Raynaud's syndrome) (Table 3.33).

Assume that patients > 40 years old presenting with unilateral Raynaud's phenomenon have underlying peripheral arterial disease unless proved otherwise.

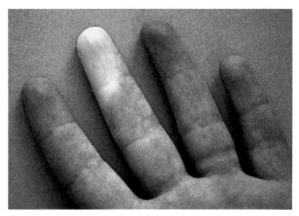

Fig. 3.40 Raynaud's syndrome in the acute phase, with severe blanching of the tip of one finger.

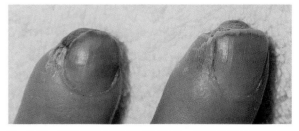

Fig. 3.41 Primary Raynaud's syndrome occasionally progresses to finger tip ulceration or even gangrene.

3.33 Diseases associated with secondary Raynaud's syndrome
• Connective tissue syndromes, e.g. systemic sclerosis, CREST (calcinosis, Raynaud's phenomenon, (o)esophageal dysfunction, sclerodactyly, telangiectasis) and systemic lupus erythematosus • Atherosclerosis/embolism from proximal source, e.g. subclavian artery aneurysm • Drug-related, e.g. nicotine, beta-blockers, ergot • Thoracic outlet syndrome • Malignancy • Hyperviscosity syndromes, e.g. Waldenström's macroglobulinaemia, polycythaemia • Vibration-induced disorders (power tools) • Cold agglutinin disorders

Investigations

Measurement of ankle : brachial pressure index

Measurement is performed using a hand-held Doppler and a sphygmomanometer. The probe is held over the three pedal arteries (posterior tibial, dorsalis pedis, perforating peroneal) in turn while a blood pressure cuff wrapped round the ankle is inflated. The pressure at which the Doppler signal disappears is the systolic pressure in that artery as it passes under the cuff. The ratio of the highest pedal artery pressure to the highest brachial artery pressure is the ankle : brachial pressure index.

In health, the ankle : brachial pressure index should be > 1.0 in the supine position. Typical values in claudication and critical limb ischaemia are < 0.8 and < 0.4 respectively. Absolute values, however, may be less informative than the trend over time.

Patients with severe lower limb ischaemia, particularly those with diabetes, may have incompressible, calcified

Examine this patient with acute pain and discoloration in his right foot
1. Feel the radial pulse for irregularity, e.g. *atrial fibrillation*. 2. Measure the blood pressure in both arms – unequal in *aortic dissection*. 3. Listen to the heart – early diastolic murmur may indicate *aortic regurgitation* due to *aortic dissection*. 4. Feel the abdomen for pulsation of *abdominal aortic aneurysm*. 5. Auscultate the abdomen for bruits of *aortoiliac disease*. 6. Look at the feet for discoloration: marbled in complete *acute ischaemia* due to embolus; fine reticular blanching mottling in early stages; coarse more fixed mottling in late stages. 7. Palpate the femoral and popliteal pulses and feel for popliteal aneurysms. 8. Squeeze the calves – tenderness suggest muscle infarction. 9. Compare the warmth of both feet with the back of your hand. 10. Palpate for the dorsalis pedis and posterior tibial pulses in both feet. 11. Ask the patient to wiggle his toes, and test fine sensation – both motor and sensory function absent in *limb-threatening ischaemia*. 12. If acute ischaemia is suspected urgently refer to vascular surgeon.

3.34 Investigations of peripheral arterial disease	
Investigation	**Common uses**
Doppler ultrasound	Ankle pressure; ankle : brachial pressure index, pulse waveform analysis
B-mode ultrasound	Abdominal aortic aneurysm, popliteal artery aneurysm
Duplex ultrasound	Carotid artery stenosis, vein bypass graft surveillance
Computerized tomography	Abdominal aortic aneurysm, detection of cerebral infarct/haemorrhage
Magnetic resonance imaging	Arteriovenous malformations, carotid artery stenosis
Angiography	Acute and chronic limb ischaemia, carotid artery stenosis

crural arteries. This produces falsely elevated pedal pressures, and ankle : brachial pressure index. In such circumstances, an alternative is to use a Doppler ultrasound probe to detect (*isonate*) the artery with the hand-held Doppler while elevating the foot. The Doppler signal disappears at a height above the bed (in centimetres) that is approximately equal to the perfusion pressure in mmHg.

Choose further tests to provide the most information at the least risk to the patient and with least expense. In most situations ultrasound techniques have replaced angiography (Table 3.34).

◆ Key points

- Widespread peripheral arterial disease may be asymptomatic for years and then present with life-threatening complications.
- Acute limb ischaemia and chronic arterial insufficiency causing rest pain and/or tissue loss needs urgent assessment.
- Use the ankle : brachial pressure index to assess the severity of chronic lower limb ischaemia.
- Patients with hemispheric or ocular transient ischaemic attacks need urgent carotid ultrasound to detect significant carotid stenosis.
- In a large patient, even a sizeable (> 6 cm diameter) abdominal aortic aneurysm may be easily missed clinically.
- Abdominal aortic aneurysm causes a pulsatile mass in the epigastrium. An expansile mass below the umbilicus is likely to be an iliac artery aneurysm.
- Actively exclude abdominal aortic aneurysm as a cause of abdominal pain, especially in men > 65 years.
- 'Renal colic' presenting for the first time in a patient > 60 years is a ruptured abdominal aortic aneurysm until proven otherwise.
- Unilateral Raynaud's phenomenon in patients > 40 years is often associated with peripheral arterial disease.

- Subclavian artery disease may present with apparent vertebrobasilar insufficiency. A systolic blood pressure difference > 15 mmHg between the arms suggests the diagnosis.
- Diabetic patients with rest pain of arterial origin may be misdiagnosed as having the pain of diabetic neuropathy.
- Visceral ischaemia is a frequently overlooked cause of 'unexplained' abdominal pain and weight loss. Consider the diagnosis especially in patients who have had multiple negative gastrointestinal investigations.
- An aneurysmal popliteal artery suggests widespread vascular disease.
- If one popliteal artery is unexpectedly easy to palpate, consider abdominal ultrasonography to exclude an abdominal aortic aneurysm.

VENOUS DISEASE

General considerations

The clinical examination is primarily concerned with determining the nature and severity of any venous problem and identifying any underlying or precipitating factors.

Venous disease is much more common in the legs than in the arms. It usually presents in one of four ways:

- deep venous thrombosis
- varicose veins
- superficial thrombosis
- chronic venous insufficiency and ulceration.

Common symptoms

The severity of symptoms (and signs) may bear little relationship to the gravity of the underlying pathology and the physical signs. For example, life-threatening deep venous thrombosis may be asymptomatic while apparently trivial varicose veins may be associated with significant discomfort.

There are four cardinal symptoms of lower limb venous disease.

Pain. Patients with uncomplicated varicose veins may complain of an aching discomfort in the leg, itching and a feeling of swelling. Symptoms are typically aggravated by prolonged standing and towards the end of the day. The pain of established deep venous thrombosis is deep-seated and associated with swelling below the level of obstruction. Superficial venous thrombophlebitis produces a red, painful area overlying the vein involved. Varicose ulceration may be painless but if there is pain it may be relieved by limb elevation.

Swelling. Swelling may be associated with varicose veins, deep venous reflux and deep venous thrombosis.

Discoloration. Chronic venous insufficiency causes pigmentation due to haemosiderin deposition in the skin leading to lipodermatosclerosis. This varies in colour from deep blue/black to purple or even bright red. It typically affects the medial aspect of the lower third of the leg but may be laterally placed if superficial reflux predominates in the short saphenous veins.

Ulceration. Patients with venous ulceration may not seek medical attention for many years. Venous ulceration is always associated with lipodermatosclerosis.

Relevant further questions depend upon the nature of the venous problem. In a patient with deep venous thrombosis remember to think about a possible pulmonary embolus and also possible causes for the development of the deep venous thrombosis, e.g. venous obstruction or compression from tumours in the pelvis or abdomen. In patients with superficial thrombophlebitis, particularly if recurrent, consider the possibility of underlying malignancy.

Questions

Deep venous thrombosis. Ask about:

- recent bed rest or operations (especially to the leg or pelvis)
- recent travel, especially long air flights
- previous trauma to the leg, especially long bone fractures, plaster of Paris splintage and immobilization
- pregnancy or features to suggest pelvic disease
- previous deep venous thrombosis
- family history of thrombosis
- recent central venous catheterization, injection of drugs etc. (in the upper limb).

The physical examination

Anatomy

In the leg the long saphenous vein passes anterior to the medial malleolus at the ankle, up the medial aspect of the calf to behind the knee, then up the medial aspect of the thigh to join the common femoral vein in the groin at the saphenofemoral junction (Fig. 3.42).

The short saphenous vein passes behind the lateral malleolus at the ankle and up the posterior aspect of the calf. It commonly joins the popliteal vein at the saphenopopliteal junction, which usually lies 2 cm above the posterior knee crease.

There are many intercommunications between the long and short saphenous systems and the venous anatomy of the leg is highly variable.

Examination of venous system

⊡ Examination sequence

→ Examine the legs with the patient standing and then lying supine.
→ Expose the patient's limbs and inspect the skin for colour changes, limb swelling and superficial venous dilatation and tortuosity.

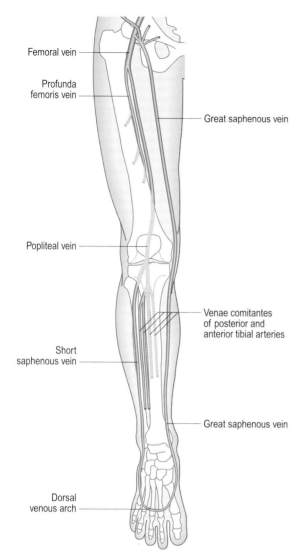

Femoral vein

Profunda
femoris vein

Great saphenous vein

Popliteal vein

Venae comitantes
of posterior and
anterior tibial arteries

Short
saphenous vein

Great saphenous vein

Dorsal
venous arch

Fig. 3.42 Veins of the lower limb.

→ Feel for any differences in temperature
→ Elevate the limb to about 15° above the horizontal and
    note the rate of venous emptying.
→ If appropriate, perform the Trendelenburg test to detect
    saphenofemoral junction incompetence.

The Trendelenburg test.   This is performed to determine
the pattern of venous incompetence in the leg.

- Ask the patient to sit on the edge of the examination
  couch.
- Elevate the limb as far as is comfortable for the patient
  and empty the superficial veins by 'milking' the leg.
- With the leg still elevated, press with your thumb over
  the saphenofemoral junction (2–3 cm below and 2–3 cm
  lateral to the pubic tubercle). If preferred, a high thigh
  tourniquet can be used instead of digital pressure.

- Ask the patient to stand while you maintain pressure
  over the saphenofemoral junction.
- If saphenofemoral junction incompetence is present the
  patient's varicose veins will not fill until your digital
  pressure, or the tourniquet, is removed.

Common abnormalities

Deep venous thrombosis.   Deep venous thrombosis
occurs most often in the leg but can affect the arm (axillary
vein thrombosis).
   The leg.   The clinical features of deep venous
thrombosis depend upon its site, extent and whether it is
occlusive or not (Table 3.35). The 'classical' features of
deep venous thrombosis relate to well-established occlusive
thrombus. Most patients who die from pulmonary embolus
have non-occlusive thrombosis and normal legs on clinical
examination. Non-occlusive thrombus poses the greatest
threat of pulmonary embolus as the clot lies within a flowing
stream of venous blood, is more likely to propagate and has
not yet induced an inflammatory response in the vein wall
to anchor it in place.
   The arm.   Deep venous thrombosis can occur as a
primary event due to repetitive trauma of the axillary or
subclavian vein, e.g. thoracic outlet syndrome. This may
follow strenuous unaccustomed use of the arm. It is more
common in body-builders perhaps because of associated
anabolic steroid use and is also seen in injecting drug users.
It can also be a complication of indwelling catheters in the
subclavian vein.
   Symptoms are arm swelling and discomfort exacerbated
by activity, especially when holding the arm overhead.
   On inspection the arm is swollen and the skin is often
cyanosed and mottled, especially on dependency. Look for
superficial distended veins (acting as collaterals) in the
upper arm, over the shoulder region and on the anterior chest
wall (Fig. 3.43).
   Superficial venous thrombophlebitis.   Inflammation
of superficial veins is associated with intraluminal, usually
sterile thrombosis. It affects up to 10% of patients with severe
varicose veins and appears to be more common during
pregnancy.

3.35 Features of deep venous thrombosis of the lower limb		
Clinical feature	**Non-occlusive thrombus**	**Occlusive thrombus**
Pain	Often absent	Usually present
Calf tenderness	Often absent	Usually present
Swelling	Absent	Present
Temperature	Normal or slightly increased	Increased
Superficial veins	Normal	Distended
Pulmonary embolism	High risk	Low risk

119

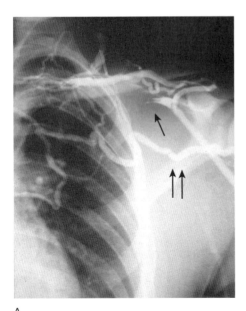

A

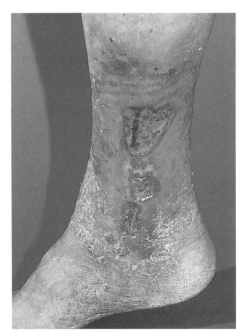

Fig. 3.44   Venous ulceration.

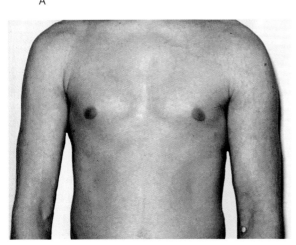

B

Fig. 3.43   Axillary vein thrombosis. (A) Angiogram. Single arrow shows site of thrombosis. Double arrows show dilated collateral vessels. (B) Clinical appearance with swollen left arm and dilated superficial veins.

Recurrent superficial thrombophlebitis may be associated with underlying malignancy. When superficial venous thrombophlebitis occurs at, or near, the saphenofemoral junction it may be associated with pulmonary embolism.

Chronic venous insufficiency.   Chronic venous insufficiency produces skin changes in the lower leg (varicose eczema, lipodermatosclerosis, ulceration) due to sustained venous hypertension which in turn is due to reflux (90%) and/or obstruction (10%) in the superficial and/or deep veins.

Chronic leg ulceration.   In developed countries, the vast majority of leg ulcers (Fig. 3.44) are caused by venous and/or arterial disease. However, 1 in 5 patients with a venous ulcer will also have significant arterial disease (Table 3.36). Bandaging for a leg ulcer is contraindicated unless there is documented evidence of the adequacy of the arterial circulation. Do this by feeling the pulses or by measuring the ankle : brachial pressure index.

◆ Key points

- The cardinal symptoms of venous disease are pain or discomfort, swelling of the limb and discoloration with ulceration.
- Life-threatening deep venous thrombosis may be asymptomatic.
- Leg ulceration in the elderly is often multifactorial. The commonest single underlying cause is chronic venous insufficiency.
- Superficial thrombophlebitis, especially in the absence of varicose veins, and where it is migratory in character, often signifies underlying malignancy.
- 1 in 5 patients with a venous ulcer has significant arterial disease. Always confirm that pedal pulses are present and the ankle : brachial pressure index is normal before prescribing graduated compression bandaging.
- The red discoloration in lipodermatosclerosis may be mistaken for soft tissue infection, especially if there is venous ulceration. Soft tissue infection, unlike lipodermatosclerosis, is associated with the other features of inflammation.

3.36	Clinical features of venous and arterial ulceration	
Clinical feature	**Venous ulceration**	**Arterial ulceration**
Age	Typically first develops at 40–45 years but many do not present until many years later; multiple recurrences are common	Typically affects patient for the first time > 60 years
Sex	Women predominate, especially in the elderly	Men predominate
Past medical history	Many have a history of deep venous thrombosis, or give a history suggestive of occult deep venous thrombosis, i.e. leg swelling after childbirth, hip/knee replacement, or long bone fracture	Most have a clear history of previous peripheral arterial disease, cardio- and cerebrovascular disease
Risk factors	Thrombophilia, family history, previous deep venous thrombosis (see above)	Smoking, diabetes, hypercholesterolaemia and hypertension
Pain	Present in about a third of patients but not usually severe; often improves with elevation	Severe pain is the rule except in diabetics with neuropathy; usually better on dependency
Site	Gaiter areas; usually medial in relation to long saphenous veins disease; 20% are lateral related to short saphenous disease	Pressure areas (malleoli, heel, 5th metatarsal base, metatarsal heads and toes)
Margin	Irregular often with neo-epithelium (appears whiter than mature skin)	Regular, indolent, 'punched out'
Base	Often pink and granulating under green slough	Sloughy (green) or necrotic (black) with no granulation
Surrounding skin	Lipodermatosclerosis always present	No venous skin changes
Veins	Full and usually varicose	Empty with 'guttering' on elevation
Swelling (oedema)	Usually present	Absent
Temperature	Warm	Cold
Pulses	Present, but may be difficult to feel	Absent

The respiratory system

GRAHAM DEVEREUX • GRAHAM DOUGLAS

RESPIRATORY EXAMINATION

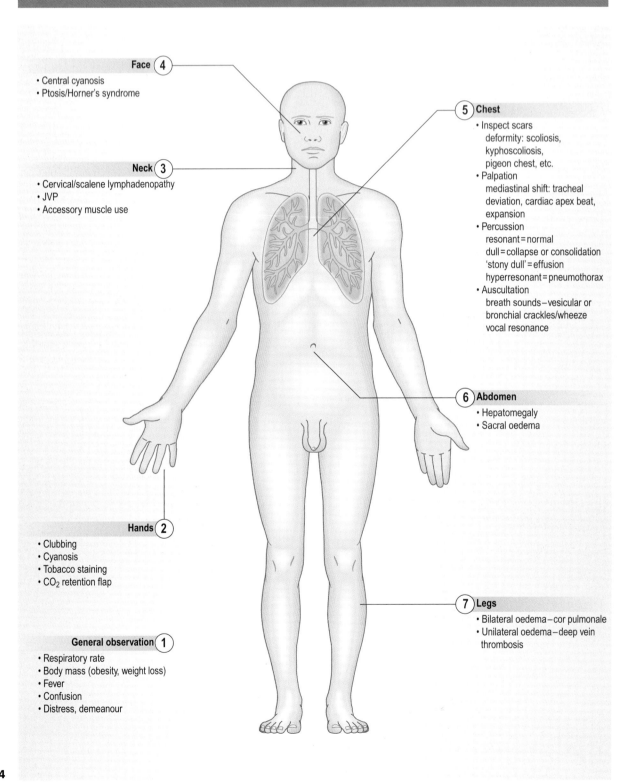

Face (4)
- Central cyanosis
- Ptosis/Horner's syndrome

Neck (3)
- Cervical/scalene lymphadenopathy
- JVP
- Accessory muscle use

Hands (2)
- Clubbing
- Cyanosis
- Tobacco staining
- CO_2 retention flap

General observation (1)
- Respiratory rate
- Body mass (obesity, weight loss)
- Fever
- Confusion
- Distress, demeanour

(5) Chest
- Inspect scars
  deformity: scoliosis,
  kyphoscoliosis,
  pigeon chest, etc.
- Palpation
  mediastinal shift: tracheal
  deviation, cardiac apex beat,
  expansion
- Percussion
  resonant = normal
  dull = collapse or consolidation
  'stony dull' = effusion
  hyperresonant = pneumothorax
- Auscultation
  breath sounds – vesicular or
  bronchial crackles/wheeze
  vocal resonance

(6) Abdomen
- Hepatomegaly
- Sacral oedema

(7) Legs
- Bilateral oedema – cor pulmonale
- Unilateral oedema – deep vein
  thrombosis

A

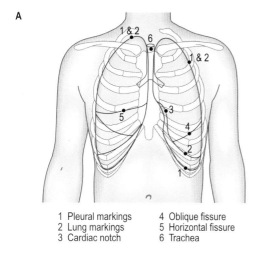

1 Pleural markings	4 Oblique fissure
2 Lung markings	5 Horizontal fissure
3 Cardiac notch	6 Trachea

B

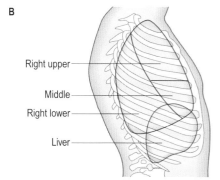

Right upper
Middle
Right lower
Liver

C

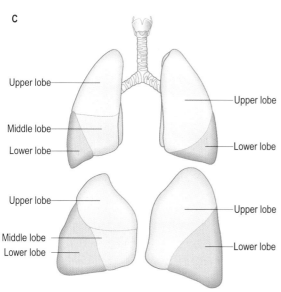

Upper lobe
Middle lobe
Lower lobe
Upper lobe
Middle lobe
Lower lobe

Upper lobe
Lower lobe
Upper lobe
Lower lobe

Fig. 4.1 Surface anatomy of the thorax. (A) Surface markings of the lungs and pleura, trachea and bronchi. The trachea is normally central and the cardiac apex beat is located at the 5th intercostal space in the midclavicular line. The bifurcation of the trachea corresponds on the anterior chest wall with the sternal angle, the transverse bony ridge at the junction of the sternum and manubrium sternum. The ribs are most easily counted downwards from the second costal cartilage at the level of the sternal angle. (B) Surface markings of the lungs and underlying viscera. (C) Lobes of the lungs: anterior view (upper) and lateral view (lower).

INTRODUCTION

Despite advances in modern medical technology, a thorough clinical history and examination are fundamental to respiratory medicine. For many common respiratory disorders a detailed history, careful examination, chest radiograph and simple tests of ventilatory function are sufficient to make the diagnosis.

A substantial proportion of emergency medicine in primary and secondary care settings involves the assessment and treatment of patients who are acutely breathless because of respiratory illnesses such as pneumothorax, pneumonia, asthma and chronic obstructive pulmonary disease (COPD). The consequences of slow and inadequate assessment of acutely breathless patients with tension pneumothorax, severe pneumonia, asthma and COPD can be fatal.

The common respiratory symptoms are breathlessness, cough, haemoptysis and chest pain. Many patients, especially smokers, are apprehensive about respiratory symptoms because they worry about the possibility of lung cancer especially if they have been referred to a specialist after an abnormal chest X-ray. These fears need to be addressed during the consultation. Simple measures at the start of the consultation such as a friendly smile, a relaxed approach, suitable arrangement of furniture and an understanding manner help put patients at ease, enabling them to give a history undistorted by their fears.

It is important to establish whether the patient has an acute respiratory illness, a chronic respiratory disorder or an acute illness superimposed on a chronic disorder. Many patients with chronic respiratory disorders adapt to their condition and regard quite marked limitations as normal and so fail to mention these during history taking. The history should enable you to understand how the patient's life differs from that of a fit individual. Ask patients to compare themselves with healthy friends. It is also useful to enquire about symptoms and illnesses during specific periods of the patient's life. Ask about symptoms and diagnoses during childhood, time off school, problems during military service, reasons for retiring and or giving up activities and hobbies such as housework, shopping, gardening, golf or football. Be aware of environmental factors that can either cause or aggravate respiratory disease (e.g. cigarette smoke, occupational exposures, pets, dusts, and allergens). Specific detailed questions about environmental exposures may help confirm a diagnosis, prevent further disease or may be the basis for compensation in cases of occupational lung disease.

COMMON SYMPTOMS

The six principal symptoms of respiratory disease are:

- cough
- sputum production
- haemoptysis
- chest pain
- breathlessness
- wheeze.

All of these can also occur in the absence of respiratory disease. For example, breathlessness, wheeze and central chest pain may be the presenting feature of an acute myocardial infarction complicated by pulmonary oedema. Diabetic ketoacidosis may present with breathlessness and weight loss.

Although many respiratory conditions share the same combination of symptoms (e.g. cough, sputum production and breathlessness are features of pneumonia, asthma, COPD, cystic fibrosis and bronchiectasis), the mode of onset, duration, progression and severity of each symptom characteristically differ. Therefore, it is not sufficient to merely ask about the presence of individual respiratory symptoms. Rather, each symptom needs careful exploration of mode of onset, duration, progression, aggravating/relieving factors and relationships with other symptoms.

COUGH

Cough is the most common symptom of respiratory disease. Most acute episodes are self-limiting and caused by infections, usually viral. Other common causes are outlined in Table 4.1. Cough is usually an involuntary reflex but may be a voluntary act. The function of cough is to remove secretions or particles from the pharynx and airways. Involuntary cough is a reflex action initiated by stimulation of sensory receptors from the pharynx to the alveoli. After a rapid increase in intrathoracic pressure caused by contraction of respiratory muscles against a closed glottis, the glottis opens with an explosive release of air into the upper airway. The sound of the cough and the circumstances in which it occurs may be helpful in making the diagnosis.

Sound of the cough

A feeble non-explosive 'bovine' cough with hoarseness may occur with respiratory muscle weakness but is more usually associated with lung cancer invading the left recurrent laryngeal nerve with resultant paralysis of the left vocal cord. A rare cause is thoracic aortic aneurysm that also damages the left recurrent laryngeal nerve. Patients with severe airflow obstruction (asthma or COPD) often have prolonged wheezy coughing, and sometimes the sustained

4.1 Causes of cough	
Sinuses	Infection

Larynx, trachea, large airways	Infection
	Tumours:
	  benign
	  malignant, primary, secondary
	Aspiration
	Gastro-oesophageal reflux
	Foreign body
	Irritant dusts

Small airways	Asthma Post-viral airway reactivity Chronic bronchitis (COPD) Bronchiectasis Bronchiolitis Irritant dusts
Alveoli	Drugs, e.g. angiotensin-converting enzyme inhibitors Infection: pneumonia, tuberculosis Alveolitis Left ventricular failure Irritant dusts

increase in intrathoracic pressure is sufficient to impair venous return to the heart, resulting in reduced cardiac output and cough syncope or near-syncope. The cough of laryngeal inflammation, infection and tumour tends to be harsh, barking or painful and may be associated with hoarseness and stridor.

A moist cough usually indicates secretions in the upper and larger airways and occurs in bronchial infection and bronchiectasis. A persistent moist 'smoker's' cough first thing in the morning is typical of chronic bronchitis. Smokers often do not mention it because it is so common they assume it is normal. Any change in the pattern of this cough may indicate the development of lung cancer.

A dry centrally painful and non-productive cough is a feature of tracheitis and pneumonia. A paroxysmal dry cough in patients with asthma may follow a viral respiratory infection and last several months. A chronic dry cough is common in interstitial disease, e.g. cryptogenic fibrosing alveolitis.

Circumstances of the cough

A nocturnal cough causing sleep disturbance is a common symptom of asthma. Occult gastro-oesophageal reflux is a common cause of daytime cough, as is chronic sinus disease with associated postnasal drip. Angiotensin-converting enzyme inhibitors used to treat left ventricular failure and hypertension may cause a dry cough, particularly in women. This is caused by peptides, e.g. bradykinin and substance P, that would normally be degraded by angiotensin-converting enzyme. Coughing during and after swallowing liquids suggests neuromuscular disease of the oropharynx. Occupational asthma and exposure to dusts and fumes are a recognized cause of chronic cough that typically lessens during weekends and holidays.

SPUTUM PRODUCTION

Expectorated respiratory secretions are known as sputum or phlegm and need to be specifically asked about. Patients may find it difficult to discuss sputum production because of a natural reluctance, and it may be regularly swallowed. There are four main types of sputum (Table 4.2).

Amount

Ask how many teaspoons of sputum are coughed up each day. Statements by patients that they cough up small (a teaspoonful) or large (a teacupful) amounts of sputum are usually helpful. Regular coughing up of large volumes of purulent sputum influenced by posture is characteristic of bronchiectasis. The sudden production of large amounts of purulent sputum on a single occasion suggests the rupture of a lung abscess or empyema into the bronchial tree. Large volumes of watery sputum with a pink tinge in an acutely breathless patient suggests pulmonary oedema, whereas large volumes of watery sputum for weeks (bronchorrhoea) is a symptom of alveolar cell cancer.

Colour

The colour of sputum is helpful (Fig. 4.2). Clear or 'mucoid' sputum is produced by patients with COPD without active infection. Yellowish sputum is found in acute lower respiratory tract infection (live neutrophils) and also in asthma (eosinophils). Green sputum (dead neutrophils) indicates chronic infection as in exacerbations of COPD,

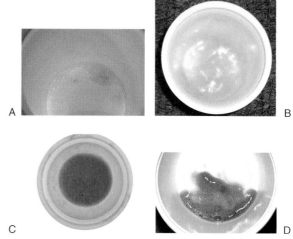

Fig. 4.2   Different colours of sputum. (A) White. (B) Yellow. (C) Green. (D) Rusty red.

bronchiectasis, etc. Purulent sputum is usually green because of the presence of lysed neutrophils and their breakdown products, specifically the green-pigmented enzyme verdoperoxidase. The first sputum produced in the morning by a patient with COPD may be green because of nocturnal stagnation of neutrophils. In the early stages of pneumococcal pneumonia sputum may be a characteristic rusty red colour as pneumonic inflammation passes through the red hepatization phase. In coal miners with pneumoconiosis the rupture of necrotic areas of pulmonary fibrosis can result in the expectoration of black sputum (*melanoptysis*).

Taste or smell

'Foul' or 'vile' tasting or smelling sputum suggests anaerobic bacterial infection and can occur in bronchiectasis, lung abscess and empyema. In some patients with bronchiectasis a change of sputum taste indicates an infective exacerbation.

Solid material

In asthma and allergic bronchopulmonary aspergillosis viscid secretions can accumulate in airways. When these are coughed up they appear as worm-like structures that are casts of the bronchi. Other recognizable solid matter that may be coughed up includes necrotic tumour and inhaled foreign bodies such as food, teeth and tablets.

HAEMOPTYSIS

Haemoptysis (coughing up blood) induces anxiety in many patients because of its association with lung cancer (Table 4.3). It is important to determine whether the blood

4.2	Types of sputum	
Type	**Appearance**	**Cause**
Serous	Clear, watery Frothy, pink	Acute pulmonary oedema Alveolar cell cancer
Mucoid	Clear, grey White, viscid	Chronic bronchitis/COPD Asthma
Purulent	Yellow, green	Bronchopulmonary infection: pneumonia bronchiectasis cystic fibrosis lung abscess
Rusty	Rusty, golden yellow	Pneumococcal pneumonia

4.3	Causes of haemoptysis

Tumour:
  malignant
  benign
	Lung cancer
	Endobronchial metastases
	Bronchial carcinoid

Infection	Bronchiectasis Tuberculosis Lung abscess Mycetoma Cystic fibrosis
Vascular	Pulmonary infarction Arteriovenous malformation
Vasculitis	Wegener's granulomatosis Goodpasture's syndrome

Trauma	Inhaled foreign body
	Chest trauma
	Iatrogenic:
	  bronchoscopic biopsy
	  transthoracic lung biopsy
	  bronchoscopic diathermy

Cardiac	Mitral valve disease Acute left ventricular failure
Haematological	Blood dyscrasias Anticoagulation

has been coughed up from the respiratory tract, been vomited from the upper gastrointestinal tract or has suddenly appeared in the mouth without coughing, suggesting a nasopharyngeal origin. Haemoptysis is an important symptom and should always be investigated.

Amount and appearance

Patients often describe whether the haemoptysis is a small or large amount of pure blood. Streaking of clear sputum with blood or the presence of blood clots in the sputum for more than a week is suggestive of lung cancer. Haemoptysis with purulent sputum suggests an infective cause such as bronchiectasis. Diffuse staining of sputum with blood (pink froth) can occur in acute pulmonary oedema. Coughing up large amounts of pure blood is fortunately rare but potentially life-threatening; the most frequent causes are bronchiectasis, tuberculosis, and lung cancer. Less frequent causes include pulmonary infarction, lung abscess, mycetoma, cystic fibrosis, aorto-bronchial fistula and Wegener's granulomatosis.

Duration and frequency

Haemoptysis occurring intermittently for a few years, usually in association with a respiratory tract infection occurs in bronchiectasis. Daily haemoptysis for a week or more is a common symptom of lung cancer, other causes include tuberculosis and lung abscess. Single episodes of

haemoptysis may need immediate investigation if they are very large or associated with symptoms, e.g. pleuritic chest pain and breathlessness suggesting pulmonary thromboembolism and infarction.

CHEST PAIN

Chest pain can originate from the pleura, the chest wall, and mediastinal structures (Table 4.4). The lungs are not a source of pain because of their exclusive autonomic innervation. A careful history of chest pain should include site, radiation, mode of onset, duration, severity, and aggravating/relieving factors including the effects of breathing and movement.

4.4	Causes of chest pain	
Non-central		

Pleural	Infection:
	  pneumonia
	  bronchiectasis
	  tuberculosis
	Malignancy:
	  lung cancer
	  mesothelioma
	  metastatic
	Pneumothorax
	Pulmonary infarction
	Connective tissue disease:
	  e.g. rheumatoid arthritis
	  systemic lupus erythematosus	

Chest wall	Malignancy:
	  lung cancer
	  mesothelioma
	  bony metastases
	Persistent cough/breathlessness
	Muscle sprains/tears
	Bornholm's disease (Coxsackie B infection)
	Tietze's syndrome (costochondritis)
	Rib fracture
	Intercostal nerve compression
	Thoracic shingles (herpes zoster)	

Central		
Tracheal	Infection Irritant dusts	
Cardiac	Massive pulmonary thromboembolism Acute myocardial infarction/ischaemia	
Oesophageal	Oesophagitis Rupture	
Great vessels	Aortic dissection	
Mediastinal	Lung cancer Thymoma Lymphadenopathy Metastases Mediastinitis	

Pleural pain

Pleuritic pain is typically sharp, stabbing and always intensified by inspiration or coughing. Irritation of the parietal pleura of the upper six ribs is perceived as a localized pain, whereas irritation of the parietal pleura overlying the central diaphragm innervated by the phrenic nerve is referred to the neck or shoulder tip. The lower six intercostal nerves innervate the parietal pleura of the lower ribs and the outer diaphragm, and hence pain from these sites may be referred to the upper abdomen.

Chest wall pain

Pain originating from the chest wall may indicate respiratory or musculoskeletal disease. Not uncommonly patients with chronic cough or breathlessness develop a generalized feeling of chest tightness or diffuse pain. Patients with asthma or COPD often mention this form of pain if asked but it is rarely a presenting complaint.

A number of features may help in differentiating chest wall from pleural pain. The sudden onset of localized pain after vigorous coughing or direct trauma is characteristic of rib fractures or intercostal muscle injury. Prevesicular herpes zoster and intercostal nerve root compression can cause chest pain in a thoracic dermatomal distribution. Malignant chest wall pain due to lung cancer, mesothelioma or rib metastases is typically dull, aching, or gnawing in nature, unrelated to respiration, progressively worsening and eventually disrupting sleep. The pain of Pancoast's tumour of the lung apex is due to erosion of the first rib and is often referred down the medial aspect of the arm because of invasion of the lower roots of the brachial plexus.

Mediastinal pain

Mediastinal pain is typically central, retrosternal and unrelated to respiration or cough. However, pain originating from the tracheobronchial tree due to infection or inhalation of irritant dusts is typically retrosternal, with a raw burning character, and is greatly worsened by cough. A dull aching retrosternal pain that progresses to disturb sleep can be a feature of malignancy invading mediastinal lymph nodes or enlarging thymoma. Massive pulmonary thromboembolism sufficient to induce an acute increase in right ventricular pressure may produce central chest pain identical to myocardial ischaemia.

BREATHLESSNESS

Breathlessness (dyspnoea) is an undue awareness of breathing. It is a natural consequence of strenuous physical exercise. Patients may use terms such as 'shortness of breath', 'difficulty getting enough air in', 'feeling puffed',

or 'tiredness'. These terms indicate that the patient is getting breathless but are usually unhelpful in elucidating possible causes (Table 4.5). A careful history of breathlessness covers mode of onset, duration, progression, variation, aggravating/relieving factors, severity and associated symptoms.

Mode of onset, duration, progression

Determine whether breathlessness has occurred suddenly and progressed rapidly over a few minutes, has occurred gradually and progressed rapidly over hours or days, or has occurred gradually and progressed relentlessly over weeks, months or years (Table 4.6). Breathlessness related to psychogenic factors often occurs suddenly at rest or while talking. The patient often complains of inability to get

4.5 Causes of breathlessness	
Non-cardiorespiratory	Anaemia Metabolic acidosis Obesity Psychogenic Neurogenic
Cardiac	Left ventricular failure Mitral valve disease Cardiomyopathy Constrictive pericarditis Pericardial effusion
Respiratory	
Airways	Laryngeal tumour Foreign body Asthma COPD Bronchiectasis Lung cancer Bronchiolitis Cystic fibrosis
Parenchyma	Pulmonary fibrosis Alveolitis Sarcoidosis Tuberculosis Pneumonia Diffuse infections, e.g. *pneumocystis jiroveci* pneumonia Tumour (metastatic, lymphangitis)
Pulmonary circulation	Pulmonary thromboembolism Pulmonary vasculitis Primary pulmonary hypertension
Pleural	Pneumothorax Effusion Diffuse pleural fibrosis
Chest wall	Kyphoscoliosis Ankylosing spondylitis
Neuromuscular	Myasthenia gravis Neuropathies Muscular dystrophies Guillain–Barré syndrome

4.6 Breathlessness, modes of onset, duration and progression	
Minutes	Pulmonary thromboembolism Pneumothorax Acute left ventricular failure Asthma Inhaled foreign body
Hours to days	Pneumonia Asthma Exacerbation of COPD
Weeks to months	Anaemia Pleural effusion Respiratory neuromuscular disorders
Months to years	COPD Pulmonary fibrosis Pulmonary tuberculosis

4.7 Severity of breathlessness: Medical Research Council classification	
Grade 1	Breathless when hurrying on the level or walking up a slight hill
Grade 2	Breathless when walking with people of own age or on level ground
Grade 3	Has to stop because of breathlessness when walking on level ground at own pace

enough air into the chest and a need to take deep breaths. This form of breathlessness may be associated with a feeling of light-headedness, dizziness, tingling in the fingers and around the mouth, chest tightness, and rarely syncope.

Variability, aggravating/relieving factors

Ask what situations or activities bring on breathlessness as this may provide clues as to the likely cause. Left ventricular failure and respiratory muscle weakness commonly present with breathlessness when lying flat (orthopnoea). This is due to inability of the left ventricle to compensate for the normal increased venous return to the heart on lying down or to embarrassment of the diaphragm in respiratory muscle weakness. However, orthopnoea can be a feature of any severe lung disease. Breathlessness that wakes the patient from sleep is typical of asthma and left ventricular failure (paroxysmal nocturnal dyspnoea). Patients with asthma are typically awoken between 3 and 5 a.m. and have associated wheezing. Breathlessness that is worst first thing on waking in the morning is more typical of COPD and may settle after coughing up sputum.

Patients with exercise-induced asthma may notice that their breathlessness continues to worsen for 5–10 minutes after stopping activity. If asthma is suspected ask directly whether exposure to allergens (e.g. animals, shaking bedding, hoovering, mowing the lawn), irritants with smoke, perfumes, fumes, cold air or drugs (e.g. aspirin) or non-steroidal anti-inflammatory drugs is associated with breathlessness. Breathlessness that improves at the weekend or on holiday is suggestive of occupational asthma or extrinsic allergic alveolitis.

Severity

It is important to determine the severity of breathlessness and the restrictions it imposes on a patient's everyday

activities. Although grading scales for breathlessness have been developed (Table 4.7), they are primarily research tools.

With milder degrees of breathlessness, ask about breathlessness during work, carrying loads, heavy exertion, walking up hills or walking with contemporaries. Breathlessness while walking on the flat, up gentle inclines, and stairs usually indicates a more severe degree of breathlessness. Severely breathless patients are dyspnoeic at rest, walking around the house, getting washed, while dressing, eating or doing light housework.

Ask how far a patient can walk before stopping to rest because of breathlessness. It is often useful to have knowledge of local geography, local shopping centres and the distance from the hospital entrance to the clinic, etc. Estimates of the time taken to walk a distance and number of stops involved, say from home to a local shop, can be a useful serial measurement of progression. Enquiring about hobbies such as golf, gardening, dancing, swimming, hill walking, etc. helps establish the severity of breathlessness and the impact on a patient's quality of life. If a patient has given up any of these activities because of breathlessness, this often suggests a longer period of limitation than the patient admits. This commonly occurs in insidious progressive diseases, e.g. COPD and pulmonary fibrosis.

Associated symptoms

Frequently a thorough history will enable you to limit the list of possible diagnoses to a few conditions by determining the association and time course of breathlessness with or without various combinations of cough, sputum, haemoptysis, chest pain and wheeze. Table 4.8 outlines some combinations of symptoms in acutely breathless patients.

WHEEZE

Wheeze is a high-pitched whistling sound produced by air passing through narrowed small airways. Typically wheeze is limited to, and louder during, expiration. Patients may use 'wheeze' to describe any noise such as rattling sounds originating from secretions in the upper airways or larynx. Wheeze on exercise is a common symptom of asthma and COPD. However, wheezing which causes night wakening is

4.8 Acute breathlessness: commonly associated symptoms
No chest pain
• Pulmonary embolism • Pneumothorax • Metabolic acidosis • Hypovolaemia/shock • Acute left ventricular failure/pulmonary oedema
Pleuritic chest pain
• Pneumonia • Pneumothorax • Pulmonary embolism • Rib fracture
Central chest pain
• Myocardial infarction with left ventricular failure • Massive pulmonary embolism/infarction
Wheeze and cough
• Asthma • COPD

4.9 The Epworth Sleepiness Scale	
For each of the situations outlined in recent everyday life, ask the patient to grade the likelihood of dozing off or falling asleep: 0 = Would never doze 1 = Slight chance of dozing 2 = Moderate chance of dozing 3 = High chance of dozing	
Situation	**Chance of dozing**
Sitting and reading Watching television Sitting inactive in a public place (e.g. a theatre or meeting) As passenger in a car for 1 hour without a break Lying down for a rest in the afternoon when circumstances permit Sitting and talking to someone Sitting quietly after a lunch without alcohol In a car, whilst stopped for a few minutes in traffic	
TOTAL	

a feature of asthma, while wheeze after wakening in the morning suggests COPD. A common mistake is failure to distinguish wheeze from inspiratory stridor caused by the partial occlusion of a large airway by tumour or foreign body.

APNOEA

Apnoea is defined as involuntary absence of breathing for 10 seconds or more. Patients with suspected sleep apnoea/hypopnoea syndrome are commonly referred to respiratory specialists. Apnoea may also be voluntary or can alternate with periods of hyperventilation in Cheyne–Stokes breathing.

The vast majority of apnoeic episodes occur during sleep when the retropharyngeal airway collapses and obstructs the upper airway. Where possible ask the bed partner about these symptoms. The usual description is of very loud snoring followed by an absence of breathing associated with increasing abdominal and thoracic movements. A grunting noise and recurrence of snoring usually accompany the end of the apnoeic episode. Nocturnal apnoea is common but when associated with daytime sleepiness consider a diagnosis of sleep apnoea/hypopnoea syndrome. Assess daytime sleepiness by asking whether patients awaken refreshed and the likelihood of their falling asleep in the morning, after meals, in public places, in meetings, in the evening watching television or when reading. The Epworth scale (Table 4.9) is used to assess daytime sleepiness. A score of 11 or greater is abnormal. Ask whether the patient drives, has fallen asleep at the wheel, has been involved or nearly involved in accidents because of sleepiness or stops frequently when driving for refreshing catnaps. Investigate patients with sleep apnoea, daytime sleepiness and problems driving as a matter of urgency, especially if they drive lorries or buses.

Rarely apnoea occurring during sleep is neuromuscular in origin. This is termed central apnoea and is not usually associated with snoring.

THE HISTORY

Past history

Information about previous respiratory and non-respiratory illnesses can help with the diagnosis and management of current respiratory conditions (Table 4.10).

Drug history

List the patient's current medications. For inhaled therapy detail the type of inhaler, dose in micrograms (not puffs) and frequency. The effects of previously prescribed medications **131**

4.10 Previous history of illness

History	Current implications
Eczema, hayfever	Allergic tendency relevant to asthma
Childhood asthma Recurrent childhood viral associated wheeze	In the past asthma was commonly termed wheezy bronchitis Relevant to adult onset (recurrence of) asthma
Whooping cough, measles	Recognized causes of bronchiectasis, especially if complicated by pneumonia
Pneumonia, pleurisy	Recognized cause of bronchiectasis Recurrent episodes may be a manifestation of bronchiectasis
Tuberculosis	Reactivation if not previously treated effectively Respiratory failure may complicate thoracoplasty Mycetoma in lung cavity may present with haemoptysis
Connective tissue disorders, e.g. rheumatoid arthritis	Lung diseases are recognized complications, e.g. pulmonary fibrosis, effusions, bronchiectasis
Previous malignancy	Recurrence, metastatic, pleural disease Chemotherapeutic agents recognized causes of pulmonary fibrosis Radiotherapy-induced pulmonary fibrosis
Recent travel, immobility,	Pulmonary thromboembolism
Recent surgery, loss of consciousness	Aspiration of foreign body, gastric contents Pneumonia, lung abscess
Neuromuscular disorders	Respiratory failure Aspiration

such as corticosteroids and inhalers on symptoms should be noted. In addition to current medications, enquire about previous medications if drug-induced respiratory disease is suspected (Table 4.11).

Family history

Cystic fibrosis and alpha-1-antitrypsin deficiency have recessive inheritance. There is an inherited predisposition for atopic asthma, and a family history of asthma, eczema and hayfever is common. Take care with 'asthma' in parents or grandparents who were smokers because it may have been misdiagnosed COPD. Diseases such as COPD, lung cancer and tuberculosis often 'run' in families. Although subtle genetic susceptibilities are possible it is more likely that a family history of COPD and lung cancer reflects the increased likelihood of children smoking when parents smoke. A family history of tuberculosis can represent significant past exposure that may reactivate later in life. In patients with asbestos-related disease without obvious occupational exposure, parental occupation may reveal that significant childhood exposure occurred either because of proximity to the parental workplace or as a result of asbestos-contaminated work clothes being brought home for cleaning.

Social history

Take a full social history as described in Chapter 1, and obtain a detailed smoking history. Cigarette smoking is the most important cause of COPD and lung cancer. A smoking history should include the ages when smoking commenced and was given up (if applicable) and average tobacco consumption over the years in terms of cigarettes per day or ounces of tobacco per week. Patients often underestimate the magnitude of their habit. Calculate pack year consumption: smoking one pack of 20 cigarettes a day for a year is equivalent to 'one pack year'. Patients with COPD usually have a consumption of greater than '20 pack years' (p. 17).

Ask about exposure to pets because of their association with asthma (dogs, cats, rodents, horses), allergic alveolitis (birds) and psittacosis pneumonia (parrots and parakeets).

Occupational history

A detailed occupational history is particularly important for respiratory disease (Table 4.12). A history of significant exposure to a recognized hazard may aid diagnosis, have implications for current employment, be the basis of compensation and lead to the prevention of further disease in work colleagues. The changing nature of industry has led to a decrease in exposure to inorganic dusts such as silica, coal dust and asbestos. Nowadays more people are exposed to chemicals, moulds, enzymes, vegetable/plant dusts, animal proteins and drug manufacture, some of which can induce asthma or allergic alveolitis. Patients with occupational lung disease need a detailed occupational history, knowledge of recognized hazardous exposures and consideration of as yet unrecognized hazards.

4.11 Examples of drug-induced respiratory conditions

Respiratory condition	Drug
Bronchoconstriction	Beta-blockers Opioids Non-steroidal anti-inflammatory drugs
Cough	Angiotensin-converting enzyme inhibitors
Bronchiolitis obliterans	Penicillamine

Diffuse parenchymal lung disease	Cytotoxic agents:
	    bleomycin
	    methotrexate
	Anti-inflammatory agents:
	    sulfasalazine
	    penicillamine
	    gold salts
	    aspirin
	Cardiovascular drugs:
	    amiodarone
	    hydrallazine
	Antibiotics:
	    nitrofurantoin
	Intravenous drug misuse
	Radiation

Pulmonary thromboembolism	Oestrogens
Pulmonary hypertension	Oestrogens Dexfenfluramine, fenfluramine
Pleural effusion	Amiodarone Nitrofurantoin Phenytoin Methotrexate Pergolide

4.12 Examples of occupational lung disease

Lung disease	Exposure	Occupation
Pulmonary fibrosis	Asbestos	Shipyard/construction workers, plumbers Boilermakers
	Quartz (silica)	Miners, quarry workers Stone masons
	Coal	Coal miners
	Beryllium	Nuclear, aerospace industries
COPD/emphysema	Coal	Coal miners
Malignancy	Asbestos	Shipyard/construction workers, plumbers Boilermakers
	Radon	Metal mining
Byssinosis	Cotton, flax, hemp	Cotton, flax, hemp manufacturing
Extrinsic allergic alveolitis	Thermophilic actinomycetes	Farmer's lung Mushroom worker's lung Air conditioner lung Humidifier fever
	Budgies, pigeons	Bird fancier's lung
Asthma	Animals	Vets, laboratory workers
	Grains, flour	Farmers, bakers, millers
	Hardwood dusts	Joiners, carpenters
	Colophony	Soldering
	Enzymes	Detergent manufacturing Pharmaceuticals
	Isocyanates	Spray painting, varnishing
	Epoxy resins	Adhesives, varnishing
	Drugs	Pharmaceutical industry
	Formaldehyde	Hospital workers
	Paraldehyde	

A thorough occupational history includes all occupations, full and part time, held since the patient left school and the number of years spent in each job. It is not sufficient to merely record job title because many innocuous titles hide significant direct or indirect hazardous exposures. For each occupation determine exactly what the job entailed and the length of any exposure. Ask about the relationship between symptoms development and the time in the job. Some occupational diseases are worse at the beginning of the working week (byssinosis, humidifier fever) while occupational asthma is characteristically worse at the end of the working week, with symptoms usually improving during holidays. Specifically ask about exposure to dust or asbestos and whether other workers have similar symptoms.

EXAMINATION OF THE RESPIRATORY SYSTEM

GENERAL EXAMINATION

Examination of the respiratory system is incomplete without a simultaneous general assessment. Observe patients as you first meet them, looking particularly for breathlessness, weight loss, mental state, etc.

Respiratory rate

Observe whether the patient is breathless at rest. Observe chest movements (surreptitiously) while feeling the pulse, and count the number of respirations per minute. Tachypnoea is a respiratory rate > 15/min and is caused by increased ventilatory drive as in fever, asthma and COPD, or reduced **133** ventilatory capacity as in pneumonia, pulmonary oedema and interstitial lung disease. A respiratory rate > 30/min is the most important prognostic sign associated with death in community-acquired pneumonia. A slow respiratory rate can occur in association with opioid toxicity, hypothyroidism, raised intracranial pressure, hypothalamic lesions, and hypercapnia.

Breathing patterns

Cheyne–Stokes breathing, or periodic respiration, is characterized by a period of increasing rate and depth of breathing followed by diminishing respiratory effort and rate, usually ending in a period of apnoea or hypopnoea. The cycle then repeats. This pattern of breathing relates to an altered sensitivity of the respiratory centre to chemical control and delay in circulation time between the lung and chemoreceptors. It is seen most frequently in stroke involving the brain stem, and in severe cardiac failure. However, it may be normal during sleep in the elderly.

Hyperventilation is a common response to acute anxiety or emotional distress and is often associated with respiratory alkalosis with low arterial carbon dioxide tension. Decreased intracellular potassium and magnesium and extracellular calcium develop because of respiratory alkalosis. Breathing is often deep, irregular and sighing, and patients often describe an inability to fill their lungs completely. When acute hyperventilation is sustained, tetany and occasionally grand mal seizure can occur.

Hyperventilation with deep, sighing respirations (Küssmaul respiration) is a response to the reduced arterial pH in metabolic acidosis. This can occur in acute renal failure, lactic acidosis, diabetic ketoacidosis and in salicylate and methanol poisoning. Although patients may not be aware of breathlessness their respiratory rate increases and they appear to have 'air hunger'.

Use of accessory muscles

While assessing the rate and pattern of breathing look to see if the accessory muscles of respiration are being used. These include the sternocleidomastoids, platysma and pectoral muscles. When the shoulder girdle is fixed they cause elevation of the shoulders with inspiration and thereby increased chest expansion. Use of accessory muscles is characteristic of patients with COPD who have hyperinflated lungs.

Stridor

Stridor is a harsh, rasping or croaking noise heard on inspiration, which may be aggravated by coughing. Common causes are foreign body or tumour partially occluding the larynx, trachea or a main bronchus. If you suspect stridor ask the patient to cough and then breathe deeply in and out with the mouth wide open. Listen carefully close to the patient's mouth. Always investigate stridor.

Hoarseness

Hoarseness is a change in quality of the voice, which may vary from slight harshness (dysphonia) to complete loss (aphonia). Usually hoarseness is due to inflammation of the larynx caused by viral infection. However, a change in voice in a patient with lung cancer suggests invasion of the left recurrent laryngeal nerve at the hilum. In such cases the left vocal cord cannot adduct to the midline, resulting in failure to produce a normal explosive cough (Fig. 4.3). The cough is then prolonged, low pitched and 'bovine'.

Cyanosis

Cyanosis is an abnormal blue discoloration of the skin and mucous membranes. Central cyanosis is seen in the lips and tongue and is usually due to arterial hypoxaemia. Methaemoglobinaemia, sulphhaemoglobinaemia and right-to-left intracardiac shunts (Eisenmenger's syndrome) are rarer possibilities. Cyanosis is defined as an absolute concentration of deoxygenated haemoglobin of > 50 g/l. In patients with a normal haemoglobin concentration central cyanosis can be detected when the arterial oxygen saturation falls below 90%, corresponding to an arterial oxygen tension of approximately 8 kPa (60 mmHg). In anaemia or hypovolaemia, patients rarely have central cyanosis because severe hypoxia is required to produce the necessary concentration of deoxygenated haemoglobin. In contrast,

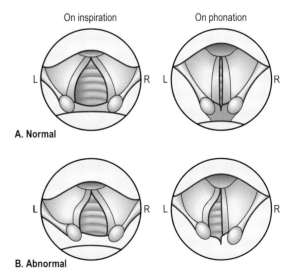

Fig. 4.3 The vocal cords. Diagrammatic representation of the laryngoscopic views of vocal cord movements showing: (A) normal movements; (B) movements in the presence of recurrent laryngeal nerve paralysis most commonly caused by lung cancer. Note that the paralysed left cord is in the cadaveric position (between inspiration and expiration).

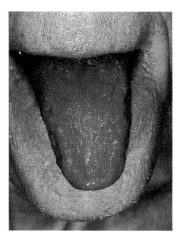

Fig. 4.4 Central cyanosis of the tongue.

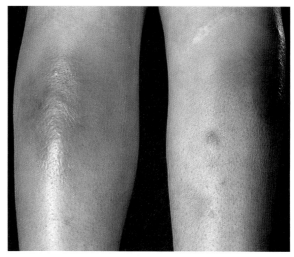

Fig. 4.5 Erythema nodosum.

patients with polycythaemia can become cyanosed at higher arterial oxygen tensions.

Cyanosis can be difficult to detect and requires good lighting conditions. It may be particularly difficult to see in black and Asian patients. Ask the patient to extend the tongue, and look carefully at the lips and tongue (Fig. 4.4).

Blood pressure

Hypotension is an important feature of septicaemia, and a diastolic pressure of 60 mmHg or less is associated with increased mortality in community-acquired pneumonia. In pneumothorax hypotension may indicate the development of tension pneumothorax with reduction in venous return to the heart and risk of cardiac arrest. Hypotension may also be a feature of life-threatening asthma.

Skin appearances

Several respiratory disorders are associated with skin changes. Acute sarcoidosis presents with the red nodular tender lesions of erythema nodosum over the shins (Fig. 4.5) and occasionally the extensor aspects of the forearms. It is often associated with bilateral hilar enlargement on chest X-ray. Lupus pernio is a waxy, purplish, maculopapular rash over the nose and cheeks seen in cutaneous sarcoidosis. Occasionally raised firm non-tender subcutaneous nodules are seen in patients with disseminated cancer (Fig. 4.6).

Hands

Finger clubbing

Clubbing of fingers and toes is an important physical sign (Fig. 4.7). Four criteria confirm clubbing:

- loss of the normal angle between the nail and nail bed
- increased nail bed fluctuation

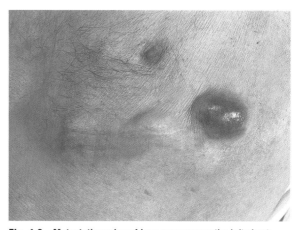

Fig. 4.6 Metastatic nodes of lung cancer over the left chest.

- increased nail curvature in later stages
- increased bulk of the soft tissues over the terminal phalanges.

To examine for finger clubbing, first look across the nail and nail bed at the 'nail bed angle'. This is normally obtuse but disappears in the early stages of finger clubbing. To detect nail bed fluctuation place both thumbs under the pulp of the terminal phalanx and attempt to move the nail within the nail bed using your index fingers (Fig. 4.8). A 'spongy feel' confirms nail bed fluctuation.

The majority of patients with clubbing have thoracic disease but it is also associated with gastrointestinal disorders and can be familial in otherwise normal subjects (Table 4.13). Rarely clubbing can develop over several weeks, as in empyema. If the underlying cause is successfully treated clubbing may resolve.

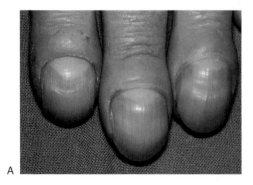

A

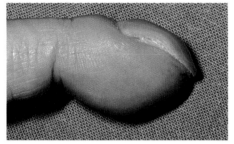

B

Fig. 4.7 Clubbing. (A) Anterior and (B) lateral view.

4.13 Causes of clubbing and hypertrophic pulmonary osteoarthropathy	
Thoracic	
Tumours: benign or malignant	Lung cancer Mesothelioma Pleural fibroma Oesophageal cancer Oesophageal leiomyoma Thymoma Atrial myxoma
Sepsis	Bronchiectasis Empyema Lung abscess Cystic fibrosis Bacterial endocarditis
Interstitial lung disease	Fibrosing alveolitis Asbestosis
Arteriovenous shunting	AV malformations in the lung Cyanotic congenital heart disease
Non-thoracic	
	Hepatic cirrhosis Coeliac disease Ulcerative colitis Crohn's disease
Familial	

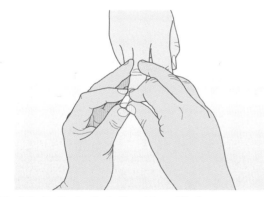

Fig. 4.8   Testing for fluctuation of the nail bed.

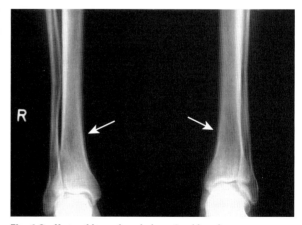

Fig. 4.9   X-ray of lower legs in hypertrophic pulmonary osteoarthropathy. Arrows show periosteal reaction.

Hypertrophic pulmonary osteoarthropathy

Very occasionally clubbing may progress to hypertrophic pulmonary osteoarthropathy. This is almost always associated with lung cancer, usually squamous cancer. Pronounced clubbing of fingers and toes is associated with pain and swelling affecting the wrists and ankles. X-rays of the distal forearm and lower legs show subperiosteal new bone formation separate from the cortex of the long bones (Fig. 4.9). Isotope bone scanning demonstrates increased activity and often the serum alkaline phosphatase is raised.

The pathogenesis of clubbing and hypertrophic pulmonary osteoarthropathy is unclear but may be neurogenic, hormonal or related to arteriovenous shunting.

Discoloration of the fingers and nails

Cigarette smoking produces a brownish stain on the fingers and nails. This discoloration is caused by tar and not by nicotine, which is colourless. Rarely nails can appear yellow or greenish as in 'yellow nails syndrome' which is associated with lymphoedema and an exudative pleural effusion (Fig. 4.10).

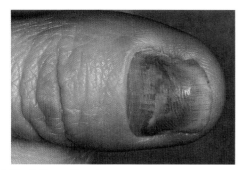

Fig. 4.10 Yellow nail syndrome.

4.14	Examples of eye conditions in respiratory disease
Condition	**Respiratory disorder**
Horner's syndrome	Apical lung cancer
Iridocyclitis	Tuberculosis Sarcoidosis
Chemosis, conjunctival and retinal vein dilatation	Carbon dioxide retention Superior vena caval obstruction
Choroidal tubercles	Miliary tuberculosis
Choroidal metastases	Disseminated cancer

Peripheral cyanosis

Peripheral cyanosis is a bluish discoloration of the fingers and toes indicating tissue hypoxia usually due to circulatory disorders or cold. Peripheral cyanosis can also occur with severe central cyanosis. Compare the colour of the patient's hands with your own.

Tremor

The commonest tremor in patients with respiratory disorders is a fine finger tremor similar to that in hyperthyroidism caused by excessive use of beta-agonist or theophylline bronchodilator drugs.

A flapping tremor (*asterixis*) is found in patients with severe ventilatory failure and carbon dioxide retention. Carbon dioxide is a vasodilator and these patients also have warm peripheries and a large-volume pulse. A similar flapping tremor can occur in other metabolic disorders such as liver failure and advanced renal failure and in acute focal parietal or thalamic lesions. It is the result of intermittent failure of the parietal mechanisms required to maintain posture. Ask the patient to hold out the arms with the hands extended at the wrists. This posture is periodically dropped, usually every 2–3 seconds, and then resumed resulting in a jerky, flapping tremor. Asking the patient to squeeze your index and middle fingers and maintain this for 30–60 seconds can also produce this tremor.

Face

The eye can be involved in respiratory disease in various ways (Table. 4.14).

Horner's syndrome (Fig. 4.11) occurs when sympathetic nerves are interrupted in the neck or brain stem. In most cases this is due to lung cancer at the apex of the lung invading the sympathetic chain at or above the stellate ganglion. This results in:

- ipsilateral partial ptosis
- ipsilateral constricted pupil (miosis)

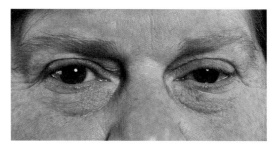

Fig. 4.11 Left Horner's syndrome.

- enophthalmos
- ipsilateral impaired sweating of the face.

Neck

Jugular venous pressure (JVP)

The JVP (p. 94) is raised in various forms of right-sided heart failure. Chronic hypoxia as in COPD leads to pulmonary arterial vasoconstriction, pulmonary hypertension, right heart dilatation and consequent elevation in the JVP. This is known as *cor pulmonale*. The JVP is also high if the intrathoracic pressure is raised as in tension pneumothorax or severe acute asthma. In major pulmonary embolism the JVP may be so elevated that it is missed in the semirecumbent position.

In superior vena caval obstruction (Fig. 4.12) the JVP is raised and non-pulsatile and the abdominojugular reflex is absent. The vast majority of cases are due to lung cancer compressing the superior vena cava. Other causes include lymphoma, thymoma and mediastinal fibrosis. Superior vena caval obstruction progresses to produce drowsiness, a sense of fullness in the head, swelling and cyanosis of the face, neck and arms, and occasionally retinal vein engorgement and papilloedema.

Constrictive pericarditis can be caused by tuberculosis and rheumatoid disease. This produces an elevated JVP with steep 'y' descent and inspiratory rise ('Küssmaul's **137**

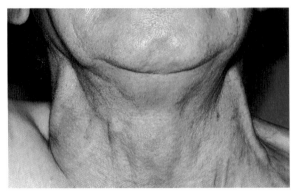

A

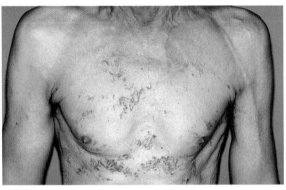

B

Fig. 4.12 Superior vena caval obstruction. (A) Distended neck veins. (B) Dilated superficial veins over chest.

sign'). Similar signs can occur in a large pericardial effusion causing cardiac tamponade.

Neck nodes

Examination of cervical and supraclavicular lymph glands in general and the scalene lymph nodes in particular is an important part of examination of the respiratory system. For instance, scalene lymph node enlargement may be the first evidence of metastatic lung cancer and localized cervical lymphadenopathy is a common presenting feature of lymphoma.

Examine neck nodes from behind with the patient sitting. The groups of cervical and supraclavicular lymph nodes are illustrated in Figure 4.13. The scalene lymph nodes are located adjacent to the first rib next to the insertion of the scalenus anterior muscle (Fig. 4.14). Palpate one side of the neck at a time using the fingers of one hand. Feel the scalene nodes with the patient's head slightly tilted to that side (see Fig. 2.22B, p. 51). Place your index finger between the clavicle and sternocleidomastoid muscle and press down gently towards the first rib. A palpable scalene node is felt as a soft mobile mass just above the hard first rib (Fig. 4.14).

Note the size and consistency of the palpable node and whether it is fixed to surrounding structures. For example in Hodgkin's disease, the lymph nodes are typically 'rubbery'; in dental sepsis and tonsillitis they are usually tender; in tuberculosis and metastatic cancer they are often 'matted' together to form a mass; and calcified lymph glands feel stony hard. Palpable lymph nodes fixed to deep structures or skin are usually malignant.

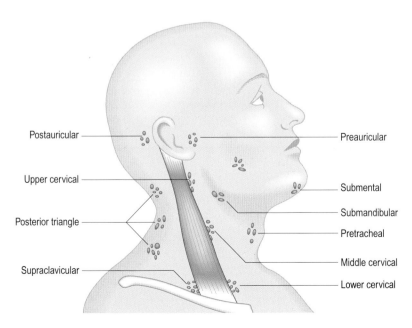

Fig. 4.13 The lymph node groupings in the neck.

Postauricular — Preauricular
Upper cervical — Submental
Posterior triangle — Submandibular / Pretracheal
Supraclavicular — Middle cervical / Lower cervical

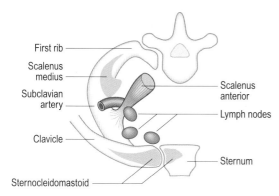

Fig. 4.14   Relation of lymph nodes to scalenus anterior.

EXAMINATION OF THE THORAX

Examine patients with their chest and upper abdomen fully exposed and evenly illuminated. If patients are not acutely ill ask them to sit over the edge of a bed or on a chair.

Inspection

Look carefully at the chest. The normal chest is bilaterally symmetrical and elliptical in cross-section. Look for scars of previous heart or lung surgery and for swellings, marks and spots on the skin. Subcutaneous lesions may be visible, including metastatic tumour nodules, neurofibromas and lipomas. Look for vascular anomalies such as spider naevi and enlarged arterial vascular channels in coarctation of the aorta and venous vascular channels in superior vena caval obstruction (Fig. 4.12B).

Abnormalities in the shape of the chest

Increase in anteroposterior diameter.   When the anteroposterior diameter is increased compared with the lateral diameter, the chest is described as 'barrel shaped'. This is associated with lung hyperinflation as seen in patients with severe COPD (Fig. 4.15A). However, the degree of chest deformity does not correlate with the severity of airways obstruction.

Kyphosis and scoliosis.   Kyphosis is an exaggerated anterior curvature of the spine and scoliosis is lateral curvature. Kyphoscoliosis involving both deformities (Fig. 4.15B) may be idiopathic or secondary to childhood poliomyelitis or spinal tuberculosis. Such deformity can be grossly disfiguring and disabling in otherwise healthy individuals. Severe kyphoscoliosis may cause reduced ventilatory capacity and increased work of breathing. These patients develop progressive ventilatory failure with carbon dioxide retention and cor pulmonale at an early age.

Pectus carinatum (pigeon chest).   This is a localized prominence of the sternum and adjacent costal cartilages often accompanied by indrawing of the ribs to form symmetrical horizontal grooves ('Harrison's sulci') above the costal margin (Fig. 4.15C). These deformities result from lung hyperinflation with repeated vigorous contractions of the diaphragm while the bony thorax is still in a pliable prepubertal state. It is most often caused by severe and poorly controlled childhood asthma but can occur in osteomalacia and rickets.

Pectus excavatum (funnel chest).   This is a developmental deformity with localized depression of the lower end of the sternum (Fig. 4.15D) or, less commonly, depression of the whole length of the sternum. The patient is usually asymptomatic but may express concern about the appearance of the deformity. In severe cases the heart is displaced to the left and the ventilatory capacity is reduced.

Palpation

Position of the mediastinum

Determine the position of the mediastinum by examination of the trachea and cardiac apex beat.

Upper mediastinal shift causes deviation of the trachea. From in front of the patient place the tip of your right index finger into the suprasternal notch and press gently against the trachea (Fig. 4.16). This can be uncomfortable, so be gentle and explain what you are doing. With the patient looking directly forwards, any deviation of the trachea from the midline is assessed using touch and vision. Slight displacement to the right is common in normal people. Causes of tracheal deviation are listed in Table 4.15.

Deviation of the cardiac apex beat indicates shift of the lower mediastinum. Displacement of the cardiac impulse without deviation of the trachea is usually due to left ventricular enlargement but can also occur in scoliosis, kyphoscoliosis, or severe pectus excavatum. The cardiac apex beat may be difficult to localize in obesity, pericardial

4.15   Causes of tracheal deviation
Towards the side of the lung lesion
• Upper lobe or lung collapse • Upper lobe fibrosis • Pneumonectomy
Away from the side of the lung lesion
• Tension pneumothorax • Massive pleural effusion
Upper mediastinal mass
• Retrosternal goitre • Lymphoma • Lung cancer

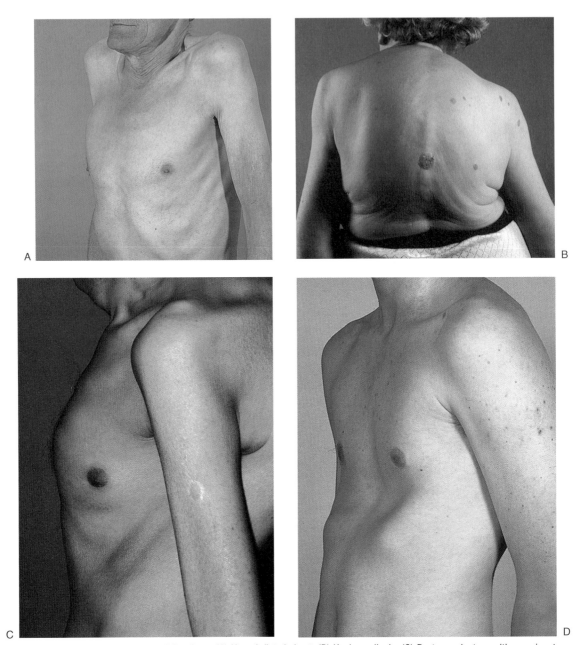

Fig. 4.15 Abnormalities in the shape of the chest. (A) Hyperinflated chest. (B) Kyphoscoliosis. (C) Pectus carinatum with prominent Harrison's sulcus. (D) Pectus excavatum.

effusion, poor left ventricular function or patients with lung hyperinflation as in COPD. The heave of right ventricular hypertrophy, found in severe pulmonary hypertension, is best felt at the left sternal edge.

The distance between the suprasternal notch and cricoid cartilage is normally three to four finger breadths. Reduction in this distance suggests lung hyperinflation. A 'tracheal tug' can be found in severe hyperinflation when fingers resting on the trachea move inferiorly with each inspiration.

Chest expansion

Both sides of the thorax should expand equally during tidal and maximal inspiration. Assess expansion of the upper

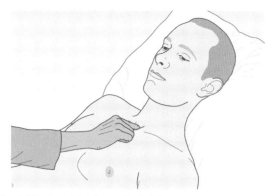

Fig. 4.16 Examining for tracheal shift.

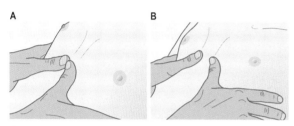

Fig. 4.17 Assessing chest expansion from front. (A) Expiration; (B) Inspiration.

lobes by observing the clavicles from behind during tidal breathing. Diminished movement on one side indicates abnormality on that side. To assess expansion of the lower lobes place your hands firmly on the chest wall with fingers extending around the sides of the chest (Fig. 4.17). Your thumbs should almost meet in the midline and should be slightly lifted off the chest so they are free to move with respiration. Ask the patient to take a deep breath. Your thumbs should move symmetrically apart at least 5 cm. Reduced expansion on one side indicates abnormality on that side, e.g. pleural effusion, lung or lobar collapse, pneumothorax and unilateral fibrosis. Bilateral reduction in chest wall movement is common in advanced COPD and diffuse pulmonary fibrosis.

With the patient supine look for paradoxical inward movement of the abdomen during inspiration, which may indicate diaphragmatic paralysis or more commonly severe COPD. Localized indrawing of the chest wall is seen in those who sustain double fractures of a series of ribs or of the sternum. The chest wall between the fractures becomes mobile or 'flail' and is sucked in with every inspiration and out during expiration producing paradoxical movement (see p. 388).

Other abnormalities on palpation of the thorax include subcutaneous emphysema, which produces a characteristic crackling sensation over gas-containing tissue. This may also cause diffuse swelling of the chest wall, neck and face. Subcutaneous emphysema is a complication of intercostal drainage of a pneumothorax. Mediastinal emphysema may complicate severe acute asthma and ruptured oesophagus. In this situation gas tracks into the mediastinum and then escapes into the soft tissues of the neck and face producing subcutaneous emphysema.

Tenderness over the costal cartilages is found in the costochondritis of Tietze's syndrome. Localized rib tenderness can be found over areas of pulmonary infarction or fracture.

Percussion

Percussion allows you to listen for the pitch and loudness of the percussed note and feel for post-percussive vibrations. It is performed in sequence over equivalent areas on the two sides of the chest (Fig. 4.18).

If you are right-handed place the palm of your left hand on the chest with fingers slightly separated (Fig. 4.19). Press the middle finger of your left hand firmly against the chest, aligned with the underlying ribs over the area to be percussed. Strike the centre of the middle phalanx of your left middle finger with the tip of your right middle finger using a loose swinging movement arising from the wrist and not the forearm. Remove the percussing finger quickly so the note generated is not dampened. Percuss the lung apices by placing the palmar surface of your left middle finger across the anterior border of the trapezius muscle, overlapping the supraclavicular fossa and directing percussion downwards. Percuss the clavicle directly within its medial third. Percussion of the clavicle more laterally merely produces dullness from the muscle masses of the shoulder. During percussion of the upper posterior chest move the scapulae laterally by asking patients to fold their arms across the front of their chest. Avoid percussing near the midline as this produces a dull note from the solid structures of the thoracic spine and paravertebral musculature. Map out abnormal areas by percussing from resonant to dull.

Percussion of normal lung produces a resonant note (Table 4.16). Pneumothorax produces a hyperresonant note. Percussion over solid structures such as the liver, heart or a consolidated area of lung produces a dull note. Find the upper level of liver dullness by percussing down the anterior wall of the right chest. Normally in adults the upper level of liver dullness is at the level of the 5th rib in the midclavicular line. Resonance below this is a sign of hyperinflation as occurs in COPD or severe asthma. The area of cardiac dullness present on the left anterior chest may be decreased when the lungs are hyperinflated. Percussion over a fluid-filled area, such as a pleural effusion, produces an extremely dull note, known as 'stony dull'. Basal dullness due to elevation of the diaphragm is easily confused with pleural fluid.

A

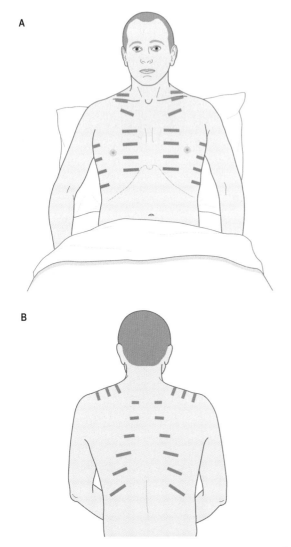

B

Fig. 4.18 **Sites for percussion.** (A) Anterior and lateral chest wall. (B) Posterior chest wall.

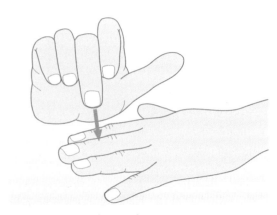

Fig. 4.19 **Technique of percussion.**

4.16 Percussion note	
Type	**Detected over**
Resonant	Normal lung
Hyperresonant	Pneumothorax
Dull	Pulmonary consolidation Pulmonary collapse Severe pulmonary fibrosis
'Stony dull'	Pleural effusion Haemothorax

⊙ Examine this patient with pleuritic chest pain

1. General examination assessing the degree and site of pain.
2. Examine for fever, confusion and raised respiratory rate – all found in *pneumonia*.
3. Look for vasculitic skin spots (*pulmonary vasculitis*).
4. Examine JVP – raised in *massive pulmonary embolism*.
5. Palpate chest wall for tenderness – found in *trauma, fractured rib* and sometimes *pulmonary embolism*.
6. Percuss the chest – area of dullness is consistent with *consolidation* (*pneumonia*) or *pleural effusion* (*pulmonary embolism*).
7. Auscultate chest – bronchial breathing found over area of *consolidation* (*pneumonia*); reduced air entry over *pleural effusion* (*pulmonary embolism*); pleural friction rub heard over *consolidation* (*pneumonia*), *pulmonary embolism* with effusion and sometimes *rib fracture*.
8. Examine lower legs for signs of deep vein thrombosis (*pulmonary embolism*).

Auscultation

The stethoscope was invented by a French physician, Laennec, who described most of the signs on auscultation of the chest in 1819.

Most sounds reaching the chest wall are low frequency and you should listen with the bell of the stethoscope. The diaphragm is best used for locating pleural or pericardial friction rubs, the high-pitched early diastolic murmur of aortic incompetence or detecting bowel sounds in the abdomen. Stretching of the skin and hairs under the diaphragm during deep breathing can produce anomalous noises like crackles, and in thin patients it may be difficult to achieve full contact between the diaphragm and skin of the chest wall.

Listen with the patient relaxed and breathing deeply through an open mouth. Avoid prolonged deep breathing as this can cause giddiness and even tetany. Auscultate both sides alternately, avoiding the midline, comparing findings over a large number of equivalent positions to ensure that localized abnormalities are not missed. Listen anteriorly from above the clavicle down to the 6th rib, laterally from the axilla to the 8th rib and posteriorly down to the level of the 11th rib. In each area listen to the quality and amplitude of the breath sounds. Identify any gap between inspiration and expiration and listen for any added sounds. Avoid auscultation within 3 cm of the midline anteriorly or posteriorly as these areas may transmit sounds directly from the trachea or main bronchi. Finally, assess the quality and amplitude of vocal resonance by asking the patient to say 'one, one, one'. In the normal lung a whispered note will not be heard but over consolidated lung, as in pneumonia, the sound is transmitted producing 'whispering pectoriloquy'.

Normal breath sounds

Normal breath sounds heard at the chest wall are caused by turbulent flow in large airways. When heard through a stethoscope these normal breath sounds have a rustling quality and are said to be 'vesicular'. The larynx makes little contribution in quiet breathing but may accentuate the noise in deep respiration.

The pattern and intensity of breath sounds reflect regional ventilation. In the normal upright lung, breath sounds are loudest at the apex in early inspiration and at the bases in mid-inspiration. During expiration, normal breath sounds rapidly fade because of decreasing airflow. In their passage through normal lungs the intensity and frequency of the sounds are decreased since normal lung parenchyma transmits sounds poorly.

Bronchial breathing

Bronchial breathing is characterized by breath sounds that are high-pitched with a hollow or blowing quality similar to those heard over the trachea and larynx during tidal breathing. The breath sounds are of similar length and intensity in both inspiration and expiration and have a characteristic pause between (Fig. 4.20). Bronchial breath sounds are found whenever normal lung tissue is replaced by uniformly conducting tissue, whether through consolidation, fibrosis or collapse *and* the relevant major bronchus is patent (Table 4.17). The presence of bronchial breathing is confirmed by finding whispering pectoriloquy. Vocal resonance is also increased over consolidated lung, which readily transmits sound.

Bronchial breathing and whispering pectoriloquy are heard most commonly over areas of pulmonary consolidation but can sometimes be heard over areas of collapse or dense fibrosis if the underlying major bronchus is patent. The presence of bronchial breathing, therefore, tends to exclude the possibility of an obstructing lung cancer. Both may also be heard at the top of a pleural effusion.

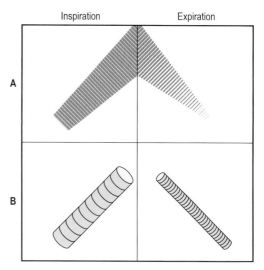

Fig. 4.20 Diagrammatic representation of breath sounds. (A) Vesicular. (B) Bronchial. Note the gap between inspiration and expiration and change in pitch and the blowing, tubular quality of bronchial breath sounds.

4.17	Causes of bronchial breath sounds
Common	
• Lung consolidation (pneumonia)	
Uncommon	
• Localized pulmonary fibrosis • At the top of a pleural effusion • Collapsed lung (where the underlying major bronchus is patent)	

The intensity of breath sounds relates to airflow and the tissue through which the sound travels. Diminished vesicular breathing therefore occurs in obesity, pleural effusion, marked pleural thickening, pneumothorax, hyperinflation due to COPD, and over an area of collapse where the underlying major bronchus is occluded (Table 4.18). If breath sounds appear reduced ask the patient to cough. If the reduced breath sounds are due to bronchial obstruction

4.18	Causes of diminished vesicular breathing
Reduced conduction	
• Obesity/thick chest wall • Pleural effusion or thickening • Pneumothorax	
Reduced air flow	
• Generalized, e.g. COPD • Localized, e.g. collapsed lung due to occluding lung cancer	

by secretions they are likely to become more audible after coughing.

Aegophony is a bleating or nasal sound heard over consolidated lung or at the upper level of a pleural effusion. It is due to enhanced transmission of high-frequency noise across abnormal lung with lower frequencies filtered out.

Added sounds

Crackles. Interrupted non-musical sounds are called crackles. The terms rales and crepitations should be abandoned. Crackles usually result from loss of stability of peripheral airways, which collapse on expiration. With high inspiratory pressures air enters rapidly into these distal airways with abrupt opening of alveoli and small bronchi, producing the characteristic crackling noise.

Note when crackles occur within the respiratory cycle. Early inspiratory crackles suggest small airways disease and can occur in bronchiolitis (Table 4.19). In pulmonary oedema crackles occur in mid-inspiration. Fine late inspiratory crackles, which sound similar to rubbing hair between the fingers, are characteristic of pulmonary fibrosis. Crackles may also be heard when air bubbles through secretions in major bronchi, dilated bronchi as in bronchiectasis or in pulmonary cavities. These crackles sound coarse, have a gurgling quality and change with coughing if the secretions are dislodged. Crackles throughout inspiration and expiration are characteristic of bronchiectasis.

Wheeze. Wheezes have a musical quality and should be timed in relation to the respiratory cycle. The term, rhonchus, should be abandoned. The sound is due to continuous oscillation of opposing airway walls and implies airway narrowing. Wheeze tends to be louder on expiration because airways normally dilate during inspiration and narrow on expiration. Inspiratory wheeze therefore implies severe airway narrowing. High-pitched wheeze arises from smaller airways and has a whistling quality, while low-pitched wheeze originates from larger bronchi. However, wheeze alone is a poor guide to the severity of airflow obstruction. In severe airways obstruction wheeze may be absent because of reduced airflow producing a 'silent chest'.

Wheeze is characteristic of asthma and COPD. A fixed bronchial obstruction, most commonly due to lung cancer, may cause localized wheeze with a single musical note that does not clear on coughing. It is very important to distinguish wheeze from inspiratory stridor.

Pleural friction rub. A pleural rub is produced when inflamed parietal and visceral pleura move over one another. This creates a creaking sound similar to that produced by bending stiff leather. It is best heard with the diaphragm of the stethoscope. It may be heard only on deep breathing at the end of inspiration and beginning of expiration. A pleural rub is usually associated with pleuritic pain and may be heard over areas of inflamed pleura in pulmonary thromboembolism, pneumonia and pulmonary vasculitis. If the pleura adjacent to the pericardium is involved a pleuropericardial rub may also be heard. Pleural friction rubs disappear if an effusion separates the pleural surfaces.

Pneumothorax click. This is a rhythmical sound synchronous with cardiac systole, produced when there is air between the two layers of pleura overlying the heart.

▶ Examination sequence

→ Note the patient's general appearance and demeanour.
→ Observe respiratory rate and pattern of breathing, and look for use of accessory muscles.
→ Listen for hoarseness and stridor.
→ Look for central cyanosis.

Examine this patient with acute breathlessness

1. Assess severity of dyspnoea and record respiratory rate per minute.
2. Look for evidence of weight loss or anaemia.
3. Examine pulse for tachycardia, arrhythmias (*cardiac disease*) or bradycardia (*cardiac disease* or severe hypoxia).
4. Measure blood pressure – hypotension found in *septicaemia* and *acute asthma*.
5. Examine tongue and lips for central cyanosis (*severe hypoxia*).
6. Examine JVP – raised in *cardiac failure*, *cor pulmonale* or *massive pulmonary thromboembolism*.
7. Palpate trachea and apex beat for mediastinal shift – displaced away from the lesion in *tension pneumothorax* or *massive pleural effusion*; toward the lesion in *lobar or lung collapse*.
8. Palpate for chest expansion – reduced in *pleural effusion*, *consolidation* (*pneumonia*), *lung or lobar collapse* or *pneumothorax*.
9. Percuss over the chest, e.g. hyperresonant note may indicate *pneumothorax*, dull note indicates *consolidation* (*pneumonia*), or *lung or lobar collapse* and a 'stony dull' note is usually found with *pleural effusion*.
10. Auscultate the chest – unilateral early inspiratory crackles (*bronchial infection* or *pneumonia*), bilateral basal medium crackles (*pulmonary oedema*), bilateral fine late inspiratory crackles (*fibrosing alveolitis*), bronchial breathing (*pneumonia*) and reduced breath sounds (*lung or lobar collapse* or *pleural effusion*).
11. Examine lower limb for pitting oedema (bilateral in *cor pulmonale* or *heart failure*; unilateral in *deep vein thrombosis*).

4.19 Causes of crackles	
Phase of inspiration	**Cause**
Early	Small airways disease as in bronchiolitis
Middle	Pulmonary oedema
Late	Pulmonary fibrosis (fine) Pulmonary oedema (medium) Bronchial secretions in COPD, pneumonia, etc. (coarse) lung abscess, tubercular lung cavities (coarse)
Biphasic	Bronchiectasis (coarse)

1. General examination looking for evidence of weight loss, anaemia, iron deficiency, and bruising.
2. Examine hands for finger clubbing (*lung cancer* or *bronchiectasis*).
3. Feel neck for lymphadenopathy, especially scalene nodes (*lung cancer* or *lymphoma*).
4. Inspect chest, e.g. for previous lung resection (*lung cancer* or *bronchiectasis*).
5. Palpate trachea and apex beat for mediastinal shift (*lung or lobar collapse* due to *lung cancer*).
6. Percuss for dullness, e.g. effusion (*lung cancer, mesothelioma, tuberculous effusion*, etc.).
7. Auscultate for biphasic crackles (*bronchiectasis*) or reduced air entry (*lung or lobar collapse* due to *lung cancer*, or *effusion* due to *lung cancer* or *mesothelioma*).

→ Measure the blood pressure.
→ Examine the skin for rashes and nodules.
→ Examine hands for finger clubbing, peripheral cyanosis and tremor.
→ Examine neck for raised jugular venous pressure (JVP) and cervical lymphadenopathy.
→ Inspect chest front and back for abnormalities of shape and scars.
→ Feel trachea and cardiac apex beat for evidence of mediastinal shift.
→ Percuss chest front and back for areas of dullness or hyperresonance.
→ Listen to chest front and back for altered breath sounds and added sounds.

INTEGRATION OF PHYSICAL SIGNS

Certain groups of physical signs are typically associated with particular pathological changes in the lungs and pleura.

However, some signs may be absent. Examine the thorax carefully before deciding which disease process is involved (Fig. 4.22).

After examination of the respiratory system a differential diagnosis can be made which will need to be confirmed or refuted by further investigations (Fig. 4.21).

◆ Key points

♦ Night-time wakening with cough and wheeze is characteristic of poorly controlled asthma.
♦ In adult-onset asthma always consider occupational causes.
♦ Consider sleep apnoea in patients who snore and have daytime sleepiness. Ask specifically about driving and occupational risks.
♦ In patients with a normal chest X-ray persistent cough is usually caused by smoking, asthma, gastro-oesophageal reflux, sinusitis or angiotensin-converting enzyme inhibitors.
♦ Patients with severe COPD may lose weight.
♦ In suspected pneumonia, respiratory rate, blood pressure and mental state are important markers of severity.
♦ Always investigate haemoptysis in a smoker by chest X-ray and, if appropriate, bronchoscopy.
♦ 'Bovine cough' or superior vena caval obstruction in a patient with lung cancer indicates that the tumour is inoperable.
♦ Bronchial breathing is unlikely in lung cancer.
♦ Distinguish stridor from wheeze, and always investigate.
♦ Pulmonary thromboembolism usually occurs in the absence of clinical signs of deep venous thrombosis.
♦ Local chest wall tenderness occurs in costochondritis, rib fracture and pulmonary infarction.
♦ Always perform pleural biopsy on initial aspiration of an undiagnosed pleural effusion.
♦ In patients with suspected pulmonary tuberculosis, arrange urgent sputum examination by Ziehl–Neelsen staining. If positive, the patient should be isolated and treated, and the disease notified.

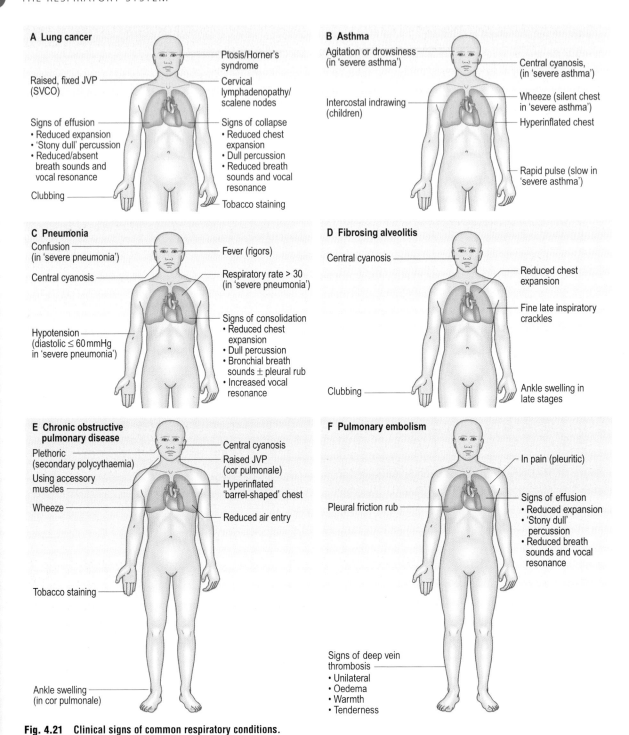

A Lung cancer

Ptosis/Horner's syndrome

Raised, fixed JVP (SVCO)

Cervical lymphadenopathy/ scalene nodes

Signs of effusion
• Reduced expansion
• 'Stony dull' percussion
• Reduced/absent breath sounds and vocal resonance

Signs of collapse
• Reduced chest expansion
• Dull percussion
• Reduced breath sounds and vocal resonance

Clubbing

Tobacco staining

B Asthma

Agitation or drowsiness (in 'severe asthma')

Central cyanosis, (in 'severe asthma')

Intercostal indrawing (children)

Wheeze (silent chest in 'severe asthma')

Hyperinflated chest

Rapid pulse (slow in 'severe asthma')

C Pneumonia

Confusion (in 'severe pneumonia')

Fever (rigors)

Central cyanosis

Respiratory rate > 30 (in 'severe pneumonia')

Signs of consolidation
• Reduced chest expansion
• Dull percussion
• Bronchial breath sounds ± pleural rub
• Increased vocal resonance

Hypotension (diastolic ≤ 60 mmHg in 'severe pneumonia')

D Fibrosing alveolitis

Central cyanosis

Reduced chest expansion

Fine late inspiratory crackles

Clubbing

Ankle swelling in late stages

E Chronic obstructive pulmonary disease

Plethoric (secondary polycythaemia)

Central cyanosis

Raised JVP (cor pulmonale)

Using accessory muscles

Hyperinflated 'barrel-shaped' chest

Wheeze

Reduced air entry

Tobacco staining

Ankle swelling (in cor pulmonale)

F Pulmonary embolism

In pain (pleuritic)

Pleural friction rub

Signs of effusion
• Reduced expansion
• 'Stony dull' percussion
• Reduced breath sounds and vocal resonance

Signs of deep vein thrombosis
• Unilateral
• Oedema
• Warmth
• Tenderness

Fig. 4.21 Clinical signs of common respiratory conditions.

A Right pleural effusion (viewed posteriorly)

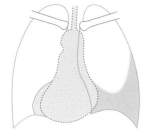

Chest expansion — Reduced
Percussion note — Stony dull
Breath sounds — Absent or decreased (occasionally bronchial)
Added sounds — None
Vocal resonance — Absent or decreased

B Right upper lobe pneumonia

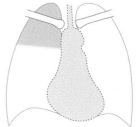

Chest expansion — Reduced
Percussion note — Dull
Breath sounds — Bronchial
Added sounds — Crackles
Vocal resonance — Increased (whispering pectoriloquy)

C Lower lobe collapse (viewed posteriorly)

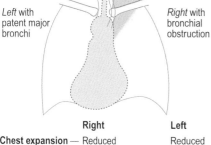

Left with patent major bronchi

Right with bronchial obstruction

	Right	**Left**
Chest expansion —	Reduced	Reduced
Percussion note —	Dull	Dull
Breath sounds —	Absent or decreased	Bronchial
Added sounds —	None	Crackles ± wheezes
Vocal resonance —	Absent or decreased	Increasing (whispering pectoriloquy)

D Right pneumothorax

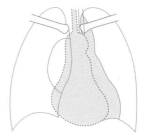

Chest expansion — Reduced
Percussion note — Hyperresonant
Breath sounds — Absent or decreased
Added sounds — Usually none
Vocal resonance — Decreased

Fig. 4.22 Integration of physical signs with examples.

COMMON RESPIRATORY INVESTIGATIONS

Chest X-ray

The chest X-ray is an important extension of the clinical examination, particularly in patients with respiratory symptoms and those with unexplained fever. The standard chest X-ray is a posteroanterior view taken with the film against the front of the chest and the X-ray source 2 m behind the patient. In an anteroposterior film the X-ray source is in front of the patient, which tends to enlarge anterior structures such as the heart.

An abnormal chest X-ray should be compared with previous films. This may indicate that abnormalities are longstanding and further investigation is unnecessary.

Interpretation of a chest X-ray requires knowledge of anatomy and pathology and appreciation of normal appearances (Fig. 4.23). A lateral film provides additional information about the nature and site of a pulmonary, pleural or mediastinal abnormality. A systematic approach is the most useful way of interpretation.

- Check name, date and orientation of the film – anteroposterior films are usually marked as such; otherwise assume posteroanterior.
- Lung fields: should be of equal translucency. Identify the horizontal fissure running from the right hilum to the 6th rib in the axillary line.
- Lung apices: look specifically for masses, cavitation, consolidation, etc. above and behind the clavicles.
- Trachea: confirm this is central, midway between the ends of the clavicles. Look for paratracheal masses, retrosternal goitre, etc.

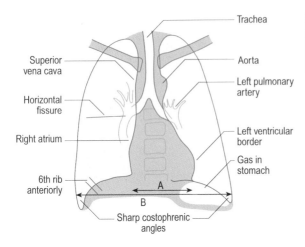

Fig. 4.23 Normal posteroanterior chest X-ray. Note vertebral outlines just seen through the heart shadow. A/B – the cardiothoracic ratio should be < 50%.

- Heart: check the heart is of normal shape and the maximum diameter is less than half the internal transthoracic diameter (cardiothoracic ratio). Look specifically for any retrocardiac masses.
- Hila: the left hilum should be higher than the right. Compare the shape and density of the two hila – both should appear concave laterally. A convex appearance suggests a mass or lymphadenopathy.
- Diaphragms: the right hemidiaphragm should be higher than the left. The anterior end of the 6th rib should cross the mid-diaphragm. If this does not reach, then hyperinflation is present.
- Costophrenic angles: these should be well-defined, acute angles. Loss of one or both suggests pleural fluid or pleural thickening.
- Soft tissues: note the presence of both breast shadows in female patients. Look around the chest wall for any soft tissue masses or subcutaneous emphysema, etc.
- Bones: step closer to the film and look at the ribs, scapulae and vertebrae. Look for fractures at the edges of each bone.

Sputum examination

The normal lung produces about 100 ml of clear sputum each day, which is transported to the oropharynx and swallowed. Coughing up sputum is always abnormal. Hospital inpatients should have a sputum pot available for inspection.

In patients with unexplained haemoptysis or suspected lung cancer, send sputum for cytological examination. In those with symptoms of lower respiratory tract infection or pneumonia, send sputum for microbiological culture. In

pneumonia a Gram stain of sputum is particularly useful in rapidly identifying the causative organism (e.g. Gram-positive – pneumococcus or staphylococcus: Gram-negative – *Haemophilus influenzae* etc.). In patients with symptoms and chest X-ray findings suspicious of pulmonary tuberculosis, Ziehl–Neelsen stains of several sputum samples must be performed. If positive, this indicates a high degree of infectivity and the patient must be urgently isolated and treated, and the condition notified.

Oximetry

An oximeter is a spectrophotometric device that measures arterial oxygen saturation (SaO_2) by determining the differential absorption of light by oxyhaemoglobin and deoxyhaemoglobin. Modern oximeters use a probe incorporating a light source and sensor that is attached to a patient's ear or finger (Fig. 4.24).

Oximeters are easy to use, portable, non-invasive and inexpensive. They are widely used for the continuous measurement of SaO_2 and to adjust oxygen therapy. An oxygen saturation of < 92% may indicate the need for oxygen therapy. It is important to appreciate the limitations of oximetry: movement artifact, arrhythmias, poor tissue perfusion, hypothermia and nail varnish can lead to spuriously low SaO_2 values, whereas dark skin pigmentation and raised levels of bilirubin or carboxyhaemoglobin can result in false increases in SaO_2. Do not use oximetry as the sole parameter to direct oxygen therapy in patients with respiratory failure.

Arterial blood gas analysis

Arterial blood gas (PaO_2, $PaCO_2$) and acid–base (pH) status is obtained from heparinized samples of arterial blood. The sample is usually taken from the radial, brachial or femoral artery. Commonly encountered patterns are (Table 4.20):

Respiratory acidosis

An acute rise in $PaCO_2$ caused by alveolar hypoventilation occurs in severe acute asthma, severe pneumonia and

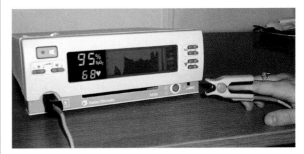

Fig. 4.24 Pulse oximeter with probe on finger.

4.20	Common causes of acid–base disturbance				
Respiratory acidosis	pH↓	CO_2↑	HCO_3↑		Acute ventilatory failure with: severe acute asthma severe pneumonia exacerbation of COPD thoracic skeletal abnormality, e.g. kyphoscoliosis neuromuscular disorders, e.g. muscular dystrophy
Respiratory alkalosis	pH↑	CO_2↓	HCO_3↓		Hyperventilation due to: anxiety/panic Central nervous system causes, e.g. stroke, subarachnoid haemorrhage salicylate poisoning
Metabolic acidosis	pH↓	CO_2↓	HCO_3↓		Increased production of organic acids: diabetic ketoacidosis acute alcohol poisoning acute renal failure lactic acidosis, e.g. shock, post-cardiac arrest Loss of bicarbonate: renal tubular acidosis severe diarrhoea Addison's disease
Metabolic alkalosis	pH↑	CO_2↑	HCO_3↑		Loss of acid: severe vomiting nasogastric suction Loss of potassium: excess diuretic therapy hyperaldosteronism Cushing's syndrome liquorice ingestion Excess alkali ingestion: milk–alkali syndrome

exacerbations of COPD and is associated with a decrease in pH. Elevation of $PaCO_2$ for more than 2–3 days may occur in COPD, respiratory muscle weakness due to neuromuscular disorders and thoracic skeletal deformities and leads to renal retention of HCO_3^- and normalization of pH. This pattern of reduced PaO_2, raised $PaCO_2$ and normal pH is known as compensated respiratory acidosis. In some patients with COPD low PaO_2 levels drive respiratory effort. Removal of this stimulus by excessive oxygen therapy may result in alveolar hypoventilation with further increase in $PaCO_2$. Unrecognized this may lead to a vicious circle resulting in death.

Respiratory alkalosis

Hyperventilation occurs with respiratory conditions (asthma, pulmonary thromboembolism, pleurisy), high altitude and acute anxiety. Alveolar hyperventilation leads to decrease in $PaCO_2$ and a consequent increase in pH. If hyperventilation persists, as occurs with stays at high altitude, renal excretion of HCO_3^- results in normalization of pH, i.e. compensated respiratory alkalosis.

Metabolic acidosis

The primary abnormality of metabolic acidosis is loss of HCO_3^- and decrease in pH. This can occur in acute renal failure, diabetic ketoacidosis, and lactic acidosis. The decrease in pH stimulates arterial chemoreceptors, resulting in alveolar hyperventilation with a consequent decrease in $PaCO_2$.

Metabolic alkalosis

The primary abnormality of metabolic alkalosis is retention of HCO_3^- (diuretic therapy, excessive ingestion) or loss of H^+ (vomiting of acidic gastric contents) resulting in an increase in pH. The increase in pH induces alveolar hypoventilation via arterial chemoreceptors with consequent increase in $PaCO_2$ (Fig. 4.25).

Spirometry

Dynamic lung volumes are measured by inhaling to total lung capacity and then exhaling into a spirometer with maximal effort to residual volume. The volume exhaled **149**

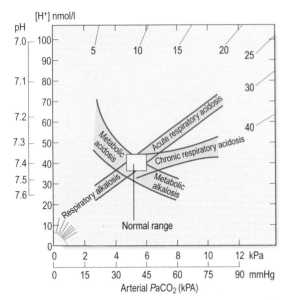

Fig. 4.25 Acid–base diagram. Relationship of arterial pH (H⁺), $PaCO_2$ and bicarbonate with disturbances in acid–base balance.

in the FEV_1/FVC ratio indicates airway obstruction. The severity of obstruction is represented by the absolute FEV_1 expressed as a percentage of predicted. Airway obstruction that reverses with inhaled beta-2-agonist or a trial of oral steroid over 5 days or more (an absolute increase in FEV_1 > 200 ml that is > 15% of baseline) favours a diagnosis of asthma over COPD.

In interstitial lung disorders such as cryptogenic fibrosing alveolitis, pulmonary sarcoidosis or extrinsic allergic alveolitis there is a decrease in FVC with preservation of FEV_1/FVC ratio, a restrictive defect (Fig. 4.26).

Peak expiratory flow

Peak expiratory flow (PEF) is measured by the subject inhaling to total lung capacity and exhaling into a peak flow meter with maximal effort. Early morning falls in PEF of > 60 l/min (> 20% maximal PEF) are very suggestive of asthma. A greater than 60 l/min fall in PEF (> 15% baseline) after exercise is diagnostic of asthma. Measurement of PEF is vital in the assessment of acute asthma and monitoring response to treatment. It is also essential for the diagnosis of occupational asthma where falls in PEF occur during the working week but resolve during weekends and holidays.

SPECIALIZED INVESTIGATIONS

Specialized investigations of respiratory disease are summarized in Table 4.21. Table 4.22 shows the techniques used in the investigation of different respiratory diseases.

in the first second and the total volume exhaled are known as the forced expiratory volume in 1 second (FEV_1) and the forced vital capacity (FVC). Normal predictive values for FEV_1 and FVC are available and are influenced by age, gender, height and race. In normal young and middle-aged adults the FEV_1/FVC ratio is usually greater than 75%, while in the elderly the ratio is usually 70–75%. A reduction

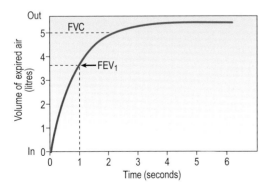

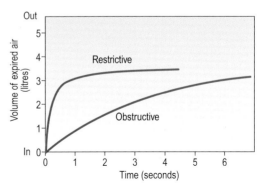

Fig. 4.26 Volume–time curves obtained using a wedge-bellows spirometer. (A) The patient takes a full inspiration and exhales forcibly and fully. Maximal flow decelerates as forced expansion proceeds. (B) Obstructive and restrictive patterns: in obstruction, FEV_1/FVC is low; in restriction, it is normal or high.

4.21 Specialized investigations of respiratory disease

Investigation	Usual respiratory indication
Blood tests	
White cell count	Lower respiratory tract infection
Haematocrit	Elevated in polycythaemia
Eosinophil count	Allergic asthma Pulmonary eosinophilia Allergic bronchopulmonary aspergillosis Churg–Strauss syndrome
C-reactive protein	Pneumonia Empyema
Serum sodium	Reduced in small cell lung cancer (inappropriate antidiuretic hormone secretion) Reduced in Legionnaire's disease and any severe pneumonia
Blood and urine osmolality	Inappropriate antidiuretic hormone secretion
Serum calcium	Elevated in bony metastases, sarcoidosis and squamous cell lung cancer
Liver function tests	Metastatic liver disease
Immunoglobulins	Deficiencies in bronchiectasis
Angiotensin-converting enzyme	Sarcoidosis
Alpha-1-antitrypsin	Hereditary panacinar emphysema
Total and specific (radioallergosorbent test) IgE	Atopic status (asthma)
Antinuclear factor	Fibrosing alveolitis
Antineutrophil cytoplasmic antibody Antiprotease III	Wegener's granulomatosis Microscopic polyarteritis nodosa
Farmer's lung and avian precipitins	Extrinsic allergic alveolitis
Cold agglutinins (IgM)	Mycoplasma infection
Serology (IgG antibodies)	Viral respiratory tract infection, e.g. influenza, respiratory syncytial virus Small bacterial infection, e.g. mycoplasma, legionella, chlamydia
D-dimer	Venous thromboembolism
Immunoreactive trypsin	Screening for cystic fibrosis
Complement-fixation transmembrane regulator (CFTR) genotyping	Cystic fibrosis

Urine tests	
Pneumococcal capsular antigen	Pneumococcal bacteraemia
Legionella urinary antigen	Legionnaire's disease

Investigation	Usual respiratory indication
Skin tests	
Heaf/Mantoux test	Exposure to *Mycobacterium tuberculosis*
Allergen skin prick tests	Atopic status (asthma)
Sweat test	Cystic fibrosis in children
Respiratory function	
Arterial blood gas tensions	Respiratory failure, acid–base balance
Spirometry	Diagnosis/monitoring of COPD
Peak expiratory flow	Diagnosis/monitoring of asthma
Carbon monoxide gas transfer	Interstitial lung disease Emphysema/COPD
Maximal mouth pressures	Respiratory neuromuscular disorders
Erect and supine FVC	Respiratory neuromuscular disorders
Exercise test	Diagnosis of asthma
Bronchial provocation studies	Asthma, especially occupational asthma
Sleep study	Sleep apnoea/hypopnoea syndrome
Radiology	
CT scan of thorax	Pulmonary or mediastinal mass Staging of lung cancer Pleural disease
High resolution CT	Interstitial lung disease Bronchiectasis
Isotope ($\dot{V}/\dot{Q}$) lung scan	Pulmonary thromboembolism
CT pulmonary angiogram	Pulmonary thromboembolism Pulmonary hypertension
Echocardiogram	Right heart dilatation (cor pulmonale)
Ultrasound of chest wall	Localization of pleural effusion
Positron-emission tomography scan	Staging of lung cancer
Invasive	
Lymph node aspiration	Cervical lymphadenopathy
Bronchoscopy	Suspected lung cancer Suspected foreign body inhalation Obtaining specimens for microbiology
Transbronchial lung biopsy	Suspected pulmonary sarcoidosis Suspected diffuse malignancy
Pleural aspiration and biopsy	Undiagnosed pleural effusion
Percutaneous fine needle lung aspiration	Peripheral lesion/suspected lung cancer
Mediastinoscopy	Staging of lung cancer Mediastinal mass
Thoracoscopy	Undiagnosed pleural disease
Lung biopsy (open or video assisted thoracoscopic surgery)	Interstitial lung disease

4.22 Useful investigations for suspected respiratory diseases

Respiratory disease	Useful investigations	Respiratory disease	Useful investigations
Asthma	PEF (diary) monitoring Reversibility to β_2-agonist, steroid trial Exercise test (PEF) Bronchial provocation studies Total and specific (radioallergosorbent test) IgE Skin prick tests	Interstitial lung disease	Chest radiograph Spirometry (FEV$_1$, FVC) Static lung volumes Carbon monoxide gas transfer High-resolution CT thorax Lung biopsy (open or video assisted thoracoscopic surgery) Antinuclear factor, antineutrophil cytoplasmic antibody and extractable nuclear antigen screen Farmer's lung and avian precipitins Angiotensin-converting enzyme
COPD	Spirometry (FEV$_1$, FVC) Carbon monoxide gas transfer Lack of reversibility to β_2-agonist, steroid 6 minute walking test Alpha-1-antitrypsin	Tuberculosis	Chest radiograph Sputum Ziehl–Neelsen stain and culture Bronchoscopy for washings
Lung cancer	Chest radiograph Sputum cytology Bronchoscopy Fine needle aspiration biopsy CT scan of thorax Mediastinoscopy	Pneumonia	Sputum Gram stain and culture Chest radiograph White cell count Blood cultures Serology for mycoplasma, legionella, chlamydia, etc. Legionella urinary antigen Pneumococcal capsular antigen in urine
Pleural effusion	Chest radiograph Pleural aspiration and biopsy CT thorax Thoracoscopy	Bronchiectasis	Chest radiograph Sputum Gram stain and culture High-resolution CT thorax Immunoglobulins
Pulmonary thromboembolism	Chest radiograph D-dimer Ventilation–perfusion ($\dot{V}/\dot{Q}$) isotope scan CT (spiral) pulmonary angiogram Pulmonary angiogram	Sleep apnoea/hypopnoea syndrome	Epworth score Sleep study

The gastrointestinal system

ALASTAIR MACGILCHRIST • ROWAN W. PARKS

GASTROINTESTINAL EXAMINATION

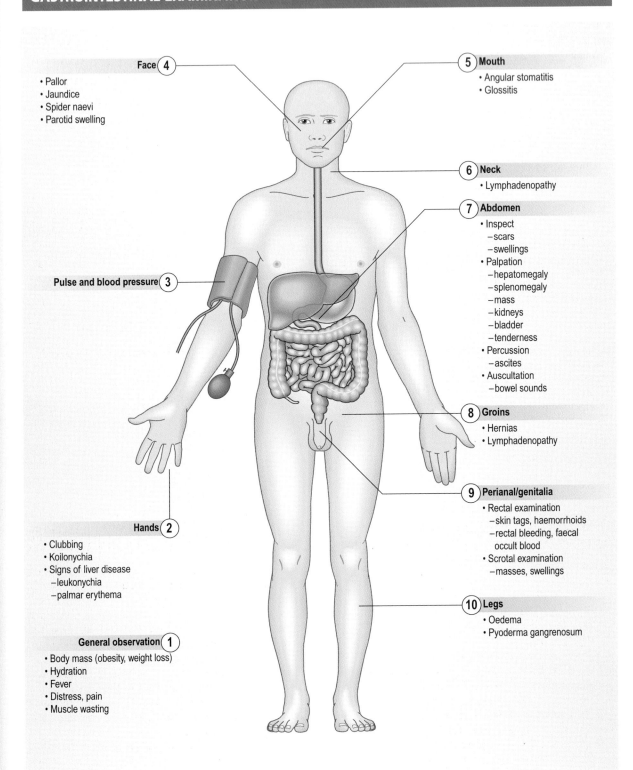

Face ④
- Pallor
- Jaundice
- Spider naevi
- Parotid swelling

⑤ **Mouth**
- Angular stomatitis
- Glossitis

⑥ **Neck**
- Lymphadenopathy

⑦ **Abdomen**
- Inspect
  - scars
  - swellings
- Palpation
  - hepatomegaly
  - splenomegaly
  - mass
  - kidneys
  - bladder
  - tenderness
- Percussion
  - ascites
- Auscultation
  - bowel sounds

Pulse and blood pressure ③

⑧ **Groins**
- Hernias
- Lymphadenopathy

⑨ **Perianal/genitalia**
- Rectal examination
  - skin tags, haemorrhoids
  - rectal bleeding, faecal occult blood
- Scrotal examination
  - masses, swellings

Hands ②
- Clubbing
- Koilonychia
- Signs of liver disease
  - leukonychia
  - palmar erythema

⑩ **Legs**
- Oedema
- Pyoderma gangrenosum

General observation ①
- Body mass (obesity, weight loss)
- Hydration
- Fever
- Distress, pain
- Muscle wasting

154

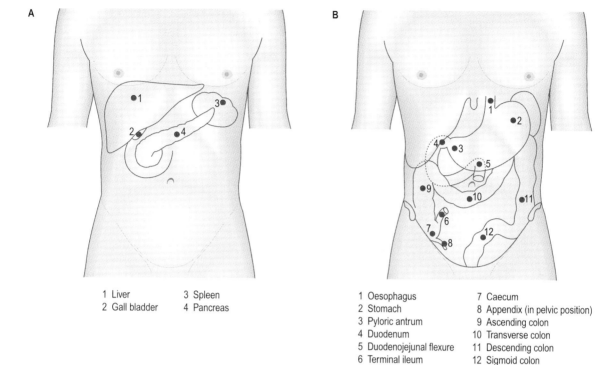

Fig. 5.1 **Surface anatomy.** (A) Surface marking of non-alimentary tract abdominal viscera. (B) Surface markings of the alimentary tract.

A	
1 Liver	3 Spleen
2 Gall bladder	4 Pancreas

B	
1 Oesophagus	7 Caecum
2 Stomach	8 Appendix (in pelvic position)
3 Pyloric antrum	9 Ascending colon
4 Duodenum	10 Transverse colon
5 Duodenojejunal flexure	11 Descending colon
6 Terminal ileum	12 Sigmoid colon

COMMON SYMPTOMS

Common symptoms of the gastrointestinal system are listed in Table 5.1.

ANOREXIA AND WEIGHT LOSS

Anorexia is loss of appetite. It is common in many upper gastrointestinal and liver diseases including malignancy and hepatitis but does not specifically indicate gastrointestinal disease. Anorexia may be expressed as a lack of interest in food. In addition to asking about appetite, ask the patient 'Do you still *enjoy* your food/meals?'

Anorexia together with weight loss should always be investigated. Patients may overestimate weight loss, so accurately record weight on more than one occasion and review the previous records. Weight loss without any other symptoms, particularly if mild (< 3 kg in 6 months), usually does *not* indicate underlying disease.

Weight loss occurs when energy expenditure exceeds calorie intake (Table 5.2). This is usually caused by reduced intake and in disease states is accompanied by anorexia. Weight loss with normal, or even increased, calorie intake is rare, but may occur in type 1 diabetes mellitus, hyperthyroidism, malabsorption, and fever. Very rapid weight loss (> 0.5 kg/day) invariably indicates fluid loss, and causes include diuretic therapy, severe diarrhoea, vomiting, heat illness or severe burns.

Weight loss is common in malignancies of the upper gastrointestinal tract, liver and pancreas, but is a late feature of colon cancer. When severe it is called cancer cachexia.

5.1	Common symptoms of the gastrointestinal system
Symptom	**Definition**
General	
Anorexia	Loss of appetite
Weight loss	
Pain	Constant, colicky, local, generalized
Abdominal distension	
Upper gastrointestinal	
Xerostomia	Dry mouth
Water brash	Sudden appearance of excessive saliva in the mouth
Painful lips, tongue and mouth	
Dysgeusia	Altered taste sensation
Dysphagia	Difficulty swallowing
Globus	Sensation of a lump in the throat
Odynophagia	Pain on swallowing
Heartburn	Burning retrosternal discomfort radiating upward
Flatulence	Belching
Dyspepsia	Indigestion
Early satiety	Premature fullness on eating
Nausea	Feeling sick
Haematemesis	Vomiting fresh or altered blood
Hiccups	
Lower gastrointestinal	
Wind	Excessive/offensive flatus, or bloating/distension
Altered bowel habit:	
diarrhoea	Abnormally soft stools and/or frequent defecation
constipation	Abnormally firm stools and/or infrequent defecation
steatorrhoea	Fatty stools, pale, greasy, difficult to flush away
Haematochezia	Rectal bleeding
Melaena	Black, tarry stools
Hepatobiliary	
Jaundice (icterus)	Yellow discoloration of skin and sclerae
Itch (pruritus)	Generalized itchiness

5.2	Energy requirements
Males	2500 kcal/day
Females	2000 kcal/day

Daily calorie deficit of 500 kcal = weight loss of 0.5 kg/week
If *no* calorie intake at all = weight loss is approximately 2 kg/wk

Inflammatory gastrointestinal disorders can also result in weight loss, e.g. pancreatitis or inflammatory bowel disease. In chronic liver disease weight loss is multifactorial; there is reduced calorie intake because of anorexia, ascites and imposed dietary restrictions on salt, malabsorption of food due to reduced bile production, and the diseased liver cannot process the absorbed nutrients.

Remember that weight loss is a common feature of many non-gastrointestinal diseases, e.g. other malignancies, chronic infections or inflammatory conditions. Mental illness such as depression is easy to overlook, especially in the elderly, and anorexia nervosa or bulimia is a common cause in adolescents. Amenorrhoea is not specific to anorexia nervosa, and menstrual irregularity is common in women who lose weight from any cause.

DYSPHAGIA

Dysphagia is difficulty swallowing and should always be investigated. Ask the patient 'Does food (or drink) stick when you swallow?' Do not confuse dysphagia with early *satiety*, the inability to complete a full meal because of premature fullness, or *globus*, the feeling of a lump in the throat. Globus does not interfere with swallowing and is not related to eating.

Normal swallowing involves the brain stem, the glossopharyngeal and vagal nerves, the enteric nervous system and oesophageal smooth muscle. The swallowing reflex begins with an oral phase which drives the food bolus into the pharynx. The pharyngeal phase then occurs with laryngeal closure (to prevent soiling of the airway) and relaxation of the upper pharyngeal sphincter (cricopharyngeus). Sequential contraction of the pharyngeal constrictors propels the bolus into the oesophagus. In the oesophagus peristaltic contractions aid distal movement and entry to the stomach is helped by relaxation of the lower oesophageal sphincter.

Dysphagia may be caused by disorders affecting any part of this sequence (Table 5.3):

- mouth (painful ulcers, mouth or throat infections, ill-fitting dentures)
- brain stem (cerebrovascular accidents, bulbar palsy)
- oesophagus (benign stricture, cancer).

Neurological dysphagia resulting from bulbar or pseudobulbar palsies is typically worse for liquids than for solids, and may be accompanied by choking, spluttering and regurgitation of fluid from the nose.

Neuromuscular dysphagia, or oesophageal dysmotility, most often presents in middle-age. It is worse for solids and may be helped by liquids and sitting upright. *Achalasia*, when the lower oesophageal sphincter fails to relax normally, leads to progressive oesophageal dilatation above the sphincter. Overflow of secretions and food into the respiratory tract may occur, especially at night when the patient lies down, and causes aspiration pneumonia. Oesophageal dysmotility may be associated with oesophageal spasm and central chest pain which may be confused with cardiac pain.

5.3   Causes of dysphagia
Oral
• Painful mouth ulcers • Mouth or throat infections, e.g. quinsy, glandular fever
Neurological
• Cerebrovascular accident • Bulbar or pseudobulbar palsy
Neuromuscular (dysmotility)
• Achalasia • Pharyngeal pouch • Myasthenia gravis
Mechanical
• Oesophageal cancer • Peptic stricture • Other benign strictures • Extrinsic compression, e.g. lung cancer • Systemic sclerosis

'Mechanical' dysphagia is often due to oesophageal stricture. When associated with weight loss, a short history, and no heartburn, suspect oesophageal cancer. Longstanding dysphagia without weight loss but accompanied by heartburn is more likely to be due to a benign peptic stricture. You cannot distinguish between the two on history alone and patients must be investigated. The site at which the patient feels the food sticking is not a reliable guide to the site of oesophageal obstruction.

Odynophagia is pain on swallowing often precipitated by drinking hot liquids. It may be present with or without dysphagia and is often an indication of active oesophageal ulceration from peptic oesophagitis or oesophageal candidiasis.

HEARTBURN AND OTHER REFLUX SYMPTOMS

Heartburn is a hot, burning retrosternal discomfort which radiates upwards. When heartburn is the principal symptom, gastro-oesophageal reflux disease is the most likely diagnosis. It is often accompanied by acid reflux due to regurgitation of acid producing a sour taste in the mouth. The burning quality and upward radiation of heartburn, and its occurrence on lying flat or bending forward help to differentiate it from retrosternal chest pain originating from the heart.

Water brash is the sudden appearance of excessive saliva in the mouth due to reflex salivation and suggests gastro-oesophageal reflux disease.

DYSPEPSIA

Indigestion is a commonly used term for ill-defined symptoms arising from the upper gastrointestinal tract.

Dyspepsia is pain or discomfort centred in the upper abdomen. There is considerable overlap in upper gastrointestinal tract symptoms, and dyspepsia is often used to encompass gastro-oesophageal reflux disease, peptic ulcer disease and non-ulcer or functional dyspepsia. Dyspepsia is very common, affecting up to 80% of the population at some time in their lives.

Pain which is worse with an empty stomach and eased by eating is the classical peptic ulcer description. This is sometimes so localized that the patient indicates a single spot where the pain occurs; the 'finger pointing' sign. Epigastric pain may be worse during or after eating, accompanied by nausea and abdominal fullness and is often worse after meals with a high spice or fat content. 'Fat intolerance' is common to all causes of dyspepsia and does not specifically suggest gall bladder disease.

NAUSEA AND VOMITING

Nausea is the sensation of feeling sick. *Vomiting* is the expulsion of gastric contents via the mouth. Both are often associated with the autonomic features of pallor, sweating and hyperventilation. Nausea and vomiting, particularly if associated with abdominal pain or discomfort, suggest upper gastrointestinal disorders. Find out what drugs the patient is taking since many medications cause nausea, and always consider pregnancy as a cause of vomiting in women of reproductive years.

Nausea without vomiting is common in dyspepsia. Peptic ulcers seldom cause painless vomiting unless complicated by pyloric stenosis causing gastric outlet obstruction. Gastric outlet obstruction causes projectile vomiting of large volumes of gastric content which is not bile stained. Obstruction distal to the pylorus produces bile-stained (green) vomit. The more distal the level of intestinal obstruction, the more marked are the accompanying symptoms of abdominal distension and intestinal colic.

Vomiting occurs in other gastrointestinal disorders, e.g. gastroenteritis, cholecystitis, pancreatitis and hepatitis but may also be a prominent feature of non-alimentary disorders (Table 5.4). In most of these, vomiting is preceded by nausea, but in some, e.g. raised intracranial pressure, the vomiting can occur without warning. Vomiting may be caused by severe pain, e.g. renal or biliary colic, myocardial infarction or from systemic disease, metabolic disorders and drug therapy.

Anorexia nervosa is an eating disorder in which patients limit calorie intake and may induce vomiting in order to

5.4 Non-alimentary cause of vomiting
Neurological
• Raised intracranial pressure, e.g. brain tumour • Middle ear disorders, e.g. labyrinthitis • Migraine
Severe pain
• e.g. myocardial infarction, renal colic
Drugs
• e.g. alcohol, opioids, theophyllines, digoxin, cytotoxic agents, serotonin specific re-uptake inhibitor antidepressants • Consider *any* drug
Metabolic/endocrine
• Pregnancy • Diabetic ketoacidosis • Uraemia • Hypercalcaemia • Addison's disease
Psychological
• Anorexia nervosa • Bulimia • Rumination

Table 5.5 Causes of upper gastrointestinal bleeding
• Gastric ulcer • Duodenal ulcer • Oesophagogastric varices • Mallory–Weiss tear • Profuse nose bleeds • Oesophagitis, gastritis, duodenitis • Oesophageal or gastric cancer • Vascular malformation

headedness and fainting, and look for pallor, tachycardia and hypotension.

Peptic ulcer is a common cause of upper gastrointestinal bleeding (Table 5.5). However, 25% of bleeding peptic ulcers present without a previous history of dyspepsia, and this proportion is higher in the elderly and patients taking non-steroidal anti-inflammatory drugs. Ask patients about recent ingestion of aspirin, non-steroidal anti-inflammatory drugs and alcohol.

Excessive alcohol ingestion may cause haematemesis:

• directly by acute alcoholic gastritis or alcohol-induced vomiting leading to a Mallory–Weiss tear
• indirectly by the development of liver cirrhosis causing portal hypertension and bleeding oesophageal varices.

lose weight. In this psychiatric condition, the vomiting is concealed and not volunteered by the patient. In bulimia, patients induce vomiting in secret after binge eating. Their weight is maintained or may increase.

Rumination is the habitual, involuntary, subconscious regurgitation of gastric contents which are then chewed and swallowed. It is uncommon and is usually brought to medical attention by the patient's family.

HAEMATEMESIS

Haematemesis is vomiting blood. The blood can be fresh and red, or degraded by gastric pepsin, when it is dark in colour and resembles 'coffee grounds'. If the source of bleeding is above the gastro-oesophageal sphincter, e.g. from oesophageal varices, fresh blood wells up in the mouth rather than being actively vomited. A lower oesophageal (Mallory–Weiss) tear due to the trauma of retching is usually associated with a characteristic history. The patient vomits forcefully several times; fresh blood only appears after the initial vomit. Upper gastrointestinal bleeding often results in melaena, the passage of altered blood per rectum. Cancers of the stomach or the oesophagus rarely present with haematemesis.

Patients find it difficult to estimate the amount of blood vomited accurately. To gauge the severity of the bleed, ask about symptoms suggesting hypovolaemia, e.g. light-

ABDOMINAL PAIN

The characteristics of abdominal pain and how these differ in biliary colic, acute pancreatitis and renal colic are shown in Tables 5.6 and 5.7.

Site of pain

Visceral abdominal pain results from distension of hollow organs, mesenteric traction or excessive smooth muscle contraction. Sympathetic innervation of the abdominal viscera (spinal cord segments T5–L2) is responsible for the conduction of pain; parasympathetic afferents do not

5.6 Characteristics of abdominal pain

• Site and radiation
• Quantity:
  – time and timing
  – speed of onset
  – duration
• Quality:
  – character
  – severity
• What makes it worse?
• What makes it better?
• Associated symptoms

5.7 Analysis of abdominal pain				
	Disorder			
	Peptic ulcer	**Biliary colic**	**Acute pancreatitis**	**Renal colic**
Main site	Epigastric	Epigastrium/right hypochondrium	Epigastrium/left hypochondrium	Loin
Radiation	Into the back	Beneath right scapula Right shoulder tip	Into the back May become generalized	Into genitalia/inner thigh
Character	Gnawing	Constant	Constant	Constant with small fluctuations
Severity	Mild to moderate	Severe	Severe	Severe
Duration	1/2–2 h	4–24 h	> 24 h	4–24 h
Frequency and periodicity	Remission for weeks/months	Unpredictable – can enumerate attacks	Unpredictable – can enumerate attacks	Usually a discrete episode
Special times of occurrence	Nocturnal Especially when hungry, e.g. between meals		After heavy drinking	Following periods of dehydration
Aggravating factors	Stress, spicy foods, alcohol, smoking, aspirin	Unable to eat during bouts of pain	Alcohol Unable to eat during bouts of pain	
Relieving factors	Food, antacids, vomiting		Eased by sitting upright	
Associated phenomena	Family history, GI bleeding, perforation	Restlessness, vomiting, jaundice	Vomiting, jaundice, paralytic ileus	Restlessness, vomiting, haematuria, dysuria
Causes	*Helicobacter pylori-* associated gastritis	Gallstones (bile salt disorders, obesity, haemolytic anaemia)	Gallstones, drugs, e.g. diuretics, alcohol Hypercalcaemia	Dehydration, hyperuricaemia, hypercalcaemia

convey pain sensation. Visceral pain is often experienced as a deep poorly localized sensation in the midline.

Somatic pain is caused by irritation of the parietal peritoneum and is usually lateralized and localized to the area of inflammation. The parietal peritoneum is innervated by the intercostal (spinal) nerves, which also innervate the overlying abdominal wall.

Pain arising from foregut structures (stomach, pancreas, liver and biliary system) is localized above the umbilicus (Fig. 5.2). Pain solely from the small intestine, e.g. small intestinal obstruction, is felt around the umbilicus (periumbilical). If the parietal peritoneum is involved, the pain will localize to that area, e.g. right iliac fossa pain in acute appendicitis and in Crohn's disease of the terminal ileum.

Colonic pain is typically felt below the umbilicus, e.g. pain in the left iliac fossa from diverticular disease of the sigmoid colon. However, it may occur in the upper abdomen, e.g. pain from the hepatic flexure can be located in the right hypochondrium.

Pain from unpaired structures such as the pancreas is usually felt in the midline and radiates through to the back. With paired structures, pain is usually felt on the affected side. The pain of renal colic classically radiates from the flank into the groin.

In young males, unilateral testicular pain strongly suggests torsion of the testis rather than epididymo-orchitis. In women always consider possible gynaecological causes such as ruptured ovarian cyst, pelvic inflammatory disease or an ectopic pregnancy. In patients of any age, with acute right iliac fossa pain, always consider appendicitis.

Radiation. The development of shoulder tip pain indicates peritoneal inflammation immediately below the diaphragm, e.g. cholecystitis (Fig. 5.3).

Nature of pain

Is the pain constant or colicky? Constant pain usually arises from a solid organ, e.g. pancreatitis. Colicky pain lasts for a short period of time (seconds or minutes), eases off and then returns. Colicky pain comes from hollow structures, e.g. small or large bowel usually in association with obstruction, or the uterus during labour. Biliary and renal 'colic' are misnamed, as the pain resulting from a stone obstructing the bile duct or ureter builds to a peak over several hours before declining.

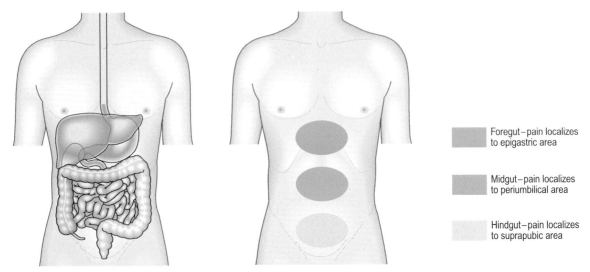

Fig. 5.2 Perception of visceral pain is localized to the epigastric, umbilical or suprapubic region according to the embryological origin of the affected organ.

Foregut—pain localizes to epigastric area

Midgut—pain localizes to periumbilical area

Hindgut—pain localizes to suprapubic area

Speed of onset

In a previously asymptomatic patient, severe sudden onset of abdominal pain, which progresses rapidly and becomes generalized in site and constant in nature, suggests perforation of a hollow viscus, a ruptured abdominal aortic aneurysm or mesenteric infarction. Accompanying or preceding symptoms may help differentiate the likely cause. Preceding constipation may suggest colorectal cancer or diverticular disease as the cause of perforation. Prior dyspepsia may suggest a peptic ulcer being the cause for perforation. Coexisting peripheral vascular disease, hypertension, cardiac failure or atrial fibrillation may suggest a vascular disorder, e.g. aortic aneurysm or mesenteric ischaemia.

The development of peripheral circulatory failure (shock) following the onset of pain may indicate intra-abdominal bleeding, e.g. ruptured aortic aneurysm or ectopic pregnancy. Torsion of an organ causes rapid onset of abdominal pain as it occludes the blood supply. Torsion of the testis or ovary produces severe abdominal pain and nausea. Torsion of the caecum or sigmoid colon (volvulus) commonly presents with sudden abdominal pain associated with the development of acute intestinal obstruction.

A slower onset and progression of abdominal pain over hours or days suggests inflammatory disorders, e.g. acute cholecystitis, appendicitis or diverticular disease.

Symptom progression

During the first hour or two after perforation, a 'silent interval' may occur when abdominal pain resolves transiently. The initial chemical peritonitis may begin to subside before bacterial peritonitis becomes established.

In appendicitis, pain is initially localized around the umbilicus (visceral pain) and spreads as the inflammatory response progresses to involve the right iliac fossa (parietal or somatic pain). If rupture of the appendix occurs, generalized peritonitis may develop. On occasions the patient may develop a localized abscess with a palpable mass associated with localized pain in the right iliac fossa.

A change in the pattern of symptoms raises the possibility that either the initial diagnosis was wrong, or that complications have developed. In acute small bowel obstruction, a change in the pain from typical intestinal colic to persistent pain with abdominal tenderness suggests intestinal ischaemia, e.g. strangulated hernia. This is an indication for urgent surgical intervention.

Accompanying features

Abdominal pain due to irritable bowel syndrome, diverticular disease or colorectal cancer, is invariably accompanied by some alteration in bowel habit.

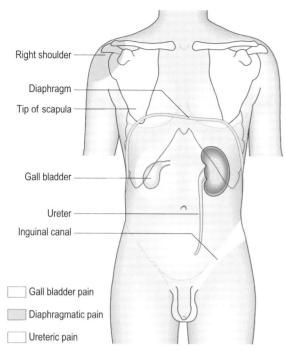

Right shoulder

Diaphragm

Tip of scapula

Gall bladder

Ureter

Inguinal canal

- Gall bladder pain
- Diaphragmatic pain
- Ureteric pain

Fig. 5.3 Characteristic radiation of pain from the gall bladder, diaphragm, and ureters. The pain is not always felt in the organ concerned.

ABDOMINAL DISTENSION

The principal causes of abdominal distension are the five Fs: *fat, flatus, faeces, fluid,* and *fetus* (Table 5.8).

Abdominal girth increasing slowly over months or years is usually due to obesity. If it occurs in a patient who is losing weight it suggests intra-abdominal disease.

Ascites is accumulation of fluid in the peritoneal cavity (Table 5.9).

Bloating is fluctuating abdominal distension which usually develops during the day and resolves overnight. It is particularly common in women and is rarely due to organic disease. It usually occurs with other symptoms of irritable bowel syndrome. Chronic simple constipation rarely produces painful distension unless associated with the irritable bowel syndrome. Painless abdominal distension in women may be the presenting symptom of ovarian pathology or a concealed pregnancy.

5.8	Causes of abdominal distension
Factor	**Consider**
Fat	Excessive alcohol consumption
Flatus	Pseudo-obstruction, obstruction
Faeces	Subacute obstruction, constipation
Fluid	Ovarian or uterine mass Bladder enlargement Ascites
Fetus	Date of the last menstrual period

WIND

Patients may call repeated belching, excessive or offensive rectal flatus, abdominal distension and *borborygmi* (audible bowel sounds) 'wind'. Ask the patient to describe what is being experienced. Belching may result from air swallowing (*aerophagy*) and is usually of no major significance. It may indicate anxiety, but sometimes occurs in an attempt to relieve abdominal pain or discomfort, and accompanies gastro-oesophageal reflux disease.

The normal volume of flatus passed per rectum varies from 200–2000 ml per day. It is a mixture of gases derived from swallowed air and from colonic bacterial fermentation of poorly absorbed carbohydrates. Excessive flatus is particularly troublesome in lactase deficiency and intestinal malabsorption. The inability to pass flatus is a feature of intestinal obstruction. Borborygmi result from the movement of fluid and gas along the bowel. Though usually just a source of embarrassment, it may indicate small bowel obstruction or dysmotility.

5.9	Causes of ascites
Common	
• Hepatic cirrhosis with portal hypertension • Intra-abdominal malignancy with peritoneal spread	
Less common	
• Nephrotic syndrome • Right heart failure • Constrictive pericarditis	
Rare	
• Budd–Chiari syndrome (hepatic venous obstruction) • Tuberculous peritonitis • Hypoproteinaemia, e.g. protein-losing enteropathy, severe malnutrition	

ALTERED BOWEL HABIT

Normal bowel movement frequency can be from three times each day to once every three days. *Diarrhoea* is the frequent passage of loose stools. *Constipation* is the infrequent passage of hard stools. Clarify what patients mean when they say they have a change in bowel habit. When they say diarrhoea do they mean a change in stool consistency from solid to liquid, an increased frequency of defecation, urgency of defecation or all three? With constipation, ask if they mean they are moving their bowels less frequently than usual, or if defecation is difficult because the stool is hard.

Constipation can result from:

- a delay in delivery of stools round the colon to the rectum, due to impaired motility (e.g. irritable bowel syndrome) or physical obstruction (e.g. colorectal cancer)
- impaired rectal sensation resulting in lack of awareness that the rectum is full, thus preventing the normal 'call to stool'
- anorectal dysfunction preventing normal defecation despite appropriate signals.

Some possible causes of constipation are given in Table 5.10, and Table 5.11 shows questions to ask patients complaining of constipation.

Diarrhoea may be high or low volume. High-volume diarrhoea (> 200 g stool/day or > 1 l per day) occurs when the water content of the stool is increased. The principal site of water absorption along the gastrointestinal tract is the colon. Diarrhoea can result from impaired water absorption in the colon or from active intraluminal secretion of fluid due to mucosal inflammation. Impaired absorption of nutrients from the small intestine leads to an increased osmolarity of the luminal contents which increases the fluid shift into the lumen across the intestinal wall. High-volume diarrhoea is divided into:

- *secretory,* due to intestinal inflammation, e.g. viral or bacterial infection, ulcerative colitis or Crohn's disease
- *osmotic*, due to malabsorption, drugs or motility disorders.

Osmotic diarrhoea stops if the patient fasts but secretory diarrhoea persists.

Causes of diarrhoea are listed in Table 5.12. The commonest cause of low-volume diarrhoea is irritable bowel syndrome, which is a common cause of disordered gastrointestinal motility in the under-50s. The diagnosis rests on a pattern of gastrointestinal symptoms because there is no confirmatory investigation. The following features are required for a diagnosis of irritable bowel syndrome:

- *abdominal pain* either accompanied by a change in bowel habit, or eased by defecation
- *alteration in bowel habit* – ranging from increased frequency with urgency to constipation, frequently alternating between the two
- *alteration in stool consistency* – ranging from liquid stools to small firm pellets or thin, 'ribbon-like' stools
- absence of 'alarm' features, e.g. rectal bleeding or weight loss
- symptoms must be *chronic*.

Abdominal distension and bloating are common, but not diagnostic.

This combination of symptoms, although consistent with a diagnosis of irritable bowel syndrome, simply indicates that the problem is colonic in origin. Ask about symptoms which suggest serious disorders, e.g. weight loss or rectal bleeding. Even in the absence of these or other 'alarm' symptoms, investigate potentially at-risk patients to exclude

5.10 Causes of constipation
• Lack of fibre in diet • Irritable bowel syndrome • Intestinal obstruction (cancer) • Metabolic/endocrine (hypothyroidism, hypercalcaemia) • Drugs (opioids, iron) • Immobility (stroke, Parkinson's disease)

5.11 Symptom checklist in patients with constipation
• Has constipation been lifelong or is it of recent onset? • How often do the bowels empty each week? • How much time is spent straining at stool? • Is there associated abdominal pain, anal pain on defecation or rectal bleeding? • Has the shape of the stool changed, e.g. become pellet-like? • Has there been any change in drug therapy?

5.12 Causes of diarrhoea
Acute
• Infective gastroenteritis • Drugs (esp. antibiotics)
Chronic
• Irritable bowel syndrome • Inflammatory bowel disease • Malabsorption • Colorectal cancer • Autonomic neuropathy (esp. diabetic) • Laxative abuse • Drug therapy • Hyperthyroidism • Constipation with overflow (spurious) • Post-bowel resection • Faecal impaction • Parasitic infestations, e.g. *Giardia lamblia*

5.13	Causes of fresh rectal bleeding

- Haemorrhoids
- Anal fissure
- Colorectal polyps
- Colorectal cancer
- Inflammatory bowel disease
- Ischaemic colitis
- Complicated diverticular disease
- Vascular malformation
- Massive upper gastrointestinal bleeding
- Aorto-enteric fistula
- Endometriosis in the rectum

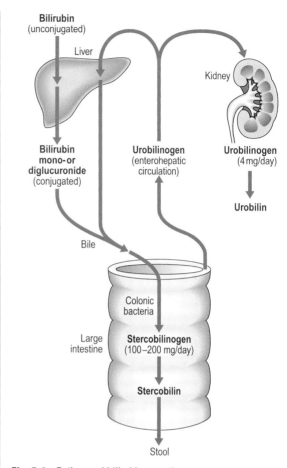

Fig. 5.4 Pathway of bilirubin excretion.

other serious disease, e.g. colorectal cancer in patients over 45 years of age.

Steatorrhoea is diarrhoea due to fat malabsorption. The stools are pale, bulky and foul-smelling. They float in the toilet pan and are difficult to flush away.

RECTAL BLEEDING

Fresh rectal bleeding indicates a disorder in the anal canal, rectum or colon (Table 5.13). Blood may be mixed with the stool, may coat the surface of otherwise normal stool, or may be seen on the toilet paper or in the pan. *Melaena* is the passage of black, tarry stools with a characteristic odour signifying blood loss in the upper gastrointestinal tract. Occasionally, with a particularly brisk or severe upper gastrointestinal bleed, blood may pass through the intestine unaltered causing fresh rectal bleeding. Such a brisk bleed will be accompanied by other features associated with severe blood loss such as shock.

JAUNDICE

Jaundice is a yellowish discoloration of the skin, sclerae and mucous membranes and is due to hyperbilirubinaemia. Normally levels of bilirubin > 50 μmol/l are needed for clinical detection in good light.

Bilirubin is a breakdown product of haemoglobin, myoglobin and haem-containing enzymes. Unconjugated bilirubin is insoluble and transported in plasma bound to albumin and so is not filtered by the renal glomeruli. Therefore if jaundice is only due to unconjugated hyper-bilirubinaemia, the patient's urine is normal in colour (acholuric jaundice).

In the liver, bilirubin is conjugated to form bilirubin mono- or diglucuronides (Fig. 5.4). These are soluble and excreted in bile giving it the characteristic green colour. With conjugated hyperbilirubinaemia, the urine will be dark. In the colon conjugated bilirubin is metabolized by the bacterial flora to stercobilin and stercobilinogen and

excreted in the stool, contributing to the brown stool colour. A small amount of stercobilinogen and stercobilin is absorbed from the bowel and, being soluble, is excreted as urobilinogen and urobilin in the urine. Urobilin is a dark-coloured compound formed by oxidation of urobilinogen, so the urine may turn darker on standing.

Jaundice may be:

- prehepatic (e.g. haemolysis)
- hepatocellular (e.g. hepatitis, hereditary liver enzyme deficiencies)
- obstructive (e.g. biliary obstruction due to gallstones, cancer of the head of the pancreas or drug-induced cholestasis) (Table 5.14).

Prehepatic

In haemolytic disorders the accompanying anaemic pallor combined with jaundice may give the patient a pale lemon complexion. The stools and urine are normal in colour.

5.14 Common causes of jaundice	
Increased bilirubin production	Haemolysis (unconjugated)
Impaired bilirubin excretion	
Congenital	e.g. Gilbert's syndrome (unconjugated)
Hepatocellular	Viral hepatitis
	Drugs
	Autoimmune hepatitis
	Cirrhosis
Obstructive (cholestatic):	
Intrahepatic	Drugs
	Primary biliary cirrhosis
Extrahepatic	Gallstones
	Cancer – pancreas, cholangiocarcinoma

5.15 Jaundice: clinical features and urinalysis

	Urine			Stools
	Colour	Bilirubin	Urobilinogen	Colour
Unconjugated	Normal	–	+	Normal
Hepatocellular	Dark	+	+	Normal
Cholestatic	Dark	++	–	Pale

The commonest hereditary enzyme defect causing hyperbilirubinaemia is Gilbert's syndrome. This autosomal dominant condition causes a defect in bilirubin conjugation and increased unconjugated hyperbilirubinaemia. It is commonly found on routine biochemical screening. Liver enzyme function is normal and any jaundice is mild (plasma bilirubin level < 100 µmol/l) but this increases on fasting or with intercurrent illness.

Hepatocellular

Hepatocellular disease causes hyperbilirubininaemia that is usually both unconjugated and conjugated. The proportion of each reflects bilirubin uptake and transport by the diseased liver, and the urine will be dark and stools will be normal in colour.

Obstructive

In biliary obstruction, conjugated bilirubin in the bile does not reach the intestine so the stools are pale. Because conjugated bilirubin is soluble, it is filtered by the kidney so the urine is dark. Obstructive jaundice is commonly accompanied by generalized itch or *pruritus*. Obstructive jaundice with abdominal pain is usually due to gallstones, and if fever or rigors are present suggests ascending cholangitis (Charcot's triad). Painless obstructive jaundice suggests malignant biliary obstruction, e.g. pancreatic cancer or cholangiocarcinoma.

THE HISTORY

Presenting complaint

Gastrointestinal symptoms are very common and often caused by functional dyspepsia and irritable bowel syndrome. Explore the patient's ideas, concerns and expectations (see Ch. 1) so that you can address these. The patient may want relief from symptoms, or reassurance that there is no serious underlying cause for the symptoms. Always investigate 'alarm symptoms' such as excessive weight loss or gastrointestinal bleeding.

Past history

History of a similar problem may suggest the diagnosis, e.g. a bleeding peptic ulcer or inflammatory bowel disease. Always ask about previous abdominal surgery.

Drug history

Ask about all prescribed medications, over-the-counter medicines, and 'alternative' medications such as herbal preparations. Almost any drug can affect the gastrointestinal tract. Aspirin and non-steroidal anti-inflammatory drugs can cause dyspepsia, gastric erosions or peptic ulcers, opioid analgesia causes nausea/vomiting and constipation, antibiotics can cause diarrhoea (with or without *Clostridium difficile* infection – pseudomembranous colitis) and many drugs can cause hepatotoxicity. Selective serotonin reuptake inhibitor antidepressants often cause nausea initially.

Family history

Many gastrointestinal conditions, including gallstones, dyspepsia, irritable bowel syndrome and diverticular disease are so common that a positive family history is not helpful. For some conditions a family history is relevant. For example, colorectal cancer in a first-degree relative < 50 years old increases the risk of colorectal cancer and polyps.

Inflammatory bowel disease is more common in patients with a positive family history, and Crohn's disease and ulcerative colitis occur more often in relatives of patients with either condition. Peptic ulcer disease often runs in families but this may be environmental due to transmission of *Helicobacter pylori* infection. Certain liver diseases are hereditary, e.g. haemochromatosis and Wilson's disease, which are both autosomal recessive disorders.

Social history

Take a dietary history (Table 5.16). Many patients assume that their symptoms are diet related. They may be correct, but establishing definite dietary links to gastrointestinal diseases has proved difficult. Nevertheless, diets lacking in fruit, vegetables and fibre increase the risk of colonic cancer and diverticular disease. Patients with diarrhoea due to lactose intolerance report worsening of their symptoms after eating dairy produce. Patients with irritable bowel syndrome often report sensitivities to dairy produce, wheat, fat and caffeine, but this is difficult to prove. True gluten enteropathy occurs in coeliac disease.

Calculate the patient's consumption in units of alcohol (1 unit = 1 glass of wine, 1 measure of spirits or ¹/₂ pint of beer). Weekly intake > 14 units in women or > 21 units in men is potentially harmful (Table 5.17) (see Ch. 1).

Ask about smoking (see Ch. 2). Smokers are at increased risk of many gastrointestinal diseases, including oesophageal cancer, colorectal cancer and peptic ulcer. Patients with

5.17 Gastrointestinal and hepatic consequences of alcohol
• Alcoholic liver disease
• Gastritis
• Pancreatitis
• Oesophageal cancer
• Diarrhoea

Crohn's disease smoke more commonly but the converse is true in those with ulcerative colitis. Patients may present with ulcerative colitis soon after stopping smoking.

Many gastrointestinal disorders, particularly irritable bowel syndrome and dyspepsia, are functional; that is, no physical abnormality can be found and the conditions may be linked to the stresses of modern life. Ask about potential sources of stress including work, home circumstances, relationships and finance as well as symptoms of anxiety and depression (see Ch. 1).

In patients with liver disease and hepatitis, ask about specific risk factors (Table 5.18).

Hepatitis C may present with chronic liver disease decades after primary infection, so enquire about drug use and other risk factors in the distant as well as the recent past.

Foreign travel is important in relation to diarrhoeal illnesses, e.g. giardiasis and amoebiasis.

5.16 The dietary history
• Fibre content (cereals, wholemeal bread, fruit and vegetables)
• Dairy products (milk, butter, cheese, yoghurt)
• Wheat (bread, pasta)
• Caffeine (tea and carbonated drinks as well as coffee)
• Alcohol

5.18 Risk factors for viral hepatitis
• Blood transfusion
• Intravenous drug use
• Tattoos
• Foreign travel
• Sex between men
• Multiple sexual partners

THE PHYSICAL EXAMINATION

GENERAL EXAMINATION

Nutritional state. Record the height, weight, waist circumference and calculate the patient's body mass index (see p. 55). Note if obesity is truncal or generalized. Look for striae, which usually indicate rapid weight gain or previous pregnancy and, rarely, Cushing's syndrome. Loose skin folds signify recent weight loss. Pallor, particularly of the conjunctivae and palmar creases, may indicate anaemia. Look for tissue stigmata of iron deficiency including koilonychia (spoon-shaped nails), angular cheilitis (painful hacks at the corners of the mouth) and atrophic glossitis

(pale, smooth tongue). The tongue has a beefy, raw appearance in folate and vitamin B_{12} deficiency. If the history suggests malabsorption look for these particularly.

Liver disease. Jaundice may be obvious, but if not, ask the patient to look up while you pull the lower eyelid down to expose the sclera and look to see if it is yellow in natural light (Fig. 5.5). Do not confuse the diffuse yellow sclerae of jaundice with the small yellowish fat pads sometimes seen at the periphery of the sclerae. Chronic liver disease (Table 5.19) produces endocrine effects because of reduced oestrogen metabolism by the liver. In men there may be a feminizing effect, with gynaecomastia (breast enlargement), loss of body hair and testicular atrophy.

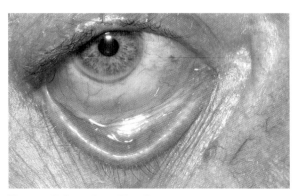

Fig. 5.5   Yellow sclera of jaundice.

5.19	Common features of chronic liver disease
Hepatomegaly (however, the liver may be small)	
Jaundice	
Ascites	
Circulatory changes	
• Spider telangiectasia, palmar erythema	
Endocrine changes	
• Loss of libido, hair loss • Men: gynaecomastia, testicular atrophy, impotence • Women: breast atrophy, irregular menses, amenorrhoea	
Haemorrhagic tendency	
• Bruises, purpura, epistaxis, menorrhagia	
Portal hypertension	
• Splenomegaly, collateral vessels, variceal bleeding, fetor hepaticus	
Hepatic (portosystemic) encephalopathy	
Other features	
• Pigmentation, digital clubbing, leukonychia, low-grade fever	

Palmar erythema and multiple *spider naevi* (isolated telangiectatic lesions found on the upper trunk, arms and face which characteristically fill from a central feeding vessel) signify chronic liver disease. Up to five spider naevi may be found in normal individuals (see Fig. 2.19, p. 50). However, women may have more if they are on oestrogen therapy or pregnant. These patients may also have palmar erythema so do not use the term 'liver palms'. Look for finger clubbing; gastrointestinal causes include cirrhosis, inflammatory bowel disease and amyloidosis. Leukonychia (white nails) are a sign of hypoalbuminaemia due to liver disease, malabsorption, protein malnutrition or nephrotic syndrome.

Dupuytren's contracture, thickening and shortening of the palmar fascia, results in flexion deformities, particularly

of the little and ring fingers (see Fig. 10.37). It was thought to be caused by alcoholic liver disease, but this association is weak. The condition has genetic and occupational factors and is more common in smokers.

Bilateral parotid swelling can occur in malnourished alcohol-dependent patients.

Gastric and pancreatic cancer may cause a palpable metastatic scalene lymph node in the supraclavicular fossa, most commonly on the left side (Troisier's sign). More widespread lymphadenopathy with hepatosplenomegaly suggests lymphoma.

The mouth and throat are part of the gastrointestinal tract and should always be assessed as part of your examination.

THE ABDOMEN

The abdomen is divided, for descriptive purposes, into nine regions by the intersection of imaginary planes, two horizontal and two sagittal (Fig. 5.6). The upper horizontal plane (transpyloric) lies at the level of the first lumbar vertebra, midway between the suprasternal notch and the symphysis pubis. The lower plane passes through the upper borders of the iliac crests. The sagittal planes are indicated on the surface by lines drawn vertically from the mid-inguinal points towards the midclavicular points.

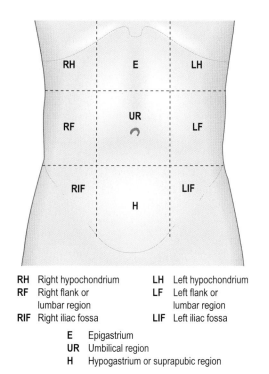

RH	Right hypochondrium	**LH** Left hypochondrium
RF	Right flank or lumbar region	**LF** Left flank or lumbar region
RIF	Right iliac fossa	**LIF** Left iliac fossa

	E	Epigastrium
	UR	Umbilical region
	H	Hypogastrium or suprapubic region

Fig. 5.6   Regions of the abdomen.

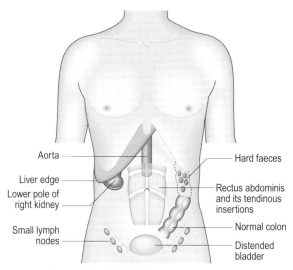

Fig. 5.7 Palpation of the abdomen. Diagram of abdomen showing palpable masses which may be physiological as opposed to pathological.

Labels on figure:
- Aorta
- Liver edge
- Lower pole of right kidney
- Small lymph nodes
- Hard faeces
- Rectus abdominis and its tendinous insertions
- Normal colon
- Distended bladder

Normal appearance

The abdomen is normally flat or slightly scaphoid and symmetrical. At rest, respiration is principally diaphragmatic and the abdominal wall moves out with inspiration. The umbilicus is usually inverted. Normally, no masses are palpable in the abdomen, but there are exceptions to this rule in thin patients (Fig. 5.7):

- the liver edge may be felt below the right costal margin
- the aorta may be palpable as a pulsatile swelling above the umbilicus
- the lower pole of the right kidney may be palpable in the right flank
- the sigmoid colon may be palpable in the left iliac fossa, particularly if loaded with faeces
- a full bladder is palpable as a mass in the suprapubic region arising out of the pelvis and dull to percussion.

The normal liver can be identified as an area of dullness to percussion over the right anterior/axillary chest between the 9th and 11th ribs.

⤏ Examination sequence

→ Whenever possible, examine the patient in good light and warm surroundings.
→ Position the patient comfortably supine with the head but not the shoulders resting on one or two pillows in order to relax the muscles of the abdominal wall.
→ Use extra pillows to support a patient with severe kyphosis.
→ Do not ask a patient with severe breathlessness to lie flat.
→ Ask the patient to remove his clothes so that there is complete exposure from the xiphisternum to the pubis.
→ Leave the chest and legs covered.

→ As well as using your eyes note any smell from the patient such as fetor hepaticus, uraemia, the characteristic smell of melaena, and ketones in fasting or ketoacidosis.

Inspection

Skin. In elderly patients seborrhoeic warts, ranging from pink to brown or black, and haemangiomas (*Campbell de Morgan spots*) are common. Think of them as normal but note any striae.

Hair. Secondary sexual hair appears at puberty. If it is absent, consider hypopituitarism or hypogonadism. Virilism in the female leads to a male distribution of pubic and body hair, whereas cirrhosis in the male may produce a female distribution of body hair.

Visible veins. Abnormally prominent veins on the abdominal wall signify portal hypertension or vena caval obstruction. In portal hypertension this results from the recanalization of the umbilical vein along the falciform ligament. Rarely this can result in distended veins flowing away from the umbilicus, the 'caput medusa'; more typically the umbilicus appears distended by blood. Do not confuse this with an umbilical hernia where the umbilicus is everted, distended, has a palpable cough impulse and does not appear vascular. Dilated tortuous veins which all flow upwards are collateral veins due to obstruction of the inferior vena cava. Rarely, obstruction of the superior vena cava will give rise to similar distended abdominal veins which all flow downwards.

Distension/swelling. Decide if the abdomen is distended and if so whether the distension is generalized or caused by a localized mass (Fig. 5.8). In obesity the umbilicus is usually sunken, whereas in the other conditions it is flat or even projecting. Localized swelling, e.g. due to massive enlargement of liver or spleen, is best seen as asymmetry when you look at the patient from the foot of the bed.

Scars and stomas. Note any surgical scars (Fig. 5.9) and clarify what they were for. They should be described in a standardized manner: vertical scars are in the midline, or paramedian to the left or right, and are above or below the umbilicus (upper or lower). An appendicectomy scar lies diagonally in the right iliac fossa. Scars from hernia repairs are also diagonal but lower in either inguinal region. A horizontal suprapubic scar, the Pfannenstiel incision, is used for gynaecological surgery. For cosmetic reasons it is often sited in a skin fold below the 'bikini line' and is easily overlooked. A right subcostal scar usually signifies an open cholecystectomy while a bilateral subcostal scar with a vertical extension to the ziphisternum – known as a 'Mercedes-Benz' scar for obvious reasons – is the result of liver surgery. A small infraumbilical incision is usually the result of previous laparoscopy. Puncture scars from the ports used for laparoscopic surgery may be visible, e.g. in the right hypochondrium for laparoscopic cholecystectomy.

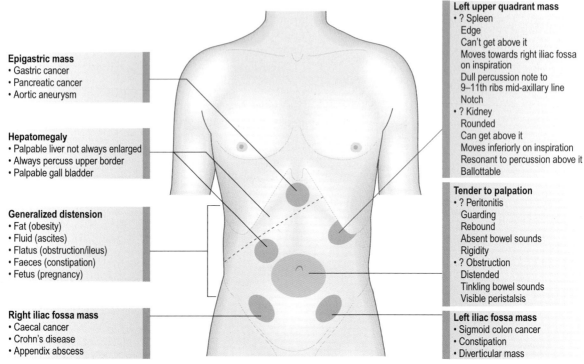

Epigastric mass
• Gastric cancer
• Pancreatic cancer
• Aortic aneurysm

Hepatomegaly
• Palpable liver not always enlarged
• Always percuss upper border
• Palpable gall bladder

Generalized distension
• Fat (obesity)
• Fluid (ascites)
• Flatus (obstruction/ileus)
• Faeces (constipation)
• Fetus (pregnancy)

Right iliac fossa mass
• Caecal cancer
• Crohn's disease
• Appendix abscess

Left upper quadrant mass
• ? Spleen
  Edge
  Can't get above it
  Moves towards right iliac fossa
  on inspiration
  Dull percussion note to
  9–11th ribs mid-axillary line
  Notch
• ? Kidney
  Rounded
  Can get above it
  Moves inferiorly on inspiration
  Resonant to percussion above it
  Ballottable

Tender to palpation
• ? Peritonitis
  Guarding
  Rebound
  Absent bowel sounds
  Rigidity
• ? Obstruction
  Distended
  Tinkling bowel sounds
  Visible peristalsis

Left iliac fossa mass
• Sigmoid colon cancer
• Constipation
• Diverticular mass

Fig. 5.8   Diagram of abdomen showing palpable abnormalities.

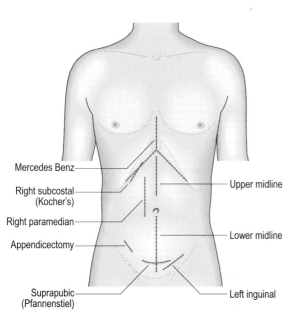

Mercedes Benz
Right subcostal (Kocher's)
Right paramedian
Appendicectomy
Suprapubic (Pfannenstiel)
Upper midline
Lower midline
Left inguinal

Fig. 5.9   Some commonly used abdominal incisions. The midline and oblique incisions avoid damage to the innervation of the abdominal musculature and the later development of incisional herniae.

Any midline scar may develop an incisional hernia. This is palpable as a defect in the abdominal wall musculature and is more obvious if the patient raises the head from the bed or coughs. A similar appearance of midline swelling in the absence of a scar is due to divarification of the rectus sheath. Stomas may be present (Fig. 5.10): usually an ileostomy is situated in the right iliac fossa; a transverse colostomy in the left hypochondrium; and a sigmoid colostomy in the left iliac fossa.

Palpation

◢ Examination Sequence

→ Ensure that your hands are warm. If the patient is in a low bed, sit on, or kneel beside, the bed on the patient's right side.
→ Ask the patient to place his arms alongside his body to help relax the abdominal wall. Placing a pillow under the patient's knees may also help by allowing flexion of the hips (Fig. 5.11).
→ Ask the patient to show you where he feels pain before you start, and to report any tenderness as you examine him.
→ Begin with gentle superficial examination of the whole abdomen. If the patient has abdominal pain, start away from the site of maximal pain and move in a systematic manner through the nine regions of the abdomen.

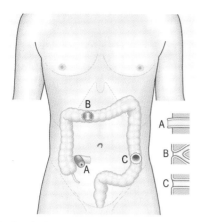

Fig. 5.10 Surgical stomas. An ileostomy is usually in the right iliac fossa and is formed as a spout (A). A loop colostomy may be created by temporary defunctioning of the distal bowel. It is usually in the transverse colon and has afferent and efferent limbs (B). A colostomy may be terminal, i.e. resected distal bowel. It is usually flush and in the left iliac fossa (C).

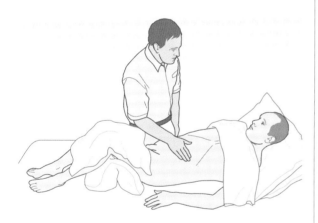

Fig. 5.11 Position of the patient and exposure for abdominal examination.

➜ Use your right hand, keeping it flat and in contact with the abdominal wall, and avoid using your finger tips. As you palpate, watch the patient's face for any sign of discomfort.
➜ Palpate lightly in each region in turn, then repeat this palpating deeply.
➜ Test muscle tone by light dipping movements with your fingers.

Abnormal findings

The abnormalities are either tenderness and/or masses.

Tenderness. Discomfort during palpation is accompanied by resistance to palpation and varies widely in severity. When deciding how severe pain and tenderness are, take into account the patient's level of anxiety, remembering that it will be heightened if the patient has abdominal pain. Apparent tenderness in several areas with minimal pressure may be due to generalized peritonitis, but is often due to patient anxiety. Severe pain with no tenderness on deep palpation, or where the tenderness disappears when the patient is distracted, suggests non-organic pathology. With these exceptions, tenderness is usually a useful indication of underlying pathology.

Palpation which elicits pain may cause the patient to voluntarily contract the overlying abdominal muscles (*voluntary guarding*). If the pain is due to inflammation, pressure of the parietal peritoneum onto the inflamed area results in a reflex contraction of the overlying muscles (*involuntary guarding*). If the whole peritoneal cavity is inflamed there will be generalized peritonitis and the muscles of the anterior abdominal wall will be held rigid (board-like rigidity). The anterior abdominal wall does not move with respiration and breathing becomes increasingly thoracic.

'*Rebound' tenderness* is a sensitive sign of intra-abdominal disease but not a reliable indicator of peritoneal irritation. Gently press your hand in, then rapidly remove it. The patient shows more discomfort as your hand is released. Ask the patient to cough, or gently percuss the abdomen and note tenderness.

Generalized severe tenderness accompanied by board-like rigidity to palpation is due to generalized peritonitis secondary to a perforated viscus, e.g. perforated duodenal ulcer or perforated diverticulum. More localized but severe tenderness may indicate localized peritonitis. The site of the tenderness is important, e.g. tenderness in the epigastrium suggests peptic ulcer; in the right hypochondrium, cholecystitis; in the right iliac fossa, appendicitis.

Palpable mass. When you feel a mass decide if it is due to enlargement of an abdominal organ, or a separate mass. If the latter, is it simply palpable faeces in a constipated patient, or is it pathological? Palpable faeces can usually be indented with your examining finger. If the mass or lump seems superficial it may be within the anterior abdominal wall rather than the abdominal cavity. Ask the patient to tense the abdominal muscles by lifting the head; an abdominal wall mass will still be palpable, whereas a deep mass will not.

Describe any mass using the basic principles from Chapter 2 (see Table 2.7, p. 54). In particular describe its site, size, surface, shape, consistency and whether it moves on respiration. If not, see if it is fixed or mobile. A pulsatile mass palpable in the upper abdomen may be normal aortic pulsation in thin people, a gastric or pancreatic tumour transmitting underlying aortic pulsation, or an aortic aneurysm.

Palpating for enlarged organs

Examine the liver, gall bladder and spleen in turn. Examination of the kidneys is covered in Chapter 6.

Hepatomegaly. Hepatic enlargement can result from chronic parenchymal liver disease from any cause. Although the liver is enlarged in early cirrhosis, it is often shrunken in end-stage cirrhosis. Fatty liver (hepatic steatosis) from alcohol or other causes can cause marked hepatomegaly. Hepatic enlargement due to metastatic tumour deposits is hard and irregular. An enlarged left lobe may be felt in the epigastrium or even the left hypochondrium. Hepatocellular cancer sometimes causes an audible bruit which can also rarely be heard in alcoholic hepatitis. In right heart failure, the liver is usually soft and may be tender. A pulsatile liver indicates tricuspid incompetence.

The aim is to feel if the lower border of the liver is palpable.

▶ Examination sequence

→ Start palpating in the right iliac fossa. If you start in the right hypochondrium, you may already be above the lower border of a massively enlarged liver.

→ Use either the radial border of your right hand, i.e. the outside edge of the forefinger, or the finger pads; in both cases keep your hand flat on the abdomen (Fig. 5.12). Do not dig in with your finger tips as you may get a false impression of the liver edge.

→ Keep your hand stationary and ask the patient to take a deep breath in. Try to feel the edge of the enlarged liver as it moves downwards on inspiration.

→ Move your hand progressively further up the abdomen a centimetre or so at a time repeating the request to breathe in until you reach the costal margin or detect the edge.

→ If you feel the liver edge, work out if it is enlarged or displaced downwards as occurs in patients with hyperinflated lungs from emphysema. The liver is dull to percussion whereas the lung is resonant, so locate the upper border of the liver by percussing over the right lateral chest wall. The lower three to four ribs are normally dull to percussion. A reduced area of dullness suggests emphysema, a shrunken liver (as occurs in end-stage

cirrhosis), or occasionally interposition of the transverse colon between the liver and the diaphragm.

→ Measure the distance below the costal margin in centimetres in the midclavicular line.

If you detect the liver edge, describe:

- size, e.g. in cm below the costal margin
- surface – smooth or irregular
- edge – smooth or irregular
- consistency – soft or hard
- if it is tender
- if it is pulsatile
- whether there is an audible bruit.

The gall bladder may be palpable in the right hypochondrium if it is swollen (Fig. 5.13A). It has a characteristic globular feel, and, unlike the liver, you can palpate above it. It becomes swollen due to obstruction either of the cystic duct (resulting in a mucocele of the gall bladder) or of the common bile duct if the cystic duct is patent, as in pancreatic cancer. A gall bladder with gallstone disease is not palpable because it becomes thickened and contracted. If the gall bladder is palpable in a jaundiced patient the obstruction is not due to gallstones but is likely to be pancreatic cancer or distal cholangiocarcinoma (Courvoisier's law).

Causes of hepatomegaly are listed in Table 5.20.

Splenomegaly. Splenomegaly refers to enlargement of the spleen. The term *hypersplenism* refers to the pancytopenia (low platelet, white cell count and haemoglobin) found in patients with chronic splenic enlargement. This is due to increased destruction of circulating blood

5.20   Causes of hepatomegaly
Chronic parenchymal liver disease
<ul><li>Alcoholic liver disease</li><li>Autoimmune hepatitis</li><li>Viral hepatitis</li><li>Primary biliary cirrhosis</li></ul>
Malignancy
<ul><li>Primary hepatocellular cancer</li><li>Secondary metastatic cancer</li></ul>
Right heart failure
Haematological disorders
<ul><li>Lymphoma</li><li>Leukaemia</li><li>Myelofibrosis</li><li>Polycythaemia</li></ul>
Rarities
<ul><li>Amyloidosis</li><li>Budd–Chiari syndrome</li><li>Glycogen storage disorders</li></ul>

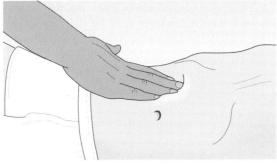

Fig. 5.12   Palpating the liver.

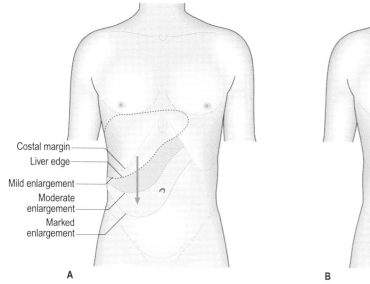
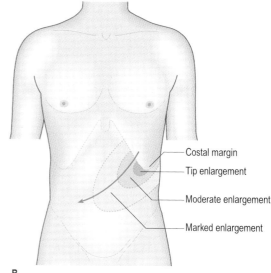

Costal margin
Liver edge
Mild enlargement
Moderate enlargement
Marked enlargement

Costal margin
Tip enlargement
Moderate enlargement
Marked enlargement

A   B

Fig. 5.13 Patterns of progressive enlargement of liver and of spleen. (A) Palpation of an enlarged liver. (B) The direction of enlargement of the spleen. The spleen has a characteristic notched shape and moves downwards and medially during full inspiration.

cells. Haematological disorders causing splenomegaly commonly, but not invariably, also cause enlargement of the liver. Haemolytic anaemia causes mild splenomegaly without hepatomegaly. Portal hypertension is usually due to cirrhosis, when the liver may or may not be enlarged.

The spleen has to increase in size threefold to be palpable, so a palpable splenic edge always indicates splenomegaly. Causes of splenomegaly are listed in Table 5.21. The spleen enlarges from under the left costal margin down and medially towards the right iliac fossa (Fig. 5.13B). If the spleen is significantly enlarged, a characteristic notch may be palpable midway along its leading edge.

⤷ Examination sequence

→ With your right hand start in the right iliac fossa and ask the patient to breathe in deeply as you press posteriorly and caudally for 1–2 centimetres (Fig. 5.14A). Try to detect the spleen as it moves down against your fingers.

→ Move your hand diagonally upwards and across the abdomen 1–2 centimetres at a time into the left hypochondrium repeating this manoeuvre.

→ Feel the costal margin along its length as the position of the spleen tip is variable.

→ If you cannot feel the splenic edge, ask the patient to roll towards you onto the right side and repeat the above.

→ Palpate with your right hand while using your left hand to press forward on the patient's left lower ribs from behind (Fig. 5.14B).

→ Feel along the left costal margin.

5.21   Causes of splenomegaly
Haematological disorders
• Lymphoma • Leukaemia especially chronic myeloid leukaemia • Myelofibrosis • Polycythaemia • Haemolytic anaemia
Portal hypertension
Infections
• Glandular fever • Malaria • Brucellosis • Kala azar (leishmaniasis) • Subacute bacterial endocarditis
Rheumatological conditions
• Rheumatoid arthritis (Felty's syndrome) • Systemic lupus erythematosus
Rarities
• Sarcoidosis • Amyloidosis • Glycogen storage disorders

Percussion

Solid or fluid-filled structures are dull to percussion. Structures containing air or gas are resonant. Normally the abdomen is resonant due to the gas content of the intestine.

171

A
B

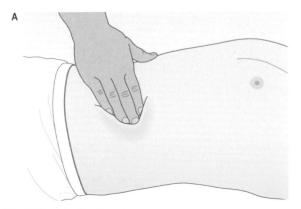
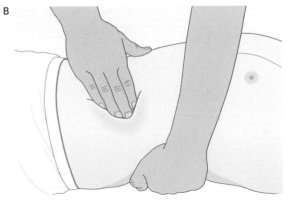

Fig. 5.14 Palpating the spleen.

- Use a lighter touch when percussing the abdomen than when you percuss the chest.
- Always percuss from the area of resonance to the area of dullness to identify the position accurately.
- Assess each organ with both palpation and percussion before moving on to the next organ.
- The kidneys are retroperitoneal and so are usually resonant because of the overlying colon.
- A palpable mass arising from the pelvis in the midline and dull to percussion is usually a full bladder, though a pregnant uterus and a pelvic tumour are other possibilities.

Shifting dullness

This test is to demonstrate the presence of ascites. With the patient supine, percuss from the midline out to the flanks (Fig. 5.15). Note any change from resonant to dull.

There are two methods :

1. Keep your finger on the site of dullness in the flank and ask the patient to turn onto the opposite side. Pause for at least 10 seconds to allow any ascites to gravitate; then percuss again and if that area is now resonant, you have demonstrated shifting dullness as the ascitic fluid became dependent.

2. Mark the point at which the percussion note changes from resonant to dull with a pen on a line parallel to the flank. Ask the patient to turn to the same side and repeat the manoeuvre: if the line has moved 'up' the abdomen towards the midline, you have demonstrated shifting dullness.

Always wait a few moments after the patient turns before repeating percussion, to allow time for the fluid to shift and settle.

Fluid thrill

If the abdomen is tense, assess for a fluid thrill. Place the palm of your left hand flat against the left side of the abdomen, flick a finger of your right hand against the right side of the abdomen. If you feel a ripple against your left hand, ask the patient (or an assistant) to place the edge of a hand

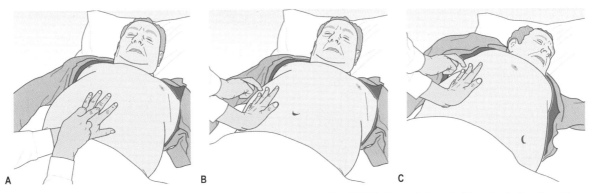

A
B
C

Fig. 5.15   Percussing for ascites. Percuss towards the flank from resonant (A) to dull (B), then ask the patient to roll onto the other side. When ascites is present, the note then becomes resonant (C).

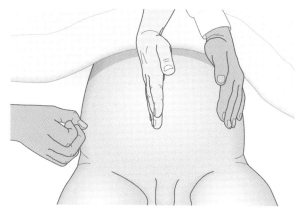

Fig. 5.16 Eliciting a fluid thrill.

on the midline of the abdomen (Fig. 5.16). This prevents transmission of the impulse via the skin. If you still feel a ripple against your left hand this is a fluid thrill. This sign is only present when ascites is obvious. If you find central dullness and lateral resonance in a woman, suspect a giant ovarian cyst.

Auscultation

With the patient lying on the back place the diaphragm of the stethoscope to the right of the umbilicus and do not move it. *Bowel sounds* are gurgling sounds caused by normal peristaltic activity of the gut. They normally occur every 5–10 seconds, but the frequency varies widely. You must listen for up to 2 minutes before concluding that they are absent. Absence of bowel sounds implies paralytic ileus or peritonitis. In intestinal obstruction, bowel sounds occur at increased frequency and have a high-pitched tinkling quality.

Listen above the umbilicus over the aorta for bruits which indicate turbulent flow from atheroma or an aneurysm. Now place the stethoscope 2–3 cm above and lateral to the umbilicus to listen for renal artery bruits as in renal artery stenosis. Listen over the liver for bruits which occur in hepatoma or acute alcoholic hepatitis. You may hear a friction rub in perihepatitis. Very occasionally you may hear a venous hum in the upper abdomen over a caput medusa.

A *succussion splash* sounds like shaking a half-filled water bottle. Shake the abdomen by lifting the patient with both hands under the pelvis. Explain first what you are going to do. An audible splash more than 4 hours after the patient has eaten or drunk anything, indicates delayed gastric emptying, e.g. pyloric stenosis.

A rectal examination (see p. 222) is an essential part of the abdominal examination and should be performed at this point together with examination of the groin and, where appropriate, of the genitalia.

Hernias

An external abdominal hernia is an abnormal protrusion of an organ or tissue, usually bowel and/or omentum, from the abdominal cavity. Hernias are common and most often occur at sites of natural openings of the abdominal wall, e.g. the inguinal, femoral and obturator canals, the umbilicus and the oesophageal hiatus. They may occur at sites of weakness, related to previous surgical incisions or stretching of the abdominal wall. *Internal hernias* occur through defects of the mesentery or into the retroperitoneal space and are not visible. *External hernias* are more prominent in the erect position, when the pressure within the abdomen rises, and during coughing when an impulse can often be felt in the hernia. This is the cough impulse.

A *reducible* hernia is one whose contents can be returned to the abdominal cavity, spontaneously or by manipulation. If not, the hernia is *irreducible*. An abdominal hernia has a covering sac of peritoneum, and the neck of the hernia is a common site of compression of the contents (Fig. 5.17). If bowel is involved in the hernia, bowel obstruction may occur. If the process leads to compression and compromise of the blood supply to the contents (bowel or omentum) the hernia is strangulated.

Hernias most commonly occur in the groins and you should examine these sites as part of your routine examination of the abdomen.

Anatomy

The inguinal canal extends from the pubic tubercle to the anterior superior iliac spine (Fig. 5.18). It has an internal ring at the mid-inguinal point and an external ring at the

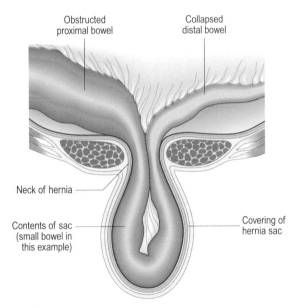

Obstructed proximal bowel

Collapsed distal bowel

Neck of hernia

Contents of sac (small bowel in this example)

Covering of hernia sac

Fig. 5.17 Hernia: anatomical structure.

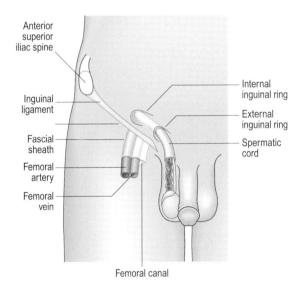

Anterior superior iliac spine

Inguinal ligament

Fascial sheath

Femoral artery

Femoral vein

Internal inguinal ring

External inguinal ring

Spermatic cord

Femoral canal

Fig. 5.18 The anatomy of the inguinal canal and femoral sheath.

pubic tubercle. Note that the mid-inguinal point is midway between the pubic symphysis and the anterior superior iliac spine *not* at the midpoint of the inguinal ligament. In males the inguinal canal contains the spermatic cord and its blood vessels.

Indirect inguinal hernias are the most common type and account for 85% of all hernias. An indirect inguinal hernia bulges through the inner ring and follows the course

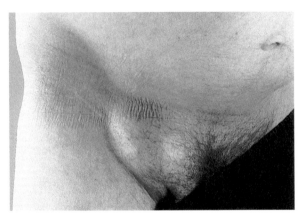

Fig. 5.19 Right inguinal hernia.

of the inguinal canal. It may extend beyond the external ring and enter the scrotum. Indirect hernias are more common in younger men.

A *direct inguinal hernia* forms at a site of weakness of the musculature of the posterior wall of the inguinal canal and will rarely extend into the scrotum. Direct inguinal hernias are more common in older men and women (Fig. 5.19).

The femoral canal lies below the inguinal ligament. A *femoral hernia* projects through the femoral ring and into the femoral canal.

- Inguinal hernias are palpable *above* and *medial* to the pubic tubercle.
- Femoral hernias are palpable *below* the inguinal ligament and *lateral* to the pubic tubercle.

Abnormal findings

Identifying a hernia from the anatomical site involved and the nature of the lump (Table 5.22) is difficult but it should be possible to differentiate between direct and indirect inguinal hernias. Bowel in a hernia may feel compressible and gurgle when palpated and you may hear bowel sounds over the swelling; omentum feels firmer.

5.22 Causes of groin lumps
• Inguinal hernia:
– indirect
– direct
• Femoral hernia
• Lymph node(s)
• Saphena varix (a varicosity of the long saphenous vein)
• Skin and subcutaneous lumps, e.g. lipoma, sebaceous cyst
• Hydrocele of spermatic cord
• Undescended testis
• Femoral aneurysm
• Psoas abscess

A strangulated hernia is a surgical emergency. It is tense and tender and shows no impulse on coughing; there may be features of bowel obstruction and later signs of sepsis and shock.

➤ Examination sequence

➔ Hernias may reduce spontaneously when a patient lies supine so, if possible, examine the patient standing.

➔ Ask the patient to stand, carefully inspect the inguinal and femoral canals and the scrotum for any lumps or bulges.

➔ Ask the patient to cough and look for any impulse over the femoral or inguinal canals and/or scrotum.

➔ Identify the anatomical relationships between the bulge, the pubic tubercle and the inguinal ligament to distinguish a femoral from an inguinal hernia.

➔ Palpate the external inguinal ring and posterior wall of the inguinal canal for possible muscle defects. Ask the patient to cough and feel for any impulse.

➔ Ask the patient to lie down and see if the hernia reduces spontaneously. If so, press with two fingers over the internal inguinal ring at the mid-inguinal point and ask the patient to cough or stand up while you continue to press over the internal inguinal ring and see if the hernia reappears. If you can prevent it from reappearing it is an indirect inguinal hernia.

➔ Always examine the opposite side as well to detect an asymptomatic hernia.

THE ACUTE ABDOMEN

The 'acute abdomen' includes a spectrum of underlying causes (Table 5.23) ranging from minor self-limiting conditions to severe life-threatening diseases that present with a history of < 1 week's duration requiring emergency admission to hospital. It commonly accounts for 50% of general surgical emergency admissions. The diagnosis and management of a patient with an acute abdomen depends on information from the history and examination, but occasionally a rapid evaluation with immediate resuscitation and intervention is required.

The most recent and severe symptoms may occupy the patient's attention to such an extent that important but apparently unrelated details of the history may be forgotten unless questioned directly (Table 5.24). If severe pain, shock or altered consciousness make it difficult to obtain an accurate history from the patient, ask partners, relatives or friends who are with the patient.

A past history of an abdominal complaint may direct your initial thoughts to specific complications of underlying disease, e.g. acute perforation in a patient with known diverticular disease. Remember that abdominal pain may be the presenting feature of disease outwith the abdomen, e.g. myocardial infarction, pneumonia, diabetic ketoacidosis, herpes zoster.

Specific abdominal signs may be masked in patients taking steroids, non-steroidal anti-inflammatory drugs or those with alcohol intoxication or a depressed level of consciousness.

The early administration of adequate opioid analgesia to a patient with severe abdominal pain is important. It will aid your clinical assessment as the patient will be more comfortable and relaxed and has no detrimental effect on clinical assessment.

5.23	Common non-traumatic causes of the acute abdomen	
Pathological process	**Organ commonly involved**	**Disease**
Inflammation	Appendix	Acute appendicitis
	Gall bladder	Acute cholecystitis
	Colon	Diverticulitis
	Fallopian tube	Salpingitis
	Pancreas	Acute pancreatitis
Obstruction	Intestine	Intestinal obstruction
	Gall bladder	Biliary colic
	Ureter	Ureteric colic
	Urethra	Acute retention of urine
Ischaemia	Intestine	Strangulated hernia
		Volvulus
		Mesenteric ischaemia
	Ovary	Torsion of ovarian cyst
Perforation	Duodenum	Perforated peptic ulcer
	Stomach	Perforated ulcer/cancer
	Colon	Perforated diverticulum
		Perforated cancer
	Gall bladder	Biliary peritonitis
Rupture	Fallopian tube	Ruptured ectopic pregnancy
	Abdominal aorta	Ruptured aneurysm

HISTORY

Pain

The commonest presenting feature is acute abdominal pain. The site of abdominal pain may indicate the likely origin of the underlying pathology. Pain experienced predominantly

175

5.24 Some typical clinical features of the important causes of an 'acute abdomen'		
Condition	**History**	**Examination**
Acute appendicitis	Nausea, vomiting, central abdominal pain which later shifts to the right iliac fossa	Fever, tenderness and guarding in the right iliac fossa, palpable mass in the right iliac fossa, pelvic peritonitis on examination
Perforated peptic ulcer with acute peritonitis	Vomiting at onset associated with acute-onset severe abdominal pain, previous history of dyspepsia, ulcer disease, non-steroidal anti-inflammatory drug or corticosteroid therapy	Shallow breathing with minimal abdominal wall movement, abdominal tenderness and guarding, board-like rigidity, abdominal distension and absent bowel sounds
Acute pancreatitis	Anorexia, nausea, vomiting, constant severe epigastric pain, previous alcohol abuse/cholelithiasis	Fever, periumbilical bruising (Cullen's sign), bruising in the loin (Grey Turner's sign), epigastric tenderness, variable guarding, reduced or absent bowel sounds
Ruptured aortic aneurysm	Sudden onset of tearing, severe back/loin/abdominal pain, circulatory collapse, history of peripheral vascular disease and/or hypertension	Shock and hypotension, pulsatile, tender, central abdominal mass with an overlying bruit, asymmetrical femoral pulses. Sometimes hypertension (renal artery involvement)
Acute mesenteric ischaemia	Anorexia, nausea, vomiting, bloody diarrhoea, constant, severe, sustained abdominal pain, previous history of cardiovascular disease	Atrial fibrillation, cardiac failure, asymmetrical peripheral pulses, absent bowel sounds, variable tenderness and guarding
Intestinal obstruction	Colicky central abdominal pain, nausea, vomiting and constipation	Surgical scars, hernias, abdominal mass, distension, visible peristalsis, increased tinkling bowel sounds
Ruptured ectopic pregnancy	Premenopausal; delayed/missed menstrual period, feeling faint, circulatory collapse, unilateral iliac fossa pain, pleuritic or shoulder-tip pain, vaginal discharge – 'late period', 'like prune juice'	Suprapubic tenderness, periumbilical bruising (Cullen's sign), pain/tenderness on vaginal examination (cervical excitation), swelling/fullness in the fornix on vaginal examination
Pelvic inflammatory disease	Sexually active female; previous history of sexually transmitted disease or pelvic inflammatory disease, recent gynaecological procedure, pregnancy or use of intrauterine contraceptive device. Irregular menstruation, dysuria, dyspareunia, lower or central abdominal pain, backache, pleuritic right upper quadrant abdominal pain (Fitz-Hugh–Curtis syndrome)	Fever, vaginal discharge, pelvic peritonitis causing tenderness on rectal examination, right upper quadrant tenderness (perihepatitis), pain/tenderness on vaginal examination (cervical excitation), swelling/fullness in the fornix on vaginal examination

in the upper abdomen arises from foregut structures, e.g. duodenal ulcer, gall bladder pathology or pancreatitis. Central abdominal pain arises from midgut structures, such as conditions affecting the small bowel and appendix. Lower abdominal pain may result from the large bowel. Gynaecological pathology may also cause lower abdominal pain (see p. 203).

Visceral pain is referred in a somatic distribution, whereas parietal pain is felt at the site of the affected organ. Therefore the classical history of a patient with acute appendicitis is that of early periumbilical pain which moves to the right iliac fossa if there is localized parietal inflammation (Fig. 5.20).

Excruciating pain unrelieved by opioids indicates a vascular lesion, e.g. bowel infarction or rupture of an abdominal aortic aneurysm. Very severe pain readily controlled by medication is more typical of acute pancreatitis or peritonitis secondary to a ruptured viscus. The pain of biliary colic or renal colic is usually promptly relieved by medication. Dull, vague and poorly localized pain is more typical of an inflammatory process or low-grade infection.

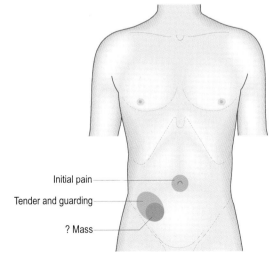

Initial pain

Tender and guarding

? Mass

Fig. 5.20 Acute appendicitis.

Sudden onset of severe pain is likely to be due to rupture of a viscus or vascular cause. Rapid onset of moderately severe pain over a short period of time may be due to renal or biliary colic, acute pancreatitis, or small bowel obstruction. Gradual onset of slowly progressive pain is more characteristic of peritoneal infection or inflammation and may be due to appendicitis or diverticular disease.

Inflammation and obstruction are the two main pathological processes accounting for acute abdominal pain. Inflammation produces a more constant pain exacerbated by movement or coughing. Patients therefore typically lie very still in order not to exacerbate the pain. Obstruction of a muscular viscus produces a colicky pain. Characteristically patients with colic move around or draw their knees up towards the chest during painful spasms.

Pain radiating from the right hypochondrium to the shoulder or interscapular region is likely to be due to gall bladder pathology, such as cholecystitis. Pain radiating from the loin to the groin is typical of renal colic due to a ureteric calculus. Central upper abdominal pain radiating through to the back which may be relieved by sitting forward is common in patients with pancreatitis. Coexistence of severe back and abdominal pain may indicate a ruptured or dissecting abdominal aortic aneurysm.

Anorexia and nausea are common but non-specific symptoms, and there may be advanced abdominal disease without these features. A history of vomiting may not, in itself, be helpful because vomiting occurs as a response to pain. However, it may indicate underlying abdominal pathology, e.g. gastroenteritis, acute gastritis, acute pancreatitis, biliary or renal colic. Severe vomiting may be due to gastric outlet obstruction or proximal small bowel obstruction. *Faeculent vomiting* is the vomiting of altered small bowel content, not of faeces. It is a late feature in distal small bowel or large bowel obstruction. In peritonitis the vomitus is usually small in volume, but persistent in nature. Severe vomiting with retching may result in a laceration at the gastro-oesophageal junction (Mallory–Weiss syndrome), or oesophageal perforation (Boerhaave's syndrome).

Other features

Ask if there have been prior similar episodes of pain and whether these have been previously investigated. The patient may have noticed swelling or pain in the groin or be aware of increasing abdominal distension. Always take a gynaecological history including a menstrual history, particularly to exclude the possibility of (ectopic) pregnancy. Ask about any purulent vaginal discharge which may indicate pelvic inflammatory disease.

Bowel habit

Alteration of bowel function is common in patients with acute abdominal emergencies. Absolute constipation, i.e.

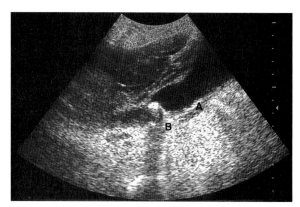

Fig. 5.21 Ultrasound scan showing thick-walled gall bladder (A) containing gallstones with posterior acoustic shadowing (B).

no gas or bowel movements, suggests intestinal obstruction and is likely to be associated with abdominal pain, vomiting and abdominal distension. Diarrhoea is the classical manifestation of gastroenteritis; however, it may also be a symptom of pelvic appendicitis. Bloody diarrhoea may be due to inflammatory bowel disease, colonic ischaemia or infective gastroenteritis.

Analgesia

Patients should always be given adequate analgesia pending formal examination. Do not withhold opioid analgesia from patients with acute abdominal pain; important clinical signs such as localized tenderness will not be masked. Analgesia relaxes the patient and aids examination with better localization of clinical signs. Do not repeatedly administer analgesia to patients with abdominal pain with no definite diagnosis without regularly reassessing their clinical state, promptly investigating them and considering surgical intervention.

PHYSICAL EXAMINATION

Inspection

Assess the general state and demeanour of the patient. Does the patient look unwell with pallor, sweating and reluctance to move? Critically ill patients may be confused and may have a depressed level of consciousness. Record the temperature, pulse rate, blood pressure and respiratory rate. Remember to examine the cardiovascular and respiratory systems, as conditions including myocardial infarction, pneumonia, pleurisy, pulmonary embolism and shingles may all present with acute abdominal pain.

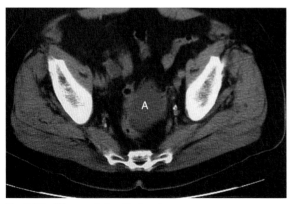

Fig. 5.22 CT scan of diverticular abscess.

Palpation, percussion and auscultation

Examine the abdomen then the back, groins, perineum, and genitalia. Perform a rectal examination (see p. 224) unless you are referring the patient urgently to a specialist where this will be repeated. Consider the patient's dignity and do not carry out assessments that will not change your management. In women, consider a vaginal examination to detect gynaecological pathology.

Gentle percussion is useful in the localization and assessment of rebound tenderness and in determining the presence of fluid within the peritoneal cavity. You may find diminished or absent liver dullness to percussion in patients with perforation of a hollow viscus and air under the diaphragm. Absent audible peristalsis, i.e. a completely silent abdomen on auscultation may indicate diffuse peritonitis. Increased peristalsis produces high-pitched 'tinkling' bowel sounds characteristic of intestinal obstruction, gastroenteritis or fulminant inflammatory bowel disease.

Named clinical signs

Murphy's sign. This is a sign of acute cholecystitis. Ask the patient to take a deep breath as you gently palpate the right upper quadrant of the abdomen. As the diaphragm descends, the acutely inflamed gall bladder comes in contact with your examining fingers causing the patient to 'catch' the inspiratory effort.

Rovsing's sign. In acute appendicitis, palpation in the left iliac fossa may produce pain in the right iliac fossa.

Iliopsoas sign. Ask the patient to flex the thigh against the resistance of your hand. A painful response indicates an inflammatory process involving the psoas muscle, e.g. retroileal appendicitis or perinephric abscess.

COMMON GASTROINTESTINAL INVESTIGATIONS

Stool

Look at the stool colour and appearance (Table 5.25).

5.25 Causes of abnormal stool appearance	
Stool appearance	**Cause**
Abnormally pale (lack of the pigment stercobilin)	Biliary obstruction
Pale and greasy	Steatorrhoea due to fat malabsorption
Black tarry stools (melaena)	Bleeding from the upper gastrointestinal tract
Grey/black colour	Oral iron or bismuth therapy
Fresh blood in or on stool	Large bowel, rectal or anal bleeding. Rarely massive upper GI haemorrhage
Stool mixed with pus	Ulcerative colitis, dysentery
Watery, odourless, flecks of mucus and epithelial cell debris (rice-water stool)	Cholera

Faecal occult blood

There are several simple methods available to test stools for the presence of blood. A positive result for faecal occult blood is produced by any cause of gastrointestinal haemorrhage, e.g. bleeding peptic ulcer, colorectal cancer, inflammatory bowel disease, etc. However, the tests are sensitive but not specific. They may be positive after vigorous tooth brushing or after eating rare steak or other red meat and may be negative even in patients with proven colorectal or gastric cancers, chronic upper gastrointestinal haemorrhage and inflammatory bowel disease.

Urinalysis

Urinalysis can confirm jaundice. Stix testing of urine at the bedside can determine the presence or absence of bilirubin and urobilinogen. Analysis of the urine can also be useful in diagnosing non-surgical causes of acute abdominal pain, e.g. diabetes mellitus and porphyria.

Ascitic fluid

A sample of the fluid should be removed for inspection and biochemical, microbiological and cytological analysis from all patients with ascites. The process is an *ascitic tap*, or *paracentesis*.

- The patient should lie flat and must have an empty bladder (by urethral catheterization if necessary). The site for aspiration is the right iliac fossa just lateral to a point midway between the umbilicus and the anterior superior iliac spine.
- Using an aseptic technique, clean the site and infiltrate the skin and down to the parietal peritoneum with local anaesthetic.
- Use a 10 ml syringe with a 19G needle to aspirate the ascitic fluid.

Ascitic fluid is usually clear and straw-coloured. Blood-stained fluid suggests intra-abdominal malignancy. Turbid fluid may indicate a high cell count due to infection, or a high protein content. Occasionally the ascitic fluid may be chylous, with a milky appearance. This is due to a high lipid content and indicates impaired lymphatic drainage.

The fluid should be analysed for protein content. A protein concentration < 25 g/l, or a gradient between the serum and ascitic albumin concentration > 11 g/l indicates a transudate. This is seen in liver disease, portal hypertension and in other hypoalbuminaemic states such as nephrotic syndrome. Fluid with a high protein content is an exudate, and suggests malignancy or infection.

Other laboratory analyses on ascitic fluid include microbiology, for cell count and culture, cytology for malignant cells and measurement of amylase (raised in pancreatic ascites) and glucose (low in tuberculous ascites).

SPECIALIZED INVESTIGATIONS

5.26   Specialized investigations in gastrointestinal and hepatobiliary disorders

Investigation	Diagnostic problem	Abnormal findings and comments
Chest X-ray	Acute abdomen, perforated viscus, subphrenic abscess	Pneumonia, free air beneath diaphragm, pleural effusion, elevated diaphragm
Abdominal X-ray	Intestinal obstruction, perforation, renal colic	Fluid levels, air above the liver, urinary tract stones
Barium meal	Dysphagia, dyspepsia	Oesophageal obstruction (endoscopy preferable if previous gastric surgery)
Small bowel barium enema	Malabsorption, subacute obstruction, unexplained GI bleeding	Duodenal diverticulosis, Crohn's disease, lymphoma
Large bowel barium enema	Altered bowel habit, iron-deficiency anaemia, rectal bleeding	Colon cancer, inflammatory bowel disease, diverticular disease
Upper abdominal ultrasound scan	Biliary colic, jaundice, pancreatitis, malignancy	Gallstones, liver metastases, cholestasis, pancreatic calcification, subphrenic abscess
Pelvic ultrasound scan	Pelvic masses, inflammatory diseases, ectopic pregnancy, polycystic ovarian syndrome	Pelvic structures and abnormalities Ascitic fluid
Upper GI endoscopy	Dysphagia, dyspepsia, gastrointestinal bleeding, gastric ulcer, malabsorption	Important in patients > 50 years even if barium meal is normal. Gastric and/or duodenal biopsies are useful
Lower GI endoscopy	Rectal bleeding, unexplained gastrointestinal bleeding, inflammatory bowel disease	Important even if the barium enema is normal. Biopsy to confirm type of colitis
Endoscopic retrograde cholangiopancreatography	Obstructive jaundice, acute and chronic pancreatitis	Diagnostic and therapeutic role Stenting strictures
Abdominal CT scan	Suspected pancreatic or renal mass, tumour staging, abdominal aortic aneurysm	Useful to confirm or exclude metastatic disease and leaking from aortic aneurysm
Laparoscopy	Acute abdomen, chronic pelvic pain, suspected ovarian disease, peritoneal and liver disease	Appendicitis, hepatic cirrhosis, ectopic pregnancy, ovarian cysts, endometriosis, pelvic inflammatory disease
Aspiration cytology	Liver metastases, intra-abdominal or retroperitoneal tumours	Tissue biopsy guided by ultrasound scanning
Liver biopsy	Parenchymal disease of liver	Tissue biopsy guided by ultrasound scanning
Pancreatic function tests	Suspected pancreatic exocrine failure	Pancreolauryl test of exocrine function requires urine samples

◆ Key points

- Common conditions, such as gastro-oesophageal reflux disease and irritable bowel syndrome, are diagnosed on history alone.
- In dysphagia, the site where the patient feels the food sticking is a poor guide to the actual level of oesophageal obstruction.
- Diagnose irritable bowel syndrome positively from the pattern of symptoms and the absence of alarm symptoms. Do not use irritable bowel syndrome as a label for 'gastrointestinal symptoms, cause unknown'.
- Patients with irritable bowel syndrome may also have other significant additional gastrointestinal disease.
- Pale stools with dark urine indicates an obstructive component to jaundice.

- In chronic liver disease the left lobe often enlarges more than the right, and may extend across the midline.
- In patients with hepatosplenomegaly, look for cutaneous signs of chronic liver disease and lymphadenopathy.
- Always consider ectopic pregnancy and pelvic inflammatory disease as a cause of abdominal pain in women of child-bearing age.
- Assess all patients with gastrointestinal bleeding for evidence of hypovolaemia.
- A palpable spleen is *always* pathological; a palpable liver may be a normal liver displaced downwards.
- Pelvic peritonitis is often best elicited by rectal examination.

The renal system

ALLAN CUMMING

RENAL EXAMINATION

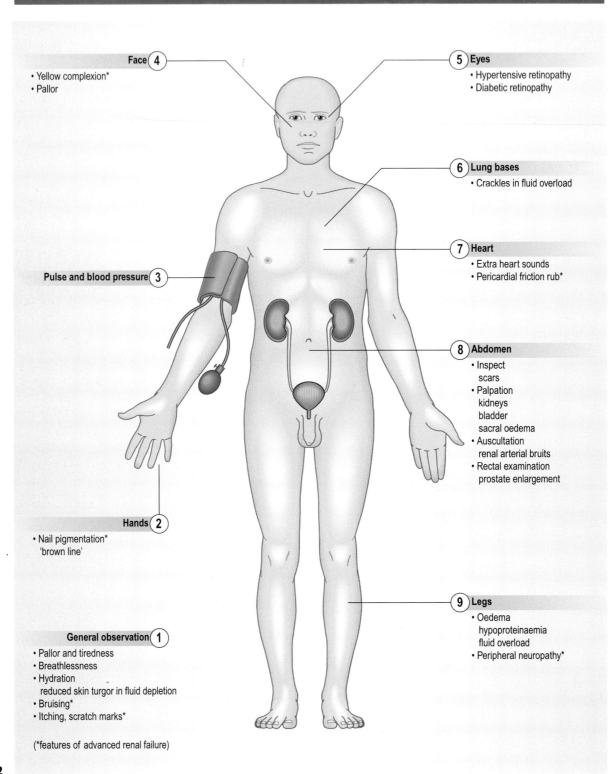

Face ④
• Yellow complexion*
• Pallor

Eyes ⑤
• Hypertensive retinopathy
• Diabetic retinopathy

Lung bases ⑥
• Crackles in fluid overload

Heart ⑦
• Extra heart sounds
• Pericardial friction rub*

Pulse and blood pressure ③

Abdomen ⑧
• Inspect
  scars
• Palpation
  kidneys
  bladder
  sacral oedema
• Auscultation
  renal arterial bruits
• Rectal examination
  prostate enlargement

Hands ②
• Nail pigmentation*
  'brown line'

Legs ⑨
• Oedema
  hypoproteinaemia
  fluid overload
• Peripheral neuropathy*

General observation ①
• Pallor and tiredness
• Breathlessness
• Hydration
  reduced skin turgor in fluid depletion
• Bruising*
• Itching, scratch marks*

(*features of advanced renal failure)

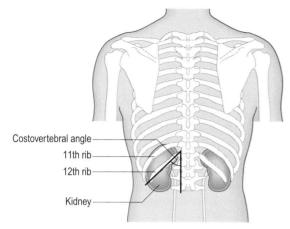

Costovertebral angle
11th rib
12th rib
Kidney

Fig. 6.1 The surface anatomy of the kidneys from the back.

INTRODUCTION

Disease of the kidneys and urinary tract is often clinically 'silent'. Detection and diagnosis often depend on bio-chemical testing of the urine for abnormal constituents or measuring the plasma creatinine concentration. These tests often detect occult renal disease in patients with diabetes mellitus, vascular disease, hypertension, or anaemia.

Severe renal disease may present with non-specific symptoms such as tiredness or breathlessness due to renal failure and its associated anaemia, or oedema due to fluid retention.

COMMON SYMPTOMS

DYSURIA AND UROGENITAL PAIN

Dysuria is pain or discomfort felt during or immediately after passing urine. It is often described as a 'burning' sensation felt at the urethral meatus, or the suprapubic region. The most common cause is infection and/or inflammation of the bladder (cystitis) and frequency is also usually present. Prostatitis and urethritis produce similar symptoms when caused by sexually transmitted infections such as gonorrhoea, often with urethral discharge. In males, dysuria with perineal and rectal pain suggest prostatic inflammation or infection and may be associated with symptoms of bladder neck obstruction.

Strangury is suprapubic pain associated with a repeated and urgent desire to urinate every few minutes, often associated with severe dysuria or inability to pass urine. It is due to acute bladder neck obstruction by a stone or blood clot.

Testicular and epididymal pain may be felt in the groin and lower abdomen to such an extent that you may overlook its testicular origin. In pubertal boys and young men this is most often the result of torsion of the testis and demands urgent intervention (See Ch. 5). The onset is frequently at night with pain in the iliac fossa. Distinguish tenderness and swelling of the testis from a strangulated hernia or acute epididymo-orchitis.

Only a minority of upper renal tract conditions are associated with pain, which is usually caused by infection, inflammation, or mechanical obstruction. Pain originating from the kidney is usually felt in the back or loin and is due to stretching of the renal capsule or renal pelvis. When constant loin pain and systemic upset, often with fever

and rigors, coexist with dysuria this suggests infection of the upper urinary tract and kidney (acute pyelonephritis) (Table 6.1).

Chronic dull aching discomfort in the loin and renal angle may occur in chronic renal infection and scarring, commonly due to vesicoureteric reflux. This kind of pain may also occur in adult polycystic kidney disease and in chronic urinary tract obstruction. Many patients with chronic

6.1 List of urinary symptoms
General
• Pain passing urine (dysuria) • Severe suprapubic pain associated with inability to pass urine (strangury) • Passing urine more often than usual (frequency) • A sudden need to pass urine (urgency) • Passing a larger volume of urine than normal (polyuria) • Passing a smaller volume of urine than normal (oliguria) • Passing urine during the night (nocturia) • Total absence of urine output (anuria) • Blood in the urine (haematuria) • Air bubbles in the urine (pneumaturia)
Females
• Stress or urge urinary incontinence
Males
• Delay in initiating urine flow (hesitancy) • Impaired urine flow • Post-micturition dribbling • Dribbling incontinence • Urethral discharge (suggesting sexually acquired infection)

obstruction are, however, pain-free and it is not a reliable symptom of this condition. More severe pain can occur intermittently in polycystic kidney disease because of infection or bleeding into a cyst.

Loin pain may be caused by other renal diseases, including stone disease and some forms of glomerulonephritis, e.g. IgA nephropathy. The dull non-localized nature of the pain may be mistaken for musculoskeletal conditions and it is often difficult to be sure that the pain is of renal origin.

Renal colic is caused by acute distension of the renal pelvis and ureter, from obstruction by calculus, blood clot, or rarely, a renal papilla in papillary necrosis. Renal 'colic' is not a true colic as the pain is unremitting. The pain is usually of sudden onset, severe and sustained. The patient is restless, nauseated and often vomits. The pain may radiate from the renal angle and loin to the iliac fossa, the groin and into the genitalia. Once the obstruction reaches the bladder, however, it is often asymptomatic until it enters the urethra and causes dysuria. In patients with urinary stones, ask about possible causes of stone formation (Table 6.2).

In the loin pain–haematuria syndrome patients complain of chronic loin discomfort which may be unilateral or bilateral and of varying severity. They consistently have microscopic haematuria and may also have attacks of frank (macroscopic) haematuria.

FREQUENCY AND URGENCY

Dysfunction of the lower urinary tract causes changes in micturition. *Frequency* is increased frequency of micturition without an increase in the total urine volume. *Urgency* is a sudden strong need to pass urine and results in incontinence if the person has no opportunity to urinate. Frequency and urgency are usually associated with disorders of the lower urinary tract – bladder, prostate and urethra – and are the dominant symptoms of lower urinary tract infection. Tumours, urinary calculi or urinary tract obstruction are less common causes.

In men > 40 years, disturbed micturition is commonly due to bladder neck narrowing and obstruction by progressive enlargement of the prostate gland. This causes frequency with the passage of small volumes of urine, impaired urinary flow, hesitancy (delay in initiating urine flow) and dribbling of urine after micturition. In women, the most common problem is weakness of the pelvic floor muscles, leading to difficulty in control of urine flow. Incontinence may occur in both these conditions.

Frequency alone, in young adults, may be due to anxiety. In the elderly, it is often the result of abnormally high bladder muscle tone (detrusor instability). Urgency alone may occur in pregnancy, due to extrinsic pressure on the bladder, or in weakness of the pelvic floor muscles or uterine prolapse. It is also a feature of neurological disease affecting the motor control of the bladder, such as multiple sclerosis. These patients may present with a false sensation of needing to pass urine.

POLYURIA, NOCTURIA, OLIGO/ANURIA, PNEUMATURIA

In healthy adults the urine output will approximate to the fluid intake minus the insensible fluid losses through the skin and respiratory tract (500–800 ml/day). Urine output is usually 2–3 l per day. *Polyuria* is the production of an abnormally large volume of urine. The most common cause is excessive fluid intake. This may be a manifestation of psychiatric disease, i.e. psychogenic polydipsia (*polydipsia* is excessive drinking), and in extreme cases may result in urine flows of up to 12 l daily.

Polyuria unrelated to fluid intake occurs when the kidneys are unable to concentrate the urine appropriately. This can result from extrarenal factors, such as the use of diuretic drugs, hyperglycaemia and glycosuria in diabetes mellitus leading to an osmotic diuresis; lack of antidiuretic hormone (ADH) from the pituitary gland in cranial diabetes insipidus, or failure of aldosterone secretion by the adrenal gland in Addison's disease.

Alternatively, impairment of concentrating ability may be due to renal causes with impaired capacity of the kidney tubules to reabsorb water in response to ADH. The most severe form is nephrogenic diabetes insipidus, which is usually genetic and due to mutations in the tubular ADH receptor. It may also reflect tubular damage by drugs such as lithium. Lesser degrees of ADH resistance causing polyuria may be seen in most types of chronic tubulointerstitial renal

6.2   Kidney stones: predisposing factors and conditions
Environmental and dietary
• Low urine volumes: high ambient temperature, low fluid intake
• Diet: high protein intake, high sodium, low calcium
• High sodium excretion
• High oxalate excretion
• High urate excretion
• Low citrate excretion
Other medical conditions
• Hypercalcaemia of any cause
• Ileal disease or resection (leads to increased oxalate absorption and urinary excretion)
• Renal tubular acidosis type I (distal) e.g. in Sjögren's syndrome
Congenital and inherited conditions
• Familial hypercalciuria
• Medullary sponge kidney
• Cystinuria
• Renal tubular acidosis type I (distal)
• Primary hyperoxaluria

damage, including reflux nephropathy and analgesic nephropathy.

Nocturia is the need to rise at night to pass urine and is a non-specific symptom of renal or urinary tract disease. This may be a matter of habit, or reflect insomnia, since the normal increase in ADH levels at night does not occur in the absence of sleep. Alternatively, it may reflect frequency or polyuria for any of the above causes. Nocturia can be a very early symptom of chronic renal failure. It is also a common symptom of cardiac failure, the diuresis resulting from the improvement in renal blood flow which occurs on lying flat.

Oliguria is a reduction in the urine volume to < 800 ml/day. Reduction in urine volume may be an appropriate response to a very low fluid intake, or may indicate loss of kidney function. The minimum urine volume needed to excrete the daily solute load varies with diet, physical activity and metabolic rate, but in general, normal kidneys do not concentrate the urine to less than 400 ml/day.

Acute renal failure is usually associated with oliguria, but 20% of patients have non-oliguric acute renal failure and this can only be diagnosed by biochemical testing of renal function.

Anuria, the total absence of urine production, is uncommon and suggests urinary tract obstruction. Obstruction is most often located in the lower urinary tract, i.e. urinary retention, as a result of bladder neck or urethral obstruction. Look for a mechanical explanation, such as marked prostatic enlargement, or a neurological cause such as spinal injury.

Pneumaturia, passing air bubbles in the urine, is very rare. It is most often caused by a fistula between the bladder and the colon, usually as a result of a diverticular abscess, Crohn's disease or cancer of the colon, bladder or female genitalia.

ABNORMAL URINE FLOW, INCONTINENCE, ENURESIS

Reduced force of the urinary stream in males suggests bladder outlet obstruction due to prostatic hypertrophy or, less commonly, a urethral stricture (Table 6.3).

Urinary *incontinence* is the involuntary passing of urine. *Urge incontinence* is when an urgent need to urinate cannot

---

6.4 Key points in a history of urinary incontinence

- Age at onset
- Number of times per day
- Occurrence during sleep (nocturnal enuresis)
- Any other associated urinary symptoms
- Provocative factors, e.g. coughing, sneezing, exercising
- Impact on daily living
- Protection/precautions required

---

be resisted, and *stress incontinence* is when leakage of urine occurs in response to situations that increase intra-abdominal pressure, such as coughing, sneezing or laughing. Some patients have both. Some relevant points to ask about in the history are listed in Table 6.4.

Many parous women experience stress incontinence because of weakness of perineal muscles, sometimes accompanied by a degree of uterine prolapse. Incontinence is also caused by neurological disorders. In sensory denervation of the bladder, e.g. diabetic autonomic neuropathy, dribbling incontinence occurs with a painless distended bladder.

Loss of motor control causes urgency. Loss of urinary control and incontinence may occur because of severe urgency, or if the subject has limited mobility. Combined motor and sensory damage occurs in spinal cord lesions, e.g. spinal trauma or multiple sclerosis. The bladder fills to a certain pressure and then empties reflexly. Some patients learn to empty the bladder by raising the intravesicular pressure by manual compression of the lower abdomen.

Causes of urinary incontinence are summarized in Table 6.5.

Nocturnal enuresis is the involuntary passage of urine while asleep ('bed-wetting'). It is common in childhood and does not necessarily indicate either physical or psychological abnormality. It may be associated with periods of emotional disturbance and persist into adult life. In a minority of cases it may indicate underlying disease of the kidneys or urinary tract and, if persistent, basic screening investigations are appropriate.

HAEMATURIA

Haematuria is the presence of red blood cells in the urine, due to bleeding from the kidneys or urinary tract (Fig. 6.2).

6.3 Features of prostatic bladder neck obstruction (prostatism)

- Reduced force of the urinary stream
- Hesitancy (difficulty in initiating the urine flow)
- Double voiding (the need to pass urine again within a few minutes of micturition)
- Urinary dribbling after micturition
- Frequency and nocturia (due to incomplete bladder emptying)
- Complete urinary retention

6.5 Causes of urinary incontinence

- Incoordination of bladder sphincter function in old age
- Spinal cord trauma or compression
- Multiple sclerosis
- Females: pelvic floor weakness following childbirth
- Males: benign prostatic hypertrophy, prostate cancer

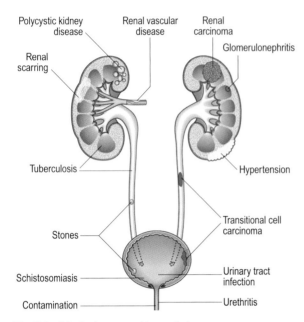

Fig. 6.2 Principal sources of haematuria.

6.7	Causes of haematuria and their relationship to pain

Painless

- Glomerulonephritis
- Tumours of the kidney, ureter, bladder or prostate[a]
- Tuberculosis[a]
- Schistosomiasis[a]
- Hypertensive nephrosclerosis
- Interstitial nephritis (unless very acute/severe)
- Acute tubular necrosis
- Renal ischaemia (renovascular disease)
- Distance running or other severe exercise
- Coagulation disorders
- Anticoagulant therapy

Painful

- Urinary tract infection
- Renal calculi with obstruction
- Loin pain–haematuria syndrome

May be either

- Urinary tract infection
- Reflux nephropathy and renal scarring
- Adult polycystic kidney disease
- Renal stones without obstruction

[a] Painless provided there is not acute obstruction of the urinary tract

Distinguish it from contamination of the urine by blood from the female genital tract during menstruation – the commonest cause of blood in the urine. Anxious patients sometimes confuse normal, concentrated urine with haematuria. Less commonly, haematuria may be confused with free haemoglobin in the urine in haemolysis, myoglobin in rhabdomyolysis, and other abnormalities of urine colour as shown in Table 6.6. Always confirm the presence of red cells by urinalysis and, to be certain, urine microscopy.

Macroscopic haematuria is visible to the naked eye and must be investigated. Painless macroscopic haematuria in an adult may be due to a benign bladder papilloma or to cancer of the kidney, bladder or prostate. It may also occur in glomerulonephritis (most commonly, IgA nephropathy), polycystic kidney disease, and chronic renal infection such as tuberculosis or schistosomiasis (Table 6.7).

Macroscopic haematuria associated with loin pain suggests a renal or ureteric origin, such as a stone, IgA

nephropathy or loin pain–haematuria syndrome. Acute bleeding from polycystic kidney disease is usually associated with pain on the relevant side.

When macroscopic haematuria is accompanied by dysuria or frequency, it is usually due to lower urinary tract infection (cystitis, urethritis) or, if there is loin pain, renal infection (pyelonephritis). Haematuria which clears rapidly during micturition usually originates from the urethra.

Almost any disease of the kidneys or urinary tract can cause microscopic haematuria. It is most often detected on routine urinalysis. Asymptomatic haematuria is a common

6.8	Causes of proteinuria

Renal disease

- Glomerulonephritis
- Diabetes mellitus
- Amyloidosis
- Systemic lupus erythematosus
- Drugs, e.g. gold, penicillamine
- Malignancy, e.g. myeloma
- Infection

Non-renal disease

- Fever
- Severe exertion
- Severe hypertension
- Burns
- Heart failure
- Orthostatic proteinuria (occurs when a patient is upright but not lying down – the first morning sample will not show proteinuria)

6.6	Abnormalities of urine colour	
Orange-brown	Conjugated bilirubin Rhubarb, senna Concentrated normal urine, e.g. very low fluid intake	
Red-brown	Blood, myoglobin, free haemoglobin, porphyrins Drugs – rifampicin, metronidazole, warfarin Beetroot, blackberries	
Brown-black	Conjugated bilirubin Drugs – L-dopa Homogentisic acid (in alkaptonuria or ochronosis)	

mode of presentation of renal or urinary tract disease, although it may be a solitary and benign finding, especially if the patient does not have associated proteinuria, hypertension or increased serum creatinine.

PROTEINURIA

Proteinuria usually indicates disease of the kidneys. Exceptions include the low-grade proteinuria seen in patients who are febrile for any reason and benign orthostatic (postural) proteinuria (Table 6.8). Patients with severe proteinuria

sometimes notice their urine is unusually frothy, but this is not a reliable symptom – even normal urine is sometimes frothy. If proteinuria is sufficient to lower the plasma albumin concentration, with resultant loss of fluid into the tissues, the patient develops generalized oedema – the *nephrotic syndrome*. Otherwise, proteinuria is asymptomatic and is detected by urinalysis.

Minor degrees of proteinuria (up to 2 g/24 h) are non-specific and may occur in any type of renal disease. Values greater than this indicate a glomerular abnormality. The most common causes are the various forms of glomerulonephritis and diabetic nephropathy.

THE HISTORY

Past history

Ask about any previous history of renal system disease. Specifically ask about:

- hypertension (which may cause, or result from, renal disease)
- diabetes mellitus (associated with diabetic nephropathy and renal vascular disease)
- vascular disease at other sites (which makes renal vascular disease more likely)
- recurrent infections (particularly urinary, which may be associated with renal scarring, and upper respiratory, which may be associated with glomerulonephritis and/or vasculitis)
- anaemia.

Growth retardation is a common feature of chronic renal failure in childhood. *Pruritus* (itch) is a prominent symptom of chronic renal failure at any age. Other symptoms include tiredness, breathlessness, poor appetite, sleep disturbance, restlessness of the legs particularly at night, muscle twitching due to hypocalcaemia and in very severe renal failure, vomiting, diarrhoea, confusion and altered consciousness.

Drug history

Renal failure has important effects on drug metabolism and pharmacokinetics, and drugs may damage the kidneys. Examples of drugs which accumulate in renal failure are digoxin, lithium, aminoglycosides, opioid analgesics and water-soluble beta-blockers such as atenolol.

A wide range of drugs may alter renal function, or cause renal failure, including angiotensin-converting enzyme inhibitors, angiotensin receptor antagonists and non-steroidal anti-inflammatory drugs. These drugs have no adverse effect on normal kidneys, but reduce glomerular filtration when the kidneys are underperfused. Non-steroidal

anti-inflammatory drugs, in particular, can dramatically reduce renal function in the presence of systemic infection or hypovolaemia. They are commonly taken as over-the-counter drugs so always ask about their usage.

Other drugs are toxic even to the normal kidneys. Examples include aminoglycosides, amphotericin, lithium, ciclosporin and tacrolimus, and in overdose, paracetamol.

Some drugs cause renal failure by indirect mechanisms. An example is rhabdomyolysis and myoglobinuric acute renal failure occurring in intravenous drug and cocaine users.

Family history

Ask the patient if any family members have renal disease. The two most important genetically determined conditions are adult polycystic kidney disease (autosomal dominant) and Alport's syndrome (X-linked). Adult polycystic kidney disease is associated with subarachnoid haemorrhage from aneurysms of the circle of Willis, while Alport's syndrome is associated with nerve deafness. Reflux nephropathy or IgA nephropathy sometimes shows familial clustering. Some patients with type 1 diabetes mellitus have a genetically determined increased susceptibility to diabetic nephropathy.

Environmental, occupational and social histories

Renal stones form more readily in concentrated urine, so that living and working in hot conditions is a risk factor. Exposure to organic solvents may be a factor in the causation of Goodpasture's syndrome and, possibly, other kinds of glomerulonephritis. Aniline dye workers have an increased incidence of urothelial tumours. Long-term exposure to lead and cadmium may cause chronic renal damage.

Social factors are always important, particularly in end-stage renal failure requiring dialysis and/or transplantation. This has major implications for lifestyle, employment and family relationships. Incontinence may also have major implications for daily living.

Smoking is a risk factor for atheromatous renal vascular disease, and for nephropathy in diabetic patients. Excess alcohol consumption is associated with hypertensive renal damage and increased incidence of IgA nephropathy.

A dietary history is important in patients who form renal stones (intake of water, calcium, oxalate). Assess dietary protein intake in patients with chronic renal failure, since a protracted high dietary protein intake may be deleterious.

Estimate sodium intake and, if necessary, this should be reduced in patients with hypertension and renal disease.

Some renal conditions are found in particular ethnic or geographical situations. Examples include Balkan nephropathy (a disease characterized by interstitial nephritis and urinary tract tumours which is probably caused by fungal toxins in grain), systemic lupus erythematosus with nephritis in the Far East, and severe hypertension or diabetes mellitus with renal failure, which are more common in patients of African origin.

THE PHYSICAL EXAMINATION

GENERAL FEATURES: SKIN, CIRCULATION, EYES

A sequence of general features to look for in patients with suspected renal disease is shown on page 182. Some features are more common in patients in end-stage chronic renal failure (Fig. 6.3).

On general observation look for fatigue, pallor and breathlessness in chronic renal failure. Increased respiratory rate and depth suggest an associated metabolic acidosis with respiratory compensation. Longstanding chronic renal failure causes a lemon-yellow complexion, and these patients also may show bruising and areas of excoriation secondary to pruritus. There may be reduced skin turgor in patients with fluid depletion, or signs of fluid overload.

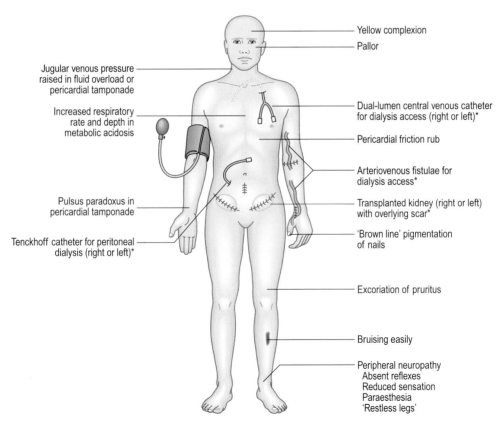

Jugular venous pressure raised in fluid overload or pericardial tamponade

Increased respiratory rate and depth in metabolic acidosis

Pulsus paradoxus in pericardial tamponade

Tenckhoff catheter for peritoneal dialysis (right or left)*

Yellow complexion

Pallor

Dual-lumen central venous catheter for dialysis access (right or left)*

Pericardial friction rub

Arteriovenous fistulae for dialysis access*

Transplanted kidney (right or left) with overlying scar*

'Brown line' pigmentation of nails

Excoriation of pruritus

Bruising easily

Peripheral neuropathy
Absent reflexes
Reduced sensation
Paraesthesia
'Restless legs'

188   Fig. 6.3   Physical signs in chronic renal failure. (* Features of renal replacement therapy.)

In the hands, a brownish discoloration of the distal nail bed is sometimes seen in longstanding renal failure.

The blood pressure is often elevated in kidney disease, but may be low in patients with tubulointerstitial disease who 'waste' sodium because of impaired tubular reabsorption. The JVP may be elevated in patients who retain salt and water. Look at the eyes for conjunctival pallor which may indicate the anaemia of chronic renal failure, and calcification at the junction of the iris and conjunctiva (limbic calcification). Examine the fundi for hypertensive changes, and retinal infarcts in severe vasculitis or systemic lupus erythematosus.

In the lungs, there may be bilateral basal lung crackles reflecting fluid overload or heart failure. On listening to the heart a midsystolic 'flow' murmur is common in patients with renal anaemia, particularly if there is a high cardiac output because of an arteriovenous fistula for dialysis access. A third or fourth heart sound may indicate fluid overload and/or heart failure. In very severe renal failure, a pericardial friction rub due to uraemic pericarditis may be heard.

ABDOMINAL EXAMINATION

Ask the patient to lie flat with his head on a pillow and his arms by his side to relax the abdominal muscles, and expose the abdomen.

Inspection

Inspect the abdomen for distension from the very enlarged kidneys of polycystic kidney disease, or occasionally in obstructive uropathy. Gross bladder distension may be seen as a suprapubic swelling. Look for scars of renal tract surgery in the loins (often missed because of their posterior site) or in the iliac fossae after renal transplant surgery. A catheter for peritoneal dialysis may be present, or may have left small scars in the midline and either hypochondrium. Absence of the abdominal wall muscles is seen in children with prune-belly syndrome, a condition associated with abnormalities of the urogenital tract.

Palpation

Palpate the abdomen gently with the fingers of your right hand. Start in the right lower quadrant and palpate each area of the abdomen systematically. Gross enlargement of the bladder or of the kidney in polycystic kidney disease (with its distinctive nodular surface) is readily detected on superficial palpation.

For lesser degrees of kidney enlargement, use a bimanual technique to feel the kidneys (Fig. 6.4). Place your left hand behind the patient's back below the lower ribs. Place your right hand over the upper quadrant anteriorly just lateral to the rectus muscle. Firmly, but gently, push your two hands together as the patient breathes out. Then ask the patient to breathe in deeply. You may feel the lower pole of the kidney moving down between the hands. If this happens, gently push the kidney back and forwards between your two hands to demonstrate its mobility. This is known as *ballotting*, and helps to confirm that the structure is the kidney. It is usually easier to feel the right kidney as it is lower than the left.

If the kidney is palpable, assess its size, surface and consistency. Polycystic kidneys have an irregular nodular surface and may vary in size from moderately enlarged to filling the whole of one side of the abdomen. Kidneys

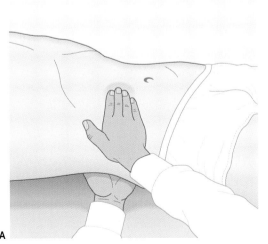
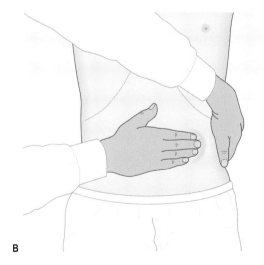

A B

Fig. 6.4 **Palpation of the kidney.** (A) Right kidney. (B) Left kidney.

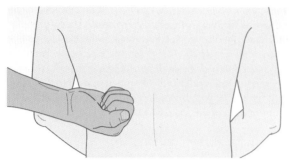

Fig. 6.5 Assessing tenderness over the renal angles.

Auscultation

Auscultate the abdomen to detect bruits possibly arising from the renal arteries. Listen carefully over both loins posteriorly and in the epigastrium using the diaphragm of the stethoscope. It is not possible to distinguish renal artery bruits from those arising in adjacent vessels, such as the mesenteric arteries, but such bruits increase the likelihood of renal vascular disease and support a decision to investigate by renal angiography. Similarly, check for diminished or absent femoral artery pulses and bruits, as both increase the probability of coexistent atheromatous renal artery disease.

containing tumours are usually firm and irregular, and sometimes tethered to surrounding structures. Enlarged obstructed or hypertrophic kidneys have a smooth surface.

Minor degrees of kidney enlargement are difficult to assess. In very thin subjects the lower pole of a normal right kidney may be palpable, but even very large kidneys may be impossible to feel in obese subjects. When the liver is markedly enlarged it may be difficult to differentiate from the right kidney, especially if polycystic kidney disease is associated with cystic disease of the liver.

Tenderness of the kidney is most obvious posteriorly in the renal angle – the angle formed between the 12th rib and the spine. Sit the patient forward and palpate firmly but gently with your fingers. If this does not cause the patient discomfort, firmly (but with moderate force only!) strike the renal angle once with the ulnar aspect of your closed fist after warning the patient what to expect (Fig. 6.5). Renal tenderness is most often due to acute pyelonephritis or acute urinary obstruction.

Enlargement of one kidney may result from compensatory hypertrophy due to renal agenesis, hypoplasia or atrophy, or surgical removal of the other kidney. It may also be due to a renal tumour or hydronephrosis. Enlargement of both kidneys occurs in polycystic kidney disease and amyloidosis, and in acute forms of glomerulonephritis. A transplanted kidney is palpable as a smooth mass in either iliac fossa with an overlying scar.

A distended bladder is palpable as a smooth firm mass arising from the pelvis. It will disappear after urethral catheterization.

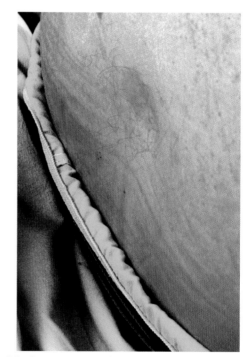

Fig. 6.6 Sacral oedema showing pitting.

Percussion

Percussion of the kidneys is generally unhelpful, although massively enlarged polycystic kidneys are dull to percussion. A distended bladder is dull to percussion in the suprapubic region. Percuss over a resonant area in the upper abdomen in the midline and then percuss downwards towards the symphysis pubis. A change to a dull percussion note indicates the upper border of the distended bladder.

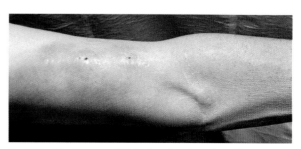

Fig. 6.7 Arteriovenous fistula showing sites of needle cannulation for dialysis.

Following examination of the abdomen, rectal examination (see Ch. 7) is used to assess the prostate for benign enlargement or malignant change. In female patients, vaginal examination may be indicated (see Ch. 7) if you suspect malignant disease involving the ureters or bladder.

Oedema may accumulate at various sites; Look for it particularly in the ankles, sacrum and, in recumbent patients, the sacrum and back of the thighs (Fig. 6.6). Patients with nephrotic syndrome classically show marked tissue oedema, but often do not have a raised JVP or added heart sounds, since the intravascular volume is normal or reduced. There may, however, be other signs of extra-vascular fluid, particularly pleural effusions and ascites.

There may be decreased peripheral reflexes indicating neuropathy in chronic renal failure. Patients undergoing dialysis for end-stage renal failure may have temporary or permanent dual-lumen catheters placed in internal jugular, subclavian or femoral veins, and arteriovenous fistulae at the wrist or elbow, to allow vascular access for haemodialysis (Fig. 6.7).

Patients with renal transplants may show features associated with immunosuppressive therapy. Steroid doses are normally low enough to avoid a Cushingoid appearance, but hirsutism and gum hypertrophy related to ciclosporin may be seen. Look carefully at the skin for warts and cancers associated with immunosuppressive therapy.

⊙ Examine this patient with haematuria

1. Measure temperature – raised in *urinary tract infection*, connective tissue disease, endocarditis with renal involvement.
2. Look for evidence of bruising or purpura (*coagulation disorder, Henoch–Schönlein purpura, vasculitis*).
3. Examine nails for splinter haemorrhages (*bacterial endocarditis* with renal involvement).
4. Measure blood pressure – elevated in *renovascular* and *chronic renal disease*.
5. Look at optic fundi for *hypertensive retinopathy*.
6. Examine abdomen for renal tenderness (*renal* or *ureteric stones* or other causes of obstruction, *renal infection* or *inflammation*).
7. Examine abdomen for enlarged, palpable kidneys – unilateral in *renal cancer, urinary tract obstruction*; bilateral in *polycystic renal disease*.
8. Assess peripheral pulses and listen for renal artery or other bruits (*renovascular disease*).
9. Palpate suprapubically for palpable bladder (*benign prostatic enlargement, prostate* or *bladder cancer*).
10. In men, perform rectal examination to assess enlargement of prostate – irregular in *prostate cancer*.

⊙ Examine this patient with loin pain

1. Measure temperature – raised in *urinary infection*.
2. Measure blood pressure – elevated in *renovascular disease* and *chronic renal disease*.
3. Look at optic fundi for hypertensive retinopathy.
4. Examine abdomen for tenderness (*renal* or *ureteric stones* or other causes of obstruction, *renal infection* or *inflammation*).
5. Examine abdomen for enlarged, palpable kidneys:
   – unilateral in *renal cancer, urinary tract obstruction*
   – bilateral in *polycystic renal disease*.
6. Look for evidence of non-renal causes of loin pain, e.g. spinal or other locomotor disease.
7. Examine urine for haematuria and proteinuria – haematuria alone is non-specific; presence of both suggests *renal inflammation*.

EXAMINATION OF THE URINE

Examination of the urine should be performed on all patients with:

- symptoms of kidney or urinary tract disease
- thirst ± polyuria
- weight loss
- abdominal pain
- jaundice
- hypertension
- pyrexia of uncertain origin.

Abnormalities may appear in the urine because the blood level of a substance is abnormally high, exceeding the ability of the tubules to reabsorb it, e.g. glucose, ketones, conjugated bilirubin, and urobilinogen. Alternatively, changes may be seen which reflect altered function of the kidney itself, e.g. protein. Finally, abnormal contents may be added to the urine at any point in its passage from the kidney to the urethra – for example, haematuria can indicate disease at any point in the urinary tract or adjacent structures. Some clinical uses of urinalysis are listed in Table 6.9 and the main components of the examination are shown in Table 6.10.

Macroscopic examination

Appearance. Normal fresh urine is clear but varies in colour. Clear urine, left to stand, may become cloudy or form fine strands of solid material due to precipitation of phosphates and urates. This is of no significance. A cloudy appearance of fresh urine is usually due to the presence

6.9	Common uses of urinalysis	
Examples		
Screening	Random	Diabetes mellitus
		Asymptomatic bacteriuria
	Selective	Antenatal care
		Hypertensive patients
Diagnosis	Primary renal disease	Glomerulonephritis
	Secondary renal disease	Bacterial endocarditis
	Non-renal disorders	Diabetes mellitus
Monitoring	Disease progression	Diabetic nephropathy
	Drug toxicity	Gold therapy
	Drug compliance	Rifampicin therapy

6.10	Elements of examination of the urine		
Macroscopic	**Biochemical**	**Microscopic**	**Microbiological**
Clarity	Specific gravity,	RBCs, WBCs	Culture and
Colour	pH	Bacteria	sensitivities
Odour	Blood, protein	Casts	Nitrites
Volume	Glucose, ketones	Crystals	
	Bilirubin,		
	urobilinogen		

of pus cells (*pyuria*), often with bacteria. A brownish and cloudy appearance may be due to the presence of blood, or pigment, as in myoglobinuria. Other colour changes suggest the presence of blood, drugs or chemicals (see Table 6.6).

Odour. An unusually strong smell suggests urinary infection. Some foods, such as asparagus, impart a characteristic smell to the urine.

Volume. Measure the urine volume over 24 hours to confirm oliguria or polyuria. The collection can also be used to measure creatinine clearance (an indicator of glomerular filtration rate), urinary protein, or excretion of sodium, potassium or calcium. In critically ill patients, hourly urine flow is a useful dynamic indicator of organ perfusion.

Collecting a 24-hour urine sample:

- Ask the patient to empty the bladder on waking, e.g. 8 a.m., and discard the urine.
- Collect all urine passed in the next 24 hours.
- Remind the patient to collect the final sample at 8 a.m. the following morning and add this to the collection.

Biochemical examination

Use *reagent strip tests* such as N-Multistix (Bayer Corporation). The technique is based on chemical reactions between constituents of urine and reagents impregnated into paper test areas on a plastic strip.

Procedure

- The urine specimen should be less than 4 hours old.
- Wear a disposable apron and gloves.
- Examine the specimen for smell, colour and other abnormalities.
- Use a watch with a second hand.
- Dip the reagent strip into the urine specimen making sure all the test areas are covered. Remove the strip after 2 seconds.
- Tap the edge of the strip against the rim of the container to remove excess urine.
- Hold the strip horizontally with test areas upward. Hold as close to the colour chart as possible and compare the test areas with the bottle label, reading each reagent at the time specified on the bottle label (Fig. 6.8).
- Dispose of apron and gloves into a clinical waste bag; wash hands.
- Document the results in the patient's clinical record.

Urinary specific gravity. Urinary specific gravity is an index of the concentration of solute (e.g. sodium, chloride, urea, glucose) in the urine. It varies in health between 1.002 and 1.035. High values suggest that the kidney is actively reabsorbing water – test this in patients with suspected fluid depletion or renal failure due to reduced renal perfusion. Abnormally low values indicate failure of the renal tubules to concentrate urine; test this in patients with unusually high urine volumes.

For definitive measurement of renal concentrating ability, urine strip testing is inadequate and precise measurement of total concentration of particles in the urine (*osmolality*) by a laboratory-based method is required. Osmolality refers to the number of solute particles/kg water. *Osmolarity* is the number of solute particles/litre of the solution. For dilute fluids such as urine the two terms are essentially synonymous.

In unexplained hyponatraemia, test for the syndrome of inappropriate ADH secretion (SIADH) by simultaneous

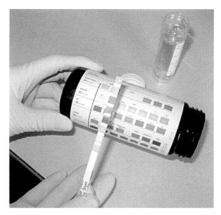

Fig. 6.8 Multistix.

measurement of plasma and urine osmolality. If the plasma osmolality is low, the urine osmolality should be lower still (< 150 mOsm/kg); any other finding is in keeping with SIADH.

In patients with unexplained polyuria, test the concentrating ability of the kidneys by an overnight fluid deprivation test. In healthy subjects, urinary osmolality should rise to > 800 mOsm/kg; any other finding suggests lack of ADH or renal tubular unresponsiveness to the hormone.

Urinary pH. In health urinary pH varies between 4.5 and 8.0. In renal tubular acidosis, either congenital or acquired, urinary acidification is impaired; urinary pH never falls below 5.3, even after an oral challenge with ammonium chloride.

Glucose. The stix test is specific for glucose. Small amounts of glucose may be excreted by the normal kidney. These amounts are usually below the sensitivity of this test but on occasion may produce a colour between the 'Negative' and 5.5 mmol/l colour blocks.

Ketones. The stix test reacts specifically with acetoacetic acid, one of the ketones found in urine. Normal urine is usually negative but false positive results may occur with highly concentrated urine specimens. Diabetic ketoacidosis is the most important cause of ketonuria, but it also occurs in starvation or very low carbohydrate diets.

Proteinuria. Use fresh urine for protein testing. A reading greater than 'trace' indicates significant proteinuria. This can occur transiently in the absence of renal disease (Table 6.11). Proteinuria < 1 g/l which disappears when lying supine (*orthostatic proteinuria*) is an occasional finding in healthy young subjects in whom protein is not detected in the first urine passed after sleeping recumbent overnight, but will be present during the day.

Proteinuria may be due to increased leakage from the glomeruli, or tubular dysfunction. Even in health some protein is filtered through the glomeruli, but most is reabsorbed and catabolized by the renal tubules. Proteinuria > 2 g per day suggests glomerular disease. Polycystic kidney disease, renal scarring and obstructive uropathy may be present without significant proteinuria.

False positive and false negative results may occur (Table 6.12). The test is relatively insensitive to Bence Jones proteins (immunoglobulin light chains, often in the urine in myeloma), which need specific laboratory testing.

6.12 Causes of misleading reagent strip test results for proteinuria	
False positive	Phenothiazine therapy Contamination with detergents, chlorhexidine Contamination with alkalis
False negative	Contamination with acid preservatives Bence Jones proteinuria

The lower limit of detection for urinary protein using reagent strips is 300 mg/l. However, urinary albumin excretion rates as low as 30 mg/day can be detected using radioimmunoassay techniques. Excretion rates of 30–300 mg of albumin per day detected by radioimmunoassay (*microalbuminuria*) occur in the early stages of diabetic nephropathy.

Haematuria. Intact erythrocytes cause green spots and free haemoglobin a green colour on the reagent area at 60 seconds. False positive findings occur (Table 6.13). The test does not differentiate between haemoglobin and myoglobin. If you suspect rhabdomyolysis measure myoglobin with a specific laboratory test.

Bilirubin and urobilinogen. Bilirubin is normally absent from urine, whereas urobilinogen may be present – up to 33 µmol/l in health. Abnormalities of either constituent in urine require investigation for possible haemolysis or hepatobiliary disease. False positive and false negative results are both possible (Table 6.14).

Urinary nitrite. Most Gram-negative bacteria convert urinary nitrate (derived from dietary nitrate) to nitrite. Although a positive result indicates bacteriuria a negative result does not exclude its presence.

6.13 Causes of misleading reagent strip test results for haematuria	
False positive	Contamination with bleach (hypochlorite) Stale urine (bacterial peroxidases)
Non-renal origin	Haemoglobinuria Myoglobinuria

6.11 Causes of transient proteinuria
• Cold exposure
• Vigorous exercise
• Febrile illness
• Orthostatic (postural) proteinuria
• Abdominal surgery
• Congestive cardiac failure

6.14 Causes of misleading urine reagent strip tests for bilirubin and urobilinogen		
	Bilirubin	**Urobilinogen**
False positive	Phenothiazines	Sulphonamides Salicylates
False negative	Vitamin C	Contamination with formalin

Microscopic examination

Most laboratories routinely examine urine for pus cells and bacteria, and comment on the presence of red blood cells. Checking for red cells by microscopy distinguishes true haematuria from haemoglobinuria and myoglobinuria, both of which give a positive test for blood on urinalysis. More detailed microscopic examination of the urine for diagnostic purposes is no longer routine in most units in the UK, since in most cases the diagnosis can be reached more easily and reliably by other means. However, it may still offer useful information in particular cases of renal disease.

Bacteria can usually be seen in an unstained film at low-power magnification. Higher magnification is necessary to distinguish erythrocytes from leucocytes, yeasts and small crystals.

Urine microscopy

- Centrifuge 10 ml of fresh urine for 5 minutes at 3000 r.p.m.
- Remove the supernatant, leaving 0.5 ml of urine and the deposit.
- Mix the sediment gently and place one drop on a clean slide.
- Overlay a cover slip and examine under the microscope with low illumination and low-power magnification.
- Examine under high-power magnification to clarify abnormalities seen.

Cells

Red blood cells (RBCs) are seen as small round cells without a nucleus. Those which have passed through the glomeruli are mostly dysmorphic (irregular in size and shape). Those from elsewhere in the urinary tract have normal morphology. Phase contrast microscopy is the best way to assess urinary red cell morphology (Fig. 6.9A).

White blood cells have lobed nuclei and granular cytoplasm. The presence of white cells with no growth of bacteria on standard culture (*sterile pyuria*) suggests renal tuberculosis, and indicates the need for mycobacterial cultures. *Renal tubular epithelial cells* are larger than white blood cells and have oval nuclei. They are seen in urinary tract infection and in inflammatory conditions such as tubulointerstitial nephritis and glomerulonephritis. Bladder epithelial cells are similar but even larger and of no clinical significance.

Expert cytological examination of an early morning specimen of urine may demonstrate *malignant cells* in cancer of the bladder, ureter or kidney.

Urinary casts

Casts are cylindrical structures which have formed in the renal tubules.

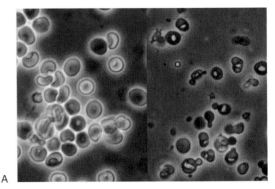

A

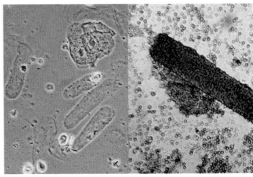

B

Fig. 6.9 Urine microscopy. (A) Phase contrast images of RBCs (×400). Right, glomerular bleeding with many dysmorphic forms including acanthocytes (teardrop forms). Left, bleeding from lower in the urinary tract. (B) Right, numerous red cells and a large red cell cast in acute glomerular inflammation (×100, not phase contrast). Left, phase contrast images show hyaline casts, a normal feature of urine (×160).

Hyaline casts (Fig. 6.9B) are relatively clear, homogeneous cylindrical structures, and consist principally of Tamm–Horsfall mucoprotein secreted by tubular cells. It is unusual to see more than one per low-power field in health. An increase in their number is non-specific, and is seen after severe exercise, during febrile illness, and in chronic renal disease.

Granular casts are hyaline casts containing granules of albumin and immunoglobulins. They may also contain cellular debris. They are pathological, and are found in disorders associated with significant proteinuria, e.g. glomerulonephritis and diabetic nephropathy.

Red cell casts are principally composed of well-defined erythrocytes, and haematuria is found on urinalysis. They indicate haematuria of glomerular origin, and are most often seen in acute disease, e.g. acute diffuse proliferative glomerulonephritis (Fig. 6.9B).

White cell casts suggest renal infection or inflammation such as acute pyelonephritis.

Crystals seen in fresh urine may indicate disease, e.g. urate crystals in gout or urate nephropathy, oxalate crystals in hyperoxaluric stone disease, cystine crystals in cystinuria.

Microbiological examination

To detect *Mycobacterium tuberculosis*, send at least three early morning urine samples to the laboratory for specific mycobacterial culture. For all other suspected bacterial infections, a fresh, clean-voided, midstream urine sample is required.

Midstream urine sample

- Give the patient a sterile urine container (a tray for a female patient).

- Ask the patient to start passing urine before collecting 10–20 ml in the container.
- Transfer urine from the tray to the laboratory container.
- Label the container with time, date and patient's name.
- Send to the laboratory without delay. If a delay is unavoidable, place the sample in a fridge (not freezer) until transport is available.
- Alternatives include suprapubic aspiration in children or non-compliant adults, and samples obtained via a urethral catheter.

COMMON RENAL INVESTIGATIONS

Biochemical assessment of renal function

Levels of urea and creatinine rise when the glomerular filtration rate is < 50 ml/min. Urea values are influenced by diet and do not measure renal function accurately. Creatinine clearance gives a more accurate measurement of glomerular filtration rate, but requires a timed urine collection – normally 24 hours – in addition to a blood sample.

Other common biochemical abnormalities in plasma of patients with renal failure include:

1. Raised potassium (decreased excretion) in acute renal failure and advanced chronic renal failure.
2. Low bicarbonate (impaired excretion of hydrogen ions, metabolic acidosis) is common in acute and chronic renal failure.
3. Low calcium (impaired activation of vitamin D_3 by the kidneys).
4. Elevated phosphate (decreased excretion).
5. Abnormalities 3 and 4 cause secondary hyperparathyroidism with elevated parathyroid hormone and alkaline phosphatase.
6. Raised urate (but seldom associated with true gout).

Other blood tests. Assessment of renal system disease commonly includes an immunology screen – including

6.15	Radiological investigations in renal system disorders	
Investigation	**Diagnostic problem**	**Look for**
Urinary tract ultrasound scan	Haematuria, proteinuria, renal failure, hypertension, renal masses, prostatism	Kidney size/shape/position; evidence of obstruction; renal cysts or solid lesions; stones; gross abnormality of bladder and post-micturition residual volume; guided kidney biopsy
Doppler ultrasound of renal arteries/veins	Possible renal vascular disease – hypertension ± renal failure Possible renal vein thrombosis	Reduced or absent renal arterial or venous blood flow
IV urography	Haematuria, renal colic, renal masses on examination	Renal, ureteric or bladder stones, cysts, tumours, hydronephrosis, other diseases
Renal angiography	Hypertension ± renal failure (especially if kidney size unequal on ultrasound or vascular disease elsewhere)	Renal artery stenosis (unilateral or bilateral); possibly proceed to angioplasty and/or stenting
Magnetic resonance imaging angiography	Possible renal vascular disease – hypertension ± renal failure	Renal artery stenosis
Renal isotope scanning	Suspected renal scarring, e.g. reflux nephropathy Divided renal function studies prior to nephrectomy	Renal uptake and excretion of radio-labelled chemicals: [99mTc] dimercaptosuccinate [99mTc] diethylene-triamine-penta-acetate [99mTc] mercapto-acetyltriglycine Check for reflux by scanning over kidneys during micturition
Abdominal CT scan	Suspected renal mass, ureteric obstruction, tumour staging	Renal, retroperitoneal or other tumour masses or fibrosis

antinuclear factor and antineutrophil cytoplasmic antibodies – to look for autoimmune diseases affecting the kidney, e.g. systemic lupus erythematosus, vasculitis.

Imaging

Renal tract imaging is indicated in all cases of renal system disease: the choice of imaging method will depend on the presenting complaint and the findings on initial assessment (Table 6.15).

Biopsy

Renal biopsy is indicated in the diagnosis and assessment of parenchymal renal disease. It is usually performed under guidance by ultrasound scanning; complication rates are low but include haemorrhage and formation of arteriovenous fistulae. Contraindications include markedly reduced kidney size, absence or inadequate function of the contralateral kidney, uncontrolled hypertension, and any clotting abnormality (including intake of aspirin or other drugs with anticoagulant effects).

◈ Key points

- ♦ Advanced renal failure may be present without any specific symptoms or physical signs. Always check blood tests to exclude renal dysfunction in patients with non-specific symptoms, e.g. tiredness.
- ♦ Haematuria combined with significant proteinuria (++ or more) usually indicates glomerular disease.
- ♦ Painless haematuria (microscopic or macroscopic) is an important presenting symptom of bladder disease. Cystoscopy is necessary to exclude papilloma or cancer.
- ♦ The oedema of nephrotic syndrome may be misdiagnosed as heart failure. Test the urine for protein; a 3–4+ positive test result confirms the diagnosis.
- ♦ Nephrotic syndrome can be associated with underlying malignancy, particularly in the elderly.
- ♦ Renal vascular disease is an important cause of hypertension and renal failure. Listen for renal artery bruits and for bruits elsewhere, e.g. femoral arteries.
- ♦ Evidence of atheromatous vascular disease elsewhere – cerebral, cardiac, or peripheral – makes renal vascular disease more likely. It is particularly prevalent in type 2 diabetes mellitus.
- ♦ Patients with multisystem, atypical or puzzling symptoms and signs, may have systemic vasculitis. Serum antineutrophil cytoplasmic antibodies may confirm the diagnosis.
- ♦ Symptoms and signs of systemic vasculitis can mimic those of subacute bacterial endocarditis.
- ♦ Negative dip stix urine testing will provide reassurance for patients concerned about the colour or the frothy nature of their urine.

The reproductive system

ELAINE ANDERSON • AILSA GEBBIE • NORMAN SMITH • PETER BERREY

Use particular care and sensitivity when examining the breasts, genitalia or rectum because these procedures may be embarrassing or intimidating for many patients. As well as remembering and using all the principles in Chapter 1, you need to have the confidence to put the patient at ease and to be able to reassure women with negative findings. Try to gauge your patient's level of anxiety. You can allay this by showing understanding, empathy and courtesy. Explain why the examination is necessary and what it involves, particularly if you need to do any additional procedures. The patient may find diagrams helpful. By doing this you will obtain informed consent. During the examination you may raise many psychological or social issues. Meet these concerns positively and non-judgementally.

Your patients should be able to change in privacy and comfort. They should undress alone but some may need help from a nurse, chaperone or relative. Do not leave your patients waiting undressed before you examine them. Examine them gently and skilfully and be alert to any discomfort or pain they experience. Stop the examination if your patient becomes distressed. Tell patients what you are doing as you carry out each step of the examination. Do not make personal remarks relating to suntans, tattoos or body piercing unless relevant and do not use phrases which may be misinterpreted as terms of endearment such as 'my dear'.

Chaperones

Whenever possible, patients should be offered a chaperone or invited to bring a friend or relative, regardless of your gender and that of the patient. The purpose is to benefit patient care and, in a minority of cases, to stop improper practitioner behaviour and rough intimate examinations. If your patient does not wish a chaperone, accept this unless you feel unhappy about it, and record it in the case notes. If there is no chaperone available, explain this and ask the patient's permission to proceed or offer another appointment time when a chaperone would be available. In primary care it is unrealistic to always have a chaperone but you should always offer one.

A family member or friend is not the same as a chaperone. In the legal sense, a chaperone is someone with nothing to gain from misrepresenting the facts. This may not always be the case with family members. Their presence may also influence patients' ability to tell you the full story, especially if there are sexual or marital problems. A chaperone acts as a support person for patients, helping them to relax during the examination and talking them through procedures. The presence of a chaperone reduces the risk of humiliation or intimidation of the patient by the doctor and protects the patient from abuse, whether real or perceived. This may save you from a false allegation of sexual abuse. However, this is extremely rare so do not let it dominate your thinking or actions.

THE BREAST EXAMINATION

Anatomy

The breasts are modified sweat glands. The nipple is usually in the fourth intercostal space in the midclavicular line, but accessory breast/nipple tissue may develop anywhere down the nipple line (axilla to groin) (Fig. 7.1).

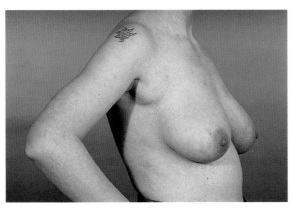

Fig. 7.1 Accessory breast tissue in the axilla.

The adult breast can be divided into the nipple, the areola and four quadrants, upper and lower, inner and outer, with the axillary tail projecting from the upper outer quadrant (Fig. 7.2).

The nipple is erectile tissue covered with pigmented skin, which also covers the areola. The openings of the lactiferous ducts are seen near the apex of the nipple but can occur anywhere on the areola.

The size and shape of the breasts in healthy women vary and are influenced by age, hereditary factors, sexual maturity, the phase of the menstrual cycle, parity, pregnancy, lactation and general state of nutrition. The amount of fat and stroma surrounding the glandular tissue determines the size of the breast, except during lactation, when the enlargement is almost entirely glandular. The breast is responsive to hormones, and its consistency varies in response to fluctuations in oestrogen and progesterone levels during the menstrual cycle and in pregnancy. Swelling and tenderness due to fluid retention and prominence of the glandular elements of the breast are more common in the premenstrual phase. With increasing age the amount of glandular tissue reduces with a corresponding increase in the relative amount

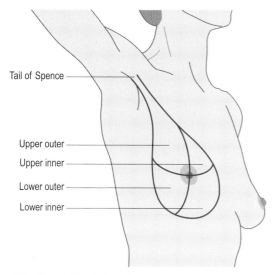

Tail of Spence

Upper outer

Upper inner

Lower outer

Lower inner

Fig. 7.2   The adult right breast.

of fat so that the breasts are softer in consistency and more pendulous. The breasts of lactating women are swollen and engorged with milk and are best examined after breastfeeding or milk expression.

Definitions and abnormalities

Breast lump

The commonest cause of a breast lump varies with age.

Breast cancer.   This is one of the commonest malignancies in the UK, affecting 1 in 10 women. The incidence increases with age, but most women regard any mass as potentially malignant and so should you until it is proved otherwise. Cancer of the male breast is uncommon with a strong genetic factor.

Characteristically cancers are solid masses with an irregular outline. They are usually, but not always, painless, firm and hard, contrasting in consistency with the surrounding breast tissue. The cancer may be contained within the breast tissue, extend directly into the overlying tissues such as skin, pectoral fascia, pectoral muscle, or metastasize to regional lymph nodes or systemic circulation.

Fibrocystic changes.   Fibrocystic changes or irregular nodularity of the breast is common, especially in the upper outer quadrant in young women. The tissue is usually rubbery in texture and varies in size with the hormonal cycle, being most prominent in the premenstrual phase. The changes are usually bilateral and benign, but any new focal change in young women which persists after menstruation should be investigated.

Fibroadenomas.   These are benign lumps due to overgrowth of parts of the terminal duct lobules. They are smooth mobile discrete rubbery lumps which occur more commonly in young women. They are the second commonest cause of a discrete breast mass in women under 35 years old.

Breast cysts.   These fluid-filled sacs are the commonest cause of a breast lump in women between the ages of 35 and 50. They present as smooth lumps, which may be soft and fluctuant when the intracystic pressure is low, becoming hard and painful if the pressure is high. Cysts may occur in multiple clusters. Most are benign but, since a cyst may be associated with malignant disease, investigate any cyst in which the aspirate is bloodstained, where there is a residual mass following aspiration or which recurs after aspiration.

Breast abscesses.   There are two types of breast abscesses:

- Lactational abscesses occur in women who are breastfeeding, and are usually peripheral.
- Non-lactational abscesses occur as an extension of periductal mastitis and are usually at the edge of, or under, the areola, and are often associated with nipple inversion. They usually occur in young female smokers. Occasionally a non-lactating abscess may discharge spontaneously through an abnormal communication between the inflamed duct and the skin. The classical position of the mamillary fistula is at the areolocutaneous border (Fig. 7.3).

Breast pain (mastalgia)

Differentiate between pain which is related to the menstrual cycle, usually worse in the latter half and relieved with the onset of menstruation – cyclical mastalgia – and persistent pain with no cyclical variation – non-cyclical mastalgia.

Most women at some time in their life will suffer cyclical mastalgia. Ascertain the severity of symptoms, how this interferes with lifestyle and when it occurs in the cycle (pain charts may be helpful).

Distinguish true breast pain from referred pain originating in the chest wall and examine other sources of pain if necessary, e.g. musculoskeletal.

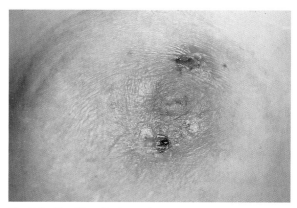

Fig. 7.3   Mamillary fistulae at the areolocutaneous border.   **199**

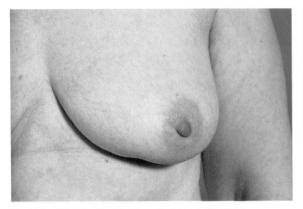

Fig. 7.4   Skin dimpling due to underlying malignancy.

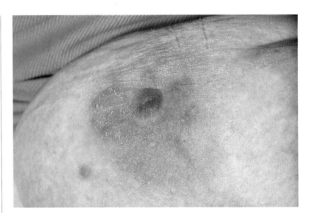

Fig. 7.6   Paget's disease of the nipple.

Skin changes

Simple skin dimpling is due to retraction of the dermis but the skin remains mobile over the cancer (Fig. 7.4).

Indrawing of the skin is due to infiltration of the dermis by tumour and the cancer is fixed to the skin.

Obstruction of the intramammary lymphatics with cancer cells causes lymphoedema of the breast. The skin is attached at the hair follicles but swollen in between, giving the appearance of the skin of an orange (Fig. 7.5). This can occur with infection but then other cardinal signs, i.e. redness, warmth and tenderness, are also present. Any 'infection' which does not respond to one course of antibiotics must be investigated to exclude an inflammatory cancer. These are aggressive tumours with a poor prognosis.

Eczematous changes of the nipple and areola may be part of a generalized skin disorder. If affecting the true nipple, it may be due to Paget's disease (Fig. 7.6). This is caused by invasion of the epidermis by cells from an underlying intraductal cancer. The diagnosis is established by a skin biopsy.

Nipple changes

Nipple inversion.   Retraction of the nipple due to shortening of the nipple ducts from periductal inflammation and fibrosis is a common finding. The characteristics of benign nipple inversion are symmetrical slit-like inversion. Nipple retraction due to malignant disease is asymmetrical and distorting, pulling the nipple away from its central position (Fig. 7.7).

Nipple discharge.   A small amount of fluid expressed from multiple ducts of the breast on massage is normal. It may be clear, yellow, white or green in colour. Persistent single duct discharge or bloodstained (macroscopic or microscopic) discharge should be investigated. The differential diagnosis includes duct ectasia, periductal mastitis, intraduct papilloma or intraduct cancer.

Galactorrhoea.   Galactorrhoea is a milky discharge from multiple ducts in both breasts and is a feature of hyperprolactinaemia. It is often accompanied by hyperplasia of Montgomery's tubercles, which are small rounded projections covering areolar glands.

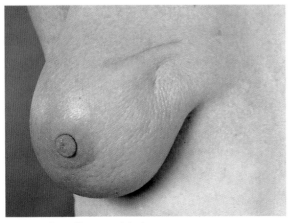

  Fig. 7.5   Peau d'orange of the breast.

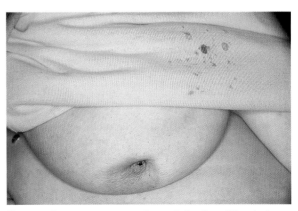

Fig. 7.7   Breast cancer presenting as indrawing of the nipple.
Note the bloody discharge on the underclothing.

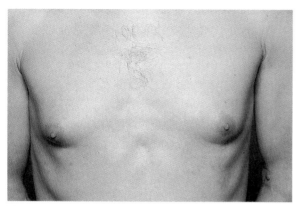

Fig. 7.8   Drug-induced gynaecomastia caused by cimetidine.

7.2 Indicators of breast cancer risk

• Female
• Increasing age
• Family history especially if associated with:
  – early age of onset
  – multiple cases of breast cancer
  – ovarian cancer
  – male breast cancer
• Early menarche
• Nulliparity or late age of first child
• Late menopause
• Prolonged HRT use
• Postmenopausal obesity
• Mantle irradiation for Hodgkin's disease especially at young age (< 30 years)

The role of the oral contraceptive pill as a major risk factor for breast cancer is still debated

7.1 Causes of gynaecomastia
Drugs including
• Cannabis • Oestrogens used in treatment of prostatic cancer • Spironolactone • Cimetidine • Digoxin
Decreased androgen production
• Klinefelter's syndrome
Increased oestrogen levels
• Chronic liver disease • Thyrotoxicosis • Some adrenal tumours

Gynaecomastia

Gynaecomastia is enlargement of the male breast and often occurs in pubertal boys (Fig. 7.8). In chronic liver disease gynaecomastia is caused by high levels of circulating oestrogens which are not metabolized by the liver. Many drugs can cause enlargement (Table 7.1).

THE HISTORY

Most breast pathology is benign, but benign and malignant conditions may present with similar symptoms including a lump, skin changes, nipple inversion, nipple discharge and pain. Acute inflammation in the breast may be benign or due to a cancer. Most women with breast symptoms are worried that they may have breast cancer; always remember this and clarify their worries so you can acknowledge and deal with them. Ask initially about the presenting complaint, including how long the symptoms have been present, what changes have occurred, any relationship to the menstrual

cycle and any specific relieving or precipitating factors. Evaluate potential risk factors (Table 7.2) and menopausal status. Remember that breast cancer may present with symptoms of metastatic disease.

Patients may attend with breast changes or because an abnormality has been detected during screening mammography. An increasing number of asymptomatic women present with mammographic abnormalities. Asymptomatic women may also present with concerns about family history and men with gynaecomastia.

EXAMINATION

➔ Examination sequence

→ Use first principles (Ch. 1) and explain the purpose of the examination. Offer a chaperone.

→ Ask the patient to sit upright on a well-illuminated chair or side of a bed, undressed to the waist and with the hands resting on the thighs, so that the pectoral muscles are relaxed (Fig. 7.9).

→ Face the patient and look at the breasts for asymmetry, local swelling or changes in the skin or nipples. Ask the patient to press her hands firmly on her hips – this contracts the pectoral muscles – and repeat the inspection.

→ Ask her to raise her arms above her head to stretch the pectoral muscles and the skin over the breast, and finally to lean forward so that the breasts become pendulous. These actions expose the whole breast and exacerbate skin dimpling.

→ Ask the patient to lie with her head supported on one pillow and put her hand under her head on the side to be examined (Fig. 7.10). You may ask her to do this on both sides at the same time.

→ With your hand held flat to the skin, palpate the breast tissue using the palmar surface of your middle three fingers and compress the breast tissue firmly against the chest wall.

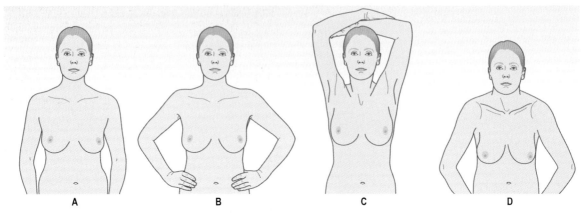

Fig. 7.9 Positions for inspecting the breasts. (A) Hands resting on thighs. (B) Hands pressed onto hips. (C) Arms above head. (D) Leaning forward with breasts pendulous.

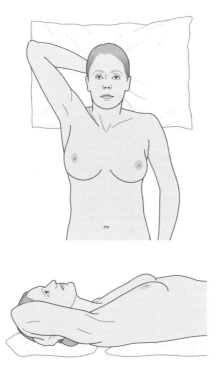

Fig. 7.10 Position for examination of the right breast.

→ Consider the breast as the face of a clock and examine each hour of the clock from the outside towards the nipple, including under the nipple. Compare the texture of one breast with that of the other. Examine all the breast tissue. Remember that the breast extends from the clavicle to the upper abdomen and the midline to the anterior

border of latissimus dorsi (posterior axillary fold). Define the characteristics of any mass (Table 7.3).

→ Tethering to the skin, where there is a fibrous connection but not direct invasion, may not be obvious on inspection but becomes apparent as dimpling overlying the tumour if you gently elevate the breast using your hand.

→ To determine if a mass is fixed to underlying tissue, ask the patient to place her hands on her hips. Hold the tumour between your thumb and forefinger and ask the patient to alternately contract and relax the pectoral muscles by pushing into her hips. Tethering to the pectoral fascia is where the tumour is solid with the chest wall when the pectoral muscle is contracted, but separate when it is relaxed. Infiltration occurs where the tumour is fixed to chest wall when the pectoral muscle is relaxed and contracted.

→ Examine the axillary tail between your finger and thumb as it extends towards the axilla.

To palpate the nipple, hold it gently between index finger and thumb and try to express any discharge. Massage the breast towards the nipple to uncover any discharge. Note the colour and consistency of any discharge along with the number and position of the affected ducts. Test any nipple discharge for blood using urine-testing sticks.

→ Palpate the regional lymph nodes, including the supraclavicular group. Ask the patient to sit, facing you, with her shoulder relaxed so you are supporting the full weight of her arm at the wrist with your opposite hand. Place the flat of your other hand high into the axilla then move it upwards over the chest to the apex. This can be uncomfortable for patients so warn them and check for

7.3 Characteristics of a breast mass
• Size (use engineer's callipers for accuracy)
• Position (as determined by clock face)
• Mobility
• Composition (i.e. fluctuant, hard, rubbery)
• Fixation to underlying tissues or skin

- any discomfort. Compress the contents of the axilla against the chest wall. Assess the size, consistency and fixation of any palpable masses.
→ Examine the supraclavicular fossa. First look for any visual abnormality then palpate the neck from behind and systematically review all cervical lymphatic chains.

INVESTIGATIONS

Accurate diagnosis of breast lesions depends on clinical assessment, backed up by mammography and/or breast ultrasound, and cytopathological diagnosis, either by fine needle aspiration cytology or core biopsy (triple assessment). Up to 10% of malignant lesions require excision biopsy to make the diagnosis. In the UK there are specific guidelines for the appropriate referral of patients with breast symptoms to specialist units where this assessment is carried out.

Fine needle aspiration

A blue (23G) or green (21G) needle (on a syringe applying suction) is passed through a breast lesion with or without anaesthetic. This immediately shows a breast cyst if it fills with fluid. Aspiration cytology will give enough cells for the diagnosis of 95% of malignancies and 85% of benign lesions. Cysts yielding bloodstained fluid or leaving a residual mass should be further investigated to exclude malignancy.

Core biopsy. Use an automatic gun which takes a matchstick-size piece of tissue under local anaesthetic. Histopathology allows differentiation of in-situ from invasive cancer and further analysis of tumour characteristics such as oestrogen receptor status.

Mammography

Mammograms are low-dose X-rays of the breasts (Fig. 7.11). Breast cancer is characteristically seen as an irregular opacity with spiculated (multiple small spikes) edges, often associated with irregular microcalcification. Mammography is more useful in older women because the breasts are less opaque and easier to interpret.

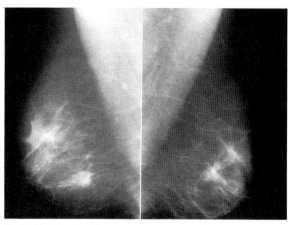

Fig. 7.11 Single oblique mammograms showing bilateral spiculate masses characteristic of cancer.

Ultrasound scanning

This differentiates solid from cystic lesions and often benign from malignant lesions. Colour Doppler further improves the sensitivity. Ultrasound is particularly helpful in women under the age of 35.

Magnetic resonance imaging (MRI)

This is useful to investigate very dense breasts or if you suspect rupture of a breast implant.

◆ Key points

- Breast cancer is very common – a lifetime risk of 1 in 10 women.
- Breast cancer risk increases with age.
- Regard any breast lump as potentially malignant until proven otherwise.
- Always inspect the breast in various positions.
- Follow this by systematic palpation of the gland and of the regional lymph nodes.
- Women over 35 with a discrete breast lump should be urgently referred to a specialist breast unit.

THE GYNAECOLOGICAL EXAMINATION

Anatomy

The female reproductive organs include the ovaries, fallopian tubes, uterus and vagina and lie within the pelvis with the rectum posteriorly and the bladder anteriorly (Fig. 7.12).

The external genitalia, or vulva, includes the labia majora, labia minora, the vaginal orifice or introitus, the urethra and clitoris. The labia minora demarcate the vestibule and this contains the urethral opening and the vaginal orifice (Fig. 7.13).

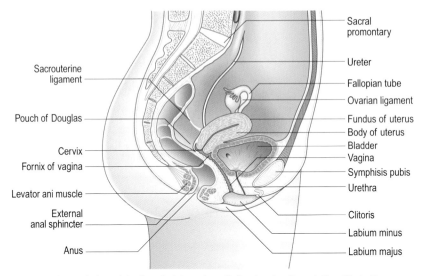

Fig. 7.12 Lateral view of the female internal genitalia showing the relationship to the rectum and bladder.

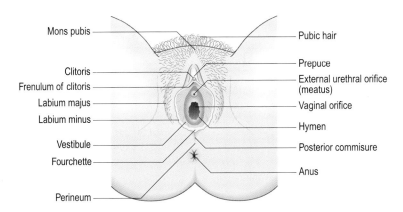

Fig. 7.13 The external female genitalia.

Bartholin's glands are pea-sized mucous glands lying deep to the posterior margin of the labia minora, which open posterolaterally into the vestibule through a duct. They provide lubrication of the introitus but may become blocked, causing swelling or pain if they are infected.

The vagina is a flattened tube, about 8–10 cm long, passing up and back from the vulva to the cervix, separated from the bladder anteriorly and the rectum posteriorly. At the top end the cervix pushes in and divides the upper vault into anterior, posterior and lateral fornices (Fig. 7.14A&B).

The uterus is a muscular pear-shaped organ divided into the cervix, body and fundus (Fig. 7.14C). It is usually angled forward from the axis of the vagina – anteverted.

However, in some women the axis may be similar to that of the vagina and the uterus is said to be retroverted (Fig. 7.15).

The adnexae are the Fallopian tubes and ovaries and their attachments. The Fallopian tubes vary in length from 8–14 cm and pass laterally from the upper outer part of the uterus (the cornu) where they open into it. They travel in the free edge of the broad ligament and curve round to meet the ovaries where each opens into a trumpet-shaped infundibulum. The infundibula are fringed by fimbriae, which are close to the ovary and help capture the ovum when it is shed at ovulation. Each ovary is oval and measures about 3×2 centimetres. It rests on the side wall of the

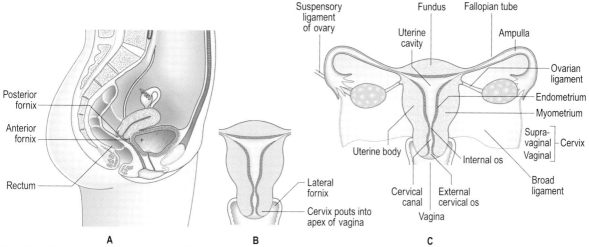

Fig. 7.14 The fornices of the vagina, and the uterus. The cervix projects into the vagina creating the anterior, posterior (A) and lateral fornices (B). (C) Section through the pear-shaped, muscular uterus (showing the cervix, body (corpus) and fundus) and the Fallopian tubes, showing the ligamentous attachments of the ovary. The uterine mucosa is the endometrium. The cervical canal has an internal and external os.

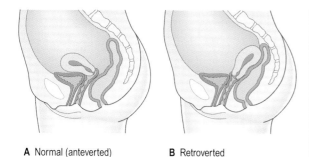

A Normal (anteverted)   **B** Retroverted

Fig. 7.15 The different anatomical positions of the uterine body within the pelvis.

pelvis and is attached to the cornu of the uterus by the ovarian ligament.

Overlying the muscular floor of the pelvis is connective tissue, which forms ligaments that help to stabilize the organs in the pelvis.

Definitions and abnormalities

Menstruation.   Menstruation (commonly called a period) normally occurs at intervals of 22–35 days, and bleeding usually lasts less than 7 days. Normal blood loss is less than 80 ml but is difficult to assess and is usually described by the woman as light, normal or heavy, although this is clearly a subjective judgement. The length of one cycle is measured from day 1 of bleeding to day 1 of bleeding in the next period. By convention, a woman who bleeds for 5 days every 29 days is recorded as K 5/29. Problems may arise with the cycle length as well as the amount and duration of blood loss.

- *Oligomenorrhoea* is when periods occur at intervals of more than 35 days.
- *Primary amenorrhoea* is when menstruation has not started by the age of 16 years.
- *Secondary amenorrhoea* occurs if periods do not occur for more than 70 days in a woman who previously menstruated. The commonest cause is pregnancy. Do not investigate this for at least 6 months in a young woman who is not pregnant because lifestyle events, such as stress and weight loss, are the commonest causes and menstruation often resumes spontaneously.
- *Menorrhagia* is an excessive amount of blood loss.
- *Flooding* is an embarrassing episode of very heavy blood loss which happens during a period. This may soak clothes, bedding or chairs. Passing clots is of no significance other than indicating very heavy bleeding.
- *Dysmenorrhoea* is painful periods. Primary dysmenorrhoea occurs between the ages of 15 and 25 and is felt in the lower abdomen, back and the inner surface of the thighs. Secondary or acquired dysmenorrhoea usually occurs after age 30.
- *Menarche* is the age at which periods start. The average age is 12–13 years.
- *Precocious puberty* is the onset of menstruation before 9 years of age and should be investigated.

- The *menopause* is the cessation of menstruation but is commonly used to describe the perimenopausal years. This time is more correctly known as the *climacteric*. The final period is only known for certain once the woman has had no further bleeding for 1 year. The menopause occurs on average at 51 years of age. The normal range is between 45–55 years. The female genital tract atrophies as circulating oestrogen levels decline following the menopause. The mucosa of the vulva and vagina atrophy and lose their normal elasticity and lubrication. The vagina narrows and sexual intercourse may become uncomfortable. Urinary symptoms such as nocturia, dysuria and urgency of micturition are common (see Ch. 6). The vulval and vaginal skin appear thin and shiny.
- *Postmenopausal bleeding* is spontaneous vaginal bleeding more than 1 year after the final menstrual period. It requires urgent investigation to exclude malignancy.

Dyspareunia. This is pain during intercourse. It may be felt superficially around the entrance to the vagina or deep within the pelvis. Young women quite commonly experience pain on intercourse due to involuntary spasm of muscles at the vaginal entrance (vaginismus). Persistent deep dyspareunia may be associated with underlying pelvic pathology. Dyspareunia may be due to vaginal dryness following menopausal changes.

Vaginal discharge. The normal physiological discharge in women of reproductive age is usually white or clear and varies in amount according to the stage of the menstrual cycle. Ask about colour, odour, heaviness, duration and associated symptoms including itching or soreness. Infection may be sexually transmitted. Non-sexually transmitted infection is usually thrush (*Candida albicans*), which gives a thick, white, curdy discharge often associated with marked vulval irritation. The other common infection is bacterial vaginosis where the usual infecting agent is *Gardnerella vaginalis*. This causes a characteristic vaginal discharge which is watery in consistency and has a fishy odour. The pH of normal vaginal secretions is usually less than 4.5 but in bacterial vaginosis it is greater than 5.

Sexually transmitted infections. Consider these in any woman with a vaginal discharge, vulval ulceration or pain, dysuria or lower abdominal pain, but remember they may occur in asymptomatic women.

Pelvic masses. Assess a pelvic mass during a vaginal examination and if it is very large you may feel it abdominally.

The pregnant uterus is the commonest cause of a mass arising from the pelvis in a woman of reproductive age. A pelvic mass may be uterine or ovarian in origin and ultrasound examination is required to differentiate between them.

Incontinence. This is common and more frequent in parous women. It may be associated with weakness of the pelvic floor support (*stress incontinence*) and present with leakage on coughing, sneezing or sudden exertion. Instability of the detrusor muscle of the bladder causes a strong desire to pass urine even when the bladder is not full (urgency) and can cause leakage (*urge incontinence*).

THE HISTORY

The *presenting complaint* needs to be clarified along with the woman's ideas, concerns and expectations.

Ask how old she was when menstruation started (menarche). Record the date of the first day of her last menstrual period. Record the number of days of bleeding and whether blood flow is normal, light or heavy. Find out how long her periods last and how often they occur. Are her periods regular and, if not, how do they vary? Women with heavy periods often have to use double sanitary protection, have flooding and pass clots. Ask about any pain associated with menstruation and if this has changed. Irregular bleeding may indicate underlying disease so ask women about bleeding between their periods or after sexual intercourse. Note what contraceptive method she is using as this can affect menstrual function. If she is not having periods, find out when they stopped and ask about other symptoms such as changes in weight or exercise.

Table 7.4 provides a checklist for taking a menstrual history.

Past history

This is relevant because the woman may have had similar problems before. Endocrine conditions may affect menstrual function so explore these possibilities.

7.4 Checklist for the menstrual history

- Age of menarche
- Date of last menstrual period
- Duration and regularity of periods
- Amount of bleeding
- Pain
- Irregular bleeding:
  – intermenstrual
  – post-coital
- Use of hormonal contraception or hormone replacement therapy
- History of any pregnancies
- Age of menopause

Drug history

Find out about any medication the woman is taking, both prescribed and from other sources. If she is menopausal ask if she is a present or past user of hormone replacement therapy. Always ask about contraception (Table 7.5), which should be used for 2 years after her periods stop before she is 50 and for 1 year if her periods stop after the age of 50.

Family history

A history of ovarian or breast cancer may be relevant.

Social history

This may include how the woman's current symptoms are affecting her relationships and her work and daily life. Sexual problems are common and can cause distress so you need to discuss her sexual history.

Sexual history

Use a simple pattern of questioning to make taking a sexual history straightforward and unambiguous (Table 7.6).
 Contact tracing. Sexual partners of patients with sexually transmitted infections must be traced and treated to prevent further transmission of the infection or re-infection of the treated person. Confidentiality is paramount so do not give information regarding any one individual to a third party.

Health education

The gynaecological consultation is an opportunity for screening and promoting health. Health education can include advice about smoking cessation, weight, breast awareness, pre-pregnancy screening, personal protection against sexually transmitted infection and domestic violence. National screening tests for women in the UK are cervical cytology and mammography. A woman needs to hear the pros and cons of these in a way that allows her to decide whether or not she wishes a particular test.

EXAMINATION

Examine the abdomen and inguinal region to detect any large masses arising from the pelvis or any lymphadenopathy before carrying out a vaginal examination.

 If a woman has never had penetrative sexual intercourse a vaginal examination is not usually undertaken, although a limited examination may be possible if she uses tampons during menstruation. Always explain the procedure fully and why it is necessary.

 Indications for a vaginal examination are:

- to take a cervical smear
- in the presence of:
  - vaginal or pelvic infection
  - menstrual dysfunction
  - lower abdominal pain
  - urogenital prolapse
  - dyspareunia
  - a mass arising from the pelvis.

Ask the woman to empty her bladder before the examination. Make sure that there is a good movable light. Ask the patient to lie on her back on an examination couch with a pillow for her head and a modesty sheet covering her chest and abdomen after she has removed clothing from these areas. Ask her to bend up both knees and, either with her heels together in the middle or separated, let her knees flop apart (Fig. 7.16).

 Women dislike having their legs 'put up in stirrups' and this is not required for a routine smear or examination. Leg supports or foot stirrups are helpful if the examination is prolonged or for minor procedures. You can use the left lateral position to examine for prolapse. In this case the patient lies on her left side with her knees drawn up slightly towards her chin.

7.5   Contraceptive methods
• Condom
• Female sheath
• Combined oral contraceptive pill
• Contraceptive skin patch
• Progestogen-only pill
• Progestogen depot injection
• Progestogen implant
• Intrauterine contraceptive device (coil)
• Intrauterine contraceptive system (slow local release of low-dose progesterone)
• Diaphragm
• Cervical cap
• Natural (rhythm)
• Sterilization, male or female

7.6   Questions to use when taking a sexual history
• Are you currently in a relationship?
• Is it a sexual relationship?
• How long have you been with your partner?
• Is your partner a man or a woman?
• When did you last have sex with anyone else?
• Are there any sexual issues that you would like to discuss?
• What do you use for contraception/protection?

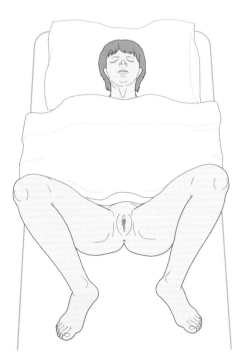

Fig. 7.16 Position for examination.

▶ Examination sequence

→ Put on gloves and apply a lubricating gel to your examining finger. Separate the labia with the forefinger and thumb of your left hand and inspect the clitoris, urethra and vaginal opening (Fig. 7.17).

→ Look for any discharge, inflammation, atrophy, ulceration or abnormalities of the Bartholin's glands. Ask the woman to cough or strain down and look at the vaginal walls for any prolapse. Note the position and extent of this and any uterine descent. Watch for involuntary leakage of urine indicating stress incontinence.

Speculum examination

→ To see further inside the vagina, use a vaginal speculum to see the cervix and the vaginal walls, to carry out a cervical smear and to take swabs if necessary. Specula are made of metal or plastic (Fig. 7.18). Metal specula require sterilization, and plastic specula are disposable but are more expensive. A metal speculum is cold and should be warmed under the hot tap. Most women find speculum examination mildly uncomfortable so always lubricate a speculum with gel even if you are carrying out a cervical smear.

→ Use your left hand to part the labia. Take the speculum in your right hand with the blades closed and the handles positioned towards the woman's left leg. Gently insert the speculum into the vaginal opening and rotate it through 90° to position the handles anteriorly. Cusco's speculum was designed for the handles to face posteriorly but it is now usual to place the handles anteriorly to avoid manipulating around the perianal region, which patients dislike. (The exception is under general anaesthetic in theatre when the speculum is used in the original way with handles posteriorly.) If a woman finds speculum examination difficult, you can ask her to insert the speculum herself.

→ Gently open the blades. Identify the cervix and note its appearance looking for an erosion, polyps or malignancy. If the cervix does not immediately come into view, withdraw the speculum slightly, close the blades and press the speculum slightly more deeply before reopening the blades. Take swabs or a cervical smear as necessary. Take the cervical smear before you perform a bimanual vaginal examination to avoid the risk of removing cellular material from the cervix during the bimanual examination. Remove the speculum and offer the woman tissues and privacy to clean herself up. Discuss your findings with her after she is dressed.

Cervical smear (Table 7.7)

→ Label a microscope slide in pencil with the patient's details before starting your examination.

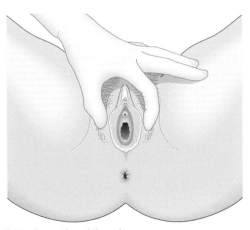

Fig. 7.17 Inspection of the vulva.

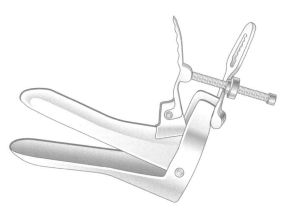

Fig. 7.18 Bivalve speculum.

7.7 Cervical smear

- Label microscope slide or cytological medium
- Visualize cervical os

Conventional smear

- Insert longer blade of spatula into os
- Rotate spatula through 360°
- Spread once across the slide
- Place slide immediately into fixative for 3 or 4 minutes
- Leave to dry in air

Liquid-based cytology

- Rotate plastic brush 5 times through 360°
- Remove brush
- Push brush 10 times against the bottom of the specimen container
- Twirl 5 times through 360° to dislodge all of the sample
- Firmly close the lid

A Using a spatula

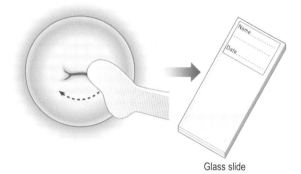

Glass slide

B Liquid-based cytology

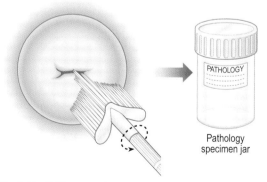

Pathology specimen jar

Fig. 7.19 Taking a cervical smear.

→ Having seen the cervix, take the spatula and put the longer end into the cervical os (Fig. 7.19A). Rotate the spatula through 360° round the cervix to scrape off a sample for cytological examination.

→ Spread the sample thinly on the slide, wiping the spatula once from one side to the other. Fix this immediately by placing the slide in a container filled with methylated spirits.

→ Liquid-based cytology (Fig. 7.19B) is widely used now instead of a spatula and glass slide. It allows increased automation to read the slides and a smaller percentage of inadequate smears. A specially designed brush is used to obtain cellular material from the cervix. The material is then transferred to a cytological medium and spun down to give the smear sample.

Bimanual examination

→ Insert your right index finger into the vagina and turn your palm upwards. If the vagina is capacious and the patient is relaxed then use your index and middle fingers (Fig. 7.20). Only use one finger if the woman is tense or experiences discomfort.

→ Feel for the cervix in the upper vagina. The cervix usually points downward and feels firm like the tip of the nose. Move the cervix from side to side and note any tenderness (cervical excitation). This can be a sign of infection.

→ With your fingers behind the cervix, place your left hand flat on the lower abdomen above the pubic symphysis (Fig. 7.21).

→ Move your vaginal fingers to push the cervix upwards and feel the fundus of the uterus with your left hand. Identify the size, shape, position and surface characteristics of the uterus and any tenderness. If you cannot feel the uterus, it may be retroverted and this is often difficult to feel easily. Put your fingers in the posterior fornix and try again.

→ Now put your fingers in each lateral fornix, one at a time, and bring your hand towards your left hand to detect any enlargement or tenderness of the ovaries or fallopian tubes (Fig. 7.22).

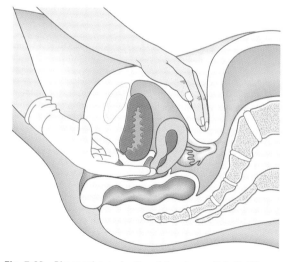

Fig. 7.20 Bimanual examination of the uterus. Note that the bladder is empty, the patient having voided just before the pelvic examination. The vaginal fingers push the cervix back and upwards so that the fundus can be reached by the abdominally located fingers.

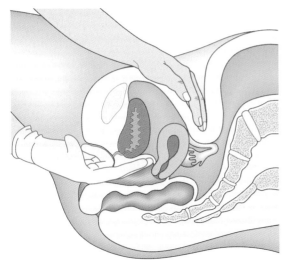

Fig. 7.21   Bimanual examination of the uterus. The vaginally located fingers now palpate the anterior surface of the uterus, which is held in position by the abdominally located fingers.

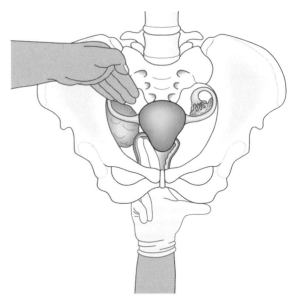

Fig. 7.22   Palpation of an ovarian mass.

◆ Key points

- Use particular care and sensitivity when taking a gynaecological history and performing a vaginal examination.
- Always offer the patient a chaperone.
- Pregnancy is the most common cause of amenorrhoea and/or a pelvic mass in a woman of reproductive age.
- If a woman finds speculum examination difficult, offer her the chance to insert the speculum herself.
- Women who have never been sexually active do not need a cervical smear.
- Sexually transmitted infections are often asymptomatic in women.
- One-third of women in their late 40s have uterine fibroids. Most are asymptomatic.
- Urgently investigate any vaginal bleeding more than 1 year following the menopause to exclude an underlying malignancy.
- Ovarian cancer often presents at an advanced stage with a large pelvic mass.

INVESTIGATIONS

7.8 Gynaecological investigations

Investigation	Diagnostic problem and comments
Vaginal pH Test using narrow range pH paper (pH 4–6)	The pH of vaginal secretions is normally < 4.5
High vaginal swab	Vaginal discharge
Endocervical swab	To exclude Chlamydia
Full blood count	Menorrhagia to check for anaemia
Thyroid function tests	Amenorrhoea (may be thyrotoxic) Heavy, prolonged periods (may be hypothyroid)
Pregnancy test (urine)	Amenorrhoea
Serum beta human chorionic gonadotrophin	Very early intrauterine pregnancy Ectopic pregnancy
Hormonal analysis: serum oestradiol, follicle-stimulating hormone/luteinizing hormone, progesterone, testosterone, prolactin	Amenorrhoea, premature menopause, hirsutism, infertility, galactorrhoea
Serum tumour markers: carcinoembryonic antigen and Ca 125	Ovarian malignancy
Pelvic ultrasound scan: abdominal Transvaginal ultrasound gives the most detailed examination of the pelvic organs	Early pregnancy, pelvic mass, abnormal menstrual bleeding, postmenopausal bleeding
Endometrial biopsy	Abnormal bleeding
Laparoscopy	Infertility, chronic pelvic pain or suspected ectopic pregnancy
Hysteroscopy A fibre-optic telescope is inserted into the uterine cavity through the cervix, allowing direct visualization of the cavity and enabling biopsies to be taken	Abnormal uterine bleeding
Urodynamic investigations Measurement of changes in intravesical and intraurethral pressures	Stress and/or urge incontinence

Examine this woman with acute pelvic pain

1. Look for signs of shock: pallor, low blood pressure, and weak, rapid pulse (*acute blood loss* or *sepsis*).
2. Record the temperature.
3. Feel lower abdomen for tenderness, guarding and rebound and check for any masses arising from the pelvis.
4. Inspect the vulva to look for any signs of bleeding.
5. Pass a vaginal speculum and look for bleeding or vaginal discharge.
6. Perform single digit examination and check for any tenderness on cervical excitation or in the fornices.
7. Take bacteriological investigations including endocervical swab for *Chlamydia* or *gonorrhoea* and a high vaginal swab.
8. Perform bimanual examination to assess the size of the uterus, any adnexal masses and elicit any tenderness of the pelvic organs.
9. Perform rectal examination if there is any suspicion of *appendicitis*.
10. Perform a pregnancy test in any woman of reproductive age. Do a serum beta human chorionic gonadotrophin if the pregnancy test is negative and there is suspicion of *ectopic pregnancy*.
11. Further investigations may be appropriate, e.g. pelvic ultrasound scan, diagnostic laparoscopy.

Examine this woman with postmenopausal bleeding

1. Look for evidence of weight loss or anaemia.
2. Feel the abdomen to detect any mass arising from the pelvis.
3. Inspect the vulva for possible malignancy.
4. Pass a vaginal speculum:
   inspect the vaginal walls for evidence of *severe atrophic change* or more rarely *vaginal cancer*
   inspect the cervix for *cancer* or *cervical polyp*.
5. Take a cervical smear if this is due or the cervix looks abnormal.
6. Perform bimanual examination to look for uterine size and to detect any adnexal mass.
7. Further investigations may be appropriate, e.g. endometrial biopsy, transvaginal ultrasound scan, examination under anaesthetic, diagnostic curettage, colposcopy and cervical biopsy.

THE OBSTETRIC EXAMINATION

Examining a pregnant patient differs from other situations because you are assessing two individuals at the same time. Women vary in how much they know about pregnancy and delivery but most want to find out more. Help your patients by freely exchanging information and helping them to access other sources. Work closely with the midwife and make sure communication with everyone is excellent by applying the principles discussed in Chapter 1.

Definitions and abnormalities

Length of pregnancy. A normal pregnancy lasts 266 days from the date of conception.

Expected date of delivery. Work out the expected date of delivery by adding 1 year 7 days and removing 3 months from the first day of your patient's last menstrual period, assuming she has a regular 28-day cycle. If her cycle is long, then ovulation is delayed because the interval between ovulation and the first day of menstruation is always 14 days. So for a 35-day cycle, the expected date of delivery is 7 days later than the normal date you calculate.

Check that the last menstrual period was normal, lasted the usual length of time and occurred after the usual interval. An implantation bleed can mimic a period, but is usually lighter and shorter, in which case the expected date of delivery will be 4 weeks earlier than anticipated. If the period occurred on stopping the oral contraceptive pill, ovulation may be delayed and the expected date of delivery will be 1–2 weeks after the date calculated. Gestation wheel calculators or the computer can be used to simplify calculation of the expected date of delivery from the last menstrual period.

Legal age of viability. The legal age of viability of the fetus in the UK is 24 weeks but occasionally a baby may be born alive before this time. The World Health Organization (WHO) recommends that a fetus should be considered viable after 22 weeks or if it weighs more than 500 g.

Abortion. An abortion is the expulsion of the fetus before it reaches viability. An abortion may be spontaneous (*miscarriage*) or induced (*termination of pregnancy*). The term abortion is now seldom used in clinical practice.

Live birth. A live birth is a fetus which, irrespective of the length of gestation, shows signs of life after delivery. These signs include beating of the heart, pulsation of the umbilical cord or definite movements of the voluntary muscles.

Stillbirth. A stillbirth is a baby delivered after 24 weeks which did not breathe or show any other sign of life.

Gestation is the duration of pregnancy from the last menstrual period.

Gravidity is the total number of present and previous pregnancies.

Parity is the number of pregnancies resulting in a live birth (at whatever gestation) together with all stillbirths *plus* the number of miscarriages, terminations and ectopic pregnancies. A multiple pregnancy is counted as one. Parity is expressed as two numbers, e.g. 2+1 (Table 7.9).

Neonatal death. A neonatal death occurs when a baby dies before 28 completed days of life. Early neonatal death occurs before 7 days and late neonatal death from then until 28 days.

Perinatal mortality rate. The *standard* perinatal mortality rate is the number of stillbirths plus the number of early neonatal deaths per 1000 total births.

The *extended* perinatal mortality rate is the number of stillbirths plus early and late neonatal deaths per 1000 total births. Factors affecting the perinatal mortality rate include maternal age, social class, lack of antenatal care and the management of labour.

Maternal mortality is the death of a woman while pregnant or within 42 days of delivery, miscarriage or termination. Her death can be from any cause but must be related to or aggravated (directly or indirectly) by the pregnancy or its management. Deaths from accidents or incidental causes are not included. Late maternal deaths are those occurring between 42 days and 1 year.

Puerperium. The puerperium is the time from the end of the third stage of labour until involution of the uterus is complete, and is approximately 6 weeks.

The fetus. The *lie* of the fetus is the relationship of its long axis to the long axis of the uterus. The lie is normally longitudinal but may be oblique or transverse.

The *presentation* describes the leading part of the fetus in the lower pole of the uterus. Normally this is cephalic, with the head presenting. It may be breech, with the bottom presenting, or shoulder, or compound when the head and a limb are present. The lie is always longitudinal when the presentation is cephalic or breech. A transverse lie is associated with a shoulder presentation (Fig. 7.23).

The *position* of the presenting part is its relationship to the maternal pelvis. You may get clues from the abdominal examination (Fig. 7.24). During labour, when the cervix

7.9 Examples of gravidity and parity
• A woman who is not pregnant and has had a single live birth, one miscarriage and one termination = gravida 3, para 1+2
• A woman who is pregnant with a singleton pregnancy and has had two previous pregnancies resulting in a live birth and a stillbirth = gravida 3, para 2
• A woman who has a singleton pregnancy and has had live twins and a previous ectopic = gravida 3, para 1+1
• A woman who is not pregnant but had a twin pregnancy resulting in two live births = gravida 1, para 1

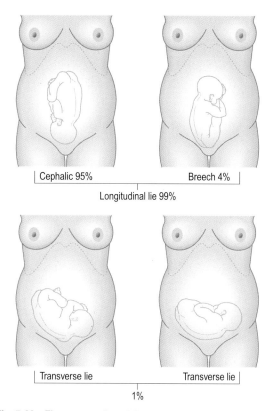

Cephalic 95%   Breech 4%

Longitudinal lie 99%

Transverse lie   Transverse lie

1%

Fig. 7.23   The presentation of the fetus.

has dilated enough to allow you to feel the suture lines on the vertex, you can confirm this by vaginal examination. Feel for the suture lines. Three suture lines run into the posterior fontanelle and four into the anterior (Fig. 7.25).

A *show* is a vaginal discharge of mucus mixed with some blood. This is due to the cervix starting to efface (shorten and be taken up) and dilate, releasing the plug of mucus which was filling it. It is a sign of the start of labour.

Polyhydramnios is an excess of amniotic fluid relative to the fetus.

THE HISTORY

A pregnant patient often has no presenting complaint and is seen routinely to monitor the progress of her pregnancy. She may complain of symptoms caused by pregnancy e.g. nausea and vomiting, constipation, haemorrhoids, urinary frequency, backache, symphyseal pain, breathlessness, ankle swelling, varicose veins and pruritus. However, any disease may occur unrelated to the pregnancy. Think of these from two points of view: the effect of the disease on the pregnancy and the effect of pregnancy on the disease.

She may complain of early symptoms of labour. These are spontaneous rupture of the membranes, a show, and the onset of regular, painful uterine contractions. Labour is established when there are three to five good-tone contractions every 10 minutes, each lasting 40–60 seconds.

It is helpful to address her ideas, concerns and expectations (see Ch. 1). Establish your patient's *age* and *parity*, and the *gestational age* of the pregnancy. Ask about her menstrual history and use of contraception. Find out about her *past obstetric history*, enquiring about all of her previous pregnancies, including miscarriages, terminations and

A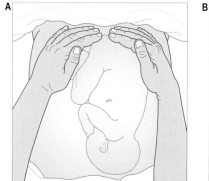 B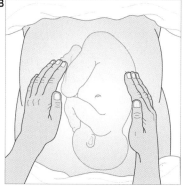 C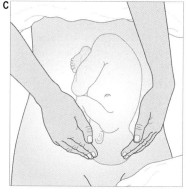

Fig. 7.24   Abdominal examination. (A) First manoeuvre – fundal palpation. The height of the fundus is estimated and the fundal area gently palpated in an attempt to identify which pole of the fetus (breech or head) is occupying the fundus. (B) Second manoeuvre – lateral palpation. The examiner's hands gently slip down the sides of the uterus with quick palpation to try to identify on which side the firm back of the fetus or the soft belly and knobbly limbs can be detected. (C) Pelvic manoeuvre. The examiner gently turns to face the patient's feet and slides the hands gently on the lower part of the uterus, pressing down on each side to determine the presenting part. If it is the fetal head it can be ballotted between the fingers.

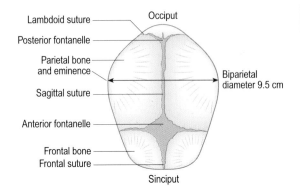

Labels: Lambdoid suture, Occiput, Posterior fontanelle, Parietal bone and eminence, Biparietal diameter 9.5 cm, Sagittal suture, Anterior fontanelle, Frontal bone, Frontal suture, Sinciput

Fig. 7.25 **Fetal skull from above – showing important obstetric diameters.**

Table 7.10 Examples of single gene disorders that can be detected antenatally
Autosomal dominant
• Huntington's chorea • Myotonic dystrophy
Autosomal recessive
• Cystic fibrosis • Sickle cell disease • Thalassaemia
X-linked
• Duchenne muscular dystrophy • Haemophilia

7.11 Age-related risk of Down's syndrome (trisomy 21)	
Maternal Age	**Risk**
20	1 in 1500
30	1 in 900
35	1 in 400
40	1 in 100
45	1 in 30

7.12 Checklist for the obstetric history
• Age • Parity • Menstrual history, last menstrual period, gestation, expected date of delivery • Presenting complaint • Past obstetric history • Past medical and surgical history • Drug history • Family history • Social history

ectopic pregnancy. Note the gestation at delivery, method of delivery and any complications she or her babies suffered.

Establish her *past history* including operations and psychiatric illnesses. Identify women with diabetes, epilepsy or other chronic conditions to give them appropriate advice about their medication and risks and to consider early referral to a specialist in that disease for shared care.

Drug history

This includes any prescribed medication, illegal drugs, her alcohol intake and smoking habits. Advise her to stop smoking and restrict her alcohol consumption to a maximum of 2 units two or three times a week. Check that she is taking 400 µg of folic acid until 12 weeks' gestation to reduce the incidence of spina bifida.

Family history

Family history is important, not only because the woman may have unwarranted anxiety about her baby but because it allows you to identify women with a high risk of having a baby with a genetic disorder (Table 7.10). They can be offered the opportunity of early diagnosis by chorion villus biopsy or amniocentesis.

Chromosomal abnormality is more common in older women. This relates to the increased risk of trisomies, with trisomy 21 (Down's syndrome) the most common (Table 7.11).

Social history

Lower socioeconomic status is linked with increased perinatal and maternal mortality. Find out who her partner is, how stable the relationship is, and if she is not in a relationship, who will give her support during and after her pregnancy. Was the pregnancy planned or not? If unplanned, find out how she feels about it.

If she is working, ask what her job entails and whether she plans to return to it. You can use this opportunity to give her advice. Encourage her to exercise regularly and to avoid certain foods such as tuna (high mercury content), soft cheeses (risk of listeria) and calves liver (high vitamin A content).

A checklist for taking an obstetric history is provided in Table 7.12.

EXAMINATION

→ Examination sequence

General principles

→ You can gain an impression of how your patient's pregnancy is proceeding by looking at her from the moment you see her. Note her demeanour, is she happy or does she appear exhausted and anxious? Note if she is pale, or breathless. Does she get up from her seat with difficulty and if so why? Offer her the chance to empty her bladder before you examine her and ask her to collect a specimen of urine for testing.

→ Measure her height and weight. Women less than 152 cm (5 feet) are more likely to have an obstructed labour and small babies. Patients over 100 kg may develop gestational diabetes and large (macrosomic) babies. Work out the body mass index (weight in kg divided by the square of the height in m). Women are at higher risk in pregnancy if the body mass index is < 20 or > 35. Serial weight measurements throughout pregnancy do not reliably predict problems such as pre-eclampsia or intrauterine growth restriction.

→ Measure her blood pressure and check a urine sample using dipstix for glycosuria and proteinuria.

→ Ask the patient to lie down on a firm but comfortable couch with her back resting at an angle of 30°. Ask her to uncover her abdomen from the lower chest to below her hips and place a sheet over any exposed underwear.

Inspection

→ Look for the abdominal distension caused by the pregnant uterus rising from the pelvis. After 24 weeks you may see fetal movements which confirm its viability. The linea nigra (black line) stretches from the pubic symphysis upwards in the midline. Striae gravidarum are the red stretch marks of this pregnancy. Striae albicantes are the white stretch marks from a previous pregnancy. Note any scars and the umbilicus, which becomes flattened as pregnancy advances and everted in polyhydramnios (excess amniotic fluid) or multiple pregnancy.

Palpation

→ Use your left hand to feel the uterus abdominally and estimate the height of the uterus above the symphysis pubis (Fig. 7.26).

→ Note any fetal movements. Facing towards the woman's head use both hands on either side of the fundus to gain an impression of which fetal part is there. Use your right hand on the woman's left side. Bring your hands down to palpate the sides of the uterus and identify which side is fuller, suggesting the back is on that side. Now turn to face the patient's feet so that your left hand is on the woman's left side. Feel the lower part of the uterus to determine the presenting part. Ballot the head by pushing it gently from one side to the other and feel it against your fingers.

→ After 20 weeks measure the fundal height in centimetres. With a tape measure, fix the end at the highest point on the fundus and measure to the symphysis pubis. The

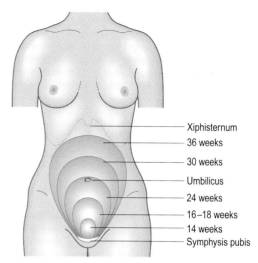

Fig. 7.26 Approximate fundal height with changing gestation.

highest point is not always in the midline. To avoid bias, do this with the blank side of the tape facing you, so that you only see the measurement on lifting the tape.

→ This measurement is equal to the gestation in weeks plus or minus 3 cm and is an indicator of growth problems in the fetus. In a tall or thin patient, the fundal height may be less than expected and in an obese patient, it may be larger.

→ You may be able to determine the position of the presenting part. When the presentation is cephalic, the vertex or top of the fetal head engages in the occipitolateral position.

→ If the presentation is cephalic, assess how far into the true pelvis the head has descended by estimating how much of the head you can feel *above* the pelvic brim. The head is divided into fifths for this (Fig. 7.27).

→ The head is fixed when it is three-fifths palpable and 'engaged' when it is two-fifths or one-fifth palpable.

Percussion

→ Percussion is unhelpful unless you suspect polyhydramnios. Confirm this by eliciting a fluid thrill but no shifting dullness (see Ch. 5).

Auscultation

→ Use an electronic hand-held Doppler fetal heart rate monitor as early as 14 weeks (Fig. 7.28A).

→ A Pinard stethoscope is not useful until after 28 weeks. Place the widest part over the anterior shoulder of the fetus (Fig. 7.28B). Facing the mother's feet put your left ear against the smaller end and press against the mother's abdomen gently to keep the stethoscope in place. Take your hands away from the stethoscope so that it is kept in place by the pressure of your head. Listen for the fetal heart. This sounds like a distant ticking noise. Imagine you are listening for a clock ticking through a pillow.

Completely above	Sinciput +++ occiput ++	Sinciput ++ occiput +	Sinciput + occiput just felt	Sinciput + occiput not felt	None of head palpable
5/5	4/5	3/5	2/5	1/5	0/5
Free, above the brim	'Fixing'	Not engaged	Just engaged	Engaged	Deeply engaged

Level of pelvic brim

Fig. 7.27 Descent of the fetal head.

Vaginal examination

In early pregnancy

A bimanual pelvic examination should only be performed if ultrasound is not available to establish gestation. Ultrasound will establish gestational age, confirm viability, exclude adnexal pathology and show multiple pregnancy.

If a vaginal examination has to be performed the size of the uterus reflects the gestation.

The pregnant uterus is equivalent to the size of an:

- apple at 6 weeks
- orange at 8–10 weeks
- grapefruit at 12–14 weeks.

Only take a cervical smear if this is clinically indicated, otherwise defer it until the postnatal check.

In late pregnancy

Vaginal examination allows you to assess cervical status before induction of labour. Feel the dilatation and length of the cervix, its consistency and position, and the station (level) of the head above or below the ischial spines (– or + respectively in cm). The cervix is most commonly located posteriorly and the head of the fetus is felt through the os.

During labour

See Table 7.13.

ANTENATAL INVESTIGATIONS

See Table 7.14.

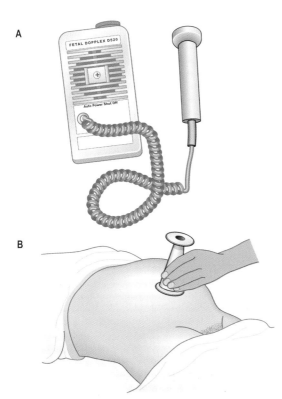

A

B

Fig. 7.28 Auscultation of the fetal heart. (A) Doppler fetal heart rate monitor. (B) Pinard fetal stethoscope. The rate varies between 110 and 150/minute and should be regular.

7.13 Vaginal examination during labour

- Date, time, examination number
- Indication (e.g. to perform artificial rupture of the membranes, to assess progress, to undertake fetal blood sample)
- Cervix – dilatation, length, effacement
- Presenting part – position, station, application to cervix, caput, moulding
- Pelvis (rarely indicated) – sacral curve, ischial spines, subpubic arch, interturberous diameter
- Fetal heart rate on completion of the vaginal examination

◆ Key Points

- ◆ Always establish maternal age, parity and gestation.
- ◆ Do not do a vaginal examination routinely in early pregnancy.
- ◆ A first trimester scan accurately determines gestational age to within a week.
- ◆ The best time to detect fetal abnormality is an ultrasound scan at 18–22 weeks.
- ◆ If the presentation is cephalic, the lie is always longitudinal.
- ◆ In antepartum haemorrhage exclude a low-lying placenta by ultrasound before carrying out a vaginal examination.

7.14 Antenatal investigations

Routine and selective investigations	Timing and/or indication	Comment
Full blood count	Booking, 28 weeks, 36 weeks	Treat if haemoglobin level falls below 100 g/l with ferrous sulphate 200 mg t.d.s.
Haemoglobin electrophoresis	Booking	For sickle cell and thalassaemias. Routine in many regions of mixed ethnicity
Blood grouping and antibody screen	Booking and as advised by laboratory	Rhesus and Kell most common cause of isoimmunization
Rubella	Booking (and after contact if not immune)	
Hepatitis B and C	Booking	If hepatitis B antigen positive, baby will require vaccination soon after birth. Breastfeeding is best avoided
HIV status	Booking (unless patient opts out)	If positive, can give mother treatment to reduce risk of vertical transmission to baby. Deliver by caesarean section. Best to avoid breastfeeding
Syphilis testing	Booking	If positive, treatment with penicillin will prevent congenital syphilis in neonate
Urinary glucose	Every visit	When positive, reduce sugar intake. If persists, carry out glucose tolerance test
Urinary protein	Every visit	Trace or +, check midstream urine specimen. ++ or more, consider pre-eclampsia
Plasma glucose	28 weeks	
Urine specimen for culture	As required	
Cervical smear	If required	
Serum screening for trisomy 21 and spina bifida	16 weeks	Detects 60% of pregnancies affected by trisomy 21
Combined biochemical screening and nuchal translucency measurement for trisomy 21	11–14 weeks	Detects 80-90% of pregnancies affected by trisomy 21
First trimester ultrasound scan	6–13 weeks	Confirms viability, gestational age within 1 week, checks for multiple pregnancy, adnexal mass
Detailed ultrasound scan	18–22 weeks	Detects 90% of major congenital abnormalities. Confirms gestation within 10 days
Ultrasound scan for placental site	Antepartum haemorrhage after 24 weeks	More reliable as gestation advances when lower segment forms. 1 in 4 patients have a low placenta at 20 weeks
Ultrasound scan for growth	When clinical suspicion, usually after 24 weeks	
Amniocentesis	15 weeks for fetal karyotype	Full karyotype takes 2-3 weeks. New methods for specific chromosomal abnormalities take 2–4 days. 0.5–1% risk of miscarriage
Chorion villus biopsy	10 weeks onwards for fetal karyotype, single gene disorders	Short-term result in 2–5 days; long-term 2–3 weeks. 1–2% risk of miscarriage

THE MALE GENITAL EXAMINATION

Male genital examination is important so you should not omit it to avoid mutual embarrassment. If you do not carry it out you may miss potentially serious disease and also leave some men inappropriately concerned about their perceived genital symptoms. As well as remembering all the principles in Chapter 1 you need to have the confidence to put patients at their ease and to be able to reassure men with negative findings, so explore their ideas, concerns and expectations when taking the history.

Anatomy

The male genitalia include the penis, scrotum, testes, epididymides, seminal vesicles and the prostate gland (Fig. 7.29).

The testes develop near the kidneys and migrate through the external inguinal ring at 8 months' gestation and into the scrotum at 9 months when the baby is born. All the structures supplying and draining the testes, including the neural, vascular and lymphatic supply, follow this route. This is clinically important, because pain in the renal tract may be referred to the scrotum and testicular cancer spreads to para-aortic nodes rather than inguinal nodes.

Puberty starts between the ages of 10 and 15, up to 2 years later than in girls (see Fig. 11.21, p. 366).

The penis. The corpora cavernosa are two cylinders on either side of the length of the penis (Fig. 7.30). They are vascular sponge-like structures, and between them on the ventral surface is the central corpus spongiosum. This is expanded at the tip into the glans penis, and the urethra passes through the centre of it. The skin covering the penis is reflected over the glans forming the prepuce (foreskin). Sexual arousal causes increased flow through the pudendal artery into the corpora and the organ becomes erect. This is under parasympathetic control. Contraction of the ejaculatory ducts and the bladder neck causes ejaculation of semen, followed by increased tone in the arterioles and diversion of blood out of the corpora and detumescence. This is under sympathetic control.

The scrotum and its contents (Fig. 7.31). The scrotum is a muscular bag with thin pigmented, rugose skin and is lined by the dartos muscle. This is highly contractile and helps to regulate the temperature of the scrotal contents, 36°C being ideal for spermatogenesis. It contains the testes separated by a septum with the left testis usually lying lower than the right. Each testicle is oval and approximately 3.5–4 cm long. Each is covered by a fibrous layer called the tunica albuginea, which is invaginated into the tunica vaginalis. Along the posterior border of each testis is the epididymis formed by the efferent tubules draining the seminiferous tubules in the testis. The head of the epididymis is about 1 cm long and lies behind the upper pole of the testis. The body and tail of the epididymis are softer and thinner and continue behind and adjacent to the testis. Lymphatics from the penis and scrotum drain to the regional inguinal nodes through the spermatic cord.

The prostate. See page 221.

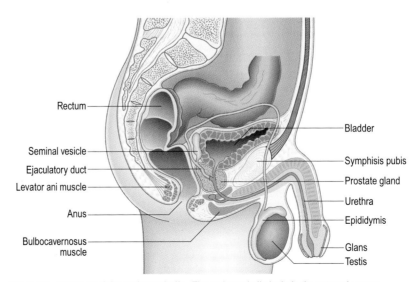

Rectum
Seminal vesicle
Ejaculatory duct
Levator ani muscle
Anus
Bulbocavernosus muscle
Bladder
Symphisis pubis
Prostate gland
Urethra
Epididymis
Glans
Testis

Fig. 7.29 Anatomy of the male genitalia. The male genitalia include the external organs, seminal vesicles and the prostate gland.

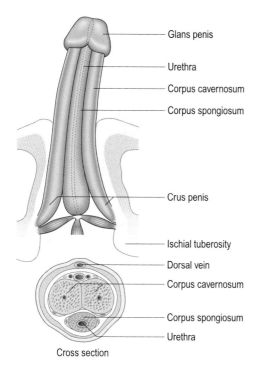

Cross section

Fig. 7.30 Anatomy of the penis. The shaft and glans penis are formed from the corpus spongiosum and the corpus cavernosum.

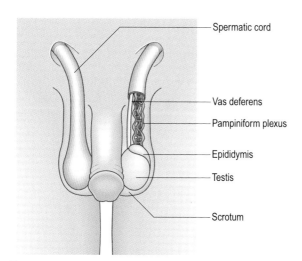

Fig. 7.31 The scrotum and its contents.

Definitions and abnormalities

Figure 7.32 shows some common abnormalities of the scrotal contents.

- *Hydroceles* are common and are an accumulation of fluid in the tunica vaginalis.
- *Spermatoceles* are smaller cysts of the epididymis.

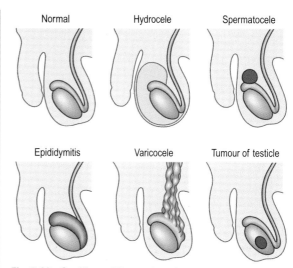

Fig. 7.32 Swellings of the scrotum. Some common abnormalities of the scrotal contents.

- *Varicoceles* are varicosities of the spermatic vein, often described as a 'bag of worms' in the scrotum.
- *Epididymitis* is painful epididymal swelling and may be due to sexually transmitted infections, e.g. *Neisseria gonorrhoeae* or *Chlamydia trachomatis*, other causes of non-gonococcal urethritis, or to urinary tract pathogens such as *Escherichia coli*.
- *Urethritis* is inflammation of the urethra and may cause *dysuria* or a *urethral discharge*.
- The most common causes of a urethral discharge are non-specific urethritis and gonococcal infection.
- *Orchitis* is a painful inflammation and swelling of the testis and is often associated with epididymitis and less commonly mumps or syphilis infection. The pain is deep and often accompanied by nausea. Painless swelling of the testes suggests a cystic lesion or malignancy.
- *Unilateral testicular atrophy* may result from mumps infection, vascular compromise after inguinal hernia repair or following a late orchidopexy for an undescended testis.
- *Bilateral testicular atrophy* suggests primary or secondary hypogonadism. Check development of secondary sexual characteristics (see p. 366), hormonal abnormalities or signs of anabolic steroid usage.
- *A single testis* may be caused by an incompletely descended testis in the inguinal canal or an ectopic testis in the groin, so check these areas. Ask the patient if he has had previous surgery for a testicular tumour or ectopic testis.
- *Phimosis* is narrowing of the preputial orifice preventing retraction of the foreskin. This may cause recurrent infection of the glans penis (*balanitis*) or of the prepuce (*posthitis*) or both (*balanoposthitis*).

- *A genital ulcer* is a break in the mucosa or skin anywhere on the genitals. If ulcers are painful then think of herpes simplex; if painless consider Reiter's syndrome, lichen simplex and rarely syphilis.
- *Erectile dysfunction* is sometimes called impotence. The man may have problems from loss of libido, being unable to achieve or maintain an erection, premature ejaculation, delayed ejaculation or failure to ejaculate and inability to achieve orgasm. Always clarify the exact problem and consider causes including psychological, alcohol, systemic disease (diabetes mellitus) and drugs; so your history needs to be wide-ranging.
- *Testicular pain* that is intense and sickening and radiates towards the groin and abdomen is usually caused by infection or trauma. Find out when the pain started and whether it is accompanied by fever and other systemic symptoms.
- *Torsion of the testis* causes sudden onset of severe testicular pain and tenderness in boys or younger men. The affected testis lies higher than the other and it is difficult to feel the epididymis separately from the testis. In epididymo-orchitis you may feel the enlarged tender epididymis separately in the early stages, and the pain usually comes on more gradually.

EXAMINATION

⏵ Examination sequence

➜ Put on gloves and ask the patient to lie down on his back on the examination couch with his genital area and upper thighs fully exposed. Look at the whole area for redness, swelling or ulcers. Note the hair distribution, in particular alopecia or infestation. Patients who shave their pubic hair may develop dermatitis (inflammation of the dermis) or folliculitis (infection around the base of the hairs causing an irritating red rash). Check the groin, perineum and scrotal skin for these rashes and intertrigo (infected eczema) in the skin creases and eczema (another name for dermatitis).

The penis
➜ *Inspection.* The penile skin has more sebaceous follicles than most other areas; enlarged follicles are sometimes mistaken for warts. Numerous uniform pearly penile papules around the corona of the glans are a common normal finding. Look at the shaft of the penis and check the position of the urethral opening.
➜ *Palpation.* Retract the prepuce to check for phimosis or adhesions. Ask the man whether this is recent and if it has caused problems such as infection, spraying during micturition or sexual difficulty. Note any rashes, abnormal curvature, pigmentation, nodules, ulcers or discharge. Remember to draw the foreskin forward after examination to avoid *paraphimosis*, which is painful oedema of the glans. Take a urethral swab if your patient has a discharge or is having sexual health screening (Table 7.15).

7.15 How to take a urethral swab
• Make sure the man has not passed urine for at least 2 hours
• Retract the prepuce
• Using a fine cotton bud or plastic loop take a sample of the discharge from the urethra
• Look at a Gram-stained smear under the microscope immediately
• Plate the swab immediately on agar plates
• If this is not possible use a charcoal transport medium
• Samples need to arrive with the laboratory within 12 hours to ensure detection of delicate organisms such as *N. gonorrhoeae*
• Send urine specimen for *Chlamydia*

The scrotum
➜ *Inspection.* Look at the scrotum for redness, swelling or ulcers; sebaceous cysts are relatively common. Remember to inspect the posterior surface.
➜ *Palpation.* If either you or the patient is cold, the cremaster muscle will contract and you will not be able to palpate the testes properly. Testicular sensitivity varies, so ask the man whether palpation is painful.
➜ Palpate the scrotum gently using both hands. Check that both testes are present in the scrotum.
➜ Place the fingers of both your hands behind the left testis to immobilize it and use your index finger and thumb to methodically palpate the body of the testis (Fig. 7.33). Feel the anterior surface and medial border with your thumb and the lateral border with your index finger.
➜ Check the size and consistency of the testis and note any nodules or irregularities. Very gently squeeze the fingers of your left hand to push the testis inferiorly and allow you to assess the upper pole of the organ. Reverse this procedure to feel the lower pole. Repeat the procedure for the right testicle. The testes are normally soft and smooth, and may be slightly different sizes. Use this opportunity to encourage all younger men to examine their testicles regularly – testicular self-examination. This helps to detect testicular tumours at an early stage.
➜ You should barely be able to feel the normal epididymis (Fig. 7.34). Note if it is enlarged or tender, or if there are any appendages.

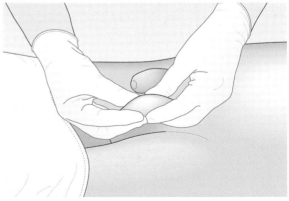

Fig. 7.33 Palpation of the testis. Gloves should be worn.

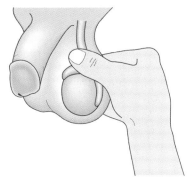

Fig. 7.34 **Palpation of the epididymis.** The epididymis is felt along the posterior pole of the testis.

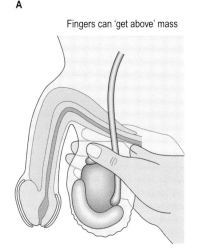

A

Fingers can 'get above' mass

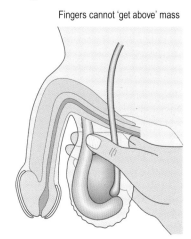

B

Fingers cannot 'get above' mass

Fig. 7.35 **Testing for scrotal swellings.** It is possible to 'get above' a true scrotal swelling (A), whereas this is not possible if the swelling is caused by an inguinal hernia that has descended into the scrotum (B).

➜ Palpate the spermatic cord with your right hand. Gently pull the right testicle downward and place your fingers behind the neck of the scrotum. Bring them forwards to your thumb which is anterior. You will be able to feel the spermatic cord and within it the vas deferens which feels like a thick piece of string (Fig. 7.35).

➜ Ask the patient to stand to look for a varicocele.

➜ If there is a bulky soft mass in the scrotum *transilluminate* it. In a darkened room hold a pen-torch against the swelling and see if light is transmitted as a bright red glow to the skin of the scrotum. This confirms it is fluid-filled, whereas no transmission of light occurs with a solid mass. Decide whether a swelling arises from within the scrotum or from an indirect inguinal hernia. Use your finger as described above to see whether you can feel above the swelling (Fig. 7.35). If so it is a true scrotal swelling, and if not it has come through the inguinal canal.

Anogenital region

The anal margin, rectum and prostate gland should all be examined as part of the male genital assessment. Perianal warts are common, often in association with genital warts (condylomata acuminata). Their presence is not always caused by sexual transmission. A rectal discharge may be due to sexually transmitted infections such as *N. gonorrhoeae* or *C. trachomatis*, and secondary syphilis may present as flat warty lesions (condylomata lata). Sexually transmitted infections are a cause of proctitis so take swabs at proctoscopy if the history suggests there is a history of anal penetration.

The prostate

The prostate can only be examined indirectly by digital examination via the rectum.

The main abnormalities are:

- benign prostatic hypertrophy
- prostatic cancer
- prostatitis:
  - acute
  - chronic:
    infected
    non-infected (inflammatory) prostatitis.

Ultrasound

Ultrasound examination of the scrotal contents is helpful in differentiating solid from cystic lesions. If you cannot palpate any abnormality then there is no point in performing an ultrasound examination, it will not reveal any more details.

◆ Key points

- ◆ Do not avoid examination of the male genitalia simply because the patient says it is all normal.
- ◆ Offer the patient a chaperone and record this if the patient declines.
- ◆ Retract the foreskin to fully examine the glans and draw it forward when you have finished to avoid causing a paraphimosis.

◆ Men who are sexually active rarely get cystitis, in contrast to women. If they have dysuria the most likely problem is a sexually transmitted infection.

◆ A urethral swab is uncomfortable; if possible send a urine sample to exclude chlamydial infection.

◆ If you cannot palpate an abnormality in the scrotum, then there is no point in carrying out an ultrasound examination since it will be normal.

◆ Do not confuse generalized skin conditions on the genitals for sexually transmitted infections.

THE RECTAL EXAMINATION

Anatomy

The anal canal is 3–4 cm long and extends from the perineum to the rectum, which is curved and about 12 cm long. The upper end of the anal canal is defined by the puborectalis muscle, which contracts if the patient coughs or consciously squeezes the pelvic muscles. The position of a lesion at the anal margin is described by using the positions of the clock face; 12 o'clock is anterior.

When the patient is lying in the left lateral position the rectum passes backwards and upwards following the curve of coccyx and sacrum posteriorly. Anteriorly, in ascending order, lie the membranous urethra, the prostate and the bladder in men; and the vagina and cervix in women (Fig. 7.36). The upper and anterior two-thirds of the rectum is covered in peritoneum reflected onto the bladder base in men and the pouch of Douglas in women.

The prostate gland surrounds the urethra and is about 3.5 cm in diameter. It sits anterior to the rectum and projects about 1 cm into it. Normally it feels rubbery and smooth and has a median groove separating symmetrical left and right lobes.

The rectum is usually empty and the rectal canal should feel smooth, uniform and elastic. The only palpable masses should be external to the rectum and normally are the prostate in men and the cervix in women.

Abnormalities

Indications for rectal examination are given Table 7.16.

Perianal skin

Excoriation is often due to infestations with worms, scabies, difficulty with hygiene because of skin tags or *haemorrhoids* (piles). These are dilated veins at the anal margin and are not palpable unless thrombosed. Perianal warts and dermatoses are also common. The perianal margin is often surrounded by sebaceous glands which, when enlarged, can be confused with perianal warts. Skin tags are common. Moist weeping perianal skin occurs in *intertrigo*, but in severe cases consider infections such as *N. gonorrhoeae* and herpes simplex virus. Intertrigo is infected, scratched, inflamed moist skin.

A

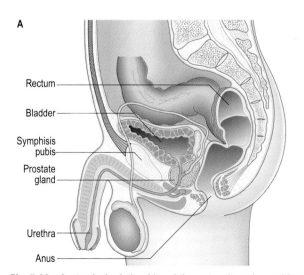

Rectum
Bladder
Symphisis pubis
Prostate gland
Urethra
Anus

B

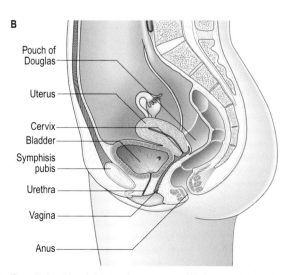

Pouch of Douglas
Uterus
Cervix
Bladder
Symphisis pubis
Urethra
Vagina
Anus

Fig. 7.36 Anatomical relationships of the rectum in males and females. The relationship of the anterior rectum to (A) the prostate gland and (B) the posterior vaginal wall and uterine cervix in women.

7.16	Indications for rectal examination

Perianal complaints

- Itching
- Pain
- Bleeding
- 'Lumps'

Alimentary complaints

- Persistent diarrhoea or constipation, altered bowel habit, mucus or blood in the stools
- 'Acute abdomen'
- A suspected lower abdominal mass, or pelvic spread from distant tumours

Genitourinary complaints

- In men when considering benign prostatic hypertrophy, acute or chronic prostatitis, prostatic malignancy
- In women when vaginal examination is difficult or anatomically impossible

Miscellaneous problems

- Unexplained prolonged backache:
  - lumbosacral nerve root pain
  - bony pain
- Unexplained iron deficiency anaemia
- Weight loss
- Pyrexia of unknown origin
- Following suspected trauma to these areas:
  - abdominal
  - pelvic
  - spinal
  - perineal including sexual assault

Anal tone varies but laxity is not necessarily a sign of abnormality.

Painful perianal lesions

Acutely thrombosed external haemorrhoids are visible distended, hard, tender, engorged veins. An anal fissure is a crack in the skin of the anal margin. This is usually small, often positioned at 6 o'clock and acutely tender on palpation so digital examination may be impossible. Abscesses are usually acutely tender, warm and fluctuant, and may be palpated (gently) between your thumb externally and index finger within the rectum.

Palpable lesions. You may mistake masses within the pelvis for faeces or vice versa. Faeces are movable and you can indent them with your finger. Rectal cancer causes a hard mucosal irregularity.

Lesions external to the rectum. Lateral tenderness suggests pelvic peritoneal infection. On the right side it may be due to appendicitis or an appendix abscess. In women acute salpingitis causes lateralized tenderness and you may palpate advanced cervical cancer. You may be confused by palpating a vaginal tampon if you do not clarify this with the patient. Peritoneal dissemination of tumours may

give the pelvic organs a rigid feel, 'frozen pelvis'. Normal seminal vesicles cannot be felt.

The prostate gland

Benign prostatic hypertrophy is common in men over 55 and feels like a smooth, symmetrical, rubbery mass, with no loss of the median sulcus. Prostate cancer feels very hard, may produce distinct craggy nodules and the median sulcus is often indistinct. You cannot use a rectal examination to detect changes confined to the anterior (median) lobe. If the gland is acutely tender and boggy this suggests acute prostatitis or an abscess.

Urinary symptoms

See Table 7.17.

Dysuria is pain around the base of the bladder, usually described as burning, which arises before, during or after micturition. If it is severe it is often accompanied by *strangury*, which is the painful need to void even after emptying the bladder. This is caused by irritation of the bladder and urethra, and causes include urinary tract infection and bladder tumours. This irritation can also cause increased *frequency* of micturition. If the patient is only passing small amounts of urine accompanied by burning pain this makes local infection very likely. If an older man has this but no pain then consider benign prostatic hypertrophy. In this case the smooth muscle of the bladder wall has hypertrophied to overcome the resistance to urine flow produced by the enlarged prostate gland. This causes

7.17	Urinary symptoms
Dysuria	Painful urination
Urgency	Unable to postpone micturition
Oliguria/anuria	Reduced/absent urine flow
Polyuria	Increased volume of urine
Frequency	Frequent passage of urine
Nocturia	Waking at night to pass urine
Haematuria	Blood in the urine
Strangury	Persistent painful feeling of needing to pass urine after micturition
Incontinence	Involuntary passage of urine Urge: when the need to micturate is felt Stress: on coughing or sneezing
Prostatism Hesitancy Slow stream Terminal dribbling	Having to wait for the urine stream to begin Poor flow rate of urine Residual urine leaks from the urethra after micturition

increased irritability of the bladder. Frequency may waken the patient at night to void and this is then called *nocturia*. Note the number of times the patients has to get up. *Urgency* of micturition is being unable to postpone micturition once the desire to pass urine has started. This may lead to immediate voiding and is called *urge incontinence*. It usually occurs at low bladder volumes because of uninhibited detrusor muscle activity (the detrusor muscle is the smooth muscle in the bladder). *Stress incontinence* where urinary flow occurs when intra-abdominal pressure is raised by coughing or exercising occurs at low bladder pressure because of sphincter incompetence. *Incontinence* is the involuntary passing of urine or faeces. If patients pass large amounts of urine (*polyuria*) with no pain then they may have excessive fluid intake or an osmotic diuresis as occurs in diabetes mellitus and insipidus.

Haematuria or blood in the urine may be visible or microscopic (see Ch. 6). Causes include tumours anywhere in the renal tract, stones or infection.

Slow stream where the rate of flow of urine is decreased in men, *hesitancy* where the man finds initiating micturition difficult and *terminal dribbling* where urine continues to leak from the meatus for a few minutes after finishing micturition are common features of prostatic hypertrophy. They reflect low residual bladder capacity. In more advanced cases there is progressive bladder enlargement with eventual overflow incontinence, which the patient experiences as continuous dribbling of urine.

EXAMINATION

Offer the patient a chaperone and record this and if the patient refuses. If there has been any kind of sexual assault defer the examination until a forensic expert is present to obtain specimens or other evidence.

Reassure the patient by explaining that the examination may be uncomfortable but should not be painful. Explain fully what is involved.

➡ Examination sequence

➔ Ask the patient to lie in the left lateral position with the buttocks at the edge of the couch, the knees drawn up to the chest and the heels clear of the perineum (Fig. 7.37).
➔ Put on gloves and have a good movable light source.
➔ Separate the buttocks and inspect the perianal skin looking for dermatological conditions, infestations, external haemorrhoids, fistulae or fissures, and signs of trauma.
➔ If you suspect a sexually transmitted infection take swabs under direct proctoscopy *before* carrying out digital examination.
➔ Lubricate your finger with water-based gel. Place the pulp of your forefinger on the anal margin with your palm facing posteriorly (Fig. 7.38). Use steady pressure on the

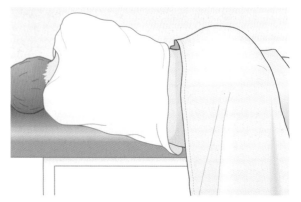

Fig. 7.37   The correct position of the patient before a rectal examination.

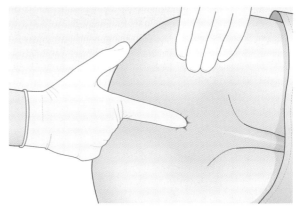

Fig. 7.38   The correct method for insertion of the index finger in rectal examination.

sphincter to pass your finger gently through the anal canal into the rectum. If there is anal spasm ask the patient to breathe out and relax. Pain and spasm are usually caused by an anal fissure. In this case try again after applying local anaesthetic gel to the anal margin for a few minutes. If the pain persists an examination under general anaesthetic may be necessary.
➔ Ask the patient to squeeze your finger to assess anal sphincter tone. Palpate round the rectum systematically. Sweep the mucosa through 360° checking for masses, stricture or points of tenderness. Note the proportion of the rectal circumference involved in any disease process, and its distance from the anus (Fig. 7.39).
➔ Identify the uterine cervix in women and the prostate in men. Prostate massage to obtain secretions is no longer advised in acute prostatitis because of the risk of septicaemia. Assess the size, shape and consistency and note any tenderness.
➔ Withdraw your finger gently to avoid sudden spasm, look at the glove for blood, mucus and stool colour. Test any stool material for blood using 'Haemoccult' test cards.

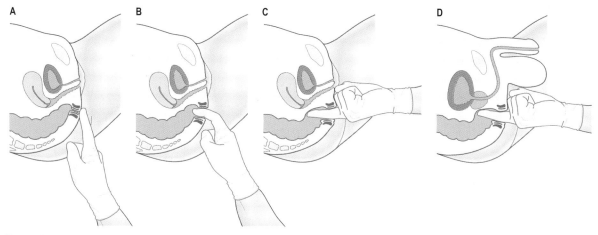

Fig. 7.39 Examination of the rectum. The finger is inserted as shown in (A) and (B). The hand is then rotated and the most prominent features are the cervix in the female (C) and the prostate in the male (D).

Proctoscopy

Proctoscopy allows you to inspect the anal canal and rectal mucosa and is the only adequate way to examine for haemorrhoids, fissures, rectal prolapse and mucosal disease. It should always be preceded by digital examination unless you suspect a sexually transmitted infection.

Proctoscopes are either metal, requiring sterilization between use, or they are plastic and disposable. They are available in standard or paediatric sizes. Some allow an internal light source to be attached and this gives better illumination than using a light directed over your shoulder. The normal rectal mucosa looks like the buccal mucosa but has prominent submucosal veins.

➡ Examination sequence

➔ Use a water-soluble gel to lubricate the proctoscope. Separate the buttocks with the forefinger and thumb of your left hand, or lift the top buttock up with your left hand. Patients may help by retracting their upper buttock with their right hand. Holding the obturator firmly in place, put the proctoscope against the anus, exert gentle sustained pressure and insert the instrument through the anal canal into the rectum in the direction of the umbilicus. Remove the obturator and attach your light source or position the lamp with your right hand while holding the proctoscope in your left.

➔ Inspect for mucosal abnormalities including masses, pus, signs of trauma or areas of inflammation or bleeding. If pus is present, or if you suspect a sexually transmitted infection, take swabs in charcoal medium and for *Chlamydia*. Ask the patient to strain down gently, and slowly withdraw the instrument. Look for significant rectal prolapse (more than 3–4 cm suggests full-thickness rectal prolapse) and haemorrhoids (usually at 3, 7 and 11 o'clock) and note their size and position.

➔ As you remove the instrument in a controlled way from the anus, look for fissures or signs of infection or trauma. Pain often causes spasm and rapid expulsion of the instrument at this point. If there are fissures and there has been anal sexual activity, take a viral swab. Herpetic vesicles are difficult to identify in this area, and herpes simplex virus is associated with recurrent or intractable fissures.

➔ Wipe the perineum to remove residual lubricant and any faecal matter and ensure that the patient can get down from the couch and get dressed with dignity.

> ● **Examine this man with rectal bleeding**
>
> 1. Look for evidence of anaemia or weight loss.
> 2. Feel abdomen for any masses or hepatomegaly.
> 3. Inspect perianal area looking for sources of bleeding and any abnormalities – skin tags or perianal fistulae in *Crohn's disease*.
> 4. If the history suggests sexually transmitted infection consider proctoscopy before digital examination.
> 5. Perform digital rectal examination:
>   - explore the anorectal canal for any masses or points of tenderness
>   - feel the prostate gland – smooth and enlarged in *benign prostatic hypertrophy* and hard and irregular in *prostate cancer*.
> 6. Withdraw your finger gently still palpating the canal systematically and check your glove for any blood.
> 7. Perform faecal occult blood test using Haemoccult test on any residue on your finger.
> 8. Perform proctoscopy and inspect the rectum looking for bleeding, *haemorrhoids*, polyps or evidence of inflammation (*ulcerative colitis* or *Crohn's disease*).
> 9. If the history suggests sexually transmitted infection take charcoal and chlamydia swabs from the rectum and look for signs of trauma, particularly if sex aids have been used.
> 10. Withdraw the proctoscope and look for signs of bleeding, fissures or *haemorrhoids*.
> 11. Further investigations may be appropriate, e.g. stool culture, sigmoidoscopy, colonoscopy and barium enema.

INVESTIGATIONS

Faecal occult blood. Use a Haemoccult card and apply a small amount of stool from your glove in both of the windows on the patient's side of the card. Shut the flap and turn the card over. Apply two drops of the manufacturer's fluid to the two windows on the other side of the card and look for development of a blue colour (due to detection of peroxidase activity of haemoglobin) after 30 seconds. This indicates occult blood.

Swabs. Take swabs for bacteria, *Chlamydia* and viruses.

◆ Key points

- Never omit the rectal examination if indicated; you will miss serious pathology.
- Do not mistake a vaginal tampon for a pelvic tumour.
- The rectal examination is an examination of the pelvis and allows you to identify pathology outside its walls.
- Rectal examination may be a more appropriate way of assessing the pelvis in some young women than vaginal examination.

The nervous system including the eye

BRIAN PENTLAND • PATRICK STATHAM • JOHN OLSON

NERVOUS SYSTEM EXAMINATION

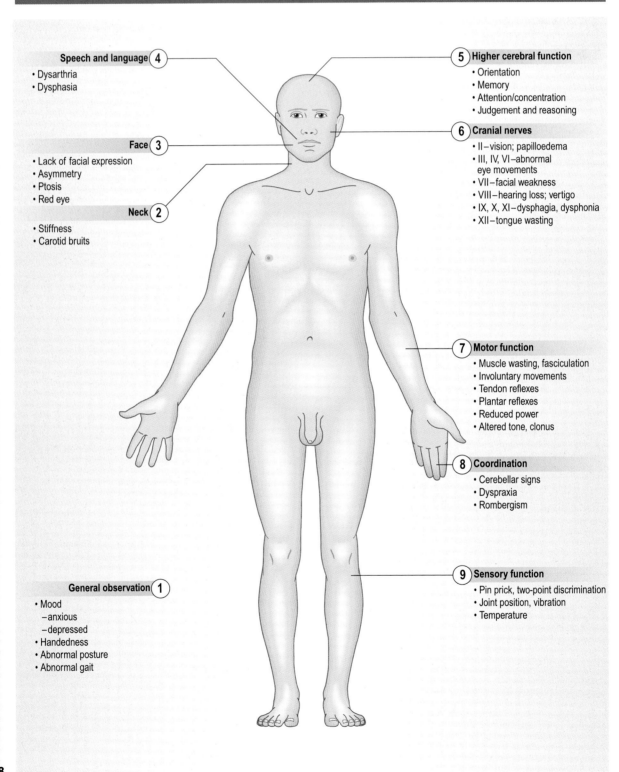

Speech and language (4)
- Dysarthria
- Dysphasia

Face (3)
- Lack of facial expression
- Asymmetry
- Ptosis
- Red eye

Neck (2)
- Stiffness
- Carotid bruits

General observation (1)
- Mood
  - anxious
  - depressed
- Handedness
- Abnormal posture
- Abnormal gait

(5) **Higher cerebral function**
- Orientation
- Memory
- Attention/concentration
- Judgement and reasoning

(6) **Cranial nerves**
- II – vision; papilloedema
- III, IV, VI – abnormal eye movements
- VII – facial weakness
- VIII – hearing loss; vertigo
- IX, X, XI – dysphagia, dysphonia
- XII – tongue wasting

(7) **Motor function**
- Muscle wasting, fasciculation
- Involuntary movements
- Tendon reflexes
- Plantar reflexes
- Reduced power
- Altered tone, clonus

(8) **Coordination**
- Cerebellar signs
- Dyspraxia
- Rombergism

(9) **Sensory function**
- Pin prick, two-point discrimination
- Joint position, vibration
- Temperature

INTRODUCTION

Neurological examination aims to determine whether a lesion of the nervous system exists and, if so, its location and likely pathology. The history is of key importance and in conditions such as epilepsy or migraine it may be the only route to diagnosis since there may be no physical signs. Encourage patients to give an unrushed account of what they feel is wrong and how their everyday activities are affected. When the individual's conscious level or cognitive function is impaired you may need a more directive approach.

COMMON SYMPTOMS

HEADACHE

Headache is the most common neurological symptom but only a proportion of sufferers consult a GP and even fewer see a neurologist. Headache is common in many non-neurological conditions (Table 8.1).

Migraine is a common cause of headache with many variants. The *classical* type is unilateral, throbbing in character and often associated with visual disturbance and nausea. Transient focal neurological deficits may accompany attacks. *Common* migraine is similar without the visual or focal symptoms. There may be triggering or aggravating factors and attacks may be cyclical. In women correlation with menstrual periods is common. Migraine lasts from less than 6 hours to 3 days. Pain-free intervals lasting weeks or months are frequent.

8.1 Onset and course of headaches
Acute single episode
• Subarachnoid haemorrhage
• Acute meningitis
• Vasodilator drugs
• Angle-closure glaucoma
Acute recurrent
• Migraine
• Cluster headache
• Neuralgias (e.g. trigeminal and post-herpetic)
• Angle-closure glaucoma
• Sinusitis
Subacute single episode
• Infections (e.g. tuberculous meningitis, cerebral abscess)
• Raised intracranial pressure (e.g. tumour, hydrocephalus)
• Benign intracranial hypertension
• Temporal arteritis
Chronic
• Tension headache
• Depression
• Cervical spondylosis
• Drugs (e.g. oral contraceptive, overuse of analgesics)

Cluster headaches (previously called migrainous neuralgia) occur in bouts lasting up to 3 months with remissions for months or years. The pain is excruciating, unilateral and often located in the cheek, temple or around the eye. It is accompanied by drooping of the eyelid (*ptosis*), a bloodshot eye and unilateral watering of the eye or nose. Episodes last from 30 minutes to about 3 hours.

Neuralgias are usually unilateral, knife-like or burning in quality and only affect single nerves. Paroxysms last only seconds at a time and recur over several minutes. In trigeminal and glossopharyngeal neuralgias, pain may be precipitated by activities, e.g. brushing teeth, shaving, or eating.

Subarachnoid haemorrhage headache classically has a very sudden 'thunderclap' or 'pistol shot' onset, often indicated by the patient with a snap of the fingers. It is usually bilateral, often worse in the occipital region and associated with nausea, vomiting, impaired consciousness and signs of meningeal irritation.

Acute meningitis usually has a less abrupt onset but otherwise has the above features. In addition it is usually accompanied by fever and sometimes intolerance of light (*photophobia*).

Raised intracranial pressure headaches are often poorly localized, worse on waking in the morning and aggravated by activities such as stooping, coughing or straining at stool. Depression and hangover headaches are worse in the morning, as are cluster headaches, but the latter usually wake the patient from sleep.

Temporal arteritis usually causes sudden onset throbbing, unilateral headache associated with general malaise. Consider the diagnosis in patients with recent onset headache aged > 55 years.

Tension headache is characteristically bilateral, often frontal, temporal or occipital or 'like a tight band'. It is usually worse towards the end of the day.

OCULAR PAIN

Pain localized to the eyes is a common variant of headache. It can range from the irritating, foreign body feeling of dry eyes to the excruciating pain of scleritis. Whether the eye on the affected side is red or not is essential to making the diagnosis.

Ocular pain with a 'white eye'

If the patient feels as though there is a foreign body, the problem involves the surface of the eye. The commonest cause is a dry eye secondary to inflammation of the skin of the eyelids, chronic *blepharitis*. Normally, secretions from three types of lid glands moisten the eye: mucin from goblet cells, aqueous from accessory lacrimal glands and oil from Meibomian glands. Inflammation in the lid leads to a dry eye. Paradoxically, overproduction of tears from the lacrimal gland, leads to the accompanying complaint of watery eyes. Blepharitis occurs in low-grade infection or inflammation of the eyelids or systemic skin conditions, e.g. atopic eczema, acne rosacea or seborrhoeic dermatitis. Dry eyes may rarely be a result of Sjögren's syndrome.

Malposition of the eyelid also causes problems. An inverted eyelid leads to painful corneal erosion and an everted eyelid exposes the eye, causing it to dry out. Rarely, watery eyes may result from a blocked drainage system. This is aggravated when the lacrimal gland is stimulated.

Foreign bodies on the surface of eye are often associated with a clear history of performing an at-risk activity, e.g. grinding metal work without eye protection. They are usually clearly obvious on examining the cornea. If no foreign body is easily seen then stain the cornea with fluorescein to reveal scratch marks or ulceration.

Fluorescein testing for corneal ulceration. Place a drop of fluorescein on the cornea. This yellow dye will reveal

8.2 Causes of corneal ulceration

Cause	History	Examination
Bacterial	Previous corneal disease Dry eyes, contact lenses	Ulcer affecting central cornea
Herpes simplex	Previous episode, general	Dendritic pattern commonest manifestation
Herpes zoster	Ophthalmic shingles affecting external nose	Crusting vesicles affecting ophthalmic division of trigeminal nerve
Acanthamoeba	Contact lens users washing lens with tap water	Severe ocular pain and photophobia
Fungal	Ocular trauma with vegetable matter or immuncompromised patient	Feathery indistinct white lesion or non-responding 'bacterial ulcer'
Neurotrophic	Previous brain stem stroke	Absent or reduced corneal sensation
Alkali burn	Injury with chemicals	Loss of adjacent conjunctival vessels indicates poor prognosis
Corneal abrasion	Trauma	A linear scratch indicates a foreign body under eyelid
Marginal keratitis	Blepharitis	Ulcer affecting peripheral cornea

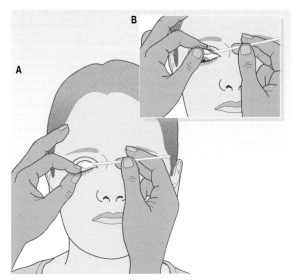

Fig. 8.1 Everting the upper eyelid, Ask the patient to look down, hold the eyelashes of the upper lid, press gently on the upper border of the tarsal plate with a cotton bud and gently pull the eyelashes up.

epithelial defects. A light with a cobalt blue filter will make any defects more obvious but is not essential.

Look under the lower and upper eyelids for a foreign body (Fig. 8.1).

Corneal ulceration is often due to herpes simplex virus (Table 8.2). In contact lens wearers, those with dry eyes or debilitated patients suspect bacterial infection. Use a dye such as fluorescein to reveal the ulcer (Fig. 8.2).

Preceding visual disturbance associated with headache or eye pain may indicate migraine. Although patients may describe flashing lights in a zig-zag pattern, many just notice blurring of vision. Cluster headaches may present as ocular pain. In subacute episodes of angle-closure glaucoma patients describe seeing haloes around lights rather than blurring of vision.

Pain on eye movement usually indicates either optic neuritis or scleritis. The eye with optic neuritis is white; the eye with scleritis is red. Pain on eye movement is so common in optic neuritis that you should review the diagnosis if it is not present.

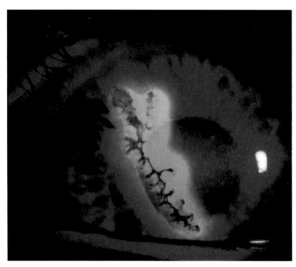

Fig. 8.2 Dendritic ulcer. Fluorescein staining showing branching dendritic ulcer.

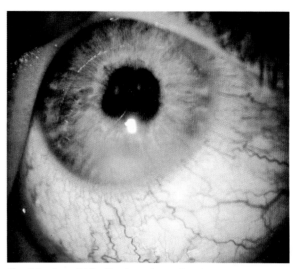

Fig. 8.3 Acute iritis. Note irregular pupil and circumciliary injection.

Ocular pain with a 'red eye'

Redness around the white of the eye just adjacent to the limbus (*circumciliary injection*) reflects involvement of the anterior ciliary arteries supplying the cornea, iris and ciliary body. More diffuse redness suggests scleritis or conjunctivitis.

Severe unilateral pain with a cloudy cornea and an oval non-reactive pupil usually indicates acute angle-closure glaucoma. Patients at risk include the long-sighted, who have a relatively shallow anterior chamber, and the elderly where thickening of the lens with age makes the anterior chamber shallower. An attack of acute angle-closure glaucoma is precipitated by pupillary dilatation, which becomes fixed by ischaemia, inducing high intraocular pressure. There is circumciliary injection. The cornea is cloudy and the underlying iris cannot be brought into focus. The pain of angle-closure glaucoma is severe and may be associated with systemic symptoms. Both eyes require treatment to prevent recurrence.

Acute iritis leads to a small irregularly shaped pupil (Fig. 8.3). Redness is centred on the limbus. The inflamed iris becomes stuck to the underlying lens. The pain is not as severe as in angle-closure glaucoma and photophobia may be the prominent feature. Recurrence is common and the patient may be HLA B27 positive with an associated condition, e.g. ankylosing spondylitis, inflammatory bowel disease or psoriasis. Rarely iritis presents bilaterally.

A *red eye with pain on eye movement indicates scleritis* (Fig. 8.4). It may be the first manifestation of a systemic or secondary vasculitis. The redness is frequently bilateral and involves all of the sclera or a sector of the sclera, unlike the circumciliary injection of iritis or angle-closure glaucoma.

In contrast, *episcleritis* is usually uncomfortable rather than painful and is not as dramatic in appearance as scleritis. Differentiate them by using topical phenylephrine; the redness of episcleritis disappears but that of scleritis does not.

Conjunctivitis is an inflammation of the conjunctivae and can be very uncomfortable. There is always an associated discharge. Unlike scleritis or episcleritis the inner eyelid is also inflamed and red (Fig. 8.5). Conjunctivitis due to bacterial infection is associated with a yellow/green discharge while chlamydial and viral infection cause a clear discharge and preauricular lymphadenopathy. Persistent watery discharge with itchy eyes in the absence of lymphadenopathy suggests an allergic cause.

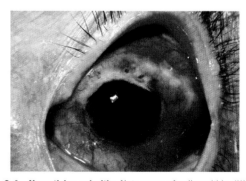

Fig. 8.4 Necrotizing scleritis. Note areas of pallor within diffuse areas of redness indicating ischaemia.

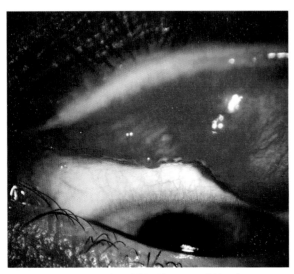

Fig. 8.5 Follicular conjunctivitis. Note upper lid has been everted showing giant papillae.

FITS, FAINTS, FUNNY TURNS AND FALLS

Transient episodes of altered (or lost) consciousness, feelings of unsteadiness or sensations of movement are common presenting symptoms, particularly in the elderly. They are commonly associated with falls. Patients find difficulty describing their experience and may use terms such as blackouts, faints, dizzy spells and funny turns. Determine exactly what patients mean from a full description of the attack(s), e.g. where and when it occurred, what they were doing at the time, how quickly was the recovery. A witness account is invaluable. Try to distinguish attacks in which consciousness is affected (fits and faints) from those characterized by dizziness or vertigo.

SYNCOPE AND SEIZURES

Syncope is alteration (or loss) of consciousness resulting from a recoverable loss of adequate cerebral blood flow. This is usually due to reduced cardiac output (*cardiac syncope*), increased peripheral vasodilatation (*vasovagal syncope*) or a combination of both. *Cardiac syncope* may be provoked by exertion (*exertional syncope*), e.g. severe aortic stenosis, or occur suddenly without warning when due to cardiac arrhythmias. Recovery is usually as rapid as the onset.

Vasovagal syncope (simple faint) has typical features:

- It usually occurs when the patient is standing.
- It may be provoked by an emotionally charged event.
- It is more common in warm environments.

- It is often preceded by a feeling of light-headedness, the vision darkens and there may be a ringing in the ears and nausea.
- Loss of consciousness is less rapid than in cardiac syncope.
- It causes skin pallor.

A *seizure* or *fit* is an alteration (or loss) of consciousness caused by sudden dysfunction of the electrical control mechanisms of the brain. Not all fits cause loss of consciousness or convulsions. An abnormal electrical discharge may arise in a localized area of the cerebral cortex resulting in a *partial seizure* or may start in both hemispheres (*generalized seizure*). Partial seizures are described as either *simple* or *complex* and both may spread to involve both hemispheres, a phenomenon described as secondary generalization.

Simple partial seizures originate from the frontal cortex. There may be no associated disturbance of consciousness, but contralateral involuntary jerking movements (motor) or unpleasant sensations (sensory) of a part of the body may occur.

Complex partial seizures usually arise from the temporal lobe. They usually cause alterations of awareness and a number of other features (Table 8.3).

Generalized seizures occur in various forms (Table 8.4). One common presentation is a tonic–clonic seizure

8.3 Features of complex partial seizures
• Dream-like states
• Disturbances of memory (déjà-vu, jamais vu)
• Hallucinations of smell, taste or auditory
• Emotional disturbance
• Abnormal behaviour

8.4 The typical pattern of a generalized seizure
Prodromal phase
• Change of mood or 'odd' feeling (aura)
Tonic phase
• Loss of consciousness • Spasm of all muscles • Cyanosis • Fall
Clonic phase
• Jerking of limbs and trunk • Tongue biting • Incontinence of urine
Post-ictal phase
• Flaccidity • Confusion • Headache • Amnesia

associated with loss of consciousness, which may be confused with syncopal attacks.

Very occasionally urinary incontinence or a few muscular twitches or even *myoclonic jerks* (sudden short-lived generalized muscle contractions) may occur in syncope, causing diagnostic confusion. However, cyanosis and tongue biting indicate a seizure. In addition, recovery from syncope is rapid, provided the patient is laid flat. After a seizure (post-ictal) phenomena of confusion and memory loss are characteristic. Occasionally, cardiac arrest presents as a seizure (Ch. 12).

DIZZINESS AND VERTIGO

Dizziness is frequently used by patients to describe a range of symptoms including syncope and seizures. It is also often used to describe an abnormal perception of movement of the environment or *vertigo*. Vertigo results from a mismatch of visual, proprioceptive and vestibular information reaching the brain. Vertigo due to vestibular causes is either peripheral (labyrinthine) or central (from a lesion affecting the vestibular nuclei in the brain stem).

In elderly people with a history of recurrent dizzy turns check for:

- *Cervical spondylosis*: dizziness associated with head movements may be accompanied by restricted neck movement on examination.
- *Postural hypotension*: light-headedness, dizziness or even collapse on standing from a sitting or lying position. Measure the blood pressure in supine and erect positions (a drop of 20 mmHg systolic or 10 mmHg diastolic is abnormal).
- *Hyperventilation*: ask the patient to pant rapidly for 2 minutes to see if this elicits dizziness.

FALLS

30% of people > 65 years fall each year. The four main groups of causes are:

- simple trip or accident
- collapse due to acute illness
- syncope
- multiple risk factors:
  - disease (e.g. cerebrovascular, Alzheimer's, Parkinson's diseases)
  - disability (e.g. impaired balance, vision, gait, cognition)
  - drugs (either a side-effect of a particular drug or due to polypharmacy).

With recurrent falls consider cardiac or vasovagal syncope and assess the multiple factors which may be contributing.

VISUAL DISTURBANCE

This can be uniocular or binocular. Double vision (*diplopia*) usually results from damage to cranial nerves II, III, IV and VI or their central connections. Other types of visual loss are discussed under the following headings:

- Blurred vision
- Sudden onset visual loss
- Gradual onset visual loss
- Distortion of vision
- Flashes and floaters
- Haloes.

Blurred vision

Ensure that it is a true blurring the whole visual field and not a central *scotoma* (a discrete defect in the visual field) or area of distortion. With a central scotoma the patient will not be able to see the examiner's face clearly but the rest of the visual field is unaffected. Distortion is best elaborated by asking the patient to look at a straight line or preferably an Amsler grid (Fig. 8.6).

An Amsler grid is used mainly for identifying defects in central vision such as central scotomas, but can be used to identify quadrantanopias or hemianopias. Instruct patients to hold the grid at a comfortable reading distance and fixate the central black spot with the eye being tested. Tell them to keep the eye still and to look at the grid using the 'sides of their vision'. Ask them to outline the affected areas.

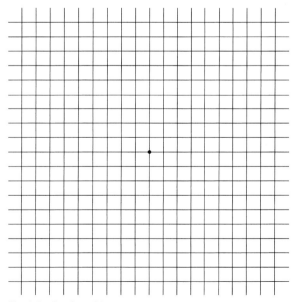

Fig. 8.6 Amsler grid.

Blurring of the whole visual field is usually due to an ocular problem, e.g. opacities in the cornea, lens, aqueous chamber or vitreous gel.

Sudden onset visual loss

Sudden onset visual loss may be temporary or permanent. Patients may complain of sudden visual loss when they close their unaffected eye if the affected eye has had gradual onset loss which they have not noticed.

Transient visual loss or disturbance is usually caused by the aura of classical migraine or transient ischaemia (*amaurosis fugax*). Increasing age and the presence of vascular risk factors increase the chance of an ischaemic cause. Absence of headache does not exclude migraine because the associated headache may be trivial or even absent. The aura of migraine is a positive phenomenon and may be white or coloured. Unlike a transient ischaemic attack it is still seen with the eyes shut. The description of zig-zag lines is virtually diagnostic of migraine and indicates occipital lobe involvement. The aura of classical migraine is always homonymous (present in both visual fields) (see Fig. 8.14, p. 242) even if the patient mistakenly attributes it to one eye. Retinal migraine, a unilateral phenomenon, may also occur, and in the absence of subsequent ocular pain or headache can be impossible to differentiate from amaurosis fugax.

Amaurosis fugax (unilateral transient ischaemia of the eye) produces a negative unilateral visual phenomenon with the patient describing the deficit as black or grey. Classically this is a short-lasting visual disturbance (minutes) appearing like a shutter coming down, up or from the side, and resolves in a similar fashion. It may be confused with the aura of migraine or the homonymous hemianopia of transient occipital lobe ischaemia.

Transient visual loss on walking suggests impaired suppression of the oculocephalic reflex (see p. 259). Normal suppression enables fixation to be maintained despite the head movements that occur on walking. Impaired suppression allows the eye to 'wobble' about. Visual loss following exercise or a hot bath is characteristic of demyelinating optic neuritis (Uthoff's phenomenon).

Permanent visual loss of sudden onset is usually caused by vascular occlusion. Establish whether the symptoms are uniocular or homonymous.

Causes of uniocular permanent sudden onset visual loss are:

- retinal artery occlusion
- anterior ischaemic optic neuropathy
- retinal vein occlusion.

Retinal artery occlusion is usually embolic, and patients have the same symptoms as in amaurosis fugax but permanently. Infarction of the optic nerve causes a visual field defect that affects the horizontal meridian. Always consider giant cell arteritis in anterior ischaemic optic neuropathy. In the absence of other symptoms, the diagnosis is more likely in the presence of a swollen and white optic nerve head and raised erythrocyte sedimentation rate (ESR) or C-reactive protein.

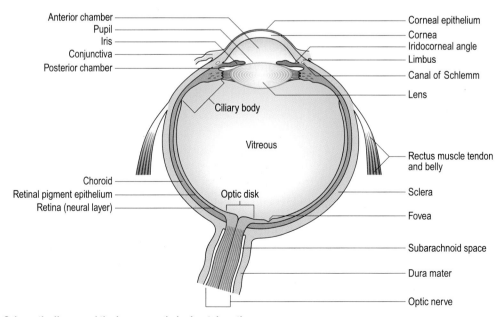

Homonymous visual loss, in the absence of hemiparesis or dysphasia, nearly always indicates occipital lobe infarction. Although the embolus is often from a proximal artery, exclude a cardiac source.

Gradual onset visual loss

Gradual onset of visual loss is commonly caused by cataract in the lens or atrophic age-related macular degeneration. In both, patients may experience glare with bright lights.

Distortion of vision

Distortion indicates disruption of the photoreceptors at the macula. In the elderly this is usually caused by macular degeneration. Untreated, central visual loss is usually rapid and irreversible. In those < 65 years it may be caused by fluid (oedema) or blood under the central retina. Scarring of the outer surface of the vitreous (epiretinal membrane) may also distort the normally smooth surface of the macula. This may occur following any insult to the vitreous, e.g. haemorrhage, inflammation or trauma.

Flashes and floaters

Flashes and floaters are common in those > 65 years and people with myopia (short-sightedness). They are caused by vitreous degeneration. The vitreous is the transparent gel in the middle of the eye (Fig. 8.7). Its base is firmly attached just behind the ciliary body, the origin of the iris. Its 'tail' is firmly attached to the optic disc. Elsewhere it is loosely attached to the major blood vessels of the retina. As the vitreous degenerates the gel liquefies and fluid escapes through perforations in the outer surface of the vitreous (posterior hyaloid surface) overlying the macula. The fluid peels the vitreous off the retina and the remaining contents

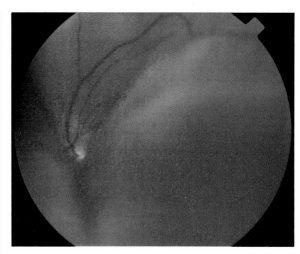

Fig. 8.8 Retinal detachment. Note the elevation of the retina around the 'attached' optic disc. The retina may be so elevated that it is visible on viewing the red reflex.

swirl about on eye movement. This is seen as something floating within the eye. If the vitreous has an abnormal attachment to the retina then, as it detaches, the retina may tear and the patient sees flashes of light. Retinal tears allow fluid from the vitreous cavity to enter the space between the retina and the retinal pigment epithelium (retinal detachment; Fig. 8.8). The patient notices visual loss starting peripherally and moving centrally.

Haloes

Haloes are coloured lights around bright lights and result from fluid in the cornea (corneal oedema) acting as a prism. They are seen with angle-closure glaucoma.

THE HISTORY

Nature and location of symptoms

Clarify the meaning of terms used by patients to describe their experience. Common sources of confusion are blackouts, vertigo and numbness, by which the patient may mean memory lapses, fear of heights and weakness rather than loss of awareness, hallucinations of movement and loss of sensation. Determine which parts of the body are affected by pain, weakness or sensory loss.

Time relationships

The onset, duration and pattern of symptoms over time often provide vital clues to the underlying pathological process.
Key prompts are:

- When did the symptoms start?
- How long did they last?
- Did they come on suddenly or gradually?

- Were they constant or did they come and go?
- Did (or do) the symptoms occur at certain times of the day/week/month?

Precipitating, exacerbating or relieving factors

- What were you doing when the symptoms occurred?
- Does any activity bring the symptoms on or make them worse when present, e.g. change of posture, exercise, sleep, coughing?
- Can you do anything to ease the symptoms when present?

Associated symptoms

Ask about other features of neurological disease which accompany the presenting symptoms, even if they are not volunteered by the patient. These include headaches, fits, faints or funny turns, memory or concentration difficulties, sensory symptoms, sphincter disturbance or sexual dysfunction, visual or hearing impairment, sleep or appetite disturbance, or mood changes.

Past history

A full past medical history is essential. Note any previous neurological events and ask about hypertension or diabetes mellitus. In younger patients take a detailed account of events surrounding birth and early development.

Drug history

Always consider a drug-related cause for symptoms. Make a complete list of recent and current medications including prescribed, over-the-counter and complementary therapies. Many neurological symptoms are caused by drugs taken for other conditions (Table 8.5). Adverse reactions may be

peculiar to an individual; some are dose-related and others occur with chronic use of medication even in low dose.

Family history

A wide range of genetic disorders affect the nervous system, e.g. neuropathies, ataxias and Huntington's disease, and many neurological diseases have genetic factors in their aetiology, e.g. epilepsy, multiple sclerosis, vascular disease. The common patterns of inheritance of some neurological conditions are shown in Table 8.6. Many conditions have a mixture of modes of inheritance, e.g. retinitis pigmentosa and the hereditary motor and sensory neuropathies. The possibility of an uncommon genetic condition should be considered in every neurological diagnosis.

Social history

Occupational factors are relevant to several neurological disorders such as peripheral neuropathies from exposure to toxins; compression or entrapment neuropathies and stress-related symptoms and syndromes. Ask about marital status and domestic circumstances. Smoking is relevant to

8.5	Neurological symptoms/syndromes due to drugs
Ataxia	Phenytoin, carbamazepine, benzodiazepines, ciclosporin, fluorouracil
Deafness	Gentamicin and other aminoglycosides, aspirin, furosemide (frusemide)
Diplopia	Carbamazepine, phenytoin
Dizziness/vertigo	Aspirin, enalapril, antihistamines, flecainide
Dysphagia	Bisphosphonates
Epilepsy	Tricyclic antidepressants, phenothiazines, fentanyl, aminophylline
Headaches	Glyceryl trinitrate, statins, sildenafil
Memory impairment	Benzodiazepine, corticosteroids, chlorpromazine, isoniazid
Myopathy	Statins, corticosteroids, bretylium tosilate, guanethidine
Parkinsonism	Chlorpromazine, haloperidol, prochlorperazine
Peripheral neuropathy	Isoniazid, metronidazole, amiodarone, procainamide, cimetidine
Tremor	Salbutamol, terbutaline, tricyclic antidepressants, amphetamines
Syncope	Antihypertensives, antiarrhythmic agents, levodopa
Visual loss	Steroids, anticholinergics, rifabutin, tamoxifen, phenothiazines, hydroxychloroquine, interferon, quinine, amiodarone, ethambutol, isoniazid

8.6	Examples of inherited neurological disorders

Autosomal dominant

- Myotonic dystrophy
- Neurofibromatosis types I and II
- Tuberous sclerosis
- Huntington's disease

Autosomal recessive

- Wilson's disease
- Friedreich's ataxia
- Tay–Sachs disease

X-linked recessive

- Duchenne muscular dystrophy
- Becker muscular dystrophy
- Fragile X syndrome

metastatic and non-metastatic manifestations of malignancy affecting the nervous system, while alcohol and drug abuse cause various neurological syndromes. As syphilis and HIV infection can result in a variety of neurological problems, it is often appropriate to take a sexual history (see p. 16).

Witness evidence

Obtain an account of the patient's symptoms from a close relative or associate in younger children, patients with cognitive impairment, and those who have had seizures, syncopal or other attacks of altered consciousness or awareness.

THE PHYSICAL EXAMINATION

Neurological assessment begins with your first contact with the patient and continues during history taking. Note facial expression, general demeanour, dress, posture, gait and speech to assess the individual's mood, and cognitive and physical state. You will often detect involuntary movements and signs of systemic disease at this stage. A detailed mental state examination (Ch. 1) and full general examination (Ch. 2) are integral parts of a neurological examination.

Vascular disease is the commonest cause of brain dysfunction in later life so measure the blood pressure and examine the heart for abnormality. Listen for cranial bruits from cerebral ateriovenous malformations by placing the stethoscope bell gently over the closed eyelid (Fig. 8.9). This is better than listening over the cranium. Systolic bruits may be heard over stenosed carotid or vertebral vessels. Carotid bruits are usually heard at the angle of the jaw, corresponding to the cervical bifurcation. Bruits from vertebral or subclavian arteries are detected at the supraclavicular fossae. Listen at and between these sites. Absence of bruits does not exclude significant stenosis.

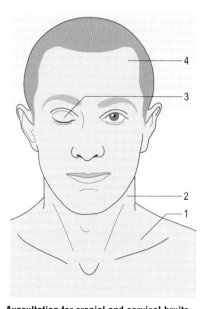

Fig. 8.9 Auscultation for cranial and cervical bruits.
(1) Supraclavicular fossa. (2) Carotid bifurcation. (3) Over closed eyes. (4) Over cranium.

ASSESSMENT OF CONSCIOUS LEVEL

Consciousness has two main components: state and content. The state of consciousness is largely dependent on the integrity of the ascending reticular activating system extending from the lower pons to the thalamus. Consciousness describes how awake a person is. The content of consciousness is how aware the person is and depends on the cerebral cortex, thalamus and their connections.

In the past, ill-defined terms such as delirium, stupor, semi-coma and deep coma were used to describe levels of consciousness. Nowadays, a reliable, standardized and reproducible method, the Glasgow Coma Scale, is used.

Glasgow Coma Scale (GCS)

Three responses are scored according to the stimulus required (Table 8.7). The response may be spontaneous;

8.7 Glasgow Coma Scale	
	Score
Eye opening	
Spontaneous	4
To speech	3
To pain	2
No response	1
Verbal response	
Orientated	5
Confused: talks in sentences but disorientated	4
Verbalizes: words not sentences	3
Vocalizes: sounds (groans or grunts) not words	2
No vocalization	1
Motor response	
Obeys commands	6
Localizes to pain: e.g. brings hand up beyond chin to supraorbital pain	5
Flexion withdrawal to pain: no localization to supraorbital pain but flexes elbow to nail bed pressure	4
Abnormal flexion to pain	3
Extension to pain: extends elbow to nail bed pressure	2
No response	1

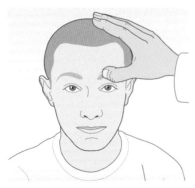

Fig. 8.10 Supraorbital nerve pressure.

elicited by questions or commands from the examiner; only occur with pain (pressure on the supraorbital nerve; Fig. 8.10); or absent.

To assess conscious level use only upper limb responses as leg responses are less consistent. The motor response may vary during examination. For instance one arm may localize to pain while the other flexes. In these cases, record the best motor response. Summation of the three responses is used. Note that the minimum GCS is 3/15, and the maximum is 15/15. In clinical practice record the responses individually, e.g. E2, V3, M4 – total 9/15. In population studies assessing severity of head injury GCS < 8 indicates severe; 9–12 moderate and > 13 mild injury.

STANCE AND GAIT

Stance and gait depend upon vision, proprioceptive, corticospinal, extrapyramidal and cerebellar pathways together with lower motor neurones and spinal reflexes. Gait disorders of non-neurological origin are discussed in Chapter 10.

➔ Examination sequence

Stance
➔ Ask the patient to stand up straight with feet close together and eyes open (preferably with bare feet).
➔ Swaying or lurching with the eyes open suggest a cerebellar defect (cerebellar ataxia).
➔ Ask the patient to close his eyes. Swaying, lurching or loss of balance indicate sensory ataxia (proprioceptive deficit) – positive Romberg's sign.

Gait
➔ Ask the patient to walk a measured 10 metres, with walking aid if needed, then turn through 180° and return.

➔ Record the time taken to complete the first 10 metres and note the length and width of steps and any tendency to veer, sway or stumble to one side.
➔ Ask the patient to walk heel to toe in a straight line (tandem gait). This emphasizes any gait instability (gait ataxia).

Common abnormalities

• Unsteadiness on standing with the eyes open is common in cerebellar disorders, particularly those involving the vermis.
• Instability which only occurs, or is markedly worse, on eye closure is indicative of proprioceptive sensory loss, referred to as *sensory ataxia* (or *Rombergism*).
• A *hemiplegic gait*, due to a unilateral upper motor neurone lesion, is characterized by the leg being extended at the knee and ankle and circumduction at the hip.
• Bilateral upper motor neurone damage leads to adduction at both hips and a scissors-like stance and gait.
• Cerebellar dysfunction leads to a broad-based, unsteady (*ataxic*) gait which usually makes tandem walking impossible.
• In Parkinson's disease initiation of walking may be delayed, the steps short and shuffling and there is loss of arm swing. The stooped posture and impairment of postural reflexes can result in a rapid short-stepped hurrying (*festinant*) gait.
• Proximal weakness associated with muscle diseases may lead to a waddling (*myopathic*) gait.
• Bizarre gaits with no other neurological signs may be psychogenic. Care should be taken, however, as conditions such as Huntington's disease can be associated with a strange walking pattern.

SPEECH

Communication difficulties will be apparent during history taking and may arise from many causes including deafness, mutism, cognitive deficits, emotional disorder and speech or language disturbance as outlined in Chapter 1.

Disturbance of articulation is *dysarthria*. Impairment of voice or sound production from the larynx is *dysphonia*. In both cases language function is intact, but patients' intelligibility may be a problem. They understand what is being said and the grammatical construction of their speech is normal.

When language areas in the dominant hemisphere are damaged, there is disturbance of understanding and/or expression of words. These disorders are *dysphasias*.

Dysarthrias and dysphonia

⮊ Examination sequence

→ Listen to the patient's spontaneous speech, noting the volume, rhythm and clarity of enunciation.

→ Ask the patient to repeat phrases such as 'yellow lorry' (to test tongue (*lingual*) sounds) and 'baby hippopotamus' (for lip (*labial*) sounds), then a tongue twister (e.g. 'the Leith police dismisseth us').

→ Ask the patient to count steadily to 30 to assess for muscle fatigue.

→ To test for dysphonia ask the patient to cough and to say 'Aaah'.

Common abnormalities

Dysarthria. Disturbed articulation may result from local lesions of the tongue, lips or mouth, ill-fitting dentures or from any disruption of the neuromuscular pathways. Lesions differ in the patterns of speech disturbance they cause and vary in their associated features.

- Bilateral upper motor neurone lesions of the corticobulbar tract lead to the confusing term of *pseudobulbar* (or spastic) dysarthria. This is characterized by a small, spastic tongue and difficulty pronouncing consonants and is often accompanied by a positive jaw jerk and emotional lability.
- *Bulbar* palsy is the result of lower motor neurone lesions affecting the same group of cranial nerves. The nature of the speech disturbance is determined by which nerves and muscles are involved. Weakness of the tongue results in difficulty with lingual sounds, while palatal weakness give a nasal quality to the speech.
- *Extrapyramidal* dysarthria causes the monotonous speech of Parkinson's disease, while *cerebellar* dysarthria may be slow and slurred similar to the speech of a drunken person.
- Myasthenia gravis is the most common cause of fatiguability of speech.

Dysphonia. This usually results from either local vocal cord pathology, as in laryngitis, or damage to the vagal nerve supply to the vocal cords. The voluntary cough in dysphonia has a 'bovine' quality.

Dysphasias

Anatomy

The language areas are located in the dominant cerebral hemisphere, which is the left in the vast majority of right-handed and most left-handed people. Other left-handers have language areas on the right (about 30%) or bilaterally.

Broca's area (inferior frontal region) is concerned with the production of words or the expression of language.

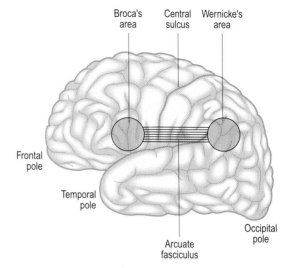

Fig. 8.11 The main language areas.

Wernicke's area (superior posterior temporal lobe) is the principal area for comprehension of spoken language. Adjacent regions of the parietal lobe are involved in the understanding of written language and numbers. The arcuate fasciculus contains the main connections between Broca's and Wernicke's areas (Fig. 8.11).

⮊ Examination sequence

→ During spontaneous speech listen to the fluency and appropriateness of the content, particularly for incorrect words (*paraphasias*) and nonsense words (*neologisms*).

→ Show the patient a common object (e.g. coin or pen) and ask its name.

→ Give a simple three-stage command (e.g. pick up the piece of paper, fold it in half and place it under the book). It is essential to give no visual clues and so it is best to give the instruction from behind the patient's head.

→ Ask the patient to repeat a simple sentence (e.g. Today is Tuesday).

→ Ask the patient to read a passage from a newspaper.

→ Ask the patient to write a sentence, and examine the handwriting.

Common abnormalities

Several forms of dysphasia have been described but four are considered here:

- *Expressive* (*motor*) dysphasia results from damage to Broca's area and is characterized by a reduction in the number of words used and non-fluent speech with errors of grammar and syntax. It has been described as of 'telegraphic' nature. Comprehension is, however, intact.
- *Receptive* (*sensory*) dysphasia occurs with dysfunction in Wernicke's area. There is poor comprehension and

although speech may be fluent it may be meaningless and contain paraphasias and neologisms.

- *Conduction* dysphasia is due to damage to the arcuate fasciculus and, while comprehension and understanding may be intact, the patient is unable to repeat words or phrases spoken by the examiner.
- *Global* dysphasia refers to a combination of expressive and receptive difficulties due to damage to both Broca's and Wernicke's areas resulting in poor comprehension and lack of fluency.
- Dominant parietal lobe lesions affecting the supramarginal gyrus and related areas may cause difficulty comprehending written language (*dyslexia*), problems with simple addition and subtraction (*dyscalculia*) and impairment of writing (*dysgraphia*).

MENINGEAL IRRITATION

Stiffness or restricted movement of the neck or lumbar region may result from various causes described in examination of the spine in Chapter 10. Inflammation or irritation of the meninges can lead to increased resistance to passive flexion of the neck and the extended leg. The corresponding signs are neck stiffness (or nuchal rigidity) and Kernig's sign. Common causes are infection in meningitis or blood in subarachnoid haemorrhage.

◢ Examination sequence

→ Position the patient supine with no pillow.
→ Expose and fully extend both legs.
→ Support the patient's head with the fingers of your hands placed at the occiput and the ulnar border of your hands against the paraspinal muscles of the patient's neck (Fig. 8.12A).
→ Flex the head gently until the chin touches the chest.
→ Ask the patient to hold that position.
→ Now flex one leg at the hip and knee with your left hand placed over the medial hamstrings.
→ Use your right hand to extend the knee while the hip is maintained in flexion. Look at the other leg for any reflex flexion (Fig. 8.12B).

If neck stiffness is present it is not possible to passively flex the neck fully and you may feel spasm in the neck muscles. Kernig's test is positive when attempts to extend the knee are resisted by spasm which is detected in the hamstrings, and the other limb may flex at the hip and knee. Kernig's sign is not present in local causes of neck stiffness, e.g. cervical spine disease or raised intracranial pressure.

A

B

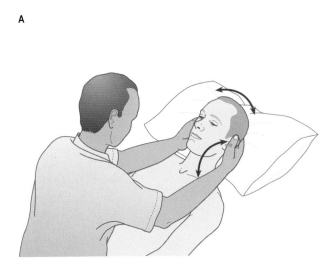
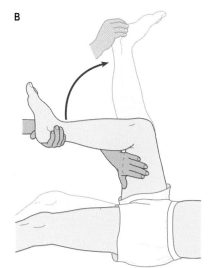
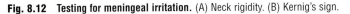

Fig. 8.12 **Testing for meningeal irritation.** (A) Neck rigidity. (B) Kernig's sign.

Examine this patient with sudden onset headache

1. Assess and record level of consciousness (intracranial lesions).
2. Measure pulse, blood pressure and temperature.
3. Look for signs of meningeal irritation: photophobia, neck stiffness and Kernig's sign (*bacterial* or *viral meningitis, subarachnoid haemorrhage*).
4. Examine the optic fundi for papilloedema (a late sign of raised intracranial pressure, and absence of papilloedema does not exclude raised intracranial pressure).
5. Examine for focal neurological signs (*cerebral haemorrhage, haemorrhage into intracranial tumour*).
6. Examine trunk and limbs for purpuric rash (*meningococcal meningitis*).
7. In those > 55 years feel for palpable temporal arteries and scalp tenderness (*temporal arteritis*).

THE EXAMINATION OF THE CRANIAL NERVES

THE OLFACTORY (I) NERVE

The olfactory nerve conveys the sense of smell. Bipolar cells in the olfactory bulb form olfactory filaments with small receptors projecting through the cribriform plate high in the nasal cavity. These cells synapse with second order neurones which project centrally via the olfactory tract to the medial temporal lobe and ipsilateral amygdaloid body.

▶ Examination sequence

➜ Check that the nasal passages are clear.
➜ Ask the patient to close his eyes and shut one nostril with a finger.
➜ Present commonly available odours such as coffee, chocolate, soap or orange peel and ask the patient to sniff.

Provided that the patient does not have nasal congestion or disease, loss of the sense of smell (*anosmia*) may result from shearing damage to the olfactory filaments after severe head injury, local compression or invasion by cancer. Patients usually complain of altered ability to taste when they have lost the sense of smell. Anosmia may also occur in Parkinson's disease and Huntington's disease. Perversion of the sense of smell (*parosmia*) is when pleasant odours are perceived as unpleasant. It is uncommon but may occur after head trauma, sinus infection or as a side-effect of drugs. Olfactory hallucinations are a feature of complex partial seizures.

THE EYE: THE OPTIC (II), OCULOMOTOR (III), TROCHLEAR (IV), ABDUCENS (VI) NERVES

Anatomy

The eye, a direct extension of the brain, is responsible for focusing an image of our external surroundings onto the photoreceptors of the neurosensory retina.

- Rod photoreceptors are responsible for night vision and detection of peripheral movement.
- Cone photoreceptors are responsible for colour vision and central vision.
- Photoreceptors synapse with the vertically orientated bipolar cells of the retina which in turn synapse with the ganglion cells of the optic nerve (Fig. 8.13).

The *optic nerve* is purely sensory. Its nuclei, the ganglion cells, are found below the horizontal nerve fibre layer of the retina. Initially unmyelinated, the nerve fibres of the optic nerve myelinate on leaving the eye through the optic disc. Passing through the orbit, the optic nerve is liable to compression from enlarged ocular muscles. The optic nerve enters the cranium through the optic canal. The two optic nerves join at the optic chiasm, where the nasal fibres, responsible for the temporal visual field, decussate. Leaving the chiasm, the optic nerve is confusingly renamed the optic tract. The optic tracts terminate by synapsing with the

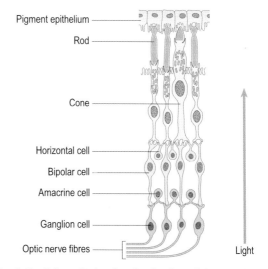

Pigment epithelium
Rod
Cone
Horizontal cell
Bipolar cell
Amacrine cell
Ganglion cell
Optic nerve fibres
Light

Fig. 8.13 Schematic drawing showing the cellular organization of the retina.

lateral geniculate bodies of the thalamus. A few fibres leave the tract before the lateral geniculate nucleus as part of the afferent limb of the pupillary reflex.

Axons of the cell bodies of the lateral geniculate nucleus make up the optic radiations. The optic radiations pass through the posterior internal capsule to enter the cerebral hemisphere via the parietal and temporal lobes to the occipital cortex (Fig. 8.14).

The oculomotor (III), trochlear (IV) and abducens (VI) nerves innervate the six external ocular muscles of each eye (Fig. 8.15A). The parasympathetic fibres from the Edinger–Westphal nucleus form part of the oculomotor nerve and are involved in the efferent supply of the pupillary reflexes (Fig. 8.15B). These three cranial nerves therefore innervate the muscles controlling eye movement and pupillary size. Although each nerve controls discrete actions they are examined together because of their close functional interrelationships.

The *oculomotor (III) nerve* nucleus lies in the ventral midbrain at the level of the superior colliculus. The nerve passes between the cerebral peduncles into the interpeduncular cerebrospinal fluid (CSF) cistern. It passes just below the free edge of the tentorium in relation to the posterior communicating artery and enters the dura surrounding the cavernous sinus. It then enters the orbital fossa

through the superior oblique fissure, where it subdivides into its terminal branches. The nerve innervates the superior, medial and inferior recti, the inferior oblique and levator palpebrae superioris muscles. These muscles open the upper lid (levator palpebrae superioris) and move the globe upwards (superior rectus, inferior oblique), downwards (inferior rectus) and medially (medial rectus). Through the parasympathetic fibres arising from the Edinger–Westphal nerves, the nerve also indirectly supplies the sphincter muscles of the iris causing constriction of the pupil, and the ciliary muscle which is responsible for focusing the lens for near vision (accommodation).

The *trochlear (IV) nerve* arises from a nucleus in the caudal midbrain at the level of the inferior colliculus. The fibres decussate before leaving the midbrain posteriorly (the left nucleus innervates the right trochlear nerve and vice versa). The nerve then passes forward and laterally in relation to the rostral pons and the free edge of the tentorium. It pierces the dura of the tentorial edge and passes through the cavernous sinus and superior orbital fissure. In the orbit it innervates the superior oblique muscle. When superior oblique contracts it causes downward movement of the globe when the eye is adducted.

The *abducens (VI) nerve* originates from a nucleus located near the midline of the caudal pons. The nerve emerges

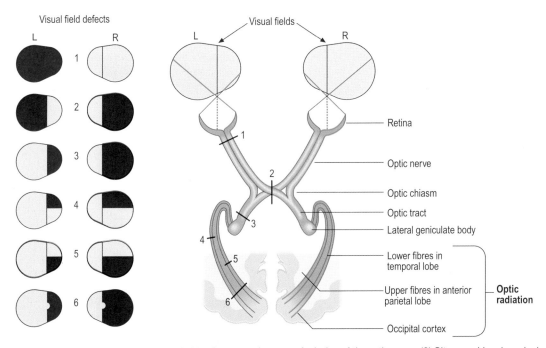

Fig. 8.14 Visual field defects. (1) Total loss of vision in one eye because of a lesion of the optic nerve. (2) Bitemporal hemianopia due to compression of the optic chiasm. (3) Right homonymous hemianopia from a lesion of the optic tract. (4) Upper right quadrantanopia from a lesion of the lower fibres of the optic radiation in the temporal lobe. (5) Less commonly a lower quadrantanopia occurs from a lesion of the upper fibres of the optic radiation in the anterior part of the parietal lobe. (6) Right homonymous hemianopia with sparing of the macula due to lesion of the optic radiation in the posterior part of the parietal lobe.

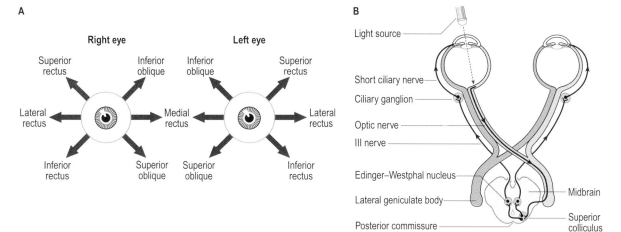

Fig. 8.15   Control of eye movement and pupil size. (A) Fields of action of pairs of extraocular muscles. This diagram will help to work out which eye muscle is paretic. For example, a patient whose diplopia is maximum on looking down and to the right has either a weak right inferior rectus or a weak left superior oblique. Cover one of the patient's eyes and ask which image disappears – the most peripheral image comes from the affected eye. (B) Pathway of pupillary constriction and the light reflex (parasympathetic).

from the ventral pontomedullary junction just lateral to the pyramid, passes through the prepontine CSF cistern and pierces the basal dura to enter Dorello's canal and then traverse the cavernous sinus. Here the nerve is in direct relation to the internal carotid artery before it passes through the superior orbital fissure to the lateral rectus muscle. Contraction of lateral rectus causes abduction of the eye.

The pupils are normally rounded, regular, equal in size and symmetrical in their responses. The autonomic nervous system and integrity of the iris determine the resting size of the pupil. The afferent limb of the pupillary reflex involves the optic nerve, bypassing the lateral geniculate nucleus to terminate in the III nerve (Edinger–Westphal) nucleus. The efferent limb involves the inferior division of the third nerve, passing through the ciliary ganglion in the orbit to terminate in the constrictor muscle of the iris. With sympathetic stimulation the pupils dilate and the upper and lower eyelids retract. With parasympathetic stimulation (the fibres of which travel with the third nerve) the opposite occurs.

Sensation from the cornea, conjunctiva and intraocular structures are conveyed by the ophthalmic branch (V_1) of the trigeminal nerve.

Nystagmus

Nystagmus is an involuntary rhythmic oscillation of the eyes. It may be horizontal, vertical or rotatory and either pendular or jerk in type. When acquired, it is usually caused by abnormalities of the vestibular system and its connections.

Pendular nystagmus is characterised by oscillations about a central point that are equal in rate and amplitude and may occur in any plane. In children it is usually congenital and may be associated with impaired vision. In adults it usually reflects brainstem or cerebellar disease and is usually associated with a head tremor.

Jerk nystagmus is characterised by oscillations which have a slow initiating phase and a fast corrective phase. The direction of the fast phase defines the direction of nystagmus. Thus 'nystagmus to the right' refers to the direction of the rapid component *not* the direction of gaze in which nystagmus occurs.

Jerk nystagmus may be peripheral or central in origin.

- Peripheral lesions affecting the vestibular apparatus or VIII nerve produce a unidirectional nystagmus away from the affected side irrespective of the direction of gaze and dampened by visual fixation. It is often aggravated by head movement and accompanied by vertigo, deafness and tinnitus.
- Central lesions in the brain stem or cerebellum produce bidirectional nystagmus (the direction of nystagmus changes with the direction of gaze) which is unaffected by visual fixation. Other causes include toxicity from alcohol or drugs, especially anticonvulsants and benzodiazepines.
- Lesions of the medial longitudinal fasciculus in the pons produce nystagmus in the contralateral abducting eye along with impaired adduction of the ipsilateral eye. When bilateral (dysconjugate or *ataxic nystagmus*) it is characteristic of demyelination due to multiple sclerosis.

EXAMINATION OF VISION

Examination of vision often involves the assessment of cranial nerves II to VIII and their central connections:

• inspection
• visual acuity
• visual fields
• ocular alignment
• pupillary examination
• colour vision
• ophthalmoscopy.

Inspection

Look at:

• head position
• position of eyelids when looking straight ahead and on eye movement
• proptosis
• periorbital appearance
• lacrimal apparatus
• eyelid margin
• conjunctiva
• sclera
• cornea
• resting appearance of pupils.

Common abnormalities

Congenital and longstanding paralytic squints often result in *abnormal head postures* with the head turned or tilted to minimize the diplopia.

Narrowing of the palpebral fissure (the gap between upper and lower eyelids) suggests ptosis or blepharospasm. If the sclera is visible above the cornea, suspect eyelid retraction or proptosis. If there is exposure below, consider ectropion.

Ptosis or droopy eyelids may result from:

• neuropathy, e.g. Horner's syndrome, III nerve palsy, Miller–Fisher syndrome variant of Guillain–Barré syndrome
• abnormal neuromuscular transmission, e.g. myasthenia gravis
• myopathy, e.g. dystrophia myotonica; chronic progressive external ophthalmoplegia
• mechanical dysfunction, e.g. senile ptosis, trauma, lid tumour.

The ptosis of Horner's syndrome (see p. 137) is partial and involves both upper and lower lids leading to a pseudo-enophthalmos (small eye). The pupil is small due to lack of sympathetic innervation to the iris.

In third nerve palsy the ptosis is often complete (Fig. 8.16). The pupil is large because of loss of parasympathetic

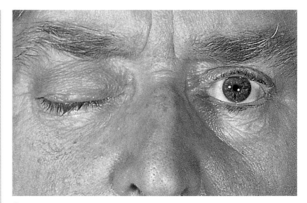

A

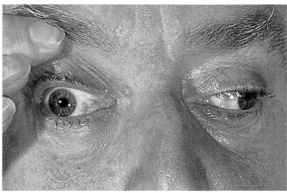

B

Fig. 8.16   Third nerve palsy. (A) Complete right ptosis. (B) Patient looking down and to the left – the right eye has rotated medially, demonstrating that the trochlear (IV) nerve is intact.

innervation of the iris and the unopposed action of cranial nerves IV and VI results in the eye looking inferolaterally.

In myasthenia gravis (Fig. 8.17), ptosis (levator palpebrae – 'third nerve') may be associated with an inability to 'bury the eyelashes' (orbicularis oculi – 'facial (VII) nerve'). This sign strongly suggests either neuromuscular junction disorder, myopathy or meningeal disorder, as it is not possible for a single lesion to affect both ipsilateral III and VII cranial nerves.

Lid lag is elicited by asking the patient to slowly look down (Fig. 8.18). The upper lid fails to cover the sclera above the iris. It is a cardinal feature of thyroid eye disease and its absence, in the presence of proptosis, should make one suspicious of another orbital cause (Table 8.8).

Proptosis localizes a problem to the orbit. Stand behind the patient and look down the front of the face from above to see if the eyeballs protrude.

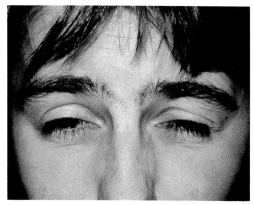

Fig. 8.17 Myasthenia gravis. The patient is attempting to open his eyelids. Note raised forehead browlines (frontalis overactivity) reflecting the effort of attempting to open the eyelids.

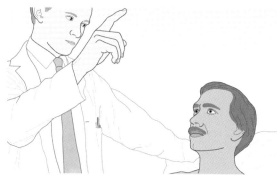

Fig. 8.18 Lid lag. With the patient sitting, position yourself on the patient's right side. Watch how the lid moves with the downward movement of the eye as the patient follows your finger moving from a point approximately 45° above the horizontal to a point below this plane. Normally there is perfect coordination as the lid follows the downward movement of the eyes.

8.8 Causes of proptosis
• Thyroid eye disease (exophthalmos) • Orbital cellulitis • Caroticocavernous fistula • Orbital metastasis • Orbital haematoma • Wegener's granulomatosis • Pseudoproptosis (pathological myopia, shallow orbits, contralateral enophthalmos)

Periorbital oedema is seen commonly with:

• allergic eye disease
• thyroid eye disease
• orbital cellulitis
• nephrotic syndrome
• cardiac failure
• angio-oedema.

Periorbital oedema may be associated with oedema of the conjunctiva (*chemosis*).

Most tear formation comes from multiple, small, accessory lacrimal glands in the lids. The lacrimal gland is situated under the lateral part of the upper lid and is responsible for secreting tears to wash away foreign bodies and to express emotion in crying. Tears drain through the lacrimal puncta and canaliculi in the medial edge of both eyelids into the lacrimal sac and thence into the nose through the nasolacrimal duct.

The lacrimal gland may become swollen through:

• inflammation (sarcoidosis)
• infection (dacroadenitis or mumps)
• malignancy (lymphoma, cancer).

The *lacrimal sac* lies between the medial canthus and the nose. Blockage of the nasolacrimal duct causes watering, sticky discharge and may result in acute dacrocystitis with abscess formation in the lacrimal sac. Blocked tear ducts often occur in infants, where they usually resolve spontaneously.

Blepharitis (inflammation of the eyelid margin) is a common cause of dry eyes. Although often isolated it may be associated with systemic skin involvement. Look for features of more widespread skin disease:

• 'ace of clubs' appearance of rosacea (erythema on forehead, cheeks and chin)
• flexural dermatitis of atopic eczema
• dandruff or seborrhoeic dermatitis.

Common lumps on the lids include:

• stye (eyelash microabscess),
• chalazion (pea-like swellings of the tarsal glands)
• basal cell cancer.

The *conjunctiva* is a transparent mucous membrane attached to the inner eyelids and outer eye. It is examined by pulling down the lower lid. If nothing is revealed, everting the upper lid may demonstrate the giant papillae of allergic eye disease or a hidden foreign body (Fig. 8.5).

Conjunctival inflammation (conjunctivitis) is considered on page 231.

The *sclera* is opaque and white. If it is thin it becomes transparent allowing the blue-green choroid to be seen. This occurs in scleromalacia, osteogenesis imperfecta and Ehlers–Danlos syndrome. The sclera are yellow in jaundice.

Scleral inflammation (*scleritis*) causes a dark-red colour, tenderness and pain on eye movement which may occur with specific eye movements or generally. White patches within red areas suggest impending necrosis and the presence of systemic vasculitis. Perform urinalysis and measure ESR or C-reactive protein in all patients with scleritis to screen for systemic vasculitis.

The *cornea* is the transparent 'window of the eye'. Opacity leads to blurred vision, haloes and 'blurring' of the

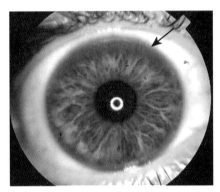

Fig. 8.19   Kayser–Fleischer ring (arrowed).

underlying iris. This can be because of epithelial damage or stromal oedema. The epithelium may be affected if the cornea is dry, traumatized or infected. Epithelial damage can be demonstrated by staining with yellow fluorescein dye. Peripheral corneal deposition is seen with hyperlipidaemia (corneal arcus) due to lipid deposition and Wilson's disease (Kayser–Fleischer ring; Fig. 8.19) due to copper deposition. Calcium may also be deposited in chronic ocular inflammation and chronic hypercalcaemia (see Ch. 6).

Visual acuity

➔ Examination sequence

→ Ask patients to use their appropriate glasses when you measure visual acuity.

→ Use good ambient lighting and a Snellen or LogMar chart (Fig. 8.20).

→ A Snellen visual acuity of 6/60 (LogMar = 1.0) indicates that at 6 metres the patient can only see letters they should be able to read 60 metres away. Normal vision is said to be 6/6 (LogMar = 0.0). In the UK you need a visual acuity of 6/10 or better to drive a car.

→ If 6/6 vision is not obtained, then a pinhole placed directly in front of the patient's glasses may correct additional refractive errors. It allows only central rays of light to enter the eye and can correct for about 4 diopters of refractive error (Fig. 8.21).

→ If patients cannot see the top line of the chart at 6 metres, bring them forward till they can and record that vision (e.g. 1/60 – can see top letter at 1 metre).

→ If patients still cannot see the top letter at 1 metre, then check whether they can count fingers, see hand movements or just see light.

→ For children use different-sized objects instead of letters. For patients complaining of central blurred vision record the near vision in each eye using reading glasses and standard charts.

Visual fields

The normal visual field extends 160° horizontally and 130° vertically. The blind spot is located 15° to the temporal side of the point of visual fixation and represents the optic nerve head. At the bedside, test visual fields by confrontation. More accurate assessments use perimetry and visual field analysers.

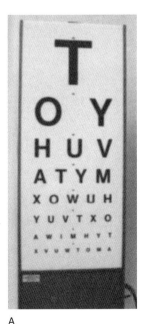

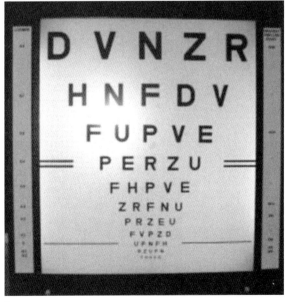

Fig. 8.20   Visual acuity charts.
(A) Snellen visual acuity chart: increasingly replaced by the LogMar visual acuity chart.
(B) Illuminated LogMar chart.

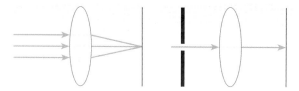

Fig. 8.21 **Pinhole.** Normally the lens focuses rays of light onto a discrete point on the retina. The pinhole partially negates the role of the lens by only allowing rays from directly in front to pass through.

→ Examination sequence

→ Sit directly facing the patient about 1 metre away.

→ Ask the patient to keep looking at your eyes.

→ Test the visual fields for homonymous defects with both your and the patient's eyes open. This is performed by small movements of the tip of your finger in each of the four outer quadrants of the patient's visual field – superotemporal, superonasal, inferotemporal, inferonasal. Ask the patient to point to the moving finger. Slowly bring your finger into the centre of the visual field until the patient detects the movement.

→ Test for sensory attention by testing both left and right fields at the same time.

→ If the homonymous hemianopia is incongruous it may be difficult to detect by confrontation and only revealed if the visual fields are examined for each eye.

→ To test the peripheral visual fields in each eye ask the patient to cover one eye and look directly into your opposite eye. Shut your eye that is opposite the patient's covered eye to leave your hands free to examine the visual fields. If finger movements are not detected then bring the finger towards the centre of vision till it is seen. Repeat for the other visual field.

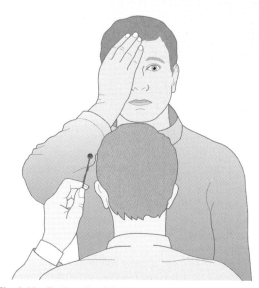

Fig. 8.22 **Testing visual fields by confrontation.**

→ To test the central visual field qualitatively in one eye use a red hatpin. Ask the patient to cover one eye and look directly at you. Shut your eye that is opposite the patient's covered eye to leave your hands free to examine the visual fields. Hold the red hatpin in the centre of the visual field as close to fixation as possible. Ask the patient to say what colour the hatpin is. If it is pale or pink this implies colour desaturation affecting usually the optic nerve. Then compare the four quadrants of the visual field centrally, enquiring again about colour desaturation (Fig. 8.22). Note that the visual field for red may be smaller than for white.

→ The hatpin can be used to examine the size of the blindspot. This is the physiological scotoma that corresponds to absence of photoreceptors at the site where the optic nerve leaves the eye. Starting from fixation, move the hatpin temporally and horizontally until it appears to disappear from your visual field. Then, while maintaining the same temporal horizontal position, move it anteriorly or posteriorly until it also disappears from the patient's visual field. Now directly compare the size of the patient's blindspot to yours.

Common abnormalities

Reduced visual acuity indicates a central visual field defect. The commonest cause is cataract. There are three retinal forms of central visual field defects:

• Lesions of the macula cause *central* scotomas. Scotomas may be incomplete and associated with distortion allowing the patient to see through them, although not clearly.

• Lesions of the peripheral retina will initially spare central vision causing *ring* scotomas.

• Lesions of the optic disc will cause horizontal or *arcuate* scotomas.

Lesions of the *optic nerve* within the orbit cause central scotomas that differ from those of macular origin in that red desaturation (red colours appear orange or pink) occurs early and there is no visual distortion.

• Unilateral optic nerve lesions cause a relative afferent pupillary defect even with apparently normal vision, whereas with macula lesions this is a late finding.

• Distension of the nerve sheath around the optic nerve, as seen with the swollen disc of papilloedema (see Fig. 8.25D, p. 251), will cause an enlarged blind spot. Optic nerve damage occurs later.

• Distortion is best assessed with an Amsler grid, a grid that is held at reading distance and assesses the central 10° of vision.

Lesions at the *optic chiasm* cause bilateral temporal visual field defects (bitemporal hemianopia) that respect the vertical meridian (see Fig. 8.14, p. 242).

• As the optic chiasm is a continuation of the optic nerve, central red desaturation is the first sign of involvement. **247**

- Initially these field defects are located centrally and only for red desaturation.
- With time they extend peripherally and become denser.

Optic tract lesions are uncommon and usually the result of suprasellar lesions such as pituitary tumours in the setting of anterior displacement of the chiasm. Asymmetrical (incongruous) homonymous visual field defects are produced.

Lesions of the *visual radiations* are common.

- Symmetrical (congruous) visual field defects are produced (homonymous hemianopia).
- Lack of awareness of visual field loss suggests parietal lobe involvement.
- As a result of the dual blood supply of the occipital cortex visual fields defects may affect only central vision.

Functional visual loss is surprisingly common and is usually 'hysterical' rather than malingering. The commonest functional visual field loss is bilateral visual field constriction that fails to expand on testing further away from the tangent screen. This tubular constriction helps to differentiate it from the funnel constriction of bilateral retinal disorders, e.g. retinitis pigmentosa (see Fig. 8.27C, p. 254) or bilateral homonymous hemianopia (cortical visual impairment).

Ocular alignment

The eyes are normally parallel in all positions of gaze except convergence. When they are not, a squint is present. Squints may be associated with:

- paresis of one of the extraocular muscles (paralytic or incomitant squint)
- defective binocular vision (non-paralytic or concomitant squints).

Acquired paralytic squints cause diplopia, the images being maximally separated and squint greatest in the direction of action of the paretic muscle. Congenital and longstanding paralytic squints often result in abnormal head postures with the head turned or tilted to minimize the diplopia. Concomitant squints are the same in all positions of gaze. They usually become manifest in childhood when they are not associated with diplopia, as this symptom is suppressed centrally in young children. Central suppression causes *amblyopia* (lazy eye).

➡ Examination sequence

➔ The examination sequence depends on whether the patient complains of double vision (diplopia) or squint.

Diplopia
➔ Look for head turns or tilts in the direction of underacting muscles.

➔ Sit directly facing the patient about 1 metre away.
➔ Ask the patient to look at the light of a pen-torch as it is moved and observe the position of the light reflexes on the cornea.
➔ The fixating (non-paretic) eye will have a light reflex in the centre, the eye with weak muscles (paretic) will have a reflex deviated from the centre.
➔ If the paretic eye has better vision than the non-paretic eye the patient will fixate with the paretic eye, leading to confusing eye movements.
➔ Look for the direction of gaze where diplopia is maximal.
➔ Ascertain whether diplopia is monocular or binocular by covering one eye.
➔ Ask whether the diplopia is horizontal, vertical, tilted or a mixture of both.
➔ If diplopia is binocular it may be obvious which muscle is involved. If not, cover one eye and examine the movement of the visible eye.
  → On horizontal movement, in the absence of proptosis, none of the ipsilateral sclera should be present on extreme gaze ('burying the white').
  → If present, it suggests ipsilateral weakness of muscle action.
➔ Weakness of up-gaze is more subjective. It is easier to assess with both eyes open for comparison of eye movement.
➔ On down-gaze you will need to hold the eyelids open.
➔ For each eye, look for nystagmus while examining the eye movements. Note the direction of any fast component and whether it changes direction with the direction of gaze.

Squint
➔ Sit directly facing the patient about 1 metre away.
➔ Examine visual acuity and the visual fields as above.
➔ Ask the patient to look at the light of your pen-torch.
➔ Cover one eye.
➔ Closely observe the uncovered eye for any movements.
➔ If it moves to take up fixation, that eye was squinting.
➔ Repeat the sequence for the other eye.

Common abnormalities

While examining eye movements always ask yourself:

- Where is the lesion?
- Does it follow the 'wiring circuitry' of a cranial nerve lesion?
- If not, then it must be a problem of either the neuromuscular junction or the muscles themselves. In myasthenia gravis there is often a combination of fatiguable ptosis ('III nerve') with weak eyelid closure ('VII nerve').

Monocular diplopia is not caused by ocular muscle imbalance but is created within the eye by 'ghosting' of an image as result of a structural abnormality. This can occur anywhere between cornea and fovea.

Pure horizontal diplopia usually results from involvement of cranial nerve VI. The symptoms are worse looking to the affected side.

- A history of orbital trauma suggests the possibility of entrapment of a medial rectus muscle.
- In demyelination the lesion is often in the pons and may be associated with ipsilateral lower motor neurone nerve palsy.
- Disruption of the neuronal connection between the medial rectus and the contralateral VI nerve palsy (median longitudinal fasciculus), as can occur in multiple sclerosis, will lead to underaction of the medial rectus and an internuclear ophthalmoparesis. Unlike VI nerve palsy, diplopia is worse on looking to the contralateral side. There is often an accompanying skew deviation giving a vertical component to the diplopia.

Other causes of impaired horizontal movement include:

- pontine gaze palsies (nuclear VI nerve palsy)
- Duane's syndrome (congenital nuclear VI nerve palsy with neuronal misdirection)
- convergence spasm (impaired uniocular lateral gaze associated with small pupils bilaterally) – miosis.

The *vertical gaze centre* is less well defined than its horizontal equivalent but is believed to involve the rostral interstitial nucleus of the median longitudinal fasciculus in the midbrain at the level of the superior colliculus. Involvement is usually due to brain stem stroke or de-myelination. In III nerve palsy, diplopia is only experienced if it is partial and involving the inferior division as the lid is not affected and there is no ptosis covering the pupil. Double vision will be worse looking down and to the side of the lesion. Thyroid eye disease is a common cause of vertical diplopia. The patient often also complains about the appearance of lid retraction or proptosis or both. Disruption of the median longitudinal fasciculus anywhere along its course within the brain stem from the vestibular nuclei to the rostral interstitial nucleus of the median longitudinal fasciculus can cause a skew deviation. This can be concomitant (equal amounts of diplopia experienced in all directions of gaze) or incomitant (variable).

Cranial nerve IV is particularly susceptible to a blow to the back of the head as it is the only nerve to emerge from the posterior aspect of the brain stem. In the setting of trauma, damage is often bilateral. Fourth nerve palsies cause vertical diplopia, particularly noticeable on down-gaze.

Myasthenia gravis can mimic any cause of diplopia. Usually the diplopia is fatiguable and worsens during the day with variable drooping of the eyelids.

If the patient's complaint is of '*squint*' rather than double vision then this suggests non-paralytic squint resulting from defective binocular vision. An amblyopic eye is often diver-gent while monocular eye movements will be intact. The cover/uncover test is particularly helpful in detecting small concomitant squints in children.

Pupillary examination

➡ Examination sequence

→ Examine the pupils for shape and symmetry, taking account of ambient lighting.

→ Ask the patient to fix the eyes on a distant point straight ahead. Bring a bright torchlight from the side to shine on the pupil. Look for constriction of the pupil shone on (*direct light reflex*) and for constriction of the opposite pupil (*consensual light reflex*).

→ With the patient's vision fixed on a distant point, present an object about 6 inches in front of the eyes and ask the patient to focus on it (convergence). Look for pupil constriction (*accommodation reflex*).

Common abnormalities

Old family photographs are frequently useful in assessing the onset of pupillary abnormalities.

Essential anisocoria where one pupil is bigger than the other, but otherwise they behave normally, is a common normal variant.

In diabetes mellitus autonomic neuropathy may lead to the presence of small pupils that respond poorly to pharmacological dilatation. They may also mimic the *Argyll Robertson* pupils of syphilis (pin-point, irregular pupils that constrict only on convergence).

An *Adie* pupil is usually mid-dilated and only poorly responds to convergence. It is a result of ciliary ganglion malfunction within the orbit. With time it may shrink in size and be confused with an Argyll Robertson pupil. It is frequently bilateral and when associated with absent neurological reflexes it is termed the Holmes–Adie syndrome.

Damage to the optic nerve results in a relative afferent pupillary defect (*Marcus Gunn* pupil). Both pupils are dually innervated at the level of the midbrain. Normally, bright lights leads to constriction of both pupils regardless of which eye is illuminated. If one optic nerve is damaged, the pupils respond differently and the undamaged optic nerve becomes dominant. Whatever lighting the dominant optic nerve is exposed to will then determine the size of both pupils.

Colour vision

Red desaturation, the impaired ability to identify red objects, is an early indicator of pathology affecting the optic nerve.

➡ Examination sequence

→ Red-green colour vision can be assessed using *Ishihara* test plates (Fig. 8.23). These consist of coloured spots forming numbers which the patient is asked to pick out. The first plate is a test plate and, if the number is not seen, it indicates poor visual acuity or functional visual loss.

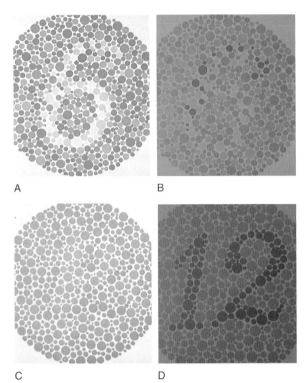

A   B

C   D

Fig. 8.23   Plates from the Ishihara series. A patient with normal vision reads both (A) and (C) without difficulty; however, a patient with red–green deficiency is unable to read the figure 6 (B) but is able to read the figure 12 (D) correctly.

Common abnormalities

- Optic nerve damage anywhere from the photoreceptors to the lateral geniculate nucleus of the thalamus causes impaired red-green colour vision that precedes loss of visual acuity.
- Congenital red-green blindness, an X-linked recessive condition that affects 7% of the male population.

Ophthalmoscopy

The eye should be examined first undilated to see the pupils and iris and then dilated using a mydriatic such as tropicamide to visualize the lens, vitreous and retina. When examining the fundus, only the optic nerve can be reliably assessed in the absence of pupillary dilatation. Many patients and clinicians have refractive errors. If patients have particularly thick lenses examine their eyes with their glasses in place. After dilating patients' eye(s) you should advise them not to drive or use machinery until the effect has completely worn off, which may take several hours.

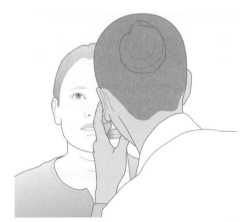

Fig. 8.24   Ophthalmoscopy: correct method. The patient's gaze is fixed on a distant point.

▶ Examination sequence

→ Start with a lens with a short focal length and advance the point of focus progressively forwards. Any abnormality will appear black within the red reflex. Unfortunately there is no standardization of the colour of the lens number for ophthalmoscopes. You cannot therefore use the colour of the lens number to indicate whether you are using a plus lens or not.

→ Examine the patient's right eye holding the ophthalmoscope in your right hand and vice versa (Fig. 8.24). Find '0' and then rotate the 'lenses' clockwise until the number 10 is obtained (plus '10'). This should be the same colour as the '1' clockwise to '0'. If not, you have gone too far. Place your other hand on the patient's forehead and ask the patient to look down.

→ Catch the lowered upper eyelid and gently retract it against the orbital rim. Holding the eyelid against the brow serves two purposes: the first to enable you to approach the patient's head as closely as possible without fear of bumping into it; and secondly to prevent the upper eyelid from obscuring your view.

→ Then ask the patient to fixate on a distant object straight ahead.

→ From a distance of about 10 cm bring the red reflex into focus.

→ Any opacity will appear black. In this way the cornea, iris and lens can be easily visualized.

→ Now come close to the patient's head such that you are touching your hand resting on the patient's forehead.

→ As you do so rotate the lenses anticlockwise, progressively increasing the focal length.

→ Observe for black opacities in the vitreous until the retina comes into focus.

Fundal examination

→ Follow the blood vessels as they extend from the optic disc in four directions: superotemporally, inferotemporally, superonasally, inferonasally (Fig. 8.25A).

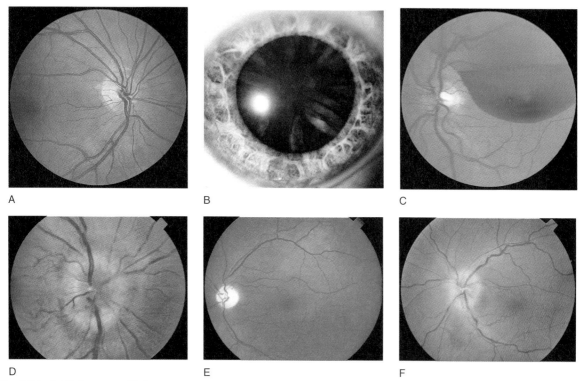

Fig. 8.25 **Ophthalmoscopy.** (A) Normal fundus. (B) Cortical cataract. (C) Preretinal haemorrhage. (D) Swollen optic disc. Papilloedema is suggested if visual acuity is unaffected, colour vision is normal and there is an enlarged blind spot. (E) Left optic atrophy. Note lack of pink neuroretinal rim. (F) Pale white swollen disc – highly suggestive of giant cell arteritis, particularly if associated with visual loss.

→ Ask the patient to look superiorly (examine horizontally), temporally (examine vertically), inferiorly (examine horizontally), nasally (examine vertically).

→ Finally locate the centre of the macula by asking the patient to look directly at the light. Ask the patient to keep the eye still while you look around the macula.

Common abnormalities

Cornea. Asymptomatic corneal scars from foreign bodies, often accompanied by remnants of rust, and previous ulceration are common.

Lens. There are three common forms of cataract:

• Peripheral cortical cataract is commonly seen in diabetes mellitus (Fig. 8.25B). It appears as incomplete black spokes coming from the periphery of the lens.

• Posterior subcapsular cataract, the typical 'steroid cataract', appears as a black opacity coming from the centre of the lens.

• Nuclear sclerosis ('ageing cataract') results in the normally transparent lens yellowing before it becomes brown, then black. It cannot usually be seen in the red reflex. Appropriate symptoms and the inability to bring the retina clearly into focus confirm its presence.

Vitreous. Vitreous haemorrhage appears as black blobs that move with eye movement (intra-gel vitreous haemorrhage). It may be the result of vitreous traction on retinal new vessels occurring in diabetic retinopathy and retinal vein occlusion. With age the vitreous detaches from the retina. Abnormal vitreous adhesion to normal retinal vessels may also cause vitreous haemorrhage. The patient may complain of 'flashes of light' which indicate that the retina may have been torn. If the haemorrhage is in the space between the retina and the posterior surface of the vitreous then a subhyaloid (preretinal) vitreous haemorrhage will be seen (Fig. 8.25C). In the setting of subarachnoid haemorrhage, subhyaloid vitreous haemorrhage is termed Terson's syndrome.

Optic disc. The optic disc enters the globe nasally and to see it you should approach the eye with the ophthalmoscope at a slight angle from the temporal side. Normally the disc is pink with a pigmented temporal margin. Pallor can be difficult to judge but if unilateral should always be accompanied by a relative afferent pupillary defect (Fig. 8.25E). Change the focus if you cannot see the disc clearly. Assess its shape and colour and vessels.

A swollen white optic disc (Fig. 8.25F) suggests arteritic anterior ischaemic optic neuropathy and is seen in giant cell arteritis and polyarteritis nodosa. Pseudophakic patients with artificial intraocular lenses following cataract extraction often have falsely pale discs. The optic neuropathy of glaucoma is associated with increased cup-to-disc ratio. Typically the vertical margins are affected first.

The optic disc is a common site for new vessel formation. Blurring of the disc margin indicates that it is raised. In the presence of an enlarged blind spot, blurring suggests distension of the optic nerve sheath. Reduced colour vision and a relative afferent pupillary response suggest an intrinsic optic nerve lesion.

Horizontal nerve fibre layer. The nerve fibre layer runs horizontally and over the retinal blood vessels. Lesions within this are therefore flat, striated and obscure retinal blood vessels.

Arteriolar occlusion (Table 8.9) causes 'cotton wool' spot formation (Fig. 8.26A) and flame haemorrhages (Fig. 8.26B).

Roth's spots are flame-shaped haemorrhages with a central cotton wool spot. They are caused by immune-complex deposition and are seen in subacute bacterial endocarditis and serum sickness (Ch. 2).

Retinitis due to infection with the herpes viruses causes a large, rapidly progressive area of 'cotton wool' spot formation. Differentiation can be difficult from the cotton wool spots caused by arterial occlusion and the two may

8.9	Common causes of arteriolar occlusion

- Accelerated hypertension,
- Retinal vein occlusion
- Diabetic retinopathy
- HIV retinopathy
- Systemic lupus erythematosus
- Systemic vasculitis

coexist in HIV infection. Cotton wool spots, however, do not enlarge over time whereas areas of retinitis do.

Retinal artery occlusion or embolism causes corresponding retinal pallor because of anterior retinal layer infarction. The optic nerve head, the fovea and the posterior retina, including the photoreceptors, are unaffected by retinal artery occlusion as their blood supply is from the short posterior ciliary arteries of the ophthalmic artery. This explains the cherry red spot sign of central retinal artery occlusion where the healthy fovea is surrounded by an oedematous retina (Fig. 8.26C). Retinal emboli may be seen at vessel bifurcations. As only the luminal contents of the vessel are normally apparent and not the wall, the embolus may appear to be paradoxically wider than the vessel it is lodged in.

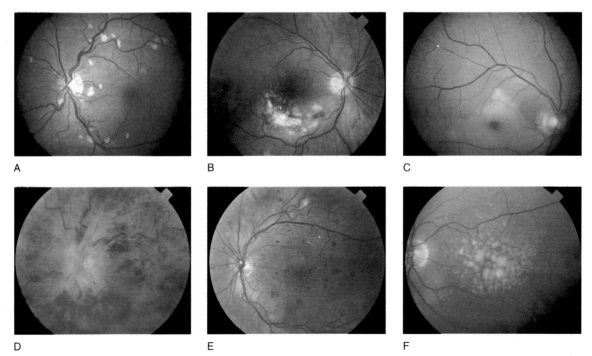

A   B   C

D   E   F

Fig. 8.26 Ophthalmoscopy. (A) Multiple cotton wool spots in HIV retinopathy. (B) Cytomegalovirus retinitis. Note: large superficial retinal infiltrate associated with flame haemorrhage. (C) Central retinal artery occlusion. Note: milky-white pale retina surrounding healthy pink fovea ('cherry red spot'). (D) Central retinal vein occlusion. Note widespread retinal haemorrhages and swollen optic disc. (E) Diabetic retinopathy. Note presence of multiple dot and blot haemorrhages indicating widespread capillary occlusion – a precursor of new vessel formation. (F) Retinal drusen. Numerous large drusen affecting the central retina (drusen maculopathy).

Vertical bipolar layer. The retinal capillaries are found in this layer. The commonest causes of capillary disease are diabetes mellitus and retinal vein occlusion (Fig. 8.26D). Capillary occlusion is also seen with HIV and radiation retinopathies. When a capillary occludes, microaneurysm formation may occur at the site. Capillaries are too small to visualize with the naked eye and on ophthalmoscopy microaneurysms appear as round dots separate from blood vessels. Microaneurysms can haemorrhage and leak leading to:

- *dot haemorrhages* – thin, vertical haemorrhages that may be difficult to differentiate from microaneurysms
- *blot haemorrhages* – larger, full-thickness bipolar layer haemorrhages that represent larger areas of capillary occlusion (Fig. 8.26E).

Intraretinal microvascular anomalies are perfused, dilated stumps of capillaries within areas of widespread capillary occlusion.

Venous beading is associated with adjacent capillary bed destruction.

Microaneurysms, dot and blot haemorrhages, intraretinal microvascular anomalies and venous beading are all surrogate markers for *capillary occlusion*. If sufficient capillaries occlude then *new vessels*, originating from postcapillary venules, will form. These new vessels grow in the potential space between the retina and the posterior vitreous surface. They can be differentiated from normal retinal vessels because instead of branching into smaller and finer vessels that eventually terminate, they form returning loops that distally are often more dilated then their proximal origins. New vessels grow intimately into the posterior surface of the vitreous and are found, unlike intraretinal microvascular abnormalities, at the border of perfused and non-perfused retina.

The vitreous is most strongly attached to the optic disc, and new vessels at this site are more likely to haemorrhage than elsewhere. New vessel formation is also commonly seen along the arcades, where the vitreous is less strongly adherent, and temporal to the macula.

Retinal veins and arteries share a common tunica adventitia where their branches cross over. Arteriosclerosis, commonly seen with hypertension, produces arteriovenous nipping, where the thickened artery, trapped by its tunica adventitia, twists and compresses the underlying vein. Arterio-sclerosis is the commonest cause of retinal vein occlusion. Raised intracapillary pressure subsequent to retinal vein occlusion results in capillary rupture and retinal haemorrhage. In central retinal vein occlusion, new vessel formation may occur on the iris (rubeosis iridis). Subsequent scarring of the drainage angle leads to rubeotic glaucoma, which is blinding and extremely painful. Eyes at risk often have a relative afferent pupillary defect and profound visual loss.

Arteriosclerotic retinal vein compression usually occurs in elderly patients or those with arteriosclerotic risk factors such as smoking, hypertension, hyperlipidaemia or diabetes mellitus. Raised intraocular pressure from chronic open-angle glaucoma is also a common cause. In younger patients, strongly consider idiopathic retinal vasculitis or thrombophilia.

Retinal pigment epithelium and photoreceptors. 90% of the blood supply to the eye goes, via the short posterior ciliary arteries, to fenestrated choroidal blood vessels that supply the retinal pigment epithelium and the posterior retina by diffusion. Disease of the retinal pigmented cells often leads to death of the overlying photoreceptors. This is seen as areas of depigmentation revealing the normally hidden choroidal vessels with adjacent clumps of precipitated pigment.

The commonest disorder of the retinal pigment epithelium is *age-related macular degeneration*. It is preceded by *drusen formation* – amorphous depositions under the retinal pigment epithelium (Fig. 8.26F). Drusen are differentiated from hard exudates, in people with diabetes mellitus, by the absence of adjacent microaneurysms. *Atrophic age-related macular degeneration* results in areas of pigment atrophy leading to gradual loss of central vision. *Neovascular age-related macular degeneration* is more severe and is associated with rapid onset visual distortion and central visual loss. Visual loss results from choroidal new vessels growing under the photoreceptors.

Hyperpigmentation of the retinal pigment epithelium (*choroidal naevi*) is a common asymptomatic finding. In contrast, *malignant melanomas* (Fig. 8.27A) are usually symptomatic, elevated, progress in size and may be associated with retinal detachment and vitreous haemorrhage.

Choroiditis (inflammation of the choroid) appears as white spots (Fig. 8.27B). When active they have a white poorly defined, fluffy edge with an overlying hazy vitreous, causing blurring of vision. When inactive, they have a well-defined pigmented edge. As the nerve fibre layer is not involved, the overlying retinal blood vessels are unaffected and clearly visible as they cross the choroiditis. Choroiditis is associated with toxoplasmosis, sarcoidosis and tuberculosis.

THE TRIGEMINAL (V) NERVE

The functions of the V nerve include sensation to the face, mouth and part of the dura and motor supply to the muscles of the jaw involved in chewing.

Anatomy

The cell bodies of the sensory fibres are located in the trigeminal (Gasserian) ganglion which lies in a cavity (Meckel's cave) in the petrous temporal dura (Fig. 8.28). **253**

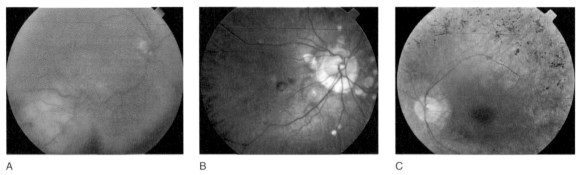

A   B   C

Fig. 8.27 Ophthalmoscopy. (A) Melanoma. Large, and more significantly, raised, pigmented lesion deep to the retinal vessels, indicating its choroid origin. (B) Choroiditis. Multiple white lesions (multifocus choroiditis). Note additional presence of greenish choroidal neovascular membrane with adjacent retinal haemorrhage. (C) Retinitis pigmentosa. A triad of optic atrophy, attenuated retinal vessels and pigmentary changes. Pigmentary changes typically start peripherally in association with a ring scotoma and symptoms of night blindness.

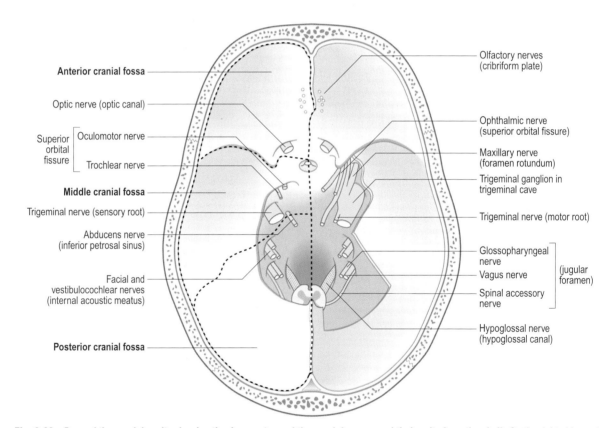

Fig. 8.28 Base of the cranial cavity showing the dura mater and the cranial nerves and their exits from the skull. On the right side, part of the tentorium cerebelli and the roof of the trigeminal cave have been removed.

Examine this patient with sudden loss of vision in one eye

1. Examine the pulse for arrhythmia (*atrial fibrillation*).
2. Measure the blood pressure (*hypertension*).
3. Listen for cardiac murmurs and carotid bruits (*valvular heart disease, carotid artery stenosis*).
4. Measure the visual acuity in both eyes.
5. Check colour vision (*optic nerve disease*).
6. Assess both peripheral visual fields for homonymous hemianopia (*cerebrovascular accident*) and the affected eye's visual field for an altitudinal or arcuate field defect (*optic nerve disease*).
7. Examine for a relative afferent pupillary defect (*optic nerve disease*).
8. Look for pain on eye movement (*optic neuritis*).
9. Perform ophthalmoscopy. The optic nerve is:
   – white and swollen in arteritic anterior ischaemic optic neuropathy (*giant cell arteritis*)
   – pink and swollen in non-arteritic anterior ischaemic optic neuropathy.
10. Look at the optic fundus:
   – numerous retinal haemorrhages indicates venous occlusion
   – pallor indicates arterial occlusion
   – retinal embolism seen at arterial bifurcations (*thromboembolic disease*).

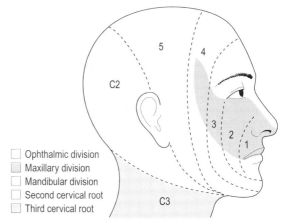

□ Ophthalmic division
□ Maxillary division
□ Mandibular division
□ Second cervical root
□ Third cervical root

Fig. 8.29 Trigeminal nerve. Areas 1 to 5 indicate distribution of pain fibres in spinal tract of V with 1 = pons and 5 = upper cervical cord.

Examine this patient with acute redness and pain in one eye

1. Assess the distribution of the redness:
   – diffuse redness suggests *conjunctivitis, episcleritis, scleritis*
   – redness of the lower inner eyelid suggests *conjunctivitis*
   – circumciliary injection suggests *keratitis, iritis* or *angle-closure glaucoma*
   – redness resolving with phenylephrine drops suggests *episcleritis*.
2. Look for evidence of ocular discharge (*conjunctivitis*).
3. Examine the clarity of the iris: a hazy iris suggests corneal oedema (*acute angle-closure glaucoma*) or aqueous chamber inflammatory cells (*acute iritis*).
4. Look for the small irregularly shaped pupil of *acute iritis*, or an oval, mid-dilated, poorly reactive pupil (*acute-angle closure glaucoma*).
5. Ask the patient to move the eye – pain indicates *scleritis*.
6. Examine the red reflex with direct ophthalmoscopy: *corneal ulceration* appears black – confirm with fluorescein dye.
7. Examine the urine for microscopic haematuria or proteinuria (*systemic vasculitis*).

The peripheral processes of these cells give rise to the three major branches of the nerve:

• ophthalmic (V_1)
• maxillary (V_2)
• mandibular (V_3).

The ophthalmic branch leaves the ganglion and passes forward to the superior orbital fissure via the wall of the cavernous sinus; the maxillary passes from the ganglion to leave the skull by the foramen rotundum; and the mandibular exits the skull via the foramen ovale.

In addition to the skin of the upper nose, upper eyelid, forehead and scalp V_1 supplies sensation to the eye (cornea and conjunctiva) and the mucous membranes of the

sphenoidal and ethmoid sinuses and upper nasal cavity. The maxillary nerve also contains sensory fibres from the mucous membranes of the upper mouth, roof of pharynx, gums, teeth and palate of the upper jaw and the maxillary, sphenoidal and ethmoid sinuses. The mandibular division supplies the floor of the mouth, common sensation (i.e. not taste) to the anterior two-thirds of the tongue, the gums and teeth of the lower jaw, mucosa of the cheek and the temporomandibular joint in addition to the skin of the lower lips and jaw area (Fig. 8.29).

From the trigeminal ganglion the V nerve passes to the pons. The central sensory connections are three nuclei: the principal sensory nucleus (touch, joint position sense); the mesencephalic nucleus (unconscious proprioception) and the spinal trigeminal tract and nucleus (pain and temperature). The latter descends from the pons to the C2 segment of the spinal cord, and the topographical arrangement of fibres within the tract is complex.

The motor fibres of V run in the mandibular branch and innervate the temporalis, masseter, medial and lateral pterygoids (muscles of mastication) and some smaller muscles not examined clinically.

Examination

There are four functions of the V nerve: sensory, motor and two reflexes.

▶ Examination sequence

Sensory
➜ Test light touch and superficial pain in the territories of V_1, V_2 and V_3.
➜ Use an orange stick to test touch sensation on the anterior two-thirds of the tongue.

Motor
→ Inspect for wasting of the muscles of mastication.
→ Feel the masseters, estimating their bulk, when the patient clenches the teeth.
→ Ask the patient to open the jaw against resistance, noting any deviation.

Corneal reflex
→ Ask the patient to look upwards to the ceiling and gently depress the lower eyelid.
→ Very lightly touch the lateral edge of the cornea with a wisp of damp cotton wool (Fig. 8.30).
→ Look for both direct and consensual blinking.

Jaw jerk
→ Ask the patient to let his mouth hang loosely open. Place your forefinger in the midline between lower lip and chin.
→ Percuss your finger with the tendon hammer (Fig. 8.31).

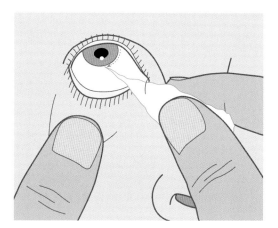

Fig. 8.30 Testing the corneal reflex.

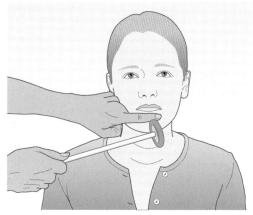

Fig. 8.31 Eliciting the jaw jerk.

Common abnormalities

• Unilateral loss of sensation in one or more branches of the V nerve may result from direct injury in association with facial fractures (particularly V_2) or local invasion by cancer.
• Lesions within the cavernous sinuses, e.g. cancer often result in loss of the corneal reflex and V_1 cutaneous sensory loss. Dysfunction of III, IV and VI may accompany such lesions.
• Herpes zoster can affect the trigeminal ganglion and result in loss of all sensory modalities.
• A brisk jaw jerk occurs with bilateral upper motor neurone lesions above the level of the pons. It is usually absent in healthy people but can be brisk in anxious individuals.

THE FACIAL (VII) NERVE

The facial nerve sends motor fibres to the muscles of facial expression and parasympathetic secretomotor fibres to the lacrimal, submandibular and sublingual salivary glands (via nervus intermedius) and receives taste sensation from the anterior two-thirds of the tongue (by its chorda tympani branch). It also provides the efferent supply to several reflexes.

Anatomy

From its motor nucleus in the lower pons, fibres of the VII nerve pass back to loop around the VI nucleus before emerging from the lateral pontomedullary junction in close association with the VIII nerve and together they enter the internal acoustic meatus. At the lateral end of the acoustic meatus the VII continues in the facial canal in the temporal bone, exiting the skull via the stylomastoid foramen and passing through the parotid gland it gives off its terminal branches. In its course in the facial canal it gives off branches to the stapedius muscle and its parasympathetic fibres as well as being joined by the taste fibres of the chorda tympani (Figs 8.32 and 8.33).

Examination

Clinical examination is usually confined to motor function and taste.

▶ Examination sequence

Motor function
→ Inspect carefully for any asymmetry of the face as a whole, or blinking or eye closure. Observe for spontaneous movement or any involuntary movements.
→ Ask the patient to wrinkle his forehead or look up above his head (which has the same effect). Then ask the patient

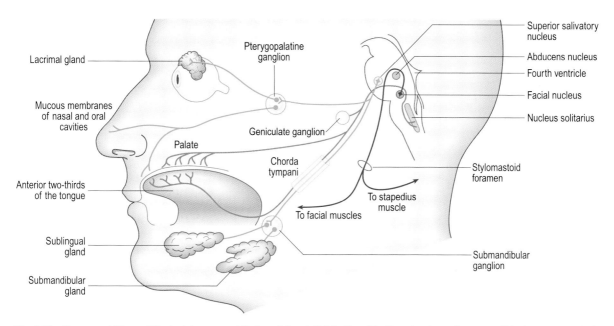

Fig. 8.32   Component fibres of the facial nerve and their peripheral distribution. [**Red**], motor; [**green**], sensory, [**blue**], parasympathetic.

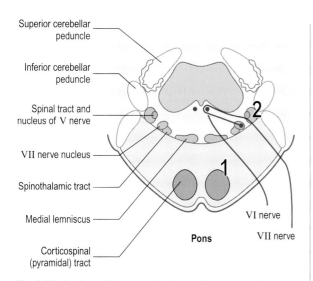

Fig. 8.33   Lesions of the pons. Lesions at (1) may result in ipsilateral VI and VII nerve palsies and contralateral hemiplegia; at (2) ipsilateral cerebellar signs and impaired sensation on the ipsilateral side of the face and on the contralateral side of the body may occur.

to bare his teeth. Demonstrating yourself and then asking the patient to mimic is often helpful. Look for any asymmetry.

→ Test power by giving the instruction 'Screw your eyes tightly shut and stop me from opening them', and then 'Blow out your cheeks with your mouth closed' (Fig. 8.34).

Taste

→ Instruct the patient not to speak during the test.

→ Ask the patient to put out his tongue.

→ Use cotton buds dipped in sugar (sweet), salt, vinegar (sour) and quinine (bitter) solutions. Apply them to the anterior two-thirds of the tongue.

→ Ask the patient to point to sweet, salt, sour and bitter on a card to indicate the response.

→ Between each test ask the patient to rinse his mouth with water.

Schirmer's test (see p. 312)

Common abnormalities

In a unilateral lower motor neurone lesion of VII, there is weakness of both upper and lower facial muscles. The inability to close the eye is often accompanied by Bell's phenomenon in which the eyeball rolls upwards. This movement is a normal response to eye closure (Fig. 8.35).

In unilateral upper motor neurone lesions, facial paresis is marked in the lower facial muscles with relative sparing of the upper face. This is because there is bilateral cortical innervation of the upper facial muscles. While the nasolabial fold may be flattened and the corner of the mouth drooping, eye closure is usually well preserved. Involuntary emotional movements, e.g. smiling, may be preserved in the presence of paresis of voluntary movement as they employ different neural pathways.

In lesions distal to the stylomastoid foramen, taste and lacrimation are preserved. Impairment (*hypogeusia*) or loss

257

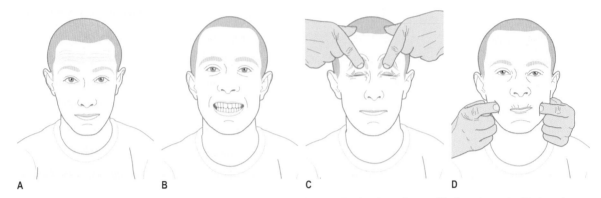

Fig. 8.34 **Testing the motor function of the facial nerves.** Ask the patient to (A) raise the eyebrows, (B) show the teeth, (C) close the eyes against resistance and (D) blow out the cheeks.

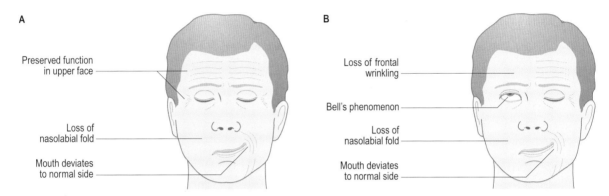

Fig. 8.35 **Types of facial weakness.** Caused in (A) by lesion of precentral area of pyramidal tract (upper motor neurone); (B) by lesion of facial nerve or nucleus (lower motor neurone), also showing Bell's phenomenon.

(*ageusia*) of taste is most commonly due to oral conditions but may accompany damage to the VII nerve in the facial canal or proximally. Damage involving the nerve to stapedius can result in sounds appearing louder than normal (*hyperacusis*).

Bilateral facial palsy is less common than unilateral lesions but both upper and lower motor neurone disorders occasionally occur. Extrapyramidal disorders, particularly Parkinson's disease, can result in a loss of spontaneous facial movements, and adverse effects of antiparkinsonian drugs include involuntary facial movements. These movements are referred to as *dyskinesias* and commonly involve the mouth and tongue (*orolingual*) or mouth and face (*orofacial*) or may take the form of facial grimacing.

Bell's palsy is an acute condition caused by swelling of the facial nerve in the facial canal resulting in lower motor neurone paralysis of VII. It may be associated with hypogeusia and hyperacusis.

Ramsay Hunt syndrome occurs when there is herpes zoster infection of the geniculate (facial) ganglion. This results in a severe lower motor neurone facial palsy and a painful vesicular eruption within the external auditory meatus.

THE VESTIBULOCOCHLEAR (VIII) NERVE

The VIII nerve has vestibular and cochlear branches largely concerned with equilibrium and hearing respectively.

Anatomy

The auditory fibres of the cochlear branch arise in the cochlea, pass along the internal acoustic meatus, join the brain stem at the pontomedullary junction and synapse in the cochlear (dorsal and ventral) nuclei. Second-order fibres ascend to the trapezoid body and lateral lemniscus, then to the inferior colliculus and medial geniculate body. Fibres from these pass to the auditory cortex in the superior temporal gyrus. As fibres cross throughout this pathway, each ear sends messages to both hemispheres.

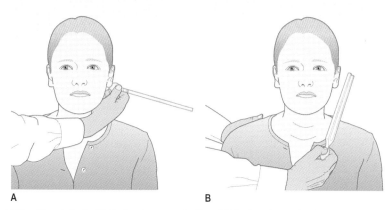

Fig. 8.36 Rinne's test. (A) Testing bone conduction. (B) Testing air conduction.

Vestibular nerve cells are bipolar with cell bodies in the vestibular ganglion. They convey impulses from the utricle, saccule and semicircular canals to a complex of four vestibular nuclei in the pons and medulla. The connections of these nuclei are numerous and complicated, with projections to the temporal lobe, cerebellum, lower motor neurones and the III, IV and VI nerve nuclei. The vestibular part of the VIII nerve, therefore, has a central role in spatial orientation and the control of body equilibrium.

Examination

Formal testing of cochlear and vestibular function requires specialist equipment but this should not detract from the value of the tests described below. Hearing loss may be suspected during history taking and a complaint of vertigo or an abnormality of posture or gait can point to a vestibular lesion. Examine the external auditory meatus (see Ch. 9) before undertaking the tests described. Exclude cervical lesions before testing for positional nystagmus or the oculocephalic reflex.

▶ Examination sequence (cochlear)

Whisper test (see p. 288)
→ Position the patient's head so that he cannot lip-read what you say.
→ Place your finger in the external auditory meatus of the patient's non-test ear and move it constantly to produce a masking noise.
→ Ask the patient to repeat words and numbers that you speak. Initially whisper but increase in volume as necessary.

Tuning fork tests (Rinne's and Weber's: see p. 288)
→ Use a 256 or 512 Hz tuning fork.
→ Rinne's test: Place the vibrating tuning fork over the mastoid process and then about 1 cm from the external auditory meatus. Ask the patient which is louder (Fig. 8.36).

→ Weber's test: Place the vibrating tuning fork in the midline high on the forehead. Ask where the sound is loudest (Fig. 8.37).

Common abnormalities (cochlear)

If deafness is unilateral the tuning fork tests determine whether it is *conductive* (due to a lesion of the external auditory meatus, tympanic membrane, middle ear cavity or ossicles interfering with sounds reaching the cochlea) or *sensorineural* (caused by damage to the cochlea or VIII nerve). Normally air conduction is better than bone conduction so that in Rinne's test the sound is louder at the external auditory meatus than at the mastoid bone. If bone conduction is better than air conduction in this test, it indicates a conductive defect. In sensorineural deafness Rinne's test is positive.

In Weber's test the sound is heard equally in both ears in normal people. In unilateral conductive deafness the sound

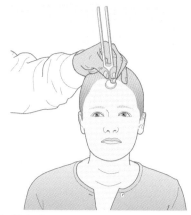

Fig. 8.37 Weber's test.

8.10 Common causes of deafness	
Cause	**Effect**
Conduction deafness	
Wax in the external ear canal Damage to tympanic membranes Fluid in inner ear Ossicular chain disruption (head injury) Otosclerosis (degenerative)	Diminished hearing on affected side Rinne's test: bone conduction louder Weber's test: louder on affected side
Sensorineural deafness	
Damage to cochlear nerve and organ of Corti Acoustic neuroma Transverse fracture of petrous temporal bone Bilaterally in the elderly (degenerative)	Rinne's test: air conduction louder Diminished hearing on affected side Weber's test: heard on unaffected side

appears louder in the deaf ear. In sensorineural deafness the sound is heard in the unaffected ear.

Common causes of conductive deafness are obstructions of the external auditory meatus, e.g. wax, otosclerosis and middle ear diseases (Table 8.10). Sensorineural deafness occurs with age (*presbyacusis*), Ménière's disease, acoustic neuroma, head injury and drug- or noise-induced damage.

▶ Examination sequence (vestibular)

Induction of positional nystagmus (Dix-Hallpike's test: see p. 289)
➡ Position the patient seated on the couch so that when supine the head and neck will overlap the end of the couch.
➡ Ask the patient to keep the eyes open throughout the test and explain what you are going to do.
➡ Quickly lower the head of the couch so the patient is supine with the head tilted 30° below the horizontal and turned 30–45° to one side.

➡ Maintain this position and look for nystagmus for 20–30 seconds.
➡ Repeat the procedure turning the head to the other side.

Oculocephalic (doll's eye) reflex
➡ With the patient supine hold his head in both hands with your thumbs holding the eyes open.
➡ Rock the head briskly from side to side, noting the movement of the eyes.

Oculovestibular reflex
➡ Examine the external auditory meatus to ensure it is free of wax and that the tympanic membrane is intact. The test should not be performed if there is tympanic perforation.
➡ Place the patient supine on the couch.
➡ Flex the patient's head to 30°.
➡ With a bowl held at the side of the head to collect the water, slowly irrigate 50 ml of iced water into the external auditory meatus. Look for deviation of the eyes for about 30 seconds.

Common abnormalities (vestibular)

Positional vertigo and nystagmus are 'peripheral' when they result from lesions of the labyrinth, such as benign paroxysmal positional vertigo, or 'central' when they are due to damage to the vestibular nerve or its connections. The latter is uncommon but may occur after trauma or with brain stem demyelination.

In normal individuals the Hallpike manoeuvre does not induce nystagmus. In peripheral lesions, vertigo and nystagmus may occur after a delay of 5–15 seconds. They decline as the position is maintained, and fatigue if the test is repeated. With central lesions there is no latency or fatigue, and vertigo is often less prominent or absent.

The normal response to the oculocephalic test is that the eyes move in the opposite direction to the head movement – as occurs in a doll (Fig. 8.38). In cases of brain stem damage this eye movement may be lost.

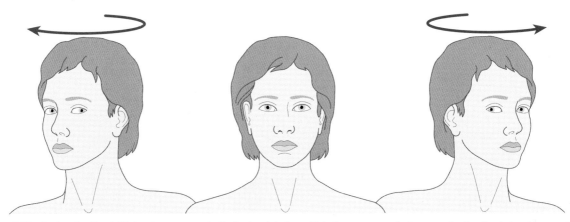

Fig. 8.38 Performing the doll's head manoeuvre in the horizontal plane. Note the eyes move in the opposite direction to head movement.

The oculovestibular reflex test is primarily used to assess for brain stem death. The normal response to ice-water irrigation in a conscious patient is nystagmus with the quick phase away from the stimulus. In a comatose patient with an intact brain stem, tonic movements occur towards the irrigated ear without the quick phase movement away. When there is severe brain damage no response occurs.

THE GLOSSOPHARYNGEAL (IX) AND VAGUS (X) NERVES

The IX and X nerves are intimately related anatomically. Both contain sensory, motor and autonomic components.

Anatomy

Both nerves arise as several roots from the lateral medulla and leave the skull together via the jugular foramen. The IX nerve passes down and forward to supply the stylopharyngeus muscle, the mucosa of the pharynx, tonsillar area and posterior third of the tongue and sends parasympathetic fibres to the parotid gland. The X nerve courses down in the carotid sheath and into the thorax, giving off several branches including pharyngeal and recurrent laryngeal branches which provide motor supply to the pharyngeal, soft palate and laryngeal muscles. The main nuclei of these nerves in the medulla are the nucleus ambiguus (motor), the dorsal motor vagal nucleus (parasympathetic) and the solitary nucleus (visceral sensation).

Examination

The glossopharyngeal nerve mainly carries sensation from the pharynx and tonsils and sensation and taste from the posterior third of the tongue. The vagus nerve carries important sensory information but also innervates upper pharyngeal and laryngeal muscles.

Testing pharyngeal sensation and the gag reflex are unpleasant for the patient and should be restricted to patients with swallowing difficulties (*dysphagia*) or nasal regurgitation.

➡ Examination sequence

- ➔ Assess the patient's speech for dysarthria or dysphonia (p. 239).
- ➔ While the patient says 'Aaah' look at the movements of the palate and uvula using a torch.
- ➔ Test pharyngeal sensation using an orange stick *gently*.
- ➔ Elicit the gag (pharyngeal) reflex by touching the posterior pharyngeal wall or faucial pillars with a tongue depressor.
- ➔ Apply the stimulus to both sides in turn.
- ➔ Ask the patient to puff out his cheeks with the lips tightly closed. Look and feel for air escaping from the nose.

Normally both sides of the palate elevate symmetrically and the uvula remains in the midline. In order to puff out the cheeks, the palate must elevate and occlude the nasopharynx. If palatal movement is weak, air will escape audibly through the nose. The gag reflex produces elevation of the palate and the pharynx, very similar to the motions seen at the beginning of vomiting.

Common abnormalities

Isolated unilateral IX nerve lesions are rare. Damage to the vagus on one side leads to deviation of the uvula when the soft palate is elevated by saying 'Aaah'. Damage to the recurrent laryngeal branch of X causes dysphonia and a 'bovine' cough. Causes include lung cancer, thyroid surgery, mediastinal tumours and aortic arch aneurysm. Bilateral X nerve lesions cause both bulbar and pseudobulbar palsies. They are associated with dysphagia, dysarthria and either lower or upper motor neurone lesions of the hypoglossal (XII) nerve. Less severe cases can result in nasal regurgitation of fluids and nasal air escape when the cheeks are puffed out.

Some clinical conditions causing IX and X nerve lesions are shown in Table 8.11.

THE ACCESSORY (XI) NERVE

The accessory nerve has two components: a cranial part closely related to the vagus and a spinal part which provides fibres to the upper trapezius and the sternocleidomastoid muscles. The spinal component is discussed here.

Anatomy

The spinal nuclei arise from the anterior horn cells of C1–5, and fibres emerge from the spinal cord, ascend through the

8.11 Common causes of IX and X nerve lesions
Unilateral of IX and X
• Skull base tumours (including meningioma) • Skull base fracture • Lateral medullary syndrome
Recurrent laryngeal
• Lung cancer • Mediastinal lymphoma • Aortic arch aneurysm • Post-thyroid surgery
Bilateral X

• Progressive bulbar palsy (motor neurone disease)
• Bilateral supranuclear lesions (pseudobulbar palsy):
  – cerebrovascular disease
  – multiple sclerosis

foramen magnum, and exit via the jugular foramen. They pass posteriorly to supply the upper half of trapezius and the sternocleidomastoid.

⮊ Examination sequence

→ Face the patient and inspect the sternocleidomastoid muscles for wasting or hypertrophy and palpate them to assess their bulk.

→ To test power in the left sternocleidomastoid, ask the patient to turn the head to the right while you provide resistance with your hand placed on the right side of the patient's chin (Fig. 8.39B). Reverse the procedure to check the right sternocleidomastoid.

→ Stand behind the patient to inspect the trapezius muscle for wasting or asymmetry.

→ Ask the patient to shrug the shoulders as you apply downward pressure with your hands (Fig. 8.39A).

Common abnormalities

Isolated XI lesions are uncommon but the nerve may be damaged during surgery in the posterior triangle of the neck, penetrating injuries or local invasion by tumour. Wasting of the upper fibres of trapezius may be associated with displacement of the upper vertebral border of the scapula away from the spine while the lower border is displaced towards it. Wasting and weakness of the sterno-cleidomastoids is characteristic of dystrophia myotonica, and weakness occurs in other myopathies and in myasthenia gravis.

THE HYPOGLOSSAL (XII) NERVE

Anatomy

The XII nerve nucleus lies in the dorsal medulla beneath the floor of the fourth ventricle. The nerve emerges anteriorly and exits the skull in the hypoglossal canal, passing to the root of the tongue where its branches innervate the tongue muscles.

⮊ Examination sequence

→ Ask the patient to open his mouth. Look at the tongue at rest for wasting, fasciculation or involuntary movement.

→ Ask the patient to protrude the tongue. Look for deviation or involuntary movement.

→ Ask the patient to move the tongue from side to side.

→ Test power by asking the patient to press the tongue against the inside of each cheek in turn while you press from the outside with your finger.

→ Assess speech (see p. 239) by asking the patient to say 'yellow lorry'.

Common abnormalities

Unilateral lower motor neurone lesions lead to wasting of the tongue on the affected side and deviation to that side on protrusion (Fig. 8.40). Bilateral lower motor neurone damage results in global wasting – the tongue lies thin and shrunken like an autumn leaf. When associated with lesions of IX, X and XI, typically in motor neurone disease, these features are called bulbar palsy.

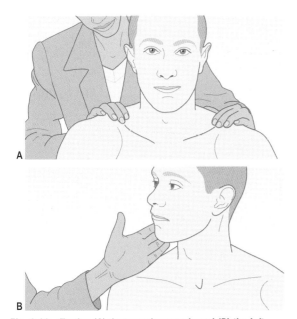

Fig. 8.39 Testing (A) the trapezius muscle and (B) the left sternocleidomastoid.

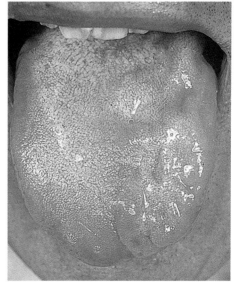

Fig. 8.40 Left hypoglossal nerve lesion.

Upper motor neurone lesions on one side are uncommon, while bilateral lesions lead to a spastic, bunched-up, almost conical or acorn-like tongue. Bilateral supranuclear lesions of IX–XII are called pseudobulbar palsy and usually result from vascular disease, motor neurone disease or occasionally multiple sclerosis.

In addition to dysarthria most cases of severe tongue weakness are associated with dysphagia.

Tremor of the resting or protruded tongue is common in Parkinson's disease. Other involuntary movements of the mouth and tongue (*orolingual dyskinesias*) are often drug induced (e.g. antiparkinsonism drugs and neuroleptics).

Examination of the cranial nerves is summarized in Table 8.12.

8.12	Cranial nerve examination at a glance
I	Sense of smell in each nostril
II	Visual acuity, visual fields, fundi and pupillary light response
III, IV and VI	Eye movements, accommodation and nystagmus
V	Facial sensation, masseters, corneal reflex and jaw jerk
VII	Muscles of facial expression and taste over anterior two-thirds of tongue
VIII	Whisper test, Rinne's and Weber's tests, and vestibular tests
IX	Pharyngeal sensation
X	Palate movements and gag reflex
XI	Trapezius and sternocleidomastoid
XII	Tongue appearance and movements

Examine this patient with suspected brain stem death

1. Confirm there is a cause of irreversible brain damage.
2. Exclude reversible causes of coma, e.g. *hypothermia, hypoglycaemia, drug overdose.*
3. Confirm patient is ventilator dependent: when disconnected, arterial PCO_2 should be > 7.0 kPa with no spontaneous respiration.
4. Examine pupillary reflexes: pupils fixed in diameter with no response to a sharp change in light intensity.
5. Examine corneal reflexes, which should be absent.
6. Irrigate the external auditory meati with iced water: oculovestibular reflexes should be absent with no nystagmus.
7. Pass a suction catheter into the oropharynx and trachea: no gag reflex should be produced.
8. The above tests should be repeated by two experienced clinicians on two occasions at least 24 hours apart.

THE EXAMINATION OF THE MOTOR SYSTEM

The assessment of the motor system is considered under the following headings:

- inspection and palpation of muscles
- assessment of tone
- examination of reflexes
- testing movement and power
- testing coordination.

Anatomy

Motor fibres together with input from other systems involved in the control of movement, including extrapyramidal, cerebellar, vestibular and proprioceptive afferents, all converge on the cell bodies of neurones in the anterior horn of the grey matter in the spinal cord. These cell bodies are referred to as the anterior horn cells of the lower motor neurones that form the final common pathway conveying impulses to the muscle (Fig. 8.41).

INSPECTION AND PALPATION

- Proper inspection of the muscles requires the fullest exposure that is in keeping with the patient's comfort and modesty.
- Look for asymmetry, inspecting both proximally and distally. Note any deformities such as clawing of the hands or pes cavus. Examine specifically for wasting or hypertrophy, fasciculation and involuntary movement.
- Palpate muscles to assess their bulk.

Common abnormalities

Muscle bulk. Lower motor neurone lesions may cause wasting in specific muscles. Longstanding or developmental upper motor neurone damage can result in disuse atrophy of muscle groups, but wasting is not seen in acute lesions. Muscle disorders may result in muscle wasting, usually

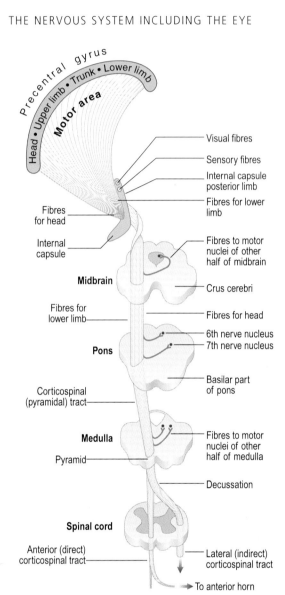

Fig. 8.41 The motor pathways.

Myoclonic jerks are sudden shock-like contractions of one or more muscles which may be focal or diffuse. They may occur singly or repetitively. Healthy individuals may experience these when falling asleep or surprised by a sudden noise. They may also occur in association with epilepsy, diffuse brain damage and dementias.

Tremor. This is an oscillatory movement about a joint or a group of joints resulting from alternating contraction and relaxation of muscles. Tremors are described according to their speed (fast or slow), amplitude (fine or coarse) and whether they are maximal at rest, on maintaining a posture or on carrying out an active movement.

Physiological tremor seen with anxiety is a fine, fast postural tremor. It occurs in hyperthyroidism and those who take alcohol or caffeine to excess.

The slow, coarse tremor of Parkinson's disease is worst at rest and reduced by voluntary movement. It is more common in the upper limbs and usually asymmetrical. The traditional description of a 'pill rolling' tremor (movement of the thumb across the finger tips) is not particularly helpful.

Cerebellar damage is the most common cause of tremor which is absent at rest but maximal on movement, so-called action or *intention* tremor.

Coarse, even violent, action tremors are associated with lesions of the red nucleus (*rubral* tremor) and subthalamic nucleus. They are most often caused by damage from vascular disease or multiple sclerosis.

Other involuntary movements. These include *dystonias*, *chorea* and *athetosis*, which are often caused by disturbance to extrapyramidal pathways. Dystonia is the slow development of an abnormal posture, often of the limb or the neck, which is maintained. Chorea and athetosis are both writhing movements; the former tends to be irregular, jerky and brief, the latter is slower, and more sustained. *Choreoathetoid* movements refer to something between the two (or uncertainty on the part of the observer!).

Dyskinesia is a group term for these types of involuntary movements, particularly when they arise as an adverse effect of neuroleptics and antiparkinsonian agents.

Tics or *habit spasms* are more stereotyped and essentially normal movements which recur involuntarily.

proximal (the notable exception is dystrophia myotonica where it is distal); rheumatoid arthritis is associated with wasting of the small muscles of the hands, and widespread wasting occurs in cachexia. Certain occupations and sports lead to muscle hypertrophy. This can also occur in muscular dystrophy but differs on palpation from healthy hypertrophic muscles with a 'doughy' feeling.

Fasciculation. These look like irregular ripples or twitches under the skin overlying muscles at rest. They occur in lower motor neurone disease, usually in wasted muscles. Flicking the skin over wasted muscle may elicit fasciculation. Non-pathological fasciculation occasionally occurs after vigorous exercise in healthy people.

Palpate muscles to confirm wasting. Wasted muscles feel 'flabby'. Inflammation of muscles (*myositis*) may be accompanied by tenderness and some forms of acute muscle necrosis (*rhabdomyolysis*) produces a firm 'woody' feel.

TONE

For clinical purposes tone is the resistance felt by the examiner when moving a joint passively through its range of movement.

Examination sequence

→ The examination room should be warm.
→ Ask the patient to lie supine on the examination couch.
→ Ask the patient to relax and 'go floppy'.
→ Passive movements of the joints should be through as full a range as possible and both slowly and quickly.
→ In the upper limb hold the patient's hand as if shaking hands, using your other hand to support the patient's elbow. Then rotate the forearm, flex and extend the wrist, elbow and shoulder, varying the speed and direction of movement.
→ With the lower limb begin by rolling or rotating the leg from side to side, then briskly lift the knee into a flexed position (Fig. 8.42A, B).
→ *Knee clonus:* with the patient relaxed and the knee extended, sharply push with your thumb and forefinger above the patella towards the foot, sustaining the pressure for a few seconds.
→ *Ankle clonus:* support the patient's leg with both the knee and ankle resting in 90° flexion. Briskly dorsiflex and partially evert the foot and sustain the pressure (Fig. 8.42C).

Common abnormalities

Muscle tone may be decreased (*hypotonia*) or increased (*hypertonia*). There are two principal types of hypertonia: *spasticity* and *rigidity*.

Hypotonia is difficult to detect in a relaxed patient and its value as a sign is open to misinterpretation. Excess hypotonia or flaccidity may occur in lower motor neurone lesions and is usually associated with muscle wasting, weakness and hyporeflexia. It may be a feature of cerebellar disease and occur in the early phases of cerebral or spinal shock when the plegic limbs are atonic prior to developing spasticity.

Spasticity is a velocity-dependent resistance to passive movement (i.e. it is detected with quick movements) and is a feature of upper motor neurone pathology. It is usually accompanied by weakness, hyperreflexia, an extensor plantar response and sometimes clonus. In mild forms it is detected as a 'catch' at the beginning or end of passive movement but in severe cases it limits the range of movement possible and may be associated with contracture. In the upper limbs it may be more obvious on attempted extension; in the legs it is more evident on flexion.

Rigidity is a sustained resistance throughout the range of movement and is most easily detected when the limb is moved slowly. In Parkinson's disease this is classically described as 'lead-pipe' or 'plastic' rigidity. In the presence of tremor there may be a regular interruption to the movement giving it a jerky feel. This is 'cog-wheel' rigidity. Other extrapyramidal conditions may also be associated with rigidity.

Clonus is a rhythmic series of contractions evoked by sudden stretch of the muscles. It can occur in healthy

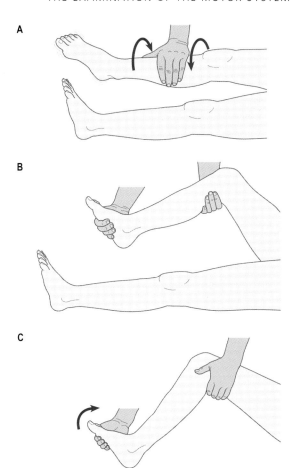

Fig. 8.42 Testing for tone. (A) Rock the leg to and fro. (B) Check the full range of movement at the knee. (C) Testing for ankle clonus.

individuals spontaneously when they are tired or apprehensive. When sustained it indicates upper motor neurone damage and is accompanied by spasticity.

DEEP TENDON REFLEXES

Anatomy

A tendon reflex is the reflex contraction of a muscle in response to stretch. It is mediated by a reflex consisting of an afferent (sensory) and an efferent (motor) neurone with one synapse between (i.e. a monosynaptic reflex). Muscle stretch activates the muscle spindles, which send a burst of afferent signals that in turn lead to direct efferent impulses, causing contraction of muscles. These stretch reflex arcs are subserved by a particular spinal cord segment which is modified by the influence of descending upper motor neurones and other neurones.

Examination

The tendon and not the muscle is struck by the hammer when testing the reflexes. The patient should be as relaxed and comfortable as possible as anxiety and pain can cause an increased response. For similar reasons deep reflexes may be performed best after testing tone and before testing power and coordination in the motor examination sequence. The technique is to flex your wrists and allow the weight of the hammer head to determine the strength of the blow. Responses are documented as:

- hyperactive (+++)
- normal (++)
- diminished (+)
- absent (−)
- when only present using reinforcement (±).

➡ Examination sequence

Principal reflexes
➔ Place the patient supine on the examination couch in a comfortable relaxed position with the limbs exposed.

➔ Check for symmetry of response by comparing each reflex with that of the other side, ensuring that both the limbs are positioned identically (Figs 8.43 and 8.44).
➔ *Reinforcement* is used whenever a reflex appears to be absent. For knee and ankle reflexes ask the patient to interlock the fingers and pull one hand against the other on your command immediately before you strike the tendon (Jendrassik's manoeuvre; Fig. 8.45). To reinforce the upper limb reflexes ask the patient to clench his teeth. If you use reinforcement, the patient must relax between repeated attempts.

Hoffman's reflex (Fig. 8.46A)
➔ Place your right index finger under the distal interphalangeal joint of the patient's middle finger.
➔ Using your right thumb flick the patient's finger downwards.
➔ Look for any reflex flexion of the patient's thumb.

Finger jerk (Fig. 8.46B)
➔ Place your middle and index fingers across the palmar surface of the patient's proximal phalanges.
➔ Tap your own fingers with the hammer.
➔ Observe for flexion of the patient's fingers.

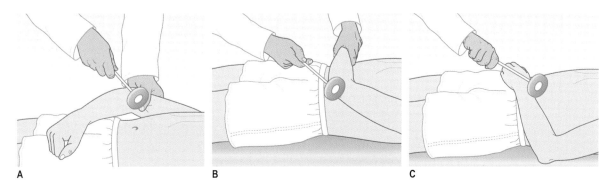

A   B   C

Fig. 8.43 **Testing the deep tendon reflexes of the upper limb.** Eliciting the (A) biceps jerk, C5 (C6); (B) triceps jerk, C6, C7; (C) supinator jerk (C5), C6.

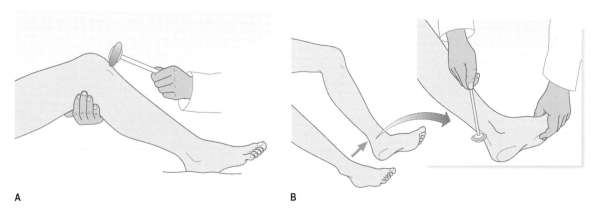

A   B

Fig. 8.44 **Testing the deep tendon reflexes of the lower limb.** Eliciting the (A) knee jerk (note that the legs must not be in contact with each other), L3, L4; (B) ankle jerk of recumbent patient, S1.

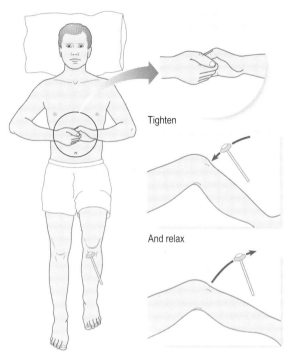

Fig. 8.45 Reinforcement while eliciting the knee jerk.

Common abnormalities

Determining whether tendon reflexes are normal or not requires practice. Abnormally brisk reflexes (hyperreflexia) are generally a sign of upper motor neurone damage. Diminished or absent jerks are most commonly due to lower motor neurone lesions but also occur in myopathies and myasthenia. In healthy elderly people the ankle jerks may be reduced or lost and in the Holmes–Adie syndrome myotonic pupils (p. 249) are associated with loss of some deep tendon reflexes. The isolated loss of a reflex may suggest a mono-neuropathy or radiculopathy (e.g. loss of ankle jerk with lumbrosacral (S1) disc prolapse). A normal reflex contraction with delayed relaxation may occur in hypothyroidism.

Positive Hoffman's (excess thumb flexion) reflex and finger jerk indicate hypertonia.

In cases of cerebellar damage the reflexes may be pendular and muscle contraction and relaxation tend to be slow.

Inverted reflexes are phenomena caused by combined spinal cord and root pathology. For example, in an inverted biceps reflex, when the biceps tendon is tapped there may be no biceps jerk but the triceps contracts (C5/6 segment lesion). In an inverted supinator reflex, when the supinator jerk is tested there is no response but finger flexion occurs (C5/6 lesion).

SUPERFICIAL REFLEXES

This group of reflexes are polysynaptic and elicited by cutaneous stimulation.

➡ Examination sequence

Plantar response (S1–2)
➔ Run a *blunt* object (car key, orange stick) along the lateral border of the sole of the foot towards the little toe (Fig. 8.47).
➔ A normal response is flexion of the large toe and adduction of the other toes.

Abdominal reflexes (T8–12)
➔ The patient should be supine and relaxed.
➔ Use an orange stick and stroke briskly but lightly in a medial direction across the upper and lower quadrants of the abdomen (Fig. 8.48).
➔ The normal response is contraction of the underlying muscle with the umbilicus moving laterally and up or down depending upon the quadrant tested.

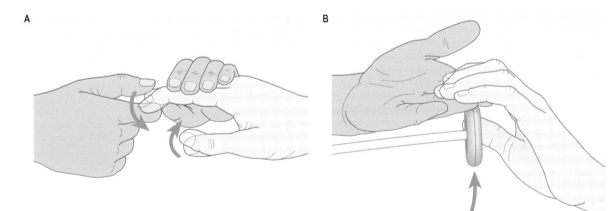

Fig. 8.46 Testing the deep tendon reflexes of the hand. (A) Hoffmann's sign. (B) Eliciting a finger jerk.

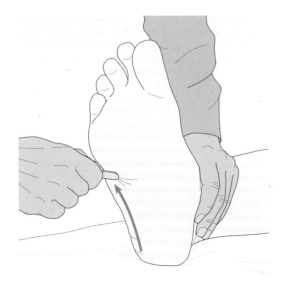

Fig. 8.47   Eliciting the plantar reflex.

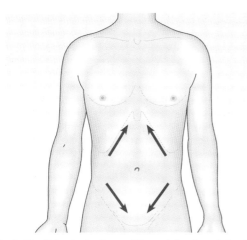

Fig. 8.48   Abdominal reflexes. Sites and direction of stimuli to elicit these.

Cremasteric reflex (L1–2)
- ➔ Abduct and externally rotate the patient's thigh.
- ➔ Use an orange stick to stroke the upper medial aspect of the thigh.
- ➔ Normally the testicle on the side stimulated will rise briskly.

Common abnormalities

An abnormal plantar response is dorsiflexion (extension) of the large toe (extensor plantar response) often accompanied by abduction of the other toes. This is an unequivocal sign of upper motor neurone damage. It will usually be associated with spasticity, clonus and hyperreflexia. The

superficial abdominal reflexes are lost in upper motor lesions but will also be affected by lower motor neurone damage affecting T8–12. They may be difficult to elicit in the obese, the elderly or those who have had abdominal surgery. The cremasteric reflex is used to assist identifying the level of spinal cord lesions, particularly after injury.

PRIMITIVE REFLEXES

The primitive reflexes (snout, grasp, palmomental and glabellar tap) have little localizing value and when present singly are of limited significance, but found in numbers they suggest diffuse or frontal cerebral damage (Table 8.13). These reflexes are present in normal neonates and young infants, indeed their absence in the 4 months after birth may indicate pathology, but they disappear as the nervous system matures. People with congenital or hereditary cerebral lesions and a few healthy individuals retain these reflexes but their return after early childhood is usually associated with brain damage or degeneration.

Common abnormalities

In adults these reflexes are often present in severe acquired brain damage from trauma, anoxia, diffuse vascular or malignant disease, encephalopathy and in dementia. Unilateral grasp and palmomental reflexes are strongly suggestive of contralateral frontal lobe pathology. The glabellar tap is positive in Parkinson's disease.

POWER

Strength varies with age, occupation, whether or not the patient exercises regularly. Muscle power is graded according to the Medical Research Council scale (Table 8.14).

In practice the majority of cases of weakness are in grade 4 range, and the use of plus or minus signs (e.g. 4+ or 4–)

8.13 Primitive reflexes	
Snout reflex	Lightly tap the lips. An abnormal response is protrusion of the mouth
Grasp reflex	Firmly stroke the palm from the radial side. In an abnormal response, your finger is gripped by the patient's hand
Palmomental reflex	Apply firm pressure to the palm next to the thenar eminence with a tongue depressor. An abnormal response is puckering of the chin.
Glabellar tap	Stand behind the patient and tap repeatedly between the eyebrows with the tip of your index finger. Normally the blink response stops after 3 to 4 times.

8.14	Medical Research Council scale for muscle power
0	No muscle contraction visible
1	Flicker of contraction but no movement
2	Joint movement when effect of gravity eliminated
3	Movement against gravity but not against examiner's resistance
4	Movement against resistance but weaker than normal
5	Normal power

8.15	Definitions of paralysis
Paresis	Partial paralysis
Plegia	Complete paralysis
Monoplegia	Involvement of a single limb
Hemiplegia	Involvement of one-half of the body
Paraplegia	Paralysis of the legs
Tetraplegia	Paralysis of all four limbs

is helpful. Use the following list of joint movements. It is also useful to record what the patient can actually do in terms of daily activities that require some muscle strength (Tables 8.15–8.17).

Upper limbs

- Shoulder: abduction, adduction, flexion and extension
- Elbow: flexion and extension
- Wrist: flexion and extension
- Finger: abduction, adduction, flexion and extension
- Thumb: extension and opposition.

Lower limbs

- Hip: abduction, adduction, flexion and extension
- Knee: flexion and extension

8.16   Patterns of motor dysfunction

- Paralysis or weakness
- Impairment of coordination
- Changes in tone and posture (dystonia)
- Involuntary movements (dyskinesia)
- Changes in the rate at which movements are performed (hypokinesis and bradykinesis)
- Loss of learned movement patterns (dyspraxia)

- Ankle: dorsiflexion, plantarflexion, inversion and eversion of foot
- Large toe: extension (i.e. dorsiflexion).

When performing a quick screening of muscle power as part of a routine assessment when no weakness is volunteered by the patient you should at least perform tests of both proximal and distal muscle groups in each limb (e.g. shoulder and finger abduction in the upper limb). For more specific complaints, and particularly in trauma, careful assessment of individual muscles is necessary.

▶ Examination sequence

→ Test the power of individual muscle groups in both limbs alternately to compare.
→ Ask the patient to contract a group of muscles to maintain a position and resist your attempt to displace the limb (*isometric* testing).
→ Ask the patient to put the joint through a movement while you try to oppose the action (*isotonic* testing).

Common abnormalities

Upper motor neurone lesions result in weakness of a relatively large group of muscles (e.g. a limb or more than one

8.17	Causes of muscle weakness		
Anatomical aetiology	**Associated features**		**Common causes**
Lower motor neurone	Muscle atrophy Fasciculation Reflexes absent or diminished Hyptonia		Peripheral neuropathies Radiculopathies Anterior horn cell damage (e.g. poliomyelitis) Motor neurone disease
Upper motor neurone	'Patterned' weakness Little or no muscle wasting Hyperreflexia Hypertonia Hypokinesis of movement		Cerebrovascular disease (e.g. hemiplegia) Spinal injury or disease (e.g. paraplegia) Multiple sclerosis
Myopathies	Muscle wasting (usually proximal) Hypotonia Tenderness (myositis)		Hereditary conditions (e.g. muscular dystrophy) Alcohol and other toxins
Psychological	Inconsistent weakness No associated features		Stress Anxiety Compensation claims

8.18	Features of motor neurone lesions

Upper motor neurone lesion

- Muscle weakness
- Increased deep tendon reflexes
- Depressed abdominal responses
- An extensor plantar response
- Spasticity

Lower motor neurone lesion

- Muscle weakness
- Depressed deep tendon reflexes
- Fasciculation
- Wasting
- Flaccidity

limb). In contrast, lower motor neurone damage can cause paresis of an individual and specific muscle (Table 8.18). In these circumstances, a more detailed examination of individual muscles is required as described in Chapter 10.

COORDINATION

The ability to perform complex movements smoothly and efficiently depends upon intact sensory as well as motor function. This section assesses cerebellar function but the tests described may be influenced by any muscle weakness, proprioceptive loss or extrapyramidal dysfunction.

Anatomy

The cerebellum consists of two hemispheres with a central vermis and lies in the posterior fossa. It is attached to the brain stem by three pairs of cerebellar peduncles. Afferent and efferent pathways convey information to and from the cerebral motor cortex, basal ganglia, thalamus, vestibular and other brain stem nuclei and the spinal cord. In general,

midline structures, e.g. vermis, are key to body equilibrium while each hemisphere controls coordination on the same (ipsilateral) side.

Examination

In addition to the following tests of limb coordination, examination of cerebellar function includes tests for dysarthria (p. 239), nystagmus (p. 260), stance and gait (pp. 238 and 314–318). In some cases dysfunction may also be accompanied by hypotonia and pendular tendon reflexes.

▶ Examination sequence

Rebound phenomenon
- → Ask the patient to stretch his arms out in front and maintain this position.
- → Push the patient's wrist quickly downward and observe the returning movement.

Finger–nose test (Fig. 8.49)
- → Ask the patient to touch his nose with the tip of the forefinger and then reach out to touch your finger tip held just within the patient's arm's reach.
- → Ask the patient to repeat the movement between nose and target finger as quickly as possible.
- → To make the test more sensitive change the position of your target finger.

Heel–shin test (Fig. 8.50)
- → Ask the patient to lie supine on the examination couch.
- → Ask the patient to raise one leg and place the heel on the opposite knee and then slide the heel tip up and down the shin between knee and ankle.

Rapid alternating movements
- → Demonstrate the act of repeatedly patting the palm of one hand with the palm and back of your opposite hand as quickly and regularly as possible.
- → Ask the patient to copy your actions.
- → Repeat with the opposite hand.

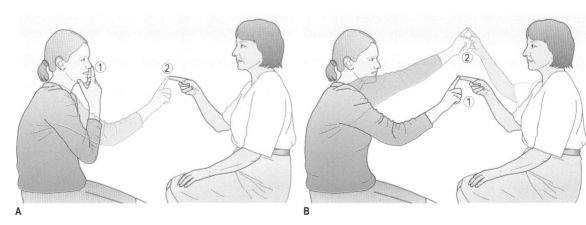

A   B

Fig. 8.49 The finger–nose test. Ask the patient to touch the tip of her nose and then your finger (A), moving your finger from one position to another, backwards and forwards as well as from side to side (B).

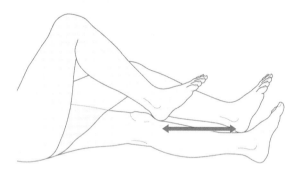

Fig. 8.50 Performing the heel–shin test with the right leg.

Common abnormalities

In cerebellar disorders the displaced outstretched arm may fly up past the original position (the rebound phenomenon); the normal response is to return to the original position.

The finger–nose test may reveal a tendency to fall short or overshoot the examiner's finger (*past-pointing*). This is *dysmetria*. In more severe cases there may be a tremor of the finger as it approaches the target finger and the patient's own nose (*intention tremor*). The movement may be slow and generally disjointed and clumsy (*dyssynergia*).

The heel–shin test is the equivalent test for the lower limbs. An abnormal finding is if the heel wavers away from the line of the shin.

Impairment of rapid alternating movements is *dysdiadochokinesis* which is evident as slowness, disorganization and irregularity of movement. Dysdiadochokinesis is typical of cerebellar disorders and is also seen in Parkinson's disease.

In disorders which predominantly affect midline cerebellar structures, e.g. tumours of the vermis and alcoholic cerebellar damage, the finger–nose, heel–shin and tests of dysdiadochokinesis may be normal. Check the stance and gait, as truncal ataxia may be the only abnormal finding.

Cerebellar dysfunction occurs in many conditions, and differential diagnosis varies with age. The most common causes of acute signs are drugs, e.g. phenytoin and alcohol, vascular lesions, trauma and demyelination (multiple sclerosis). Alcohol also causes a chronic cerebellar syndrome.

APRAXIA

Dyspraxia or *apraxia* is difficulty or inability to perform a motor action despite the patient understanding the task and in the absence of motor weakness, cerebellar, extrapyramidal or sensory impairment. If, after formal motor and sensory examinations are normal, you suspect that the patient has difficulty formulating and executing skilled movements perform the following tests.

➔ Examination sequence

➔ Ask the patient to perform an imaginary act, e.g. drinking a cup of tea; combing the hair; folding a letter and placing it in an envelope.

➔ Ask the patient to draw a geometrical figure and to write a sentence.

➔ Ask the patient to put on a pyjama top or dressing gown, one sleeve of which has been pulled inside out.

Common abnormalities

In *ideational* apraxia the patient may explain the nature of the task but cannot initiate it. In *ideomotor* apraxia the patient may perform it in an odd or bizarre fashion. Both types are associated with either frontal or parietal lesions. *Constructional* apraxia (difficulty drawing a figure) is a feature of parietal disturbance. *Dressing* apraxia, which is often associated with spatial disorientation and neglect, is usually due to non-dominant hemisphere parietal lesions.

THE EXAMINATION OF THE SENSORY SYSTEM

Detailed examination of sensation can be time-consuming and unnecessary unless the patient volunteers sensory symptoms or you suspect a specific pathology such as spinal cord compression, syringomyelia, peripheral nerve disorder or parietal lesion. Sensory symptoms include pain, spontaneous abnormal sensations usually of 'tingling' or 'pins and needles' (*paraesthesia*), and loss of sensation or numbness. *Neurogenic* pain is often particularly unpleasant, difficult to describe and may not conform to a dermatomal or peripheral nerve distribution. Ensure that by numbness the patient means lack of sensation rather than weakness or clumsiness. Reduced ability to feel pain (*hypoalgesia* or *hypoaesthesia*) or temperature (*thermoanaesthesia*) on testing may be accompanied by scars from injuries or burns which have gone unnoticed. Touch or other simple sensory stimuli may be perceived by the patient as heightened (*hyperalgesia* or *hyperaesthesia*) or unpleasant or painful (*hyperpathia* or *allodynia*).

271

Anatomy

Conscious proprioception (joint position sense) and vibration are conveyed in large, fast-conducting fibres in the posterior (dorsal) columns. Pain and temperature sensation are carried by small, slow-conducting fibres of the spinothalamic tract. The posterior column remains ipsilateral from the point of entry up to the medulla but most pain and temperature fibres cross within one or two segments of entry to the contralateral spinothalamic tract. All sensory fibres relay in the thalamus before sending information to the sensory cortex in the parietal lobe (Fig. 8.51).

THE SENSORY MODALITIES

In addition to the modalities conveyed in the principal ascending pathways (touch, pain, temperature, vibration and joint position sense) sensory examination includes tests of discriminative aspects of sensation which may be impaired by lesions of the sensory cortex. Assess these cortical sensory functions after you have shown the main pathway sensations are intact. This is usually only required for cases where a parietal lesion is suspected. Clear explanation of precisely what is required is vital and avoid repetition of testing. In general it is better to ask patients to avert their gaze rather than close their eyes. The exceptions are tests of joint position and cortical sensation and where psychological disturbance is suspected. When mapping out an area of altered sensation it is best to move from reduced to higher sensibility (i.e. from hypoaesthesia to normal or normal to hyperaesthesia).

➡ Examination sequence

Light touch
→ Use a wisp of cotton wool (or lightly apply your finger) and ask the patient to respond to each touch.
→ Time the stimuli irregularly and make a dabbing rather than a stroking or tickling stimulus.
→ Compare each side for symmetry.

Superficial pain
→ Use a fresh neurological pin, e.g. Neurotip™. Do not use a hypodermic needle. The pin must be disposed of after each patient to prevent transmitting infection.
→ Explain and demonstrate that the ability to feel a sharp pinprick is being tested.
→ Follow the testing points in Figure 8.52, comparing for symmetry.
→ Map out the boundaries of any area of reduced, absent or increased sensation.

Deep pain
→ Explain the test and ask the patient to report as soon as he feels discomfort.
→ Squeeze the muscle bellies, e.g. calf, biceps, or apply pressure to finger or toe nail beds. Do not apply pressure with an instrument, e.g. pen.

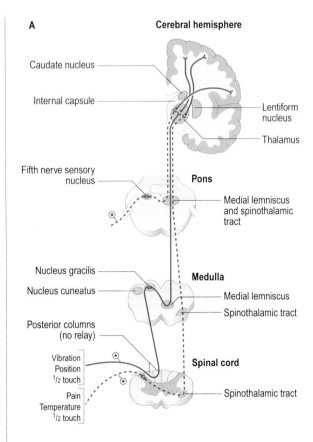

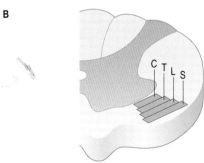

Fig. 8.51   (A) The main sensory pathways. (B) Spinothalamic tract. To show layering of the spinothalamic tract in the cervical region: C represents fibres from cervical segments which lie centrally; fibres from thoracic, lumbar and sacral segments (labelled T, L and S respectively) lie progressively more laterally.

Temperature
→ Touch the patient with a cold metallic object, e.g. tuning fork, and ask if it feels cold. More sensitive assessment requires tubes of hot and cold water at controlled temperatures but this is seldom performed.

Vibration
→ Place a vibrating 128 Hz tuning fork over the sternum. Ask the patient 'Do you feel it buzzing?'

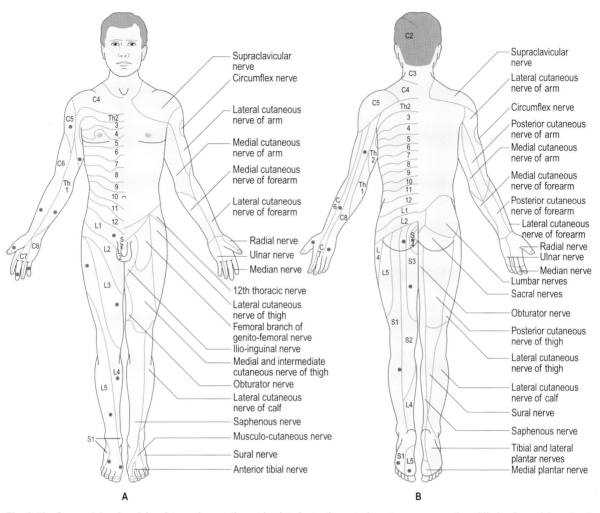

Fig. 8.52 Segmental and peripheral nerve innervation and points for testing anterior cutaneous sensation of limbs. By applying stimuli at the points marked, both the dermatomal and main peripheral nerve distributions are tested simultaneously.

→ Now place it on the tip of the large toe (Fig. 8.53). If sensation is impaired, place it on the interphalangeal joint and progress proximally – the medial malleolus, tibial tuberosity and anterior iliac spine depending upon the response.

→ Repeat the process in the upper limb. Start at the distal interphalangeal joint of the forefinger and if sensation is impaired proceed proximally – radial styloid, olecranon, acromion.

→ If in doubt as to the accuracy of the response, ask the patient to close the eyes and report when you stop the fork vibrating with your fingers.

Joint position sense

→ With the patient's eyes open demonstrate the procedure. Hold the distal phalanx of the patient's large toe at the sides to avoid giving information from pressure (or middle finger) and move it up and down (Fig. 8.54).

→ Ask the patient to respond with 'up' or 'down' as you make these movements without the patient assisting or resisting. Now ask the patient to close the eyes and identify the directions in a random sequence of small movements (e.g. up, down, down, up).

→ Test both large toes (or middle fingers). If impaired, move to more proximal joints in each limb.

Two-point discrimination

→ Use a two-point discriminator (an instrument like a pair of blunt-tipped school compasses) or an opened-out paper clip.

→ Ask the patient to look away or close the eyes.

→ Apply either one or two points to the pulp of the patient's forefinger and ask whether one or two stimuli were felt.

→ Then adjust the distance between the two points to determine the minimum separation at which they are felt separately.

→ Test both fingers and thumbs.

273

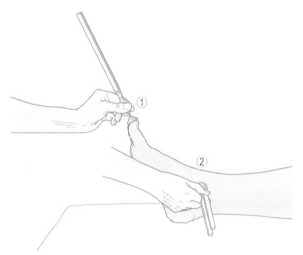

Fig. 8.53 Testing vibration sensation at (1) the big toe and (2) the ankle.

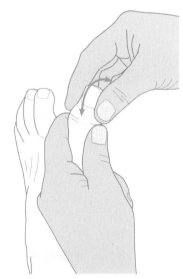

Fig. 8.54 Testing for position sense in the big toe.

Point localization

→ With the patient's eyes closed, lightly touch various body parts, e.g. hand, finger, shoulder, and ask which part has been touched and whether on the right or left side.

→ Repeat touching individual fingers asking the patient to identify which is touched. (It is often wise to ensure that the patient knows the names of the fingers first.) Inability to do so is finger agnosia.

Stereognosis and graphaesthesia

→ Ask the patient to close the eyes.

→ Place familiar small objects (e.g. coin, key, matchstick) in the patient's hand and ask the patient to identify what they are after feeling them (stereognosis).

→ Use the blunt end of a pencil or orange stick and trace letters or digits on the patient's palm. Ask the patient to identify the figure (graphaesthesia).

Sensory inattention

→ Ask the patient to close the eyes. Touch the back of each of the patient's hands in turn and ask which has been touched.

→ Now touch both hands simultaneously and ask whether the left, right or both sides were touched.

Common abnormalities

Abnormalities on sensory testing are best considered according to whether the lesion(s) is in the peripheral nerve(s), dorsal root(s), spinal cord or intracranial (Table 8.19).

Peripheral nerve and dorsal root. A large number of pathological processes affect peripheral nerves, generally resulting in peripheral neuropathies or polyneuropathies. Peripheral neuropathies tend to affect the lower limbs first and more prominently. In many case touch and pinprick sensation are lost in a 'stocking and glove' distribution (Fig. 8.55A).

In some large fibre peripheral neuropathies, vibration and joint position sense are disproportionately affected. Patients may report staggering when they close their eyes during hair washing (Rombergism, see p. 238). Occasionally when such patients are asked to close their eyes and hold their hands outstretched, their fingers will make involuntary slow wandering movements (*pseudoathetosis*).

Injuries and other damage to individual nerves lead to loss of all modalities in that nerve's territory. Sensory root damage leads to dermatomal sensory loss (see Fig. 8.52).

Polyneuropathies may be classified by (1) mode of onset (acute, subacute or chronic), (2) pathology (axonal or demyelinating), (3) principal function disturbed (motor, sensory, autonomic or mixed) or (4) aetiology (Table 8.20).

Spinal cord. Traumatic and compressive lesions of the spinal cord cause loss or impairment of sensation in a dermatomal distribution below the level of the lesion. A zone of hyperaesthesia may be found immediately above the level of sensory loss.

8.19 Tests of sensation	
Modality	**Pathway**
Light touch Proprioception Vibration Two-point discrimination	Large fast-conducting axons Dorsal columns Medial lemniscus
Pinprick (superficial pain) Deep pain Temperature	Smaller slower-conducting axons Spinothalamic tracts
Stereognosis Graphaesthesia Two-point discrimination	Parietal cortex (only valid if peripheral sensory function intact)

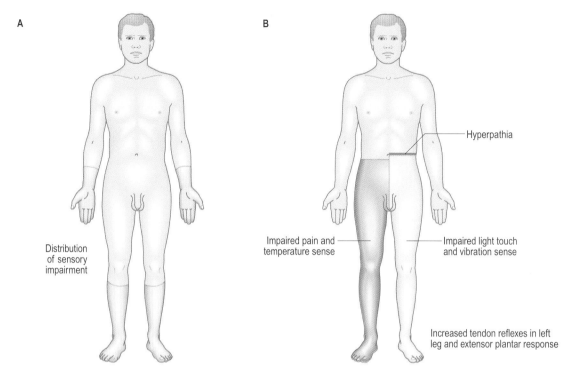

Fig. 8.55   Patterns of sensory loss. (A) In peripheral neuropathy. (B) Brown–Séquard syndrome. Note the distribution of corticospinal, posterior column and lateral spinothalamic tract signs. The cord lesion is on the right.

8.20 Causes of polyneuropathies	
Genetic	**Inflammatory**
• Hereditary motor and sensory neuropathies • Hereditary sensory and autonomic neuropathies • Refsum's disease	• Acute inflammatory or idiopathic (Guillain–Barré syndrome) • Chronic idiopathic • Connective tissue disorders (rheumatoid arthritis, systemic lupus erythematosus, polyarteritis nodosa, scleroderma)
Drugs and toxins	**Systemic medical conditions**
• Alcohol • Isoniazid, metronidazole, amiodarone, perhexiline, phenytoin • Lead, arsenic, mercury • Solvents, carbon disulphide, herbicides, pesticides	• Diabetes mellitus • Renal failure • Hypothyroidism • Acromegaly • Critical illness neuropathy • Sarcoidosis
Vitamin deficiencies	
• Vitamins B_1, B_6, B_{12} • Vitamin E	**Malignant disease**
Infections	• Cancer (paraneoplastic) • Lymphoproliferative disorders
• Leprosy • HIV • Diphtheria	**Others**
	• Amyloidosis • Paraproteinaemias

Anterior spinal artery syndrome usually results in loss of spinothalamic sensation and motor function, with sparing of dorsal column sensation. A similar pattern of pain and temperature loss and sparing of dorsal column sensation (dissociated loss) occurs in syringomyelia.

When one half of the spinal cord is damaged the Brown-Séquard syndrome may occur. This is characterized by ipsilateral motor weakness and loss of vibration and joint position sense with contralateral loss of pain and temperature (Fig. 8.55B).

Intracranial. Brain stem lesions are often vascular in origin and determining the site of the lesion relies on understanding the relevant anatomy (Fig. 8.56). *Alternating analgesia* is a term for the loss of pain and temperature sensation on one side of the face (V nerve nucleus damage) and the opposite side of the body (spinothalamic tract damage) and occurs in lower brain stem lesions.

Thalamic lesions may cause a patchy sensory impairment on the opposite side with a very unpleasant, poorly localized pain often of a burning quality.

Cortical lesions in the parietal lobe lead to impairment of some of the principal presenting pathway sensations, particularly joint position sense, but are more likely to result in the abnormalities described above.

CORTICAL FUNCTION

Thinking, emotions, language, behaviour, planning and initiating movements and perceiving sensory information are functions of the cerebral cortex and are central to awareness of and interaction with the environment. Certain areas of the cortex are associated with specific functions so that particular patterns of dysfunction can help localize the site of an intracranial pathology (Fig. 8.57). Our understanding of the relationships between structure and function in the cerebral cortex is incomplete but improving rapidly, especially due to advances in neuroradiology.

Frontal lobe. The posterior part of the frontal lobe is the precentral gyrus (or *motor strip*) which controls voluntary movement. It is organized with the lower limbs represented superiorly and the head inferiorly. Unless a cortical lesion is very large it results in upper motor neurone signs in one limb or one side of the face in contrast to lesions deeper within the cerebrum which cause hemiplegia and facial weakness.

The area anterior to the precentral gyrus is concerned with personality, social behaviour, emotions, cognition and expressive language, and contains the frontal eye fields and

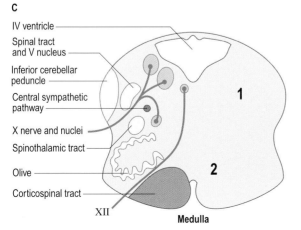

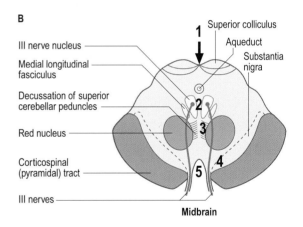

Fig. 8.56 Anatomy of brain stem lesions. (A) Arteries at the base of the brain. (B) Lesions of the midbrain: according to lesion site (1) weakness of upward gaze and vertical nystagmus; (2) bilateral III nerve palsies and internuclear ophthalmoplegia; (3) ipsilateral III nerve palsy, contralateral cerebellar signs and rubral tremors; (4) ipsilateral III nerve palsy and contralateral hemiplegia; (5) quadriparesis. (C) Lesions of the medulla: (1) ipsilateral cerebellar signs, jerking nystagmus on turning the eyes to the side of the lesion, impaired sensation on the ipsilateral face and contralateral body, Horner's syndrome, dysphonia and dysphagia; (2) crossed paralysis with ipsilateral wasting and weakness of tongue and contralateral hemiplegia.

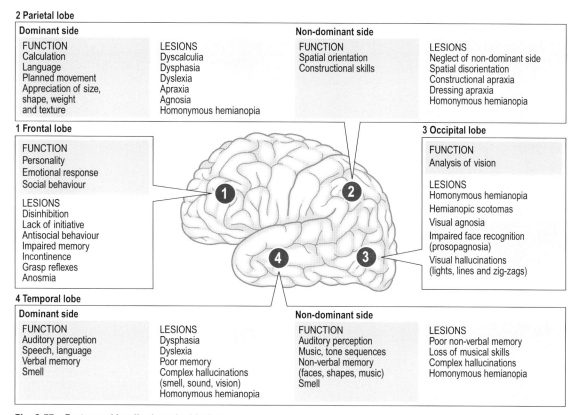

2 Parietal lobe

Dominant side		Non-dominant side	
FUNCTION Calculation Language Planned movement Appreciation of size, shape, weight and texture	LESIONS Dyscalculia Dysphasia Dyslexia Apraxia Agnosia Homonymous hemianopia	FUNCTION Spatial orientation Constructional skills	LESIONS Neglect of non-dominant side Spatial disorientation Constructional apraxia Dressing apraxia Homonymous hemianopia

1 Frontal lobe

FUNCTION
Personality
Emotional response
Social behaviour

LESIONS
Disinhibition
Lack of initiative
Antisocial behaviour
Impaired memory
Incontinence
Grasp reflexes
Anosmia

3 Occipital lobe

FUNCTION
Analysis of vision

LESIONS
Homonymous hemianopia
Hemianopic scotomas
Visual agnosia
Impaired face recognition
(prosopagnosia)
Visual hallucinations
(lights, lines and zig-zags)

4 Temporal lobe

Dominant side		Non-dominant side	
FUNCTION Auditory perception Speech, language Verbal memory Smell	LESIONS Dysphasia Dyslexia Poor memory Complex hallucinations (smell, sound, vision) Homonymous hemianopia	FUNCTION Auditory perception Music, tone sequences Non-verbal memory (faces, shapes, music) Smell	LESIONS Poor non-verbal memory Loss of musical skills Complex hallucinations Homonymous hemianopia

Fig. 8.57 Features of localized cerebral lesions.

cortical centre for micturition. The range of findings in frontal lobe damage include:

- changes of personality and behaviour (e.g. apathy or disinhibition)
- loss of emotional responsiveness or emotional lability
- cognitive impairments (particularly memory, attention and concentration)
- expressive dysphasia (dominant lobe) (see p. 239)
- conjugate gaze deviation to the side of the lesion
- urinary incontinence
- primitive reflexes (e.g. grasp).

Temporal lobe. Both temporal lobes are important for memory and the perception of smell, and damage to either may result in a form of epilepsy with complex partial seizures characterized by hallucinations and memory disturbances. The lower fibres of the optic radiation are located in this lobe and it is the area of auditory perception. Dysfunctions of the temporal lobe may manifest with:

- memory impairment
- complex partial seizures

- contralateral upper quadrantanopia
- receptive dysphasia (dominant lobe).

Parietal lobe. The postcentral gyrus (*sensory strip*) is the most anterior part of the parietal lobe and is the principal destination of conscious sensations. The upper fibres of the optic radiation pass through it. The dominant hemisphere contains aspects of language function and the non-dominant lobe is concerned with spatial awareness. Damage to the parietal lobes is often associated with re-emergence of primitive reflexes. Signs of parietal lobe dysfunction include:

- cortical sensory impairments
- contralateral lower quadrantanopia
- dyslexia, dyscalculia, dysgraphia
- apraxia
- primitive reflexes.

Occipital lobe. The main function of the occipital lobe is the analysis of visual information. Visual field defects with hemianopia or scotoma may occur. Other abnormalities are the inability to recognize visual stimuli (*visual agnosia*) and distorted perceptions of visual images. Examples of **277** the latter are seeing things larger (*macropsia*) or smaller (*micropsia*) than in real life. Visual hallucinations may also be found. Occipital damage may be associated with:

- visual field defects
- visual agnosia
- disturbances of visual perception
- visual hallucinations.

Common abnormalities

Frontal lobe damage is common in cases of severe head injury, other forms of severe acquired brain injury (e.g. subarachnoid haemorrhage, anoxia, hypoglycaemia) and in dementias. The temporal and occipital lobes may also be affected in severe traumatic brain injury Localizing damage to a particular lobe or lobes can be helpful in situations where a space-occupying lesion (e.g. tumour or abscess) is present or a particular arterial territory is involved in a vascular incident.

PERIPHERAL NERVE DAMAGE

Single nerve lesions (*mononeuropathies*) are uncommon. However, some nerves are particularly liable to damage in cases of trauma or in syndromes where the nerve is compressed (*compression* or *entrapment neuropathies*). Five nerves are considered: the radial, ulnar and median in the upper limb, and lateral cutaneous nerve of thigh and common peroneal in the leg.

Median nerve (Fig. 8.58A). This may be compressed as it passes between the flexor retinaculum and the carpal bones at the wrist (carpal tunnel syndrome) and is the most common entrapment neuropathy. The diagnosis is principally made from the history (Table 8.21).

- Test for weakness of thumb opposition and abduction. Test opposition by asking the patient to touch the thumb and fifth finger tip together while you attempt to break them apart with your finger. Test for abduction with the patient's hand held palm up on a flat surface. Ask the patient to move the thumb vertically against your resistance.

Causes of carpal tunnel syndrome are listed in Table 8.22.

Radial nerve. This may be compressed by a crutch as it runs through the axilla, or injured in fractures of the humerus.

- Test for weakness of extensors of arm (especially the wrist and fingers).
- There is sensory loss over the dorsum of the hand (Fig. 8.58B) and loss of triceps tendon jerk.

Ulnar nerve. This is most often affected at the elbow by external compression or injury, e.g. dislocation.

- Test for weakness of abduction and adduction of the fingers. These tests are done on a flat surface. Test adduction by placing a card between the patient's fingers and pulling it out against resistance.
- Look for wasting of small muscles of the hand supplied by the nerve (can result in *claw* or *benediction* hand) and sensory loss on the ulnar side of the hand (Fig. 8.58C).

Common peroneal nerve. This is most commonly damaged in fractures of the head of the fibula but can also be compressed by tight bandages, plaster of Paris or as a

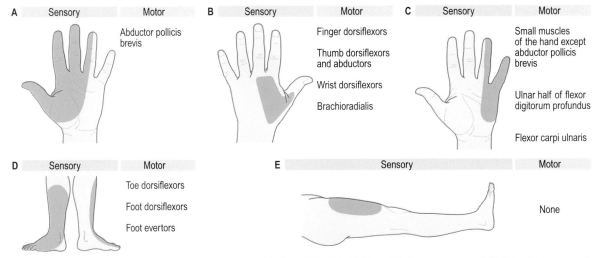

Fig. 8.58 **Sensory and motor deficits in nerve lesions.** (A) Median. (B) Radial. (C) Ulnar. (D) Common peroneal. (E) Lateral cutaneous of the thigh.

8.21	Common features of carpal tunnel syndrome

- More common in women
- Paraesthesiae and/or pain in the hand (usually spares the little finger)
- May radiate up arm to elbow
- Weakness in hand
- Symptoms commonly occur at night
- May wake the patient from sleep
- Patient may hang the hand and arm out of the bed to get relief
- Thenar muscle wasting (in longstanding cases)

8.22	Causes of carpal tunnel syndrome

- Idiopathic
- Pregnancy, oral contraceptive pill and premenstrual
- Rheumatoid arthritis
- Distal radial fractures, e.g. Colles' fracture
- Hypothyroidism
- Acromegaly
- Amyloidosis
- Nephrotic syndrome
- Mucopolysaccharidosis V (Scheie's syndrome)

result of repetitive kneeling or squatting. This damage may result in foot drop.

- Test for weakness of dorsiflexion and eversion of the foot and sensory loss over the dorsum of the foot (Fig. 8.58D).

Lateral cutaneous nerve of thigh. The lateral branch of this purely sensory nerve may be trapped or kinked as it passes through the inguinal ligament, giving rise to unpleasant paraesthesiae in the lateral thigh, especially when walking (Fig. 8.58E). This condition, which is most common in obesity or pregnancy, is known as *meralgia paraesthetica*.

- Test for loss of or heightened sensation over the lateral aspect of the thigh.

THE DIAGNOSTIC PROCESS: PUTTING IT TOGETHER

The first stage in neurological diagnosis is to decide whether a lesion has occurred within the nervous system. Then you need to determine the site(s) of damage and the underlying pathology. This process is not necessarily linear, and interpretation of history and examination findings is often an exercise in pattern recognition.

Many patients present with symptoms, but no signs, of neurological dysfunction. Resist the temptation to attribute the complaint to psychological disorder. Many patients with serious pathology, e.g. epilepsy, spinal cord compression, Guillain–Barré syndrome or post-traumatic intracranial haematoma are erroneously diagnosed as suffering from anxiety or hysteria. Underlying psychological factors are important, but a diagnosis of psychological disturbance should be considered only after confidently excluding neurological disease.

The history often provides the best clue to the pathology of any lesion and guides subsequent examination. Deciding whether there is a single lesion, multiple sites of damage or diffuse disorder in the nervous system is useful. For instance, tumours and strokes may lead to damage at a specific site; multiple sclerosis is characterized by lesions scattered in site and time; and chronic alcohol misuse can lead to widespread cerebral, brain stem, spinal cord and peripheral nerve disturbances.

COMMON NERVOUS SYSTEM INVESTIGATIONS

Neurological symptoms and signs often result from systemic disorders. Baseline investigations include blood tests of haematological, renal and hepatic function; urinalysis and chest X-ray. HIV antibody testing may be indicated. More specialized tests include lumbar puncture to examine the cerebrospinal fluid, electrical recordings of brain, muscle, nerve, etc. (*clinical neurophysiology*), radiological procedures (*neuroradiology*), automated visual field analysis, fundal photography and specific genetic tests (*neurogenetics*). Before ordering such investigations, discuss with the appropriate specialist.

SPECIALIZED INVESTIGATIONS

Table 8.23 outlines some of the specialized investigations done in neurology with examples of indications for them. It is by no means comprehensive. Some invasive tests, e.g. brain biopsy and myelography, are now done very infrequently owing to rapid advances in scanning techniques.

Some of the more commonly used clinical neurophysiology tests are as follows:

- *Electroencephalography* records the spontaneous electrical activity of the brain using electrodes placed on the scalp and occasionally with a needle electrode passed percutaneously through the foramen ovale to record activity from the temporal lobe. *Telemetry* is a technique of 24- to 48-hour electroencephalography recording. Electroencephalography is principally used in the investigation of epilepsy but is also used in some cases of encephalitis or dementia. In addition, electroencephalography is used in the investigation of sleep disorders.
- *Evoked potentials*. There are three main forms of evoked potential recording: visual, auditory and somatosensory in which the cortical response to stimuli (visual, auditory and sensory) are recorded with electrodes positioned at specific points on the scalp. Such tests are valuable in the investigation of various conditions including multiple sclerosis, hearing impairments, suspected brain stem tumours and brachial plexus injuries.
- *Electromyography* is used to investigate disorders affecting muscles, using a concentric needle electrode inserted into the muscle. The electrical activity is displayed on an oscilloscope and an audio-monitor, allowing the neurophysiologist to see and hear the pattern of activity.
- *Nerve conduction studies* involve applying electrical stimuli to nerves and measuring the speed of conduction of the impulse along them. The technique is used for both motor and sensory nerves and is helpful in diagnosing peripheral nerve disorders such as nerve compressions or polyneuropathies.

Table 8.24 identifies specialized investigations employed in visual disorders.

8.23 Specialized investigations of the nervous system

Investigation	Usual indication
Invasive	
Nerve biopsy	Peripheral neuropathies
Muscle biopsy	Muscular dystrophy Myopathies
Brain biopsy	Neurodegenerative conditions Encephalitis
Needle aspiration of brain	Cerebral abscess
Needle aspiration of spine	Tuberculosis
Liver biopsy	Wilson's disease
Renal biopsy	Polyarteritis nodosa
Rectal biopsy	Amyloidosis
Bone marrow aspiration	Vitamin B_{12} deficiency Myeloproliferative disorders
Lumbar puncture	Meningitis, encephalitis Multiple sclerosis Malignant infiltration
Intracranial pressure monitoring	Trauma Normal pressure hydrocephalus
Radiology	
Chest X-ray	Source of cerebral metastases Tuberculosis Sarcoidosis
Skull X-ray	Fracture Bone erosion, e.g. tumour Calcification, e.g. tumour, Sturge–Weber syndrome
CT brain scan	Trauma: fractures, intracranial haematoma Stroke and subarachnoid haemorrhage Tumours, tuberculoma Cerebral atrophy
MR brain scan	Multiple sclerosis Infection Metastases Infiltrative malignancy Pontine myelinolysis
MR spine	Tumours Prolapsed intervertebral disc Syringomyelia Vascular malformations
SPECT scan	Dementia Malignancy
PET scan	Parkinson's disease
Ultrasound of extracranial arteries	Atherosclerotic stenosis
Transcranial ultrasound	Hydrocephalus (in infants)

8.23 Specialized investigations of the nervous system (*cont'd*)

Investigation	Usual indication
Radiology	
Echocardiogram	Stroke: source of embolism
Angiography	Atheroma of extracranial vessels Aneurysms Arteriovenous malformations
Myelography	Spinal compression
Neurophysiology	
EEG	Epilepsy Encephalopathy/encephalitis Sleep disorders
EMG	Myopathy Muscular dystrophy Motor neurone disease
Single-fibre EMG	Myasthenia gravis
Nerve conduction studies	Entrapment neuropathy Peripheral neuropathy
Visual evoked potentials	Multiple sclerosis
Brain stem auditory evoked potentials	Acoustic neuroma
Somatosensory evoked potentials	Brachial plexus lesions
ECG	Epilepsy/syncope Stroke Muscular dystrophy
Blood tests	
Haemoglobin	Syncope, seizures Stroke
MCV	Vitamin B_{12} deficiency
White cell count	Infection (e.g. meningitis)
Blood film	Neuro-acanthocytosis
Blood culture	Meningitis Endocarditis-stroke
Erythrocyte sedimentation/ C-reactive protein	Cranial arteritis
Vitamin B_{12} and folic acid	Peripheral neuropathy Dementia
Red cell thiamine	Wernicke–Korsakoff syndrome
Clotting/thrombophilia screen	Stroke
VDRL-TPHA	Neurosyphilis
HIV	Central nervous system involvement

Angiotensin-converting enzyme	Sarcoidosis
Antinuclear factor and dsDNA	Stroke
Rheumatoid factor Antiphospholipid antibody	Peripheral neuropathy Stroke
Acetylcholine receptor antibodies	Myasthenia gravis
Anti-Hu/anti-Yo antibodies	Encephalitis
Anti-calcium-channel antibodies	Myasthenic (Eaton–Lambert) syndrome
Serum immunoglobulins	Myeloma
Thyroid function test	Tremor Carpal tunnel syndrome
GH; ACTH; FSH/LH; Prolactin; TSH	Pituitary tumour
Liver function tests	Ataxia Peripheral neuropathy
Urea/creatinine	Encephalopathy Peripheral neuropathy
Electrolytes	Diabetes insipidus/SIADH Periodic paralysis
Glucose	Coma Stroke Neuropathies
Serum lipids and cholesterol	Stroke
Calcium	Epilepsy Tetany
Drug/toxin screen	Coma Epilepsy Peripheral neuropathy
Caeruloplasmin/serum copper	Wilson's disease
Creatine phosphokinase	Muscular dystrophy, myopathy
Lactate	Myophosphorylase deficiency (McArdlc's syndrome)
DNA analysis	Huntington's disease Hereditary ataxias and neuropathies
Edrophonium test	Myasthenia gravis
Urine tests	
Glucose Ketones Bence Jones protein Porphobilinogen Copper	Peripheral neuropathy Diabetic coma Myeloma Porphyria Wilson's disease

ACTH, adrenocorticotrophic hormone; EEG, electroencephalography; EMG, electromyography; FSH/LH, follicle-stimulating hormone/luteinizing hormone; GH, growth hormone; MCV, mean corpuscular volume; PET, positron-emission tomography; SIADH, syndrome of inappropriate antidiuretic hormone; SPECT, single photon emission computerized tomography; TSH, thyroid-stimulating hormone; VDRL-TPHA, Venereal Disease Research Laboratory – *Treponema pallidum* haemagglutination

8.24	Specialized investigations of visual disorders
Condition	**Investigation**
Retinal artery occlusion	Electrocardiogram Carotid ultrasound Echocardiography
Retinal vein occlusion	Lipid profile Blood glucose Fundal photography Fluorescein angiography
Age-related macular degeneration	Amsler grid Fluorescein angiography
Non-resolving conjunctivitis	Swab for Chlamydia
Corneal ulcer	Scrape for microscopy and culture
Recurrent acute or chronic iritis	HLA B27 typing X-ray sacroiliac joints Chest radiograph Syphilis serology Angiotensis-converting enzyme

Posterior uveitis	Chest radiograph
	Syphilis serology
	Antinuclear factor, antineutrophil
	   cytoplasmic antibody and
	   extractable nuclear antigen screen

Scleritis	Urinalysis
	C-reactive protein
	Antinuclear factor, antineutrophil
	   cytoplasmic antibody and
	   extractable nuclear antigen screen
	Chest radiograph

Atypical optic neuritis	Automated visual fields
	MR scan of orbit
	Lumbar puncture
	Urinalysis
	C-reactive protein
	Antinuclear factor, antineutrophil
	   cytoplasmic antibody and
	   extractable nuclear antigen screen
	Chest radiograph
	DNA analysis for Leber's hereditary
	   optic neuropathy

◆ Key points

Nervous system

◆ Headaches present on waking and aggravated by change of posture may be due to raised intracranial pressure.

◆ If a patient cannot talk properly consider the five Ds: Deafness, Dementia, Dysphasia, Dysarthria and Dysphonia.

◆ Dysphasia is often mistaken for confusion.

◆ Eyewitness accounts are invaluable in determining the nature of blackouts.

◆ Most cases of loss of smell (anosmia) and deafness are due to local disorders of the nose and ear respectively.

◆ The sensory loss in V nerve lesions does not extend onto the pinna or beyond the angle of the mandible.

◆ Solitary lesions of IX and X are uncommon.

◆ Severe muscle wasting is usually due to a lower motor neurone lesion.

Eye

◆ Blepharitis is a common cause of dry eyes and ocular discomfort.

◆ Pain on eye movement suggests optic neuritis or scleritis.

◆ Circumciliary injection indicates inflammation that affects the iris root/ciliary body, e.g. iritis, keratitis, angle-closure glaucoma.

◆ Amaurosis fugax is unilateral visual loss. The patient describes the deficit as black or grey.

◆ The aura of migraine is a positive visual phenomenon that may be white, coloured or scintillating.

◆ Sudden onset permanent visual loss is usually caused by vascular occlusion.

◆ A white, swollen optic disc with visual loss suggests giant cell arteritis.

◆ Distortion of vision suggests disruption of the macular photoreceptors by blood, fluid, scar or traction.

◆ Flashes and floaters are forerunners of retinal detachment.

◆ Haloes are associated with angle-closure glaucoma.

◆ Unilateral optic nerve lesions cause a relative afferent pupillary defect even with apparently normal vision, whereas with macular lesions this is a late finding.

◆ In oculomotor (III) nerve palsy in a comatose patient the pupil is usually spared in metabolic conditions but is involved in structural lesions.

The ear, nose and throat

FIONA NICOL • KIM AH-SEE

Acute diseases of the ears, nose and throat are very common in a fit individual or someone with chronic disease elsewhere. These areas are also affected by systemic disease and so you must become familiar with their normal appearance and competent in assessing their function.

THE EAR

Anatomy

The ear is divided into external or outer, middle and inner ear.

Outer ear. The outer ear consists of the pinna, external auditory meatus and the lateral surface of the tympanic membrane (Fig. 9.1). The pinna is fibrocartilage tightly covered by skin, while the ear lobe is simply fat with no cartilage. The ear canal or external auditory meatus is cartilaginous in the outer third and bony in the inner two-thirds. The skin of the outer third contains hair, sebaceous and ceruminous glands but these are absent in the bony meatus. Squamous debris from the outer part of the drum migrates to the outside and is mixed with cerumen and sebum to become wax.

Middle ear. The middle ear is formed by the medial surface of the tympanic membrane, the tympanic cavity, the mastoid air cells and the eustachian tube. The three auditory ossicles traverse the cavity and transmit sound from the external ear to the inner ear. The eustachian tube equalizes pressure between the middle ear and the atmosphere.

The tympanic membrane or eardrum lies obliquely across the external auditory meatus. It is normally grey and semitranslucent and is in two parts. The *pars tensa* consists of an outer layer of squamous epithelium, a middle fibrous layer and an inner layer of mucous membrane. This is continuous with the epithelium of the middle ear cavity. The *pars flaccida* lacks the middle fibrous layer and is easily retracted in patients with negative middle ear pressure. The part of the middle ear cavity above the bony roof of the external auditory meatus is called the *attic*.

A fibrous ring circles the tympanic membrane and fixes it into the surrounding bone. The handle of the malleus attaches onto the fibrous layer of the *pars tensa*. Both this and the short process can be seen through the auriscope (Fig. 9.2).

The malleus articulates with the incus medially and this in turn articulates with the stapes. This joint is the weakest link in the ossicular chain and is liable to disruption from trauma or prolonged infection.

The *chorda tympani*, a branch of the facial VII nerve passes horizontally medial to the malleus and lateral to the long process of the incus. It carries taste fibres from the anterior two-thirds of the tongue and may be damaged by severe trauma to the ear.

Inner ear. The inner ear or labyrinth is in two parts, the cochlea and the vestibule. It communicates with the middle ear through the oval and round windows.

The hair cells in the cochlea convert the mechanical energy from sound into electrical impulses, which are transmitted in the cochlear division of cranial nerve VIII.

The vestibule deals with balance and consists of the lateral, superior and posterior semicircular canals, which are arranged at right angles to each other. These open out

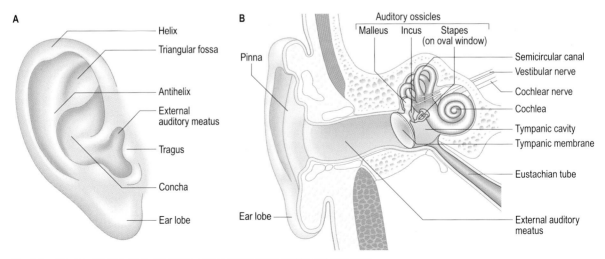

284 **Fig. 9.1** **The ear.** (A) The pinna. (B) Cross-section of the outer, middle and inner ears.

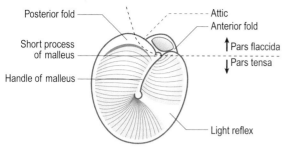

Posterior fold — — Attic
— — Anterior fold
Short process — ↑ Pars flaccida
of malleus — ↓ Pars tensa
Handle of malleus —
— Light reflex

Fig. 9.2 Structures visible on auriscopic examination of the right ear.

9.1 Causes of earache (otalgia)
Otological
• Acute otitis externa
• Acute otitis media
• Perichondritis
• Trauma
• Herpes zoster (Ramsay Hunt syndrome)
• Tumour
Non-otological
• Tonsillitis
• Dental disease
• Temporomandibular joint dysfunction
• Cervical spine disease
• Cancer of the pharynx or larynx

into a vestibule which contains the utricle and the saccule. Within these are specialized areas called the maculae. When the head moves, movement of the endolymph stimulates small calcific particles and the hair processes embedded in the membrane at the maculae. At one end of each semicircular canal is a receptor organ, the *crista ampularis*. This is lined by cells with hair processes which are stimulated by the endolymph. The vestibular division of the vestibulocochlear (VIII) nerve innervates the utricle and semicircular canals, while the saccule part of the posterior semicircular canal is innervated by the cochlear division. This provides information on head posture and movement.

These structures are held in a bony framework, the osseous labyrinth. The membranous labyrinth within this holds two fluid-filled compartments. The perilymph has a composition similar to that of extracellular fluid, and the endolymph, with a higher potassium concentration, is more similar to intracellular fluid.

COMMON SYMPTOMS

The main symptoms associated with the ear are:

• pain (otalgia)
• discharge (otorrhoea)
• hearing loss
• tinnitus (hearing noises in the absence of an obvious source)
• a sensation of abnormal movement (vertigo).

Otalgia

Pain may be referred from other sites, and problems in the nose, sinuses, mouth and cervical spine can cause earache. The characteristics of the pain help diagnose its cause (Table 9.1).

Otorrhoea

A discharge may be:

• mucopurulent
• serous
• bloodstained.

The character of the discharge gives a clue as to the pathology. Profuse, inoffensive mucoid otorrhoea suggests a perforation of the tympanic membrane and infection from the middle ear. A chronic offensive scanty discharge may be a sign of a cholesteatoma caused by infected keratin forming in a pocket behind the tympanic membrane. The onset of bleeding or pain in chronic discharge may indicate malignant change, but acute bleeding after trauma suggests the two are related. In severe trauma the temporal bone may be fractured and leakage of cerebrospinal fluid will be watery.

Hearing loss

Hearing loss may be:

• conductive
• sensorineural
• mixed.

Conductive hearing loss is due to any process which disrupts conduction of sound energy from the outer ear, through the tympanic membrane and ossicular chain to the inner ear (Table 9.2). Speech is retained and hearing is good if sounds are amplified.

Sensorineural hearing loss is due to cochlear or neurological damage, and speech may be impaired. Small degrees of amplification may cause unpleasant distortion. This is known as recruitment and is due to damage to the hair cells of the cochlea.

Deafness or total hearing loss is unusual, so hearing loss is usually described as being mild, moderate, severe or

9.2 Causes of hearing loss
Conductive
• Wax
• Otitis externa
• Middle ear effusion
• Trauma to the tympanic membrane/ossicles
• Otosclerosis
• Chronic middle ear infection
• Tumours of the middle ear
Sensorineural
• Genetic, e.g. Alport's syndrome, Jerrell–Lange–Neilson syndrome
• Prenatal infection, e.g. rubella
• Birth injury
• Trauma
• Infection:
– meningitis
– measles
– mumps
– syphilis
• Degenerative (presbyacusis)
• Occupation or other noise induced
• Acoustic neuroma
• Idiopathic: Ménière's disease, sudden deafness

profound. Any hearing loss should be quantified formally by an audiologist.

Most hearing loss is gradually progressive and related to ageing (presbyacusis). Ask about the age and speed of onset: people who develop hearing loss before they acquire speech have unusual speech that is vowel based and lacking in the clear articulation of specific consonants. Family history is important since some syndromes are inherited. Otosclerosis, a cause of conductive deafness where the stapes footplate becomes fixed, is also hereditary. Other causes include infection and trauma, which may be accompanied by bleeding and discharge. This may be accompanied by the accumulation of debris, perforation of the tympanic membrane and, sometimes, disruption of the ossicular chain. Some drugs are ototoxic, e.g. aminoglycosides, and there are associations between hearing loss and some neurological and renal conditions. Occupation and leisure activities may be important since prolonged exposure to loud noise causes sensorineural hearing loss.

Tinnitus

The *subjective* sensation of sound with no auditory stimulus can be caused by almost any pathology in the auditory apparatus. It is usually a rushing, hissing or singing sound. Contrast this with *autophony*, which is abnormal perception of one's own voice, or *objective* tinnitus where patients may hear internal body noises such as the sound of blood-flow through the middle ear.

Tinnitus is often accompanied by hearing loss. It can be difficult to find the cause and offer a cure for subjective tinnitus. Remember that tinnitus may have causes unrelated to the ear, e.g. carotid artery bruits, intracranial aneurysms, arteriovenous malformations or tumours.

Vertigo

This is an hallucination of movement. You must distinguish it from dizziness or light-headedness. Vertigo usually feels to patients as though they or their surroundings are moving. It may be intermittent or constant. The latter is more likely to be central and progressive, whereas intermittent and paroxysmal vertigo is usually vestibular and may be accompanied by nausea and vomiting as occurs in travel sickness.

Deformity of the ear

Congenital deformities include underdevelopment of the pinna (microtia) and an absent pinna (anotia). These may be associated with middle and inner ear abnormalities. Accessory auricles are seen in front of the tragus, as is a preauricular sinus. Sometimes children have markedly protruding ears – 'bat ears'. These can be surgically corrected if children are unhappy with their appearance.

In Down's syndrome the auricles are usually small and the lobule may be rudimentary or absent.

The helix of the ear is a site for gouty tophi – white chalky deposits of sodium biurate crystals. Redness and swelling of the pinna occurs in soft tissue infection usually due to acute otitis externa in the ear canal.

Injury to the ear

Trauma to the pinna can cause a haematoma. If this is extensive or repeated it may result in a 'cauliflower ear'. Damage to the external auditory meatus is caused by a variety of objects, many of which, people insert themselves. These include cotton buds, paper clips and pencils. These often damage the skin of the external auditory meatus and cause infection. They may also damage the middle ear, but rarely the inner ear. Blunt trauma such as a blow to the side of the head may rupture the tympanic membrane, dislocate the ossicles and damage the inner ear. This may be accompanied by hearing loss, vertigo and damage to the *chorda tympani*.

EXAMINATION

➔ Examination sequence

➔ Look at the pinna, noting its shape, size and any deformity.
➔ Look behind the ears for any scars from surgery and see if the patient wears a hearing aid. Ask the patient to remove it before you go any further.
➔ Gently pull on the pinna and ask the patient if it is sore. Tenderness on palpation of the tragus suggests infection of the external auditory meatus or temporomandibular joint problems.

➜ Look at the size of the meatus. If it is very wide this suggests previous mastoid surgery. Note any discharge or colour change in the skin.

➜ Use an auriscope with the largest speculum that will comfortably fit the external auditory meatus and check that it produces a good light. Explain to the patient what you are going to do.

➜ Hold the auriscope in a pen grip between your index finger and thumb with the ulnar border of your hand against the patient's cheek (Fig. 9.3). If the patient moves his head during your examination your hand will move too and limit any trauma to the ear. Use your left hand for the patient's left ear and your right hand for the patient's right ear.

➜ Gently pull the pinna upwards and backwards to straighten the cartilaginous external auditory meatus. Introduce the speculum and inspect the skin of the external auditory meatus for infection, wax and foreign bodies. In severe otitis externa or furunculosis where a boil is present the external auditory meatus may be completely occluded. You can remove wax by gentle syringing with warm water to fully inspect the deeper structures. However, do not syringe any ear with a history of perforation or infection. If in doubt refer to ENT for microsuction.

➜ Look at the tympanic membrane. You should be able to see a cone of light as the concave surface of the tympanic membrane reflects the light forwards – the light reflex. Look for the anatomical features in a systematic fashion. There are a wide variety of normal appearances so practise to gain experience. Note the pearly grey translucent appearance of the normal drum (Fig. 9.4). White patches are tympanosclerosis and indicate previous scarring from perforation. Notice any current perforation and its site and size. Marginal defects extend to the annulus but central perforations retain membrane around them (Fig. 9.5). Their position is described in relation to the handle of the malleus. If the perforation includes most of the tympanic membrane it is described as being subtotal.

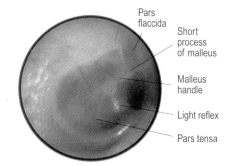

Fig. 9.4   A normal right eardrum.

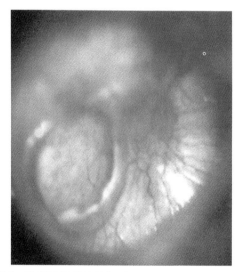

Fig. 9.5   Healing central perforation.

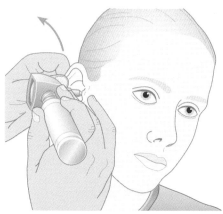

Fig. 9.3   Examination of the ear using an auriscope.

There may be a flush of blood vessels over the handle of the malleus, this occurs in early otitis media. If the drum is bright red then otitis media is more advanced. Look for an effusion behind the tympanic membrane. This may be visible because of a fluid level but can be indicated by a retracted dull tympanic membrane. Acute effusions can occur in acute upper respiratory tract infections. Acute otitis media typically results in mucopurulent middle ear fluid which invariably releases itself by perforating the tympanic membrane, leading to a profuse discharge from the ear (Fig. 9.6A). If persistent, the fluid becomes thick leading to *glue ear* – otitis media with an effusion (Fig. 9.6B). You may see a grommet in situ (Fig. 9.6C) if this has been treated surgically.

In eustachian tube dysfunction there may be absorption of the air in the middle ear and the drum will become retracted. This gives undue prominence to the short process of the

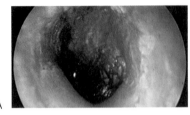

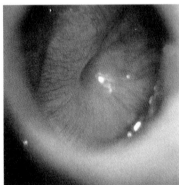

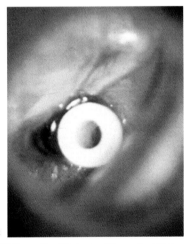

Fig. 9.6 Otitis media. (A) Acute otitis media. (B) Secretory otitis media ('glue ear' showing fluid level). (C) A grommet in place.

> **○ Examine this patient who complains of a sore ear**
>
> 1. General examination looking for evidence of systemic upset (*acute otitis media*).
> 2. Inspect and palpate the pinna and surrounding area (*acute mastoiditis, acute otitis externa, trauma* (*haematoma*), *previous surgery*).
> 3. Inspect both external auditory meati for signs of discharge, crusting, excoriation (*acute otitis media, acute otitis externa*).
> 4. Feel the tragus for tenderness (*acute otitis externa*).
> 5. Using the otosope, examine the external auditory meati (remember to lift the pinna upwards and backwards to straighten the canal).
> 6. Inspect the tympanic membrane for surface appearance and integrity. If the view is obscured with wax/debris consider syringing or microsuction.
> 7. Palpate the temporomandibular joints for tenderness and crepitus (*temporomandibular joint dysfunction*).
> 8. Examine the throat (referred pain from oropharynx).
> 9. Consider other investigations such as audiology (hearing test).

Whispered voice test

Stand behind the patient. Start with your mouth about 15 cm from the patient's ear and mask hearing in the other ear by rubbing the tragus. Ask the patient to repeat back the words you say. Use a combination of numbers and letters. Start at 15 cm with a normal speaking voice to confirm the patient understands the test. Repeat, but this time at arms-length from the patient's ear. Typically, if a patient can hear a whispered voice at 60 cm, the patient's hearing is better than 30 dB, i.e. normal.

This test is difficult in a noisy environment or with patients whose first language is not English. Further near-patient tests are done with a tuning fork of 512 Hz.

Weber's test (p. 259)

Place the base of the vibrating tuning fork on the top of the patient's head or in the middle of the forehead; ask the patient where he hears the noise. If hearing is normal or hearing loss is symmetrical, then he will hear the noise in the middle or equally in both ears.

If hearing loss is due to a conductive problem in one ear, he will hear the sound loudest in that ear because outside sounds are not interfering with it. If the hearing is reduced by sensorineural deafness then the sound will be loudest in the unaffected ear. Note which side Weber's test lateralizes to. To clarify the type of hearing loss you must carry out Rinne's test.

Rinne's test (p. 259)

Place the base of the vibrating tuning fork on the patient's mastoid process. Ask patients to let you know when they cannot hear it any more. Immediately place the tuning fork prongs close to the external auditory meatus on the same side and ask patients if they can hear it now. If they can, it

malleus. Ask the patient to perform a Valsalva manoeuvre (forced expiration against a closed glottis) while you observe the tympanic membrane. In the normal ear you should see the tympanic membrane move outwards and if you ask patients they will confirm that their ears 'popped'.

Testing hearing

Make a crude assessment of hearing from the history. The phone or doorbell is louder than conversation in a quiet room. The need to raise your voice in this situation implies a degree of hearing loss, while failing to hear the bell or phone suggests more severe loss.

implies that air conduction is better than bone conduction and so there is no conductive deafness. Carry out the same process for the opposite ear.

Rinne's test is negative when conductive deafness is present, i.e. bone conduction is better than air conduction. Note this in the record as BC > AC.

One exception to this is when one ear has no hearing at all. The test may be negative as sound is conducted through the skull bones to the 'good' ear – a false-negative Rinne's test.

Testing vestibular function

Information from the vestibular apparatus is integrated through central nervous pathways with eye movements and postural adjustments. Balance also relies on eyes, muscle, joint and skin receptors. All are processed in the cerebellum (see p. 270).

Dix–Hallpike's positional test

This is used for patients with benign paroxysmal positional vertigo. Explain to patients what you are going to do and what to expect (dizziness). Ask them to sit upright close to the edge of the couch. Turn their head 45° to one side and then rapidly lower them so that their head is now 30° below the horizontal (Fig. 9.7). Ask them to keep their eyes open and to report any vertigo they experience. Watch their eyes carefully for nystagmus. In benign paroxysmal positional vertigo there is a latent period of up to 20 seconds before they experience vertigo and you will see rotatory nystagmus which beats towards the lower ear. This response fatigues, so if you repeat it immediately there will be a lesser response. This is called adaptation. Other conditions including Ménière's disease, vestibular neuronitis, head injury and brain tumour can mimic benign paroxysmal positional vertigo symptoms.

Central pathology produces immediate nystagmus not necessarily with vertigo and shows no adaptation. Causes

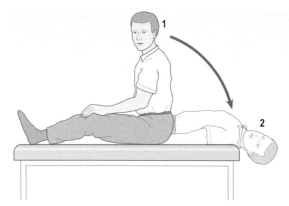

Fig. 9.7 Dix–Hallpike position test.

include cerebrovascular disease, multiple sclerosis and brain tumours.

Repeat the test, turning the patient's head to the other side.

Fistula test

If the patient has middle ear disease and vertigo, repeatedly compress the tragus against the external auditory meatus to occlude the meatus. If this produces a sense of imbalance or vertigo it suggests an abnormal communication between the middle ear and the vestibular apparatus, e.g. erosion due to cholesteatoma.

Other investigations

Audiometry

This takes different forms depending on the age of the patient. It includes pure tone and speech testing. Objective pure tone testing helps to eliminate variability. The audiology department may also carry out caloric tests and electronystagmography and posturography to assess vestibular function.

THE NOSE

Anatomy

The nose is formed from two nasal bones that articulate with the maxilla on each side. The shape of the nose is determined by the cartilages that form the lower two-thirds of the nose and attach to the nasal bones. The septal cartilage divides the nose into two nasal cavities and fuses posteriorly with the bony septum (the perpendicular plate of the ethmoid and vomer bones). The outer skin of the nose continues just into the opening of the nasal cavities (nasal vestibule) where it contains hair and sebaceous glands.

The nasal cavities open to the exterior through the nostrils (anterior nares). On the lateral wall of each cavity are paired *turbinates* (conchae) that project into it (Fig. 9.8). These are the superior, inferior and middle turbinates (occasionally a fourth, the supreme, is present). These divide the cavity into superior, inferior and middle meati.

Inferior view of nose　　　**External nose**

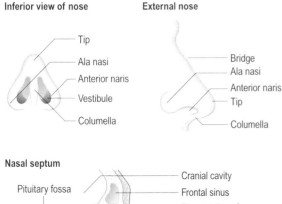

Nasal septum

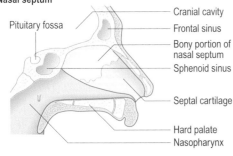

Lateral wall of nose

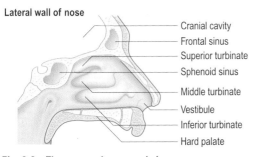

Fig. 9.8　The nose and paranasal sinuses.

The paranasal sinuses – maxillary, frontal, ethmoid and sphenoid – are air-filled spaces in the bones of the skull which open through ostia into the nasal cavity. The posterior ethmoid and sphenoid sinuses drain into the superior meatus, the anterior ethmoid, frontal and maxillary sinuses drain into the middle meatus, and the nasolacrimal duct into the inferior meatus. The mucous membrane of the nose and the sinuses is ciliated columnar epithelium rich in mucous glands. It warms and humidifies the air. Mucus is secreted into the sinuses and swept by the cilia through the ostia into the nasal cavity. It is then moved to the posterior part of the nose where it is swallowed.

COMMON SYMPTOMS

The important symptoms of nasal and sinus disease are:

- nasal obstruction

- rhinorrhoea (discharge):
  - blood (epistaxis)
  - watery (e.g. rhinitis, cerebrospinal fluid)
  - purulent
- sneezing and coughing
- disturbance of smell
- nasal deformity
- sinus pain causing facial pain or headache.

Nasal obstruction

A blocked nose may be unilateral or bilateral. If it is long-standing it suggests a structural deformity such as a deviated nasal septum that may be congenital or follow trauma. Other mechanical problems include polyps or enlarged turbinates. If the blockage varies, it suggests mucosal changes such as occur in seasonal or perennial rhinitis due to allergy or viral infection as in a 'cold'.

Nasal discharge

Discharge may be unilateral or bilateral. A watery discharge suggests allergic rhinitis but purulent discharge is secondary to infection as occurs in the later stages of a 'cold', sinus infection or with a foreign body.

Epistaxis

A nosebleed (epistaxis) varies from an infrequent minor problem to a life-threatening major haemorrhage. There is a rich blood supply to an area of the anterior nasal septum (Little's area) that is easily traumatized and is a common site for bleeding, especially in children. Causes include trauma from nose picking, surgery or infection. Prolonged bleeding is associated with, but not caused by, hypertension, anticoagulants and recent alcohol consumption.

Sneezing

This is the protective sudden expulsive effort, which clears the nasal passages of irritants. It is common in viral upper respiratory infection and allergic rhinitis. The latter may be associated with rhinorrhoea, palatal and conjunctival itching and nasal obstruction.

Disturbance of smell

Patients may complain of no sense of smell (*anosmia*) or a reduced sense of smell (*hyposmia*). Anosmia may follow trauma (head injury) or can occur after a viral upper respiratory tract infection (viral neuropathy). Mechanical obstruction of the nose by nasal polyps or mucosal oedema and swelling in allergic rhinitis usually causes hyposmia but may cause anosmia. *Casosmia* is an unpleasant smell due to chronic sepsis in the nose.

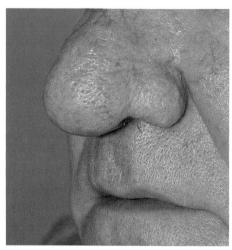

Fig. 9.9   Rhinophyma as a complication of rosacea.

Nasal deformity

This may be acute in trauma with pain and swelling and usually epistaxis. Once any swelling has settled, the shape of the nose may remain deformed if the nasal bones have been displaced. Reduction of a nasal fracture should be attempted within 2 weeks of the injury before the bones begin to set. If the skin is affected by acne rosacea for many years, the nose may be enlarged, red and bulbous (*rhinophyma*; Fig. 9.9). Destruction of the nasal septum due to local trauma may produce flattening of the bridge and a 'saddle' deformity. Other causes include Wegener's granulomatosis, congenital syphilis and chronic snorting of cocaine. Widening of the nose is an early feature of acromegaly and a late feature of neglected nasal polyposis.

Nasal and facial pain

Nasal pain is extremely rare except following trauma. Pain over the sinuses usually indicates infection. However, other causes of facial pain are common and include migraine, dental sepsis and trigeminal neuralgia.

EXAMINATION

➔ **Examination sequence**

Inspection

→ Look at the external surface and appearance of the nose. Note any skin disease, or deformity.

→ Deviation of the nose is best appreciated by standing behind the patient and looking down the nose from above while asking the patient to look upwards (sky-line view).

→ Note any periorbital swelling or conjunctival injection that may help to confirm sinus infection or allergic rhinitis.

→ To see the anterior nares clearly, especially in children, press on the tip of the nose to elevate it (Fig. 9.10). In children you will see the nasal vestibule, the anterior end of the septum and the anterior end of the inferior turbinates. In adults use a nasal speculum or a large-bore speculum on an auriscope to get the same view. .

→ Look for the septum, which should be in the midline. If it deviates to one side, the inferior turbinate on the other side may be hypertrophied causing bilateral blockage. Look at the nasal septum for bleeding points, clots where bleeding has recently stopped, crusting and perforations which may occur with nose picking, granulomatous disease such as Wegener's granulomatosis, cocaine use and inhalation of industrial dusts, e.g. nickel and chromium.

→ On the lateral wall inspect the anterior end of the inferior turbinate. This is hypertrophied in allergic rhinitis and its mucosa is pale and moist. In vasomotor rhinitis, the mucosa is swollen and red. A pale grey moist swelling blocking the nostril may be a polyp (Fig. 9.11).

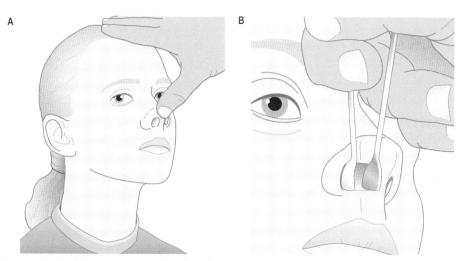

Fig. 9.10   (A) Elevating the tip of the nose to give a clear view of the anterior nares. (B) Anterior rhinoscopy using a Thudicom's nasal speculum.

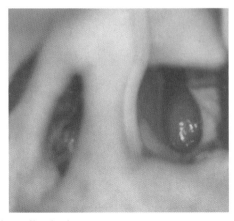

Fig. 9.11 Nasal polyp.

Palpation

→ Feel the nasal bones gently to help distinguish bony from cartilaginous deformity.

→ Feel any facial swelling and note tenderness. Facial swelling is unusual in sinusitis but occurs with a dental root abscess, and cancer of the maxillary antrum.

→ Block each nostril in turn and ask the patient to breathe in to assess nasal obstruction. If you probe a polyp in the nasal cavity, it is soft, mobile and pain free. This is difficult to do without using a head-light and both hands.

→ A more detailed examination of the nasal cavity extending back to the nasopharynx can be performed using fine-bore endoscopy.

→ You can see the postnasal space using a small mirror inserted through the mouth and passed beyond the soft palate. This is called posterior rhinoscopy.

THE MOUTH AND THROAT

Anatomy

The mouth or oral cavity extends from the lips anteriorly, up to but not including the tonsils posteriorly. Within it are the anterior two-thirds of the tongue, the lips, the hard palate, the teeth and the alveoli of the maxilla and mandible. The gums are closely adherent to the alveolus and related to the teeth. The throat includes the pharynx (subdivided into nasopharynx, oropharynx, and hypopharynx) and the larynx (subdivided into the supraglottis, glottis and subglottis).

The mouth. The lips form a seal for the oral cavity and play a role in articulation and visual signalling. The tongue is a mass of interlaced muscle covered with squamous epithelium. Its normal appearance varies greatly from pink through red to very dark brown. The normal surface of the tongue has a velvety texture because of the filiform papillae. There are also pink fungiform papillae which contain salivary glands. At the junction of the anterior two-thirds of the tongue and the posterior third are the circumvallate papillae, which also contain taste buds (Fig. 9.12). These are larger and round and appear a darker red, standing out against the paler surroundings. They are arranged in a wide V with the apex pointing posteriorly. The tongue contains numerous taste buds and is essential for articulation, mastication, and swallowing.

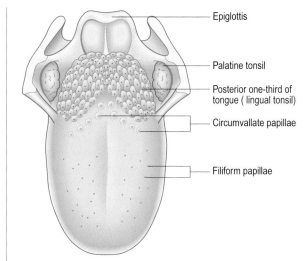

Fig. 9.12 Anatomy of the tongue.

The base of the tongue has the anterior and posterior tonsillar, or faucial, pillars laterally with the palatine tonsils located between them (Fig. 9.13).

The parotid, submandibular and sublingual salivary glands secrete saliva into the oral cavity. The parotid gland produces

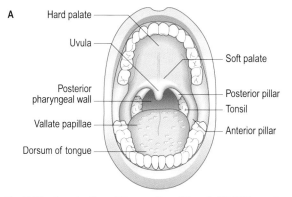

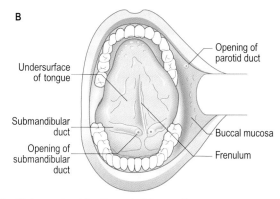

Fig. 9.13 Examination of the mouth and throat. (A) With mouth open; (B) with tongue touching the roof of the mouth.

a serous secretion and the submandibular a seromucinous one. The parotid gland sits in front of the ear and is traversed by the facial nerve. It opens into the mouth (Stensen's papilla) on the buccal mucosa opposite the second upper molar. The submandibular gland lies anterior and medial to the angle of the jaw and its duct (Wharton's) opens into the floor of the mouth next to the frenulum of the tongue. Saliva is essential to keep the mouth moist; it lubricates food, and helps articulation, mastication and taste. This also helps the first stage of swallowing and oral hygiene since saliva contains IgA.

Teeth.   In children the primary dentition is complete by 3 years and consists of 20 'milk' teeth. Secondary dentition starts at around 6 years and is complete by the late teens. Adults have 32 permanent teeth (Figs 9.14 and 9.15).

The throat.   The *pharynx* consists of the upper parts of the digestive and respiratory tract and stretches from the base of the skull to the cricopharyngeal sphincter. The *nasopharynx* lies behind the choanae of the nose above the soft palate. The *oropharynx* is bounded by the uvula above and the upper surface of the epiglottis below and contains the tonsils.

The *hypopharynx* is the posterior pharyngeal wall, the piriform fossae and the post-cricoid area. The piriform fossae are the lateral walls of the pharynx adjacent to the larynx and they channel food into the upper oesophagus.

The *larynx* consists of several muscles and cartilage. Its functions are to prevent food and saliva entering the respiratory tract, and voice production. Its sensory supply is via the superior and recurrent laryngeal branches of cranial nerve X (vagus). Its motor supply is mainly from the recurrent laryngeal nerve which loops round the arch of the aorta on the left and the subclavian artery on the right before entering the larynx inferiorly.

SYMPTOMS OF MOUTH AND THROAT DISEASE

Common symptoms are:

- mouth pain
- odynophagia (pain on swallowing)
- stridor (noisy breathing)
- dysphonia (difficulty in voice production)
- dysphagia (difficulty swallowing)
- lump, swelling or other changes in appearance
- halitosis (bad breath).

Pain

Sore mouth

The commonest cause is local pain from dental caries or periodontal infection. Inflammation of the gums (gingivitis) may cause a narrow red line at the border of the gums, swollen interdental papillae and bleeding of the gums with

Fig. 9.14 Primary and secondary dentition.

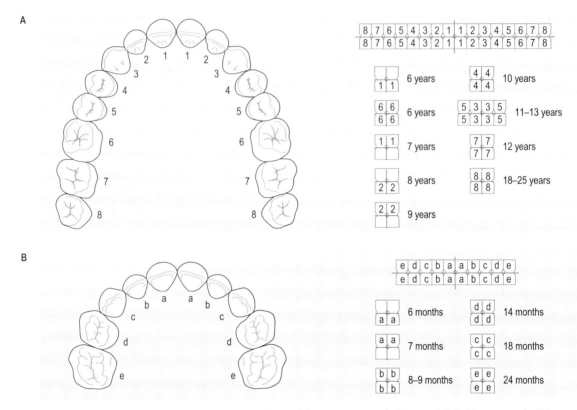

Fig. 9.15   (A) Permanent upper arch and average eruption times of the permanent teeth. An upper left deciduous central will be designated | a; a lower right permanent lateral incisor 2 |, a lower left permanent third molar | 8, etc. **(B) Primary upper arch and average eruption times of the deciduous teeth.**

9.3 The gums in systemic conditions	
Phenytoin treatment	Firm and hypertrophied
Scurvy	Soft, haemorrhagic
Acute leukaemia	Hypertrophied and haemorrhagic
Cyanotic congenital heart disease	Spongy and haemorrhagic
Chronic lead poisoning	Punctate blue line

minor trauma, e.g. brushing teeth. As this progresses, food debris, bacteria and pus accumulate between the teeth and gums causing halitosis and eventually leading to the teeth becoming loose and falling out. Teeth brushing or dental manipulation can cause transient bacteraemia which in turn may cause infective endocarditis in patients with valvular heart disease. Other changes in the gums occur in certain systemic conditions (Table 9.3). Ulceration on the gums, tongue or buccal or lingual surfaces may be due to trauma, vitamin and mineral deficiency (anaemia), or lichen planus. Infection from bacteria (Vincent's angina), yeast (thrush) or

viruses (herpes simplex) also cause characteristic changes. Painful vesicles on the palate can be caused by herpes zoster. Diffuse oral thrush should make you think of antibiotic therapy, use of inhaled steroids and immunodeficient states, e.g. HIV infection or leukaemias.

Sore throat

This is one of the most common symptoms presented to doctors. Patients may use this to describe pain anywhere in the mouth or throat so clarify exactly where they feel the pain. Many viruses cause acute inflammation of the pharynx, while acute follicular tonsillitis (Fig. 9.16) may be caused by streptococcal infection. In both there may be a pustular exudate on the tonsils and associated systemic features of fever, malaise, anorexia and cervical lymphadenopathy. Viral sore throat is a self-limiting condition treated symptomatically but bacterial tonsillitis may require antibiotics.

In glandular fever, palatal petechiae can be seen and the tonsil may be covered in a white pseudomembrane (Fig. 9.17). Diphtheria caused by *Corynebacterium diphtheriae* causes

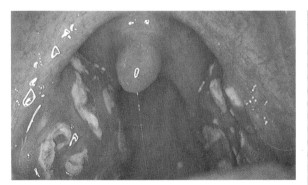

Fig. 9.16   Acute tonsillitis.

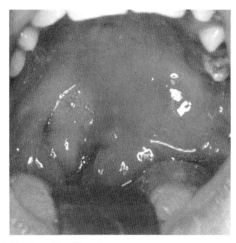

Fig. 9.18   A peritonsillar abscess

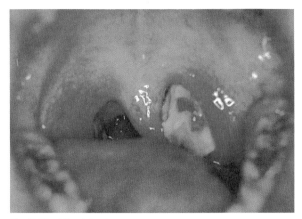

Fig. 9.17   Glandular fever

9.4   Causes of stridor
Neonate
• Laryngomalacia (commonest) • Congenital tumours
Child
• Infection • Croup (viral) • Epiglottitis (bacterial) • Laryngitis • Foreign body
Adult
• Infection • Epiglottitis • Laryngitis • Trauma • Cancer of the larynx • Cancer of the trachea or main bronchus

a true grey membrane over the tonsil but is rarely seen these days because of childhood immunization.

A peritonsillar abscess (quinsy; Fig. 9.18) causes extreme pain so that the patient dribbles saliva out of his mouth rather than swallowing it. Trismus (spasm of the pterygoid muscles preventing the jaw from fully opening) is present and the uvula is often displaced to the opposite side. Any persistent mass or ulcer on the tonsil associated with pain may be a squamous cancer. Throat pain often radiates to the ear because of the dual innervation of the pharynx and external auditory meatus via the vagus nerve.

Stridor

Stridor is a noise from the upper airway on inspiration, caused by narrowing. Noise present on both inspiration and expiration (biphasic stridor) indicates narrowing at the level of the vocal cords or trachea, while noise on expiration (wheeze) indicates narrowing of the smaller, peripheral airways.

Causes of stridor are listed in Table 9.4.

> **Examine this patient who complains of a sore throat**
>
> 1. General examination looking for evidence of systemic upset (pyrexia, flushing, tachycardia, drooling).
> 2. Palpate the neck for lymphadenopathy, especially tender jugulodigastric nodes (*bacterial tonsillitis* or *glandular fever*).
> 3. Inspect the oral cavity and oropharynx with dentures removed, using a bright light source and a wooden tongue depressor looking for surface appearance and asymmetry in the tonsils.
> 4. Ask the patient to open his mouth: difficulty (trismus) indicates inflammation affecting muscles of mastication.
> 5. Using a gloved finger, feel the oral cavity especially the tongue.
> 6. Look into the nostrils using the broad auriscope attachment, for evidence of inflammation (*rhinitis* and *postnasal drip*).
> 7. Consider further examination of the larynx and hypopharynx (specialist examination).
> 8. Consider further investigations (blood film and monospot for *glandular fever*), allergy testing if seasonal symptoms (*allergic rhinitis*), throat swab (for *bacterial tonsillitis*).

Epiglottitis usually presents with rapidly progressive airway obstruction occurring within a few hours, sore throat, fever and drooling and is most common in small children.

Acute laryngotracheobronchitis (*croup*) in infants usually has a longer history (24–48 hours) and the airway obstruction is less severe.

Do not try to examine the throat in a patient with stridor as this may induce laryngospasm and total airway obstruction.

Snoring is caused by an obstruction to the upper airway while asleep. This may be due to enlarged adenoids and tonsils in children. In adults, snoring is more common in older and overweight patients. If severe, it may be associated with apnoeic episodes during sleep. This in turn causes daytime sleepiness, producing the condition obstructive sleep apnoea.

Dysphonia

Dysphonia is a change in the quality of the patient's voice. Anyone with hoarseness for more than 4 weeks should have the larynx examined by direct laryngoscopy to exclude cancer since most other causes remit spontaneously. If dysphonia is associated with stridor then refer urgently for specialist assessment.

Dysphonia is caused by the smooth edges of the vocal cords not meeting in close apposition. The speed of onset and quality of the voice will give you clues as to the cause since any acute vocal cord insult may cause dysphonia (Table 9.5). The cause is usually obvious in those who have had an upper respiratory tract infection or who abuse their voice. Some people develop functional dysphonia for which no physical cause is found. This tends to vary over time and is associated with a normal cough confirming good

9.5	Causes of dysphonia
Neonate	
• Congenital abnormality • Neurological disorder	
Child	

• Infection:
  – croup
  – laryngitis
• Voice abuse (screamer's nodes)	

Adult	

• Infection:
  – upper respiratory tract infection
  – laryngitis
• Trauma
• Vocal cord nodules (singer's nodes)
• Neurological
• Cancer of the larynx
• Functional	

apposition of the vocal cords. Smoking, excess alcohol or poor dental hygiene, however, raises the possibility of malignancy. Causes of recurrent laryngeal nerve damage with vocal cord palsy, e.g. lung cancer, cancers of the oesophagus or thyroid and aortic or subclavian aneurysm produce progressive hoarseness with features of the underlying disease.

Dysphagia

This is difficulty in swallowing (see Ch. 5). Malignancy of the postcricoid area is more common in women with Paterson–Brown–Kelly (Plummer–Vinson) syndrome. Pain on swallowing (odynophagia) usually indicates inflammation but also occurs in cancer of the oropharynx, hypopharynx, larynx and cervical oesophagus.

Lumps and other changes

In the neck

These may be noticed by the patient or by another person. The most common cause is an enlarged lymph node and the source may be in the head, neck, chest or abdomen. Generalized lymphadenopathy may be associated with hepatosplenomegaly and lymphadenopathy in other regions. Ask about systemic features such as fever, sweats and malaise (see Ch. 2). Tenderness in a node usually indicates inflammation due to infection. In a sore throat from any infective cause, the jugulodigastric nodes can often be palpated. These lie posterior to the angle of the mandible and anterosuperior to the internal jugular vein. They are often tender but settle quickly as the infection resolves (Table 9.6).

In the face

Stones may block the ducts causing painful swelling of the salivary glands. Other causes of enlargement of the salivary glands include mumps, sarcoidosis, bacterial infection (suppurative parotitis; Fig. 9.21) or tumour.

Reduced flow of saliva as occurs in Sjögren's syndrome or as a side-effect of anticholinergic drugs leads to a dry mouth (*xerostomia*). This may result in overgrowth of oral bacteria, sore throat, ulceration and halitosis.

In the oral cavity

Lips. The colour of the lips gives an indication of both blood oxygenation and temperature. Hypoxia or cold causes central cyanosis or blue discoloration. Cold exposure causes desquamation and cracking of the lips. Riboflavine deficiency may produce red cracking at the line of closure of the lips. Inflamed painful cracking of the skin at the corners of the mouth (*angular stomatitis*; Fig. 9.22) may be due to

9.6   Causes of neck lumps

Midline structures

- Thyroid isthmus swelling – commonest cause in adults (see Ch. 2)
- Thyroglossal cyst (Fig. 9.19) – commonest cause in children (lump moves when patient sticks out tongue)
- Laryngeal swellings
- Submental lymph nodes
- Dermoid cysts

Lateral structures

In the anterior triangle
(bounded by the midline, the anterior border of sternocleidomastoid muscle and body of mandible; Fig. 9.20)
- Thyroid lobe swellings
- Pharyngeal pouch
- Submandibular gland swelling
- Branchial cyst
- Lymph nodes:
  - malignant: lymphoma, metastatic disease
  - infection:
    any bacterial infection of head/neck (including teeth)
    viral infection, e.g. infectious mononucleosis, HIV
    tuberculosis
- Parotid gland swelling, e.g. mumps, parotitis, stones, autoimmune disease, benign and malignant tumours

In the posterior triangle
(bounded by posterior border of sternocleidomastoid muscle, trapezius and the clavicle; Fig. 9.20)
- Lymph nodes:
  - malignant: lymphoma, metastatic cancer
  - infection:
    any bacterial infection of head/neck (including teeth)
    viral infection, e.g. infectious mononucleosis, HIV
    tuberculosis
- Carotid artery aneurysm
- Carotid body tumour
- Cystic hygroma
- Cervical rib

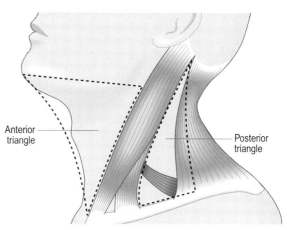

Fig. 9.20   Sites of swellings in the neck.

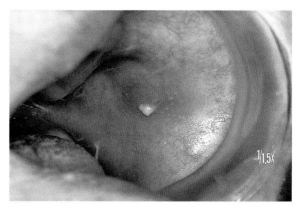

Fig. 9.21   Pus discharging from parotid duct.

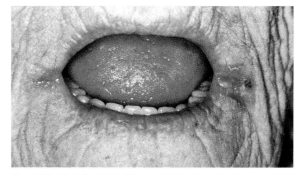

Fig. 9.22   Angular stomatitis.

local irritation from excess saliva or poorly fitting dentures but may also indicate iron deficiency. The lips are a common site for localized malignancy, e.g. squamous and basal cell cancers. The former are associated with smoking, especially pipe, the latter with sun exposure.

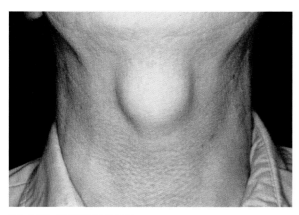

Fig. 9.19   Thyroglossal cyst.

Melanin deposition on the buccal mucosa is normal in black people. Abnormal buccal pigmentation is found in Addison's disease (see Fig. 2.8B, p. 44), haemochromatosis or the rare Peutz–Jeghers syndrome (polyposis of the small intestine with pigmentation on the fingers and lips and in the mouth).

Lumps in the mouth. The patient may not notice a lump if it is behind the tongue but any painless persistent mass should be assumed to be an oral cancer and referred to an oral surgeon. Even if the patient has only just noticed it, the lump may have been present for some time.

Mucous retention cysts occur on the mucosa of the cheeks and lips as bluish domes less than 1 cm diameter, and often burst spontaneously. They usually occur in younger people. A dental surgeon should assess any mass associated with the teeth.

Some patients present with the feeling of a lump in the throat (*globus pharyngeus*). Look for postnasal drip and gastro-oesophageal reflux. Occasionally it is a sign of underlying malignancy. Warning signs are progressive symptoms and associated features including dysphagia, hoarseness, odynophagia and weight loss. In most cases examination is normal and the symptom is associated with anxiety. The condition generally remits spontaneously but may recur.

Tongue. Areas of changing denuded smooth mucosa (geographic tongue) or of excessive furring can be found in normal subjects. Black discoloration can be seen in heavy smokers while a smooth red tongue due to diffuse atrophy of the papillae may indicate iron or vitamin B_{12} deficiency (Fig. 9.23). The tongue may be enlarged (macroglossia) in Down's syndrome, acromegaly, hypothroidism and amyloidosis. Wasting and fasciculation of the tongue are features of motor neurone disease. Both lower motor neurone lesions of the hypoglossal nerve (cranial nerve XII) and stroke (upper motor neurone lesion) cause the extended tongue to deviate towards the side of the lesion.

White patches on the tongue or oral mucosa are usually due to thrush, a candidal yeast infection (Fig. 9.24), or leukoplakia, a premalignant condition that requires excision biopsy (Fig. 9.25). The white patches of thrush can be easily scraped off with a tongue depressor while leukoplakia cannot. Aphthous ulcers are small and painful on the inner sides of the lips, the edges of the tongue and the insides of the cheeks (Fig. 9.26). They occur in crops and usually

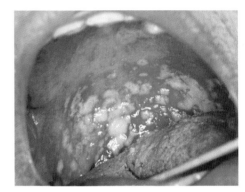

Fig. 9.24   Oral thrush.

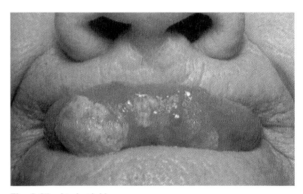

Fig. 9.25   Leukoplakia.

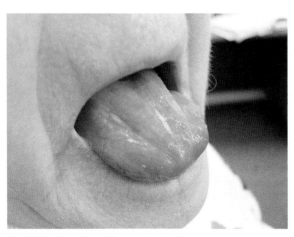

Fig. 9.23   Smooth, red tongue of glossitis.

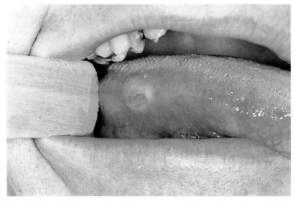

Fig. 9.26   Aphthous stomatitis causing a deep ulcer in a patient with inflammatory bowel disease.

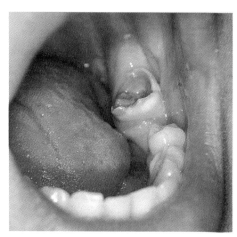

Fig. 9.27 Dental caries.

heal within a few days. Mouth ulcers may be the first presentation of inflammatory bowel disease, e.g. Crohn's disease or ulcerative colitis. Any mouth ulcers persisting for over 3 weeks require biopsy to exclude oral cancer.

Rotten teeth (dental caries; Fig. 9.27) are common in patients with poor oral hygiene.

Offensive smell

Halitosis is usually associated with dental caries and gingivitis but may be caused by tonsillar infection, or paranasal sinus infection with a purulent postnasal drip.

EXAMINATION

→ Examination sequence

→ Have a good light source. A head mirror or head-light allows both hands free to manipulate instruments.

Inspection
→ Observe the patient's demeanour and face for obvious abnormalities. These include skin disease, scars, lumps, signs of trauma, deformity and asymmetry of the face.
→ Look at the lips, then ask the patient to open his mouth. Inspect the buccal mucosa, gums and teeth. If dentures are being worn, ask the patient to remove them and offer a pot or paper tissue to put them in. Note the patient's dental hygiene, and any gingivitis.
→ Ask the patient to evert the lips. Look for areas of discoloration, inflammation, ulceration or nodules.
→ Look at the hard palate. Note any cleft, abnormal arched palate or telangiectasia.
→ Look at the tongue, first with it inside the mouth then ask the patient to put it out, and look at the lateral borders. Neurological disease, painful mouth, or a tight frenulum may all limit its protrusion. This gives a better view of the posterior of the tongue and also allows you to assess the

XII nerve (hypoglossal) function. Ask the patient to touch the roof of the mouth with the tongue, and inspect the floor of the mouth. Note any changes and the punctum of the submandibular glands.
→ Look at the posterior aspect of the oral cavity and the oropharynx. Ask the patient to say 'Aaah'. Some patients open wide enough to allow a good view of all the structures, but to obtain a clear view use a tongue depressor. These are usually made of wood and disposable. Place it firmly on the patient's tongue as far back as the posterior third of the tongue and ask the patient to say 'Aaah' again as you hold the tongue down.
→ Look at the uvula and see if it moves symmetrically.
→ Look at the soft palate for any cleft or structural abnormality. Note any telangiectasia, which are common in viral infections. Look at the tonsillar pillars and tonsils and note their size, colour, any discharge or membrane and whether they are symmetrical in shape and size. Tonsils are maximal in size around the age of 8. Thereafter they involute, and may be difficult to see in adults.
→ Use the tongue depressor to gently scrape off any white plaques that you see. Thrush comes away easily but leukoplakia is not removed. Some people are very sensitive to the tongue depressor and even a gentle examination stimulates their gag reflex. Check for symmetrical movement of the soft palate and limit any further examination to avoid discomfort for the patient. Deliberately touch the posterior pharyngeal wall or tonsillar pillars to stimulate the gag reflex.
→ Ask the patient to put out his tongue and move it to the left; use the tongue depressor to see into the right posterolateral edge of the tongue. This is a site for many cancers and any changes here should prompt further investigation. The patient may not have noted any symptoms. Repeat this for the other side.

Palpation
→ If you have noted any lesion in the mouth put on a pair of gloves and palpate it with one hand outside on the patient's cheek or jaw and a gloved finger inside the patient's mouth. Feel the lesion and identify its characteristics. Use a similar technique for the salivary glands if they are affected. Rarely you may feel a stone in the parotid duct in a patient with sudden onset of swelling of this gland. Stones in the submandibular duct are more common and usually easily palpated along the floor of the mouth.
→ Finally palpate the cervical lymph nodes systematically (see pp. 51 and 52).

◆ Key points

♦ Hold the auriscope like a pen to avoid hurting the patient and to give you fine control over the speculum.
♦ Pain when you retract the pinna suggests infection in the external auditory meatus.
♦ If patients can hear a whisper at arm's length, their hearing is likely to be normal.
♦ Do not syringe an ear that may have a perforated tympanic membrane; use microsuction to clear wax.

- Use the auriscope to visualize the internal nares.
- Look for nasal deviation from above the patient.
- A pearly grey mass obstructing a nostril that is painless if probed is a polyp.
- Most patients, particularly children, open their mouth wide enough for a good view without you using a tongue depressor.

- Palpate any masses in the mouth with your gloved finger inside the oral cavity.
- Always examine the lateral borders of the tongue (using a depressor if necessary) so that you do not miss hidden cancer.

The musculoskeletal system

JIM S. HUNTLEY • DAVID M. REID • A. HAMISH R. W. SIMPSON

MUSCULOSKELETAL EXAMINATION

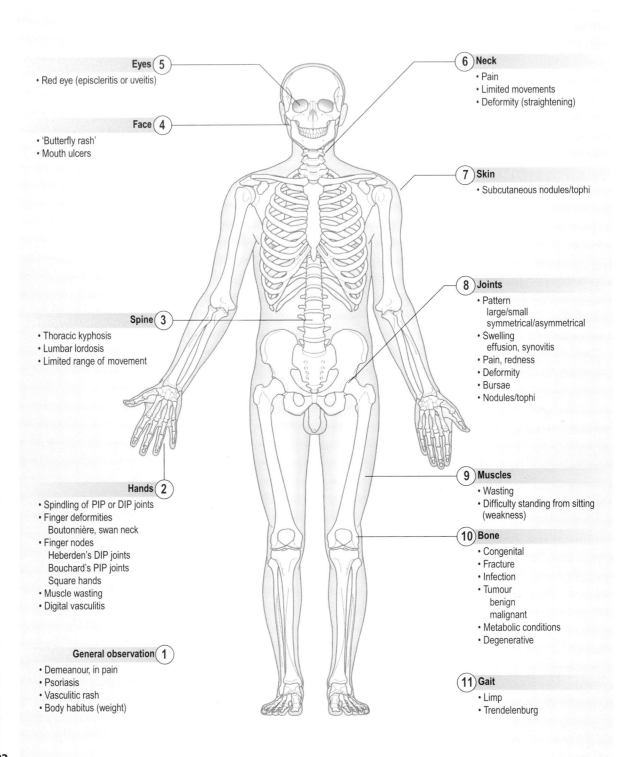

Eyes ⑤
- Red eye (episcleritis or uveitis)

Face ④
- 'Butterfly rash'
- Mouth ulcers

Spine ③
- Thoracic kyphosis
- Lumbar lordosis
- Limited range of movement

Hands ②
- Spindling of PIP or DIP joints
- Finger deformities
  Boutonnière, swan neck
- Finger nodes
  Heberden's DIP joints
  Bouchard's PIP joints
  Square hands
- Muscle wasting
- Digital vasculitis

General observation ①
- Demeanour, in pain
- Psoriasis
- Vasculitic rash
- Body habitus (weight)

⑥ **Neck**
- Pain
- Limited movements
- Deformity (straightening)

⑦ **Skin**
- Subcutaneous nodules/tophi

⑧ **Joints**
- Pattern
  large/small
  symmetrical/asymmetrical
- Swelling
  effusion, synovitis
- Pain, redness
- Deformity
- Bursae
- Nodules/tophi

⑨ **Muscles**
- Wasting
- Difficulty standing from sitting
  (weakness)

⑩ **Bone**
- Congenital
- Fracture
- Infection
- Tumour
  benign
  malignant
- Metabolic conditions
- Degenerative

⑪ **Gait**
- Limp
- Trendelenburg

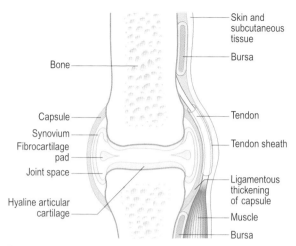

Bone

Capsule
Synovium
Fibrocartilage pad
Joint space

Hyaline articular cartilage

Skin and subcutaneous tissue
Bursa

Tendon

Tendon sheath

Ligamentous thickening of capsule
Muscle
Bursa

Fig. 10.1 Structure of a joint and surrounding tissues.

10.1	Causes of joint pain (arthralgia)
Generalized	
Infective	Viral, e.g. rubella, mumps, hepatitis B Bacterial, e.g. staphylococci, tuberculosis, *Borrelia* Fungal
Post-infective	Rheumatic fever, reactive arthritis
Inflammatory	Rheumatoid arthritis, systemic lupus erythematosus, ankylosing spondylitis, scleroderma
Degenerative	Osteoarthritis
Tumour	Primary, e.g. osteosarcoma, chondrosarcoma Metastatic, e.g. from lung, breast, prostate Systemic tumour effects, e.g. hypertrophic pulmonary osteoarthropathy
Crystal formation	Gout, pseudogout
Others	Trauma Fibromyalgia syndrome Sjögren's syndrome Hypermobility syndromes
Localized	
Tendonitis	e.g. shoulder rotator cuff lesions, such as supraspinatus tendonitis, Achilles tendonitis
Enthesopathies	e.g. tennis elbow, golfer's elbow
Bursitis	e.g. trochanteric bursitis
Nerve entrapment	e.g. carpal tunnel syndrome

INTRODUCTION

To examine the musculoskeletal system you need to know the anatomy (Fig. 10.1), normal function and common pathologies. Several systemic disorders may affect the musculoskeletal system, so be aware of patterns of features. For example psoriasis affects the skin, nails and sometimes the joints, and joint symptoms and erythema nodosum may occur in sarcoidosis.

Clinical examination can be more relevant than advanced investigations such as magnetic resonance imaging. This is because you can assess the *functional* significance of any abnormality, e.g. the degree of ligamentous laxity at a joint.

There are a large number of conditions affecting the musculoskeletal system but if you follow a simple system it is possible to narrow down the possibilities.

- Was the problem caused by, or related to, an injury? If it was, follow the guidance in chapter 12.
- If not, are the joints affected? If they are then you may be dealing with a type of arthritis, or one of the causes of arthralgia (Table 10.1). The term *arthritis* implying joint inflammation may be a misnomer, e.g. as in osteoarthritis. *Arthralgia* means joint pain. Almost all patients with arthritis have arthralgia, but only a minority of patients with arthralgia have arthritis. If you suspect arthritis you need to establish whether it is an 'inflammatory' or 'non-inflammatory' process.
- Inflammatory conditions produce pain at rest and on movement, and symptoms are often worse in the morning. Inflammatory arthritis is characteristically worse in the morning or after periods of inactivity. Stiffness tends to ease with movement or after a warm bath or shower. Inflammatory arthritis may be seropositive or seronegative.

- Seropositive arthritis is associated with autoantibodies, e.g. rheumatoid factor. About 80% of cases of rheumatoid arthritis are positive for IgM rheumatoid factor. However, low titres can occur in other conditions and occasionally in the general population.
- Causes of seronegative arthritis are ankylosing spondylitis, psoriatic arthritis, the reactive arthritides also called *Reiter's syndrome* (which follow bacterial dysentery caused by *Salmonella*, *Shigella*, *Campylobacter* or *Yersinia* infections, or sexually acquired infection with *Chlamydia*), crystal arthritis (gout and pseudogout) and septic arthritis.
- How many joints are involved? If only one, it is a *monoarthritis*, two to four joints constitute *oligoarthritis* and more than four, *polyarthritis* (Fig. 10.2 and Table 10.2).
- Are the joints affected symmetrically or asymmetrically? Rheumatoid arthritis and systemic lupus erythematosus tend to produce symmetrical forms of arthritis, whereas seronegative arthritis is more often asymmetrical.
- Are the small or large joints of the arms or legs affected? Rheumatoid arthritis characteristically affects small joints in the early stages, while seronegative arthritis most often affects the larger joints.

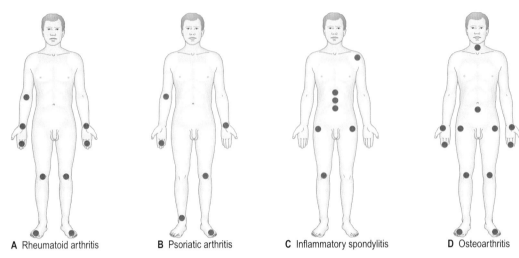

A Rheumatoid arthritis   **B** Psoriatic arthritis   **C** Inflammatory spondylitis   **D** Osteoarthritis

Fig. 10.2 Contrasting patterns of involvement in polyarthritis. (A) Rheumatoid arthritis (symmetrical, small and large joints, upper and lower limbs). (B) Seronegative psoriatic arthritis (asymmetrical, large > small joints, associated periarticular inflammation giving dactylitis). (C) Seronegative inflammatory spondylitis (axial involvement, large > small joints, asymmetrical). (D) Osteoarthritis (symmetrical, small and large joints).

10.2 Differential diagnosis of mono- oligo- and polyarthritis

Type	Examples	Type	Examples
Monoarthritis (single joint involvement)		Inflammatory	Infective: bacterial endocarditis, *Neisseria gonorrhoea*, mycobacteria Sarcoidosis
Infective	*Staphylococcus aureus*, *Staph. epidermidis*, *Salmonella*, tuberculosis, *Neisseria gonorrhoea*, *Escherichia coli*, *Haemophilus*	Polyarthritis presenting as oligoarthritis	
Traumatic	e.g. haemarthrosis	**Polyarthritis (involvement of five or more joints)**	
Bleeding diathesis	Haemarthrosis such as in haemophilia	Inflammatory: inflammatory	e.g. rheumatoid arthritis, systemic lupus erythematosus
Post-traumatic			
Degenerative	Acute exacerbation of underlying state, Charcot joint	infective: bacterial viral	Lyme disease, subacute bacterial endocarditis Rubella, mumps, glandular fever, chickenpox, hepatitis B and C, HIV
Metabolic	Crystal arthropathies – gout, pseudogout	post-infective	Rheumatic fever
Polyarthritis presenting as monoarthritis	e.g. rheumatoid arthritis	Non-inflammatory: osteoarthritis metabolic other	Nodal with Heberden's/Bouchard's nodes Haemochromatosis Hypertrophic pulmonary osteoarthropathy
Oligoarthritis (involvement of two to four joints)			
Degenerative	Osteoarthritis		
Inflammatory	Seronegative conditions: reactive arthritis psoriatic arthropathy ankylosing spondylitis		

If the joint problem is non-inflammatory it may be caused by a degenerative or, rarely, a neoplastic process. Some musculoskeletal cancers, especially if rapidly growing, may have an inflammatory type of presentation.

If joints are not involved, the problem may involve the surrounding tissues or be referred from another site. Surrounding structures include ligaments, tendons, tendon sheaths, bursae, muscle and bone (see Fig. 10.1), and the process may be inflammatory due to infective or non-infective causes, or non-inflammatory.

When examining the patient distinguish between:

- focal pathology (e.g. lateral epicondylitis of the elbow ('tennis elbow'), medial meniscal tear of the knee, osteoarthritis at the hip)
- systemic conditions with (one or more) local manifestations (e.g. rheumatoid arthritis, systemic lupus erythematosus, psoriasis)

- referred pain from a different site, e.g. diaphragmatic irritation causing shoulder-tip pain
- radicular pain, e.g. pain felt down the back of the leg from an intervertebral disc protruding onto a nerve root.

COMMON SYMPTOMS

PAIN

Determine whether the pain originates from a joint (*arthralgia*), muscle (*myalgia*) or other soft tissue structure. The site may be well localized and suggest the diagnosis, e.g. the first metatarsophalangeal joint in gout (Fig. 10.3). If, however, pain is referred, it may be difficult to determine the exact source (Tables 10.3 and 10.4).

Determine whether the pain is mechanical or non-mechanical. Is it present at rest or aggravated by movement? Pain caused by a mechanical problem is worse on movement and eases with rest. Pain present at rest may be due to a process such as inflammation, infection or tumour and is often aggravated by movement.

The onset and timing of pain give clues to the diagnosis. For instance, pain from traumatic injury is usually immediate but is also exacerbated by movement or if bleeding occurs into the affected joint (*haemarthrosis*).

10.3 Assessing musculoskeletal pain (*mnemonic SOCRATES*)
Site
Onset
Character
Radiation
Associated factors
Timing (frequency, duration, periodicity)
Exacerbating features (exercise, use, etc.)
Severity

10.4 Common patterns of referred and radicular musculoskeletal pain	
Site of pathology	**Perceived at**
Cervical spine	Occiput, vertex of head Shoulders, arms
Thoracic spine	Chest
Lumbar spine	Buttocks, knees. legs
Shoulder	Lateral aspect of upper arm
Elbow	Forearm
Hip	Anterior thigh, knee
Knee	Thigh, hip

The onset of arthralgia and the pattern of joints involved suggests the disease process.

- Crystal arthritis (gout and pseudogout) causes acute, sometimes extreme, pain which develops quickly and is often associated with redness (*erythema*) of the affected joint.
- Joint sepsis causes pain that develops over a day or two.
- Episodic pain lasting for 1–2 days in one or more joints is sometimes called *palindromic rheumatism.*
- Flitting joint pain which starts in one joint and moves to affect others over a period of days is a feature of rheumatic fever and gonoccocal arthritis.

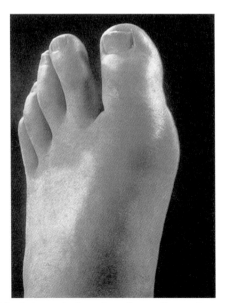

Fig. 10.3 Podagra. Acute gout causing swelling, erythema and extreme pain and tenderness of the first metatarsophalangeal joint.

10.5 Causes of muscle pain (myalgia)	
Infective	
Viral	Coxsackie, CMV, ECHO
Bacterial	*Streptococcus pneumoniae*, *Mycoplasma*
Parasitic	Schistosomiasis, toxoplasmosis
Inflammatory	Polymyalgia rheumatica, myositis, dermatomyositis, temporal (giant cell) arteritis
Traumatic	Tears, haematoma, rhabdomyolysis
Drugs	e.g. alcohol, statins, zidovudine
Neuropathic	

Pain is subjective and patients often have difficulty expressing its character. Chronic pain is commonly associated with anxiety and depression, which may worsen the patient's perception and response. Ask if pain disturbs sleep by preventing patients getting to sleep or by waking them.

- Bone pain is often described as penetrating, deep or boring and is characteristically worse at night. Localized pain suggests tumour, chronic infection (*osteomyelitis*), avascular necrosis or osteoid osteoma (a benign bone tumour).
- Generalized bony conditions such as osteomalacia and Paget's disease usually cause diffuse pain.
- Muscle pain (Table 10.5) is usually described as stiffness and is poorly localized, deep and aggravated by use of the muscle. It is associated with muscle weakness in some cases, e.g. polymyositis, but not in polymyalgia rheumatica.
- Partial muscle tears may be painful, but complete rupture may be relatively pain-free.
- Fracture pain is sharp and stabbing, aggravated by attempted movement or use and relieved by rest and splintage.
- 'Shooting' pain is often caused by mechanical trapping of a peripheral nerve, e.g. buttock pain which 'shoots' down the back of the leg, caused by lumbar intervertebral disc protrusion.
- Chronic joint pain in patients > 40 years old with progression over years is commonly caused by osteoarthritis. These patients often say that their symptoms vary, with 'good' and 'bad' days.
- Neurological involvement in diabetes mellitus, leprosy, syringomyelia and syphilis (*tabes dorsalis*) may cause loss of pain from joints, or pain that is disproportionately less than you would expect from examination. Even grossly abnormal joints may be pain-free (*Charcot joint*).
- Pain that is disproportionately *greater* than expected is seen in *compartment syndrome* (increased pressure in a fascial compartment, which compromises the perfusion and hence viability of the compartmental structures) and *reflex sympathetic dystrophy*, also called *algodystrophy*.

This poorly understood condition develops after injury, illness or spontaneously and is characterized by severe 'burning' pain, local tenderness, oedema, abnormal sweating and colour, temperature changes and localized osteoporosis.

STIFFNESS

Establish what the patient means by stiffness; is it:

- a restricted range of movement?
- difficulty moving, but with a normal range of movement?
- painful movement?

Ask whether stiffness is localized to a particular joint or is more generalized, as in ankylosing spondylitis and rheumatoid arthritis.

If stiffness predominates over pain, suspect *spasticity* (increasing muscle contraction in response to stretch) or *tetany* (involuntary sustained contraction), and examine for the increased tone characteristic of an upper motor neurone lesion (see Ch. 8).

Stiffness may relate to the soft tissues rather than the joint itself. In polymyalgia rheumatica stiffness commonly affects the shoulder and pelvic areas. Other common soft tissue causes are:

- inflammation at tendon insertion sites (*enthesopathies*), e.g. at the medial and lateral epicondyles of the elbow ('golfer's' and 'tennis' elbow respectively)
- calcific tendinitis, e.g. supraspinatus tendonitis (Fig. 10.4)
- myalgia
- reflex sympathetic dystrophy.

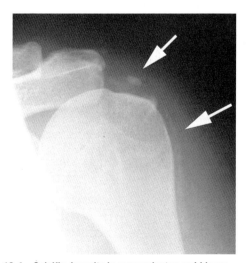

Fig. 10.4   Calcific deposits in supraspinatus and biceps tendons.

There are characteristic differences between inflammatory and non-inflammatory presentations of joint stiffness:

- Inflammatory arthritis presents with early morning stiffness that takes at least 1 hour to wear off with activity.
- Non-inflammatory, mechanical arthritis tends to occur after resting, and stiffness lasts only a few minutes on movement. There may be pain on movement. This typically eases with rest, but may return later in the day.

REDNESS (ERYTHEMA) AND WARMTH

Erythema and warmth over a joint are seen in acute inflammatory arthritis. Erythema is common in infective, traumatic and crystal-induced conditions. It is unusual in seropositive rheumatoid arthritis or systemic lupus erythematosus, and if present may suggest coexisting joint infection.

SWELLING

Establish the site, localization, extent and time course of any swelling. Swelling may be diffuse soft tissue oedema or localized and caused by a discrete collection of fluid in a joint, bursa or tendon sheath (Fig. 10.5A). The time course is especially important when considering joint swelling caused by intra-articular fluid.

The knee is particularly prone to swelling. When vascular structures such as bone and ligament are injured, rapid tense swelling develops within minutes because of bleeding into the joint (Fig. 10.5B). This process is even more rapid and severe if the patient is taking anticoagulants or has an underlying bleeding disorder, e.g. haemophilia. If avascular structures such as the menisci are torn or articular cartilage is abraded, a reactive effusion may take hours or days to form and produce joint swelling.

WEAKNESS

Weakness suggests a joint disorder, peripheral nerve lesion, e.g. median nerve compression in carpal tunnel syndrome, or muscle disease. Establish if the problem is secondary to pain, and whether it is focal or generalized.

The location of weakness is important. Predominantly proximal weakness suggests a primary muscle disease such as immune-mediated inflammatory muscle disease, e.g. dermatomyositis or polymyositis, or a non-inflammatory myopathy, e.g. secondary to chronic alcohol use, steroid therapy or thyrotoxicosis.

Distal weakness is more likely to be neurological such as the peripheral neuropathy of thiamine or vitamin B_{12} deficiency, connective tissue disorders, or peroneal muscular atrophy (*Charcot–Marie–Tooth disease*). Peroneal muscular

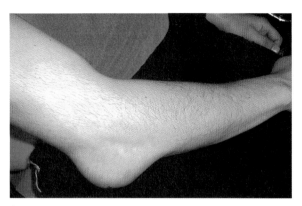

A

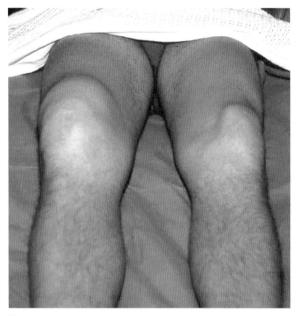

B

Fig. 10.5   Joint swelling. (A) Olecranon bursitis. (B) Right knee haemarthrosis.

atrophy is the most common inherited neuromuscular condition and causes progressive wasting of the distal musculature with weakness and loss of reflexes.

If the weakness is intermittent and worsens during activity, then consider myasthenia gravis. Slowly progressive generalized weakness is a feature of motor neurone disease. Other primary muscle diseases include the heritable muscular dystrophies (Table 10.6 and Fig. 10.6).

LOCKING AND TRIGGERING

Locking is an incomplete range of movement at a joint because of an anatomical block. It may be associated with **307**

10.6 The muscular dystrophies		
	Inheritance	Gene product
Duchenne	X-linked	Dystrophin
Becker	X-linked	Dystrophin
Dystrophia myotonica	Autosomal dominant	Myotonin
Fascioscapulohumeral	Autosomal dominant	
Limb girdle	Autosomal recessive	

pain. Patients use 'locking' to describe a variety of problems, so establish precisely what they mean.

True locking is a block to the usual range of movement caused by a mechanical obstruction (such as a loose body or torn meniscus) within the joint. This prevents the joint reaching the extremes of the normal range of movement. The patient may be able to 'unlock' the joint by trick manoeuvres. This is characteristic of true locking.

Pseudo-locking is a loss of range of movement due to pain rather than a mechanical block. For instance, some patients with patellofemoral pain (typically teenage girls with chondromalacia) hold the knee in full extension and will not flex it.

Sometimes when extending a finger from a flexed position there is a block to extension, which then 'gives' suddenly. This is *triggering*. It results from nodular tendon thickening or a fibrous thickening of the flexor tendon sheath. In adults it usually affects the ring or middle fingers. It can be congenital, usually affecting the thumb.

DEFORMITY

Acute deformity may occur when there is a fracture, dislocation, or alteration of the external skin contour due to swelling, e.g. haemarthrosis or intramuscular haematoma (Fig. 10.7). Chronic joint deformity results in malalignment of the bones forming the joint, or malapposition of the joint surfaces which may be partial (*subluxation*) or complete (*dislocation*). Establish if the joint deformity is fixed or mobile (*passively correctable*).

EXTRA-ARTICULAR MANIFESTATIONS

Inflammatory arthritis is commonly associated with extra-articular features (Tables 10.7 and 10.8). The pattern of the joint condition (symmetric/asymmetric/flitting) and extent (mono-, oligo-, or polyarthritis) may suggest both the diagnosis and the extra-articular features to be sought.

Skin, nail and soft tissue features

The skin and related structures are the commonest sites of associated lesions. Skin rashes, often aggravated by exposure to light, are common in vasculitis, e.g. systemic lupus erythematosus. The skin and nail appearances in psoriasis are usually obvious (see Figs 2.17B, p. 49, and 2.40B, p. 68) but may be hidden by clothing.

In scleroderma the thickened, tight skin produces a characteristic appearance of the face (see Fig. 2.12D, p. 47).

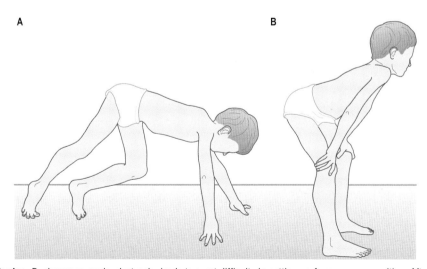

A   B

Fig. 10.6   Gower's sign. Duchenne muscular dystrophy leads to great difficulty in getting up from a prone position. After rolling over, the affected individual walks the hands and feet towards each other (A), then uses his hands to climb up his legs (B), he reaches an upright position by swinging the arms and trunk sideways and upwards.

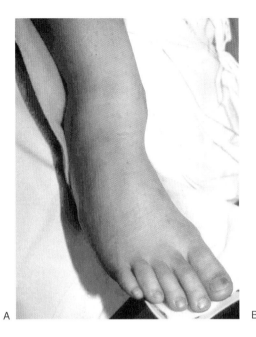 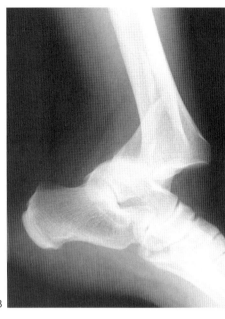

A   B

Fig. 10.7 Ankle deformity. (A) Clinical appearance. (B) Lateral X-ray view showing tibiotalar fracture dislocation.

10.7	Arthritis and other manifestations outwith the musculoskeletal system
Felty's syndrome	Rheumatoid arthritis with splenomegaly, lymphadenopathy, and neutropenia
Sjögren's syndrome	Arthritis with 'dry eyes' (keratoconjunctivitis sicca), xerostomia (reduced or absent saliva production), salivary gland enlargement and Raynaud's phenomenon
Enteropathic arthritis	Associated with inflammatory bowel disease – ulcerative colitis and Crohn's disease
Psoriatic arthritis	With skin and nail features of psoriasis
Haemophilia	Associated with (especially knee) arthropathy because of recurrent haemarthroses
Sickle cell disease	Associated with osteonecrosis of the hip due to bone infarction
Still's disease	Juvenile idiopathic arthritis
Reiter's syndrome	Urethritis, conjunctivitis, and inflammatory oligoarthropathy about 1–3 weeks after sexually transmitted *chlamydial* infection or infective gastroenteritis

10.8	Association of arthropathy with extra-articular features		
Type of arthropathy	**Symmetry**	**Condition**	**Extra-articular features**
Monoarthropathy		Septic arthritis	Fever, malaise, source of sepsis, e.g. skin, throat, gut
		Gout	Tophi, signs of renal failure (see p. 188)
		Osteoarthritis	
Oligoarthropathy	Asymmetrical	Reiter's syndrome	Urethritis, mouth and/or genital ulcers, conjunctivitis, iritis, enthesopathy, e.g. Achilles tendinopathy/plantar fasciitis, skin rash (keratoderma blenorrhagica)
		Ankylosing spondylitis	Enthesopathy, iritis
		Psoriatic	Psoriasis, nail pitting
		Osteoarthritis	
Polyarthropathy	Symmetrical	Rheumatoid arthritis	Raynaud's phenomenon, subcutaneous rheumatoid nodules, episcleritis, dry eyes, pleurisy
		Systemic lupus erythematosus	Raynaud's phenomenon, photosensitive rash especially on face, alopecia, fever, episcleritis
		Osteoarthritis	

In the hands, flexion contractures, calcium deposits in the finger pulps (Fig. 10.8) and tissue ischaemia leading to ulceration may occur.

Subcutaneous skin nodules in rheumatoid arthritis occur characteristically over the extensor surface of the forearm (Fig. 10.9). The nodules are firm and non-tender and may be felt at sites of pressure or friction, e.g. the sacrum. Achilles tendons and toes are sites where ulceration and infection may develop. Rheumatoid nodules are strongly associated with a positive rheumatoid factor and can occur at other sites such as the lungs. Similar skin

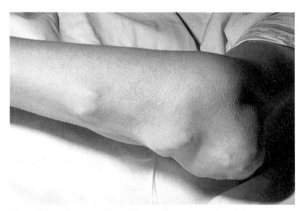

Fig. 10.9   Rheumatoid nodules and olecranon bursitis.

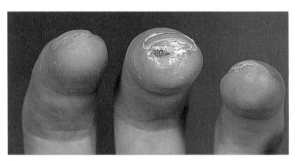

A

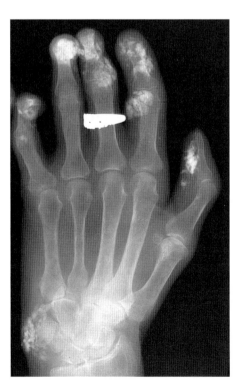

B

Fig. 10.8   Scleroderma in the hand. (A) Calcium deposits ulcerating through the skin. (B) X-ray showing calcium deposits.

nodules are found in systemic lupus erythematosus, rheumatic fever and scleroderma.

Reiter's syndrome is a form of reactive arthritis with extra-articular features (Fig. 10.10A). It is often associated with skin and nail changes identical to those of psoriasis, together with conjunctivitis, circinate balanitis (lesions on the prepuce and glans which form painless superficial ulcers; Fig. 10.10B), urethritis and superficial mouth ulcers (Fig. 10.10C).

Bony nodules occur in osteoarthritis affecting the hand. They are smaller and harder than rheumatoid nodules and located on the dorsal aspect of the interphalangeal (IP) joints of the fingers. At the distal interphalangeal (DIP) joints they are called *Heberden's nodes* (Fig. 10.11A), and at the proximal interphalangeal (PIP) joints, *Bouchard's nodes* (Fig. 10.11B).

Gouty tophi are firm, white, irregular subcutaneous crystal collections (monosodium urate monohydrate). Common sites are the helix of the ear and extensor aspects of the fingers, hands and toes (Fig. 10.12). The skin overlying tophi may ulcerate discharging urate crystals and become secondarily infected.

Small dark red vasculitic spots due to small skin infarcts occur in many systemic inflammatory disorders, including rheumatoid arthritis, systemic lupus erythematosus (see Fig. 2.17E, p. 49) and polyarteritis nodosa, and indicate active disease. Common sites for these lesions are the nail folds, finger and toe tips and other areas exposed to pressure.

Raynaud's phenomenon is episodic ischaemia of the fingers precipitated by stimuli such as cold, pain and stress. There is a typical progression of colour change. Blanching (white) leads to cyanosis (blue) and is followed by reactive hyperaemia (red) associated with altered sensation (*dysaesthesia*) and pain. Raynaud's phenomenon is common in otherwise healthy individuals but is frequently present in scleroderma and systemic lupus erythematosus.

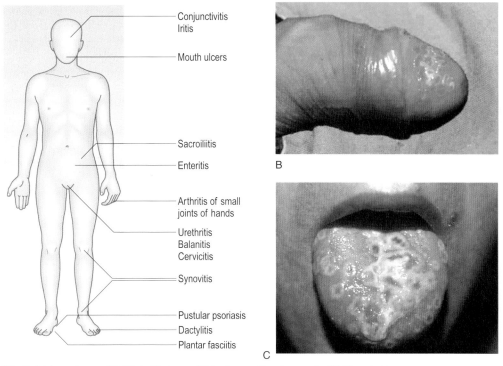

Fig. 10.10   Reiter's syndrome. (A) Clinical features. (B) Lesions on the glans penis. (C) Ulcerated tongue.

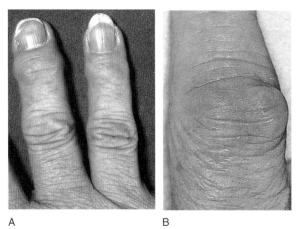

Fig. 10.11   Osteoarthritis of the hand. (A) Heberden's nodes. (B) Bouchard's nodes.

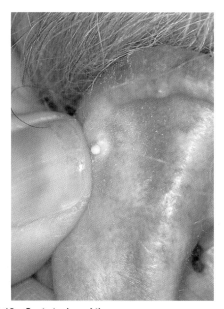

Fig. 10.12   Gouty tophus of the ear.

Eye features

The eyes are affected in many inflammatory musculo-skeletal conditions.

- Conjunctivitis is a feature of reactive arthritis and ankylosing spondylitis.
- Reduced tear production with 'dry eyes' (*keratoconjunctivitis sicca*) may contribute to conjunctivitis and inflammation of the eyelids (blepharitis) (see p. 230). This occurs in many inflammatory conditions including Sjögren's syndrome, rheumatoid arthritis and systemic lupus erythematosus.
- Scleritis and episcleritis (Fig. 10.13) can be seen in rheumatoid arthritis and other vasculitic disorders.
- Anterior uveitis (*iritis*) is seen in about 25% of patients with ankylosing spondylitis and reactive arthritis.
- The sclera are blue in osteogenesis imperfecta (see Fig. 2.12C, p. 47).

The *Schirmer tear test* is used to diagnose keratoconjunctivitis sicca. Hook small strips of notched blotting paper about 40 mm long over the lower eyelids while the patient looks upwards. The notch is ~ 5 mm from one end of the strip and is the point at which the strip is bent over the

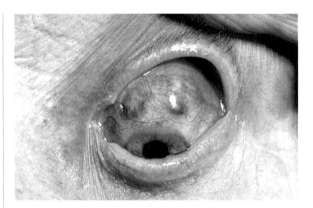

Fig. 10.13   Scleritis and scleromalacia.

eyelid. Ask patients to close their eye and sit comfortably for exactly 5 minutes, then remove the strips. Measure the distance that tears travel down the strip from the notch with a millimetre rule. > 15 mm is normal, 5–15 mm equivocal and < 5 mm abnormal.

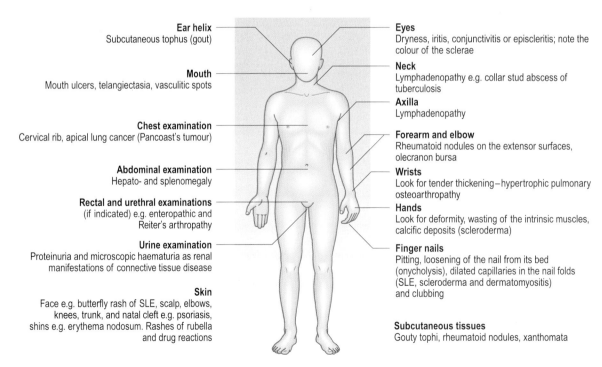

Ear helix
Subcutaneous tophus (gout)

Mouth
Mouth ulcers, telangiectasia, vasculitic spots

Chest examination
Cervical rib, apical lung cancer (Pancoast's tumour)

Abdominal examination
Hepato- and splenomegaly

Rectal and urethral examinations
(if indicated) e.g. enteropathic and Reiter's arthropathy

Urine examination
Proteinuria and microscopic haematuria as renal manifestations of connective tissue disease

Skin
Face e.g. butterfly rash of SLE, scalp, elbows, knees, trunk, and natal cleft e.g. psoriasis, shins e.g. erythema nodosum. Rashes of rubella and drug reactions

Eyes
Dryness, iritis, conjunctivitis or episcleritis; note the colour of the sclerae

Neck
Lymphadenopathy e.g. collar stud abscess of tuberculosis

Axilla
Lymphadenopathy

Forearm and elbow
Rheumatoid nodules on the extensor surfaces, olecranon bursa

Wrists
Look for tender thickening – hypertrophic pulmonary osteoarthropathy

Hands
Look for deformity, wasting of the intrinsic muscles, calcific deposits (scleroderma)

Finger nails
Pitting, loosening of the nail from its bed (onycholysis), dilated capillaries in the nail folds (SLE, scleroderma and dermatomyositis) and clubbing

Subcutaneous tissues
Gouty tophi, rheumatoid nodules, xanthomata

Fig. 10.14   Extra-articular manifestations of musculoskeletal conditions.

THE HISTORY

Presenting complaint

Record the categories of pain (use the SOCRATES format, p. 305), stiffness, swelling, weakness, locking and the duration of each. Instability, deformity, sensory disturbance and loss of function may also be presenting complaints.

If the problem relates to an injury, obtain an exact account of the mechanism and subsequent events, e.g. development of swelling.

Identify functional difficulties, including ability to hold and use items such as pens, tools and cutlery. How does the condition affect activities of daily living (Table 10.9) such as washing, dressing, toileting? Can they use stairs, and do they need aids to walk? Ask about functional independence, especially cooking, housework and shopping.

Past history

Note any past history that might contribute to the complaint, e.g. pain and restricted movement in a joint that had been dislocated. Identify co-morbid factors, diabetes mellitus, steroid therapy, ischaemic heart disease, stroke and obesity.

Drug history

Many drugs have side-effects that may either worsen or precipitate musculoskeletal conditions (Table 10.10).

Family history

A single gene defect (monogenic inheritance) is found in peroneal muscular atrophy (Charcot–Marie–Tooth disease), osteogenesis imperfecta, Ehlers–Danlos syndrome, Marfan's syndrome and the muscular dystrophies. Osteoarthritis, osteoporosis and gout are heritable in a variable polygenic fashion. Seronegative spondyloarthritis is more common in patients with HLA B27 (Table 10.11). Rheumatoid arthritis is also associated with a familial tendency.

Environmental, occupational and social histories

These may be relevant in the aetiology and in assessing how the patient is affected. They may also lead to litigation, e.g. in occupation-related complaints such as repetitive strain injury, hand-vibration syndrome, and fatigue fractures. Army recruits, athletes and dancers are at particular risk of fatigue fractures.

Some conditions are seen in certain ethnic groups: sickle cell disease may present with bone and joint pain; osteomalacia is more often seen in Asian patients; bone and

10.9	Joints involved in activities of daily living		
Activity	Joint(s) involved	Function required
Pinch grip	Thumb, index finger	Opposition and flexion of thumb (note: sensation is also required for optimal function)
Key grip	Thumb, index finger	Adduction and opposition of thumb
Gripping taps, handles, bottle tops	Hand, wrist	Grasp
Eating, cleaning teeth and face	Hand, elbow	Grasp, elbow flexion
Dressing, washing, hair care	Hand, elbow, shoulder	Pinch, grasp, elbow flexion, shoulder abduction/rotation
Toileting, cleaning perineum	Hand, wrist, elbow, shoulder	Grasp, wrist/elbow flexion, forearm supination, internal shoulder rotation

10.10	Drugs associated with adverse musculoskeletal effects	
Drug	Possible adverse musculoskeletal effects
Corticosteroids	Osteoporosis, myopathy, avascular necrosis, infections
Statins	Myalgia, myositis, myopathy
Angiotensin-converting enzyme inhibitors	Myalgia, arthralgia, positive antinuclear antibody
Antiepileptics	Osteomalacia, arthralgia
Immunosuppresant/ cytotoxic	Infections
Quinolones	Tendonopathy, tendon rupture

10.11 Conditions linked to human leucocyte antigen (HLA B27 type)

- Ankylosing spondylitis
- Reactive arthritis (Reiter's syndrome)
- Psoriatic arthritis (some forms)
- Enteropathic arthritis – associated with ulcerative colitis and Crohn's disease

joint tuberculosis is more common in African and Asian patients.

Take a sexual history (p. 16) since sexually transmitted disease may be relevant, e.g. Reiter's syndrome, gonococcal arthritis and hepatitis B.

Table 10.12 identifies social factors that may contribute to musculoskeletal conditions.

10.12	Social factors and musculoskeletal conditions
Alcohol	Trauma, myopathy, rhabdomyolysis, nerve palsies
Smoking	Lung cancer with bony metastases, hypertrophic pulmonary osteoarthopathy
Drugs of misuse	Trauma, hepatitis B, HIV
Diet	Vitamin deficiencies, e.g. osteomalacia (vitamin D), scurvy (vitamin C) Anorexia nervosa. e.g. osteoporosis

THE PHYSICAL EXAMINATION

It is difficult to describe dynamic tests in pictures and text, so get an experienced clinician to check your technique. Practise examining as many normal joints as possible so that you become familiar with normal appearances and ranges of movement.

Basic principles

- Observe the general appearance of the patient.
- Do not cause the patient additional pain.
- When examining a limb compare it with the opposite side.
- Assess active before passive movements.
- Use standard terminology when describing joint and limb positions and movement.

Movements are always described from the neutral position (Fig. 10.15). The commonly used terms are:

- *Flexion:* bending at a joint from the neutral position.
- *Extension:* straightening of a joint back to the neutral position.
- *Hyperextension:* movement beyond the normal neutral position, most commonly because of a torn ligament or an underlying ligamentous laxity, e.g. Ehlers–Danlos syndrome.
- *Adduction:* movement towards the midline of the body (for the fingers, adduction is movement towards the axis of the limb).
- *Abduction:* movement away from the midline.

Two additional terms are used to describe the position of a limb because of deformity at an affected joint or bone:

- *Valgus:* the part distal deviates away from the midline.
- *Varus:* the part distal deviates towards the midline.

The following equipment is needed to perform a musculoskeletal examination:

- tape measure
- tendon hammer
- blocks for assessing leg-length discrepancy
- goniometer (a protractor for measuring the range of joint movement) (Fig. 10.16).

Hypermobility

Some patients have a greater than normal range of joint movement. They may present with recurrent dislocations or sensations of instability if severe, but frequently just with arthralgia. Mild hypermobility is a normal variant but two inherited conditions affecting connective tissues – Marfan's syndrome and Ehlers–Danlos syndrome – cause hypermobility.

Hypermobility is assessed using the scoring system shown in Table 10.13.

THE GALS SCREEN

The GALS (gait, arms, legs, spine) screen is a useful rapid screen for musculoskeletal and neurological deficits as well as functional ability (Fig. 10.17).

Screening questions

- Do you have any pain or stiffness in your muscles, joints or back?
- Can you dress yourself without difficulty?
- Can you walk up and down stairs without difficulty?

If all three replies are negative the patient is unlikely to have a significant musculoskeletal problem. If the patient answers positively carry out a more detailed assessment.

➡ Examination sequence

→ Ask patients to undress to their underwear and stand in front of you. It may help to demonstrate some actions rather than simply telling them what to do.

Gait
→ Ask the patient to walk ahead in a straight line for several steps, then turn and walk back towards you. Look for smoothness and symmetry of the gait.

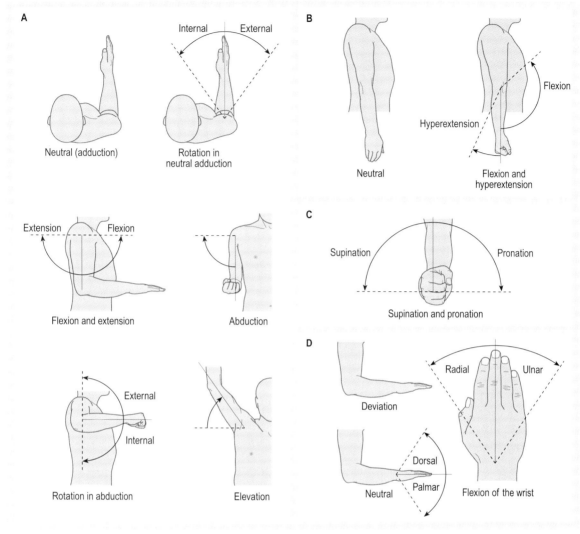

Fig. 10.15A–D Upper limb. Joint positions and movements.

Arms

→ Stand in front of the patient to carry out the tests.

→ Gently press the midpoint of each supraspinatus to detect the hyperalgesia of fibromyalgia (Fig. 10.17A).

→ Ask the patient to:

  → Put his hands behind his head, with the elbows going back (Fig. 10.17B). This tests abduction and external rotation of the glenohumeral joint. Getting your hand to your head is functionally important and is essential for feeding, washing and dressing.

  → Place the elbows by the side of the body and bend them 90°. Turn the palms up and down (Fig. 10.17C). This tests pronation and supination at the wrist and elbow.

  → Bend the arms up to touch the shoulders. This tests elbow flexion.

→ Make a 'prayer sign' bending the wrist back as far as possible. Put the backs of the hands together in a similar fashion. This tests wrist flexion and extension.

→ Put the arms straight out in front of the body. This tests elbow extension.

→ Clench the fists (Fig. 10.17D), and then open the hands flat. This tests both wrists and hands. Inspect the dorsum of the patient's hands and check for full finger extension at the metacarpophalangeal, proximal and distal interphalangeal joints.

→ Squeeze your index and middle fingers. This tests the strength of the power grip.

→ Touch each finger tip with his thumb. This tests precision grip and problems in coordination or concentration.

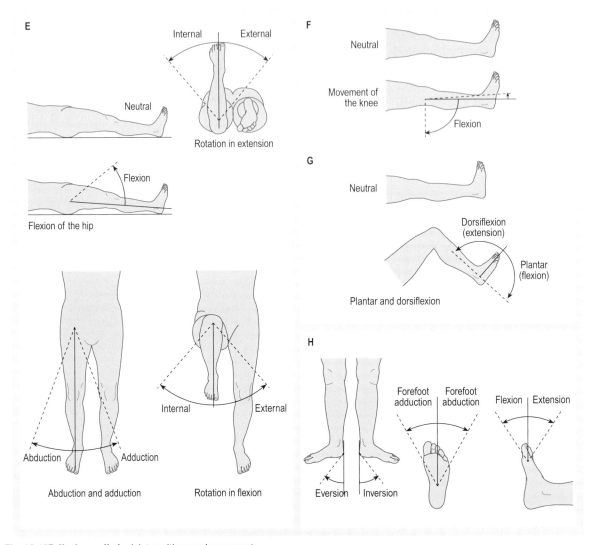

Fig. 10.15E–H **Lower limb.** Joint positions and movements.

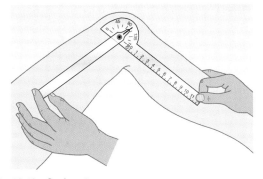

Fig. 10.16 **Goniometer.**

10.13 Assessing hypermobility	
Ask the patient to:	**Score**
Bring the thumb back to touch the forearm	1 point each side
Extend the little finger > 90°	1 point each side
Extend the elbow > 10°	1 point each side
Extend the knee > 10°	1 point each side
Touch the floor with palms of hands and knees straight	1 point
A score of 6 or more indicates hypermobility	

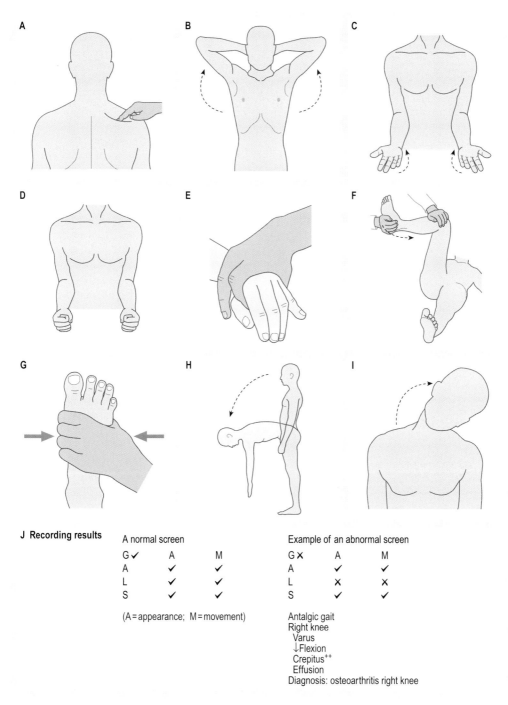

A

B

C

D

E

F

G

H

I

J **Recording results**

A normal screen

G	✔	A	M
A		✔	✔
L		✔	✔
S		✔	✔

(A = appearance; M = movement)

Example of an abnormal screen

G	✘	A	M
A		✔	✔
L		✘	✘
S		✔	✔

Antalgic gait
Right knee
  Varus
  ↓Flexion
  Crepitus++
  Effusion
Diagnosis: osteoarthritis right knee

Fig. 10.17   The GALS screen.

➔ Gently squeeze the patient's metacarpal heads (Fig. 10.17E). Tenderness may indicate an inflammatory condition, e.g. rheumatoid arthritis involving the metacarpophalangeal and proximal interphalangeal joints.

Legs

➔ Do Thomas's test for fixed flexion deformity on both hips (pp. 336–337) (if there is no contraindication).
➔ Flex each hip and knee with your hand on the patient's knee, feeling for crepitus in patellofemoral joint, knee and hip flexion (Fig. 10.17F).
➔ Flex the patient's knee and hip to 90°, passively rotate each hip internally and externally, noting pain or limited movement. This tests hip rotation (internal and external).
➔ Palpate each knee for warmth and swelling. Check for patellar tap. These detect inflammation and effusions.
➔ Look at the feet for any abnormality. Examine the soles looking particularly for calluses and ulcers, indicative of abnormal load bearing.
➔ Gently squeeze the metatarsal heads for tenderness, found in inflammatory conditions such as rheumatoid arthritis (Fig. 10.17G).

Spine

➔ Stand behind the patient and assess the straightness of the spine, muscle bulk and symmetry in the legs and trunk. Look for any asymmetry at the level of the iliac crests (indicating unilateral leg shortening), and swelling or other abnormality of the gluteal, hamstring, popliteal and calf muscles. Look at the Achilles tendons and hindfoot regions for swelling or deformity.
➔ Stand beside the patient and ask him to bend down and try to touch his toes (Fig. 10.17H). This allows you to see any abnormal spinal curvature or limited extension at the hips.
➔ Stand behind the patient and ask him to:
  ➔ Turn from side to side (while holding the pelvis) without moving the feet. This tests mainly thoracolumbar rotation.
  ➔ Slide the hand down the leg towards the knee. This tests lateral lumbar flexion.
➔ Stand in front of the patient and ask him to:
  ➔ Put his ear on his shoulder (Fig. 10.17I). This tests

lateral cervical flexion, the first movement affected in cervical spine spondylosis.
➔ Look up and at the ceiling and then down at the floor. This tests cervical flexion and extension.
➔ Let the jaw drop open and move it from side to side. This tests both temporomandibular joints.
➔ Ask the patient to lie supine on the couch. This tests the patient's ability to do this.

GAIT

Gait is the cyclical pattern of musculoskeletal motion that carries the body forwards. Normal gait is smooth, symmetrical and ergonomically economical with each leg 50% out of phase with the other.

For each leg, gait has two phases: *swing* and *stance*. The swing phase is from toe-off to heel-strike, when the foot clears the ground. The stance phase is from heel-strike to toe-off, when the foot is on the ground and load bearing (Fig. 10.18). When both feet are on the ground this is *double stance*.

A *limp* is an abnormal gait due to pain, structural change (e.g. lower limb length discrepancy), tone abnormality, or weakness (Fig. 10.14).

Pain

An *antalgic* gait is one which is altered to reduce pain. Painful conditions in a lower limb are usually aggravated by weight-bearing so the patient minimizes the time spent in the stance phase on that side. This results in a 'dot–dash' mode of walking.

In contrast, if the source of pain is in the spine, then axial rotatory movements are minimized resulting in a slow gait with small paces. Paradoxically, patients with hip pain may lean towards the affected side as this decreases the compression force on the hip joint.

Stance phase	Swing phase

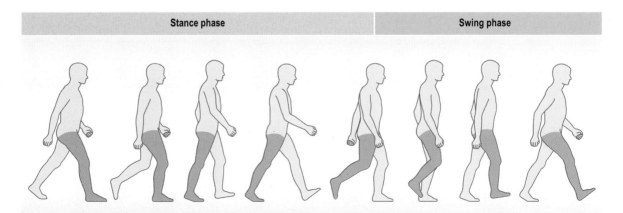

Fig. 10.18 Phases of the normal gait cycle.

Structural change

This is most obvious in limb-length discrepancy. A patient may walk on tiptoe on the shorter side, and have compensatory hip and knee flexion on the longer side. In addition there may be pelvic tilting on block testing (p. 335). Other structural changes producing an abnormal gait include deformities such as joint fusions, bone malunions and contractures.

Weakness

This may be due to nerve or muscle pathology or alteration in muscle tone. In a normal gait the hip abductors of the stance leg raise the contralateral hemipelvis.

In *Trendelenburg gait*, abductor function is poor when weight-bearing on the affected side, so the contralateral hemipelvis falls. This effect may be reduced by a truncal lurch over the affected hip (*Duchenne sign*) (see Fig. 10.43).

Common causes of a Trendelenburg gait are:

- weakness of the hip abductors, e.g. in polio or paresis of the superior gluteal nerve after total hip replacement
- structural hip joint problems, e.g. congenital dislocation of the hip
- painful hip joint problems, e.g. oesteoarthritis.

Another abnormal gait due to weakness is *'drop-foot'*. This occurs in common peroneal nerve palsy. The gait is high stepping to allow clearance of the 'flapping' foot.

Increased tone

This commonly occurs following an upper motor neurone lesion, e.g. cerebrovascular accident (stroke) or cerebral palsy. The gait produced depends on the specific lesion, contractures and compensatory mechanisms. A common pattern in cerebral palsy is the energy-inefficient *crouch gait*, resulting from gastrocnemius and soleus weakness in which the hips and knees are always flexed.

The limping child

The age of the child is important in determining the likely cause (Table 10.14). In acute limp consider trauma and infection. Ask about recent vaccinations, infections and antibiotic treatment. Ask about pyrexia, early-morning stiffness and pain to help diagnose inflammatory conditions such as juvenile idiopathic arthritis.

⇨ Examination sequence

➔ Watch the patient walking in a straight line, initially barefoot, and then in shoes. For children it may help to ask them to walk fast or run as this tends to unmask any abnormality.
➔ Observe the patient from behind, in front, and the side.
➔ Evaluate what happens at each level (foot, ankle, knee, hip and pelvis, trunk and spine) during both stance and swing phases.

The procedure for examination of the joints is given in Table 10.15.

10.14 'The limping child' – age-related conditions that cause a limp	
1–3 years	Developmental dysplasia of the hip Neuromuscular disease e.g. muscular dystrophy Juvenile idiopathic arthritis Limb length discrepancy Child abuse Septic arthritis
4–10 years	Transient synovitis – 'the irritable hip' Perthes' condition Limb length discrepancy Juvenile idiopathic arthritis Septic arthritis Tumour
> 10 years	Slipped upper femoral epiphysis Osgood–Schlatter's condition 'Shin splints' Tarsal coalition Heel pain Kohler's disease

10.15 Joint examination		
Look		
Skin	Colour	
	Scars	
	Rashes	
Shape	Swelling, bony or soft tissues	
	Muscle wasting	
Position	Deformity	
Feel		
Skin	Temperature	
Soft tissues	Swelling:	
	hard	
	soft	
	fluctuant	
	Texture:	
	supple	
	indurated	
	Tenderness	
Bones and Joints	Tenderness	
Move		
Active movements	What the patient can do	
Passive movements	What you can do to the patient	
Abnormal movements	e.g. increased anterior–posterior movement at the knee due to cruciate ligament rupture	
Special tests	As appropriate	

THE REGIONAL EXAMINATION

THE SPINE

The spine is divided into the cervical, thoracic, lumbar and sacral segments. Remember that most spinal diseases are not confined to one segment and often cause alteration in the posture or function of the whole spine. Spinal disease may occur without local symptoms and present with pain, neurological symptoms or signs in the trunk or limbs. The key to accurate diagnosis depends on knowledge of the underlying bony and neurological anatomy (Fig. 10.19), a careful history and eliciting signs and symptoms which help to differentiate between mechanical (non-inflammatory) and inflammatory causes (Table 10.16).

10.16 Common spinal problems
• Mechanical back pain • Prolapsed intervertebral disc • Spinal stenosis • Ankylosing spondylitis • Compensatory scoliosis resulting from leg-length discrepancy • Cervical myelopathy • Pathological pain/deformity (e.g. osteomyelitis, tumour, myeloma) • Osteoporotic vertebral fracture resulting in kyphosis (or rarely lordosis), especially in the thoracic spine with loss of height • Cervical rib • Scoliosis • Spinal instability (e.g. spondylolisthesis)

Nomenclature in spinal disease

- *Scoliosis:* lateral curvature of the spine (Fig. 10.20).
- *Kyphosis:* curvature of the spine in the sagittal (anterior–posterior) plane with the apex posterior (Fig. 10.20) (the thoracic spine normally has a mild kyphosis).
- *Lordosis:* curvature of the spine in the sagittal (anterior–posterior) plane with the apex anterior (Fig. 10.20) (the cervical and lumbar spines normally have a lordosis).
- *Gibbus:* spinal deformity caused by an anterior wedge deformity localized to a single vertebra producing an increase in forward flexion (Fig. 10.20).

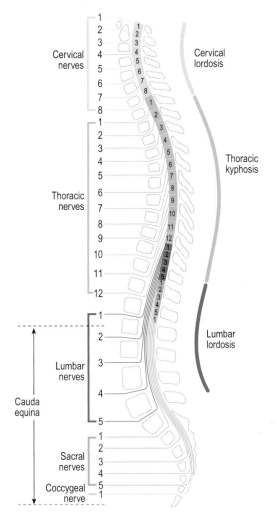

Fig. 10.19   The normal spinal curves.

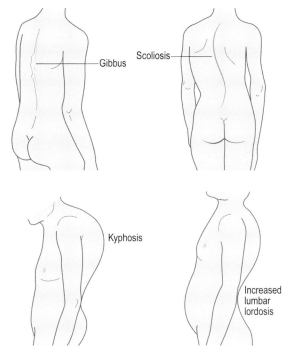

Fig. 10.20   Spinal deformities.

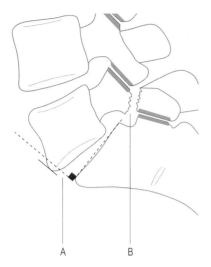

Fig. 10.21 Lumbosacral junction showing (A) anterior translation of L5 on S1 (spondylolisthesis) and (B) defect in pars interarticularis (spondylolysis).

- *Spondylosis:* degenerative change in the spine.
- *Spondylolysis:* defect in the pars interarticularis of a vertebral arch (Fig. 10.21).
- *Spondylolisthesis:* the anterior slip of one vertebra on an inferior vertebra (Fig. 10.21).
- *Retrolisthesis:* the posterior slip of one vertebra on an inferior vertebra.

Cervical spine

Anatomy

Nodding of the head occurs at the atlanto-occipital joints, and rotational neck movements mainly at the atlantoaxial joint. Flexion, extension and lateral flexion occur mainly at the midcervical level.

The neural canal contains the spinal cord and the emerging nerve roots, which pass through exit foraminae bounded by the facet joints posteriorly and the intervertebral discs and neurocentral joints anteriorly. The nerve roots, particularly in the lower cervical spine, may be compressed or irritated by lateral disc protrusion or osteophytes arising from the facet or neurocentral joints. A central disc protrusion may press directly on the cord.

History

The commonest symptoms are pain and difficulty turning the head and neck. This may lead to an inability to turn the head fully to left or right. Patients may complain of difficulty when driving, especially when attempting to reverse.

Neck pain is usually felt posteriorly but may be referred to the head, shoulder, arm or interscapular region. Cervical disc lesions cause radicular pain in one or other arm, roughly following the dermatomes of the nerve roots affected.

Disease of the upper cervical spine affecting the atlanto-occipital joints produces pain radiating to the occiput in the C2 nerve root distribution. Spondylosis of the middle and lower cervical spine tends to cause pain radiating to the upper border of trapezius, the interscapular region or the arms, and is often associated with local tenderness. Irritation of the C6 and C7 nerve roots can give rise to widely referred pain in the interscapular region or the radial fingers and thumb. Irritation of C8 can cause pain on the ulnar side of the forearm, ring and little fingers.

If the spinal cord is compromised then lower limb weakness, difficulty walking, loss of sensation and sphincter disturbance may occur.

It is imperative that you observe the following:

- In patients with rheumatoid arthritis be particularly careful during examination as atlantoaxial instability can lead to spinal cord damage when the neck is flexed.
- In patients with a history of neck injury never elicit the range of movements. Splint the neck and check for abnormal posture. Check neurological function in the limbs and X-ray to assess bony injury.

◢ Examination sequence

→ Ask the patient to remove enough clothing for you to see the neck and upper thorax, then to sit on a chair.

Look

→ Face the patient. Observe the posture of the head and neck and note any abnormality or deformity, e.g. loss of lordosis (usually due to muscle spasm) (Table 10.17).

Feel

→ The midline spinous processes from the occiput to T1 (the process of T1 is usually the most prominent).
→ The paraspinal soft tissues.
→ The supraclavicular fossae – for cervical ribs or enlarged cervical lymph nodes.
→ The anterior neck structures including the thyroid.
→ Note any tenderness in the spine, trapezius, interscapular and paraspinal muscles.

10.17 Causes of abnormal neck posture	
Loss of lordosis or flexion deformity	Acute lesions, rheumatoid arthritis
Increased lordosis	Ankylosing spondylitis
Torticollis (wry neck)	Sternocleidomastoid contracture
Lateral flexion (cock robin position)	Erosion of lateral mass of atlas in rheumatoid arthritis

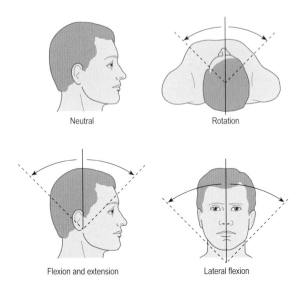

Fig. 10.22 Movements of the cervical spine.

10.18 Causes of pain in the thoracic spine

Adolescents and young adults

- Scheuermann's disease
- Ankylosing spondylitis
- Disc protrusion (rare)

Middle-aged and elderly

- Degenerative change
- Osteoporotic fracture

Any age

- Tumour
- Infection

Move

→ Assess active movements first (Fig. 10.22). Ask the patient to:
  → 'Put your chin onto your chest' to assess forward flexion. The normal range is 0 (neutral) to 80°. Record a decreased range as the chin–chest distance.
  → 'Look upwards at the ceiling as far back as you can' to assess extension. The normal range is 0 (neutral) to 50°. Thus the total flexion–extension arc is usually around 130°.
  → 'Put your ear onto your shoulder' to assess lateral flexion. The normal range is 0 (neutral) to 45°.
  → 'Look over your right/left shoulder'. The normal range of lateral rotation is 0 (neutral) to 80°.
→ Gently perform passive movements if there are reduced active movements and see if the end of the range has a sudden or a gradual resistance and whether it is pain or stiffness that restricts movement. Note any pain or paraesthesiae in the arm on passive neck movement, suggesting nerve root involvement.
→ Perform a neurological assessment of the upper and lower limbs (see pp. 263–276).

Thoracic spine

Anatomy

This segment of the spine is the least mobile and maintains a physiological kyphosis throughout life. Movement is mainly rotational with only a very limited amount of flexion, extension and lateral flexion.

History

The presenting symptoms in the thoracic spine are localized spinal pain (see Table 10.18), pain radiating round the chest wall or, less frequently, symptoms of paraparesis including sensory loss, leg weakness, and loss of bladder or bowel control. Disc lesions are rare but may be accompanied by pain radiating around the chest (*girdle pain*) mimicking cardiac or pleural disease.

Pain arising from the thoracolumbar junction can occur in ankylosing spondylitis and may be confused with pulmonary, renal or cardiac problems. Patients with vertebral collapse due to malignancy may have associated spinal cord compression. Consider infection as a cause of acute pain especially if systemic upset or fever is present. When thoracic pain is poorly localized consider intrathoracic causes such as myocardial ischaemia or infarction, oesophageal or pleural pain and aortic aneurysm.

▶ Examination sequence

→ Ask the patient to undress to expose the neck, chest and back.

Look

→ With the patient standing, inspect posture from behind, the side and the front, noting any deformity, e.g. rib hump or abnormal curvature.

Feel

→ The midline spinous processes from T1 to T12. Feel for increased prominence of one or more posterior spinal processes implying anterior wedge-shaped collapse of the vertebral body – often related to osteoporosis.
→ The paraspinal soft tissues for tenderness.

Move

→ Ask the patient to sit with arms crossed. Ask the patient to twist round and look at you.

Lumbar spine

The normal lordosis may be lost in disorders such as ankylosing spondylitis and lumbar disc protrusion. The surface markings are the spinous processes of L4/5, which are level with the pelvic brim, and the 'dimples of Venus', which overlie the sacroiliac joints.

The principal movements are flexion, extension, lateral flexion and rotation. Most patients can bring the tips of their fingers at least to the level of the knees in forward and lateral flexion. Extension should be approximately 10–20°. In flexion, the upper segments move first, followed by the lower segments to produce a smooth lumbar curve. However, even with a rigid lumbar spine, if the hips are mobile, patients may be able to touch their toes.

In the adult, the spinal cord ends at the L2 level. Below this the spinal nerve roots may be injured or compressed by disc protrusion, whereas above this level the spinal cord itself may be involved.

History

Low back pain is an extremely common complaint responsible for many days lost from work. Most low back pain is 'mechanical' due to degenerative disease. The common distribution of radicular back pain due to nerve root compression is down the posterior aspect of the leg to the ankle (*sciatica*). Pain due to inflammation of the sacroiliac joints may be referred down both legs to the knees.

An important objective of the history is to recognize patients with significant spinal pathology (*red flag features*) (Table 10.19). Consider also abdominal and retroperitoneal pathology, e.g. abdominal aortic aneurysm, pancreatitis, peptic ulcer, renal pathologies.

Important spinal conditions are acute disc protrusion, spinal stenosis, ankylosing spondylitis, osteoporotic fracture, infection and tumours. Infection and tumours are likely to be associated with symptoms such as weight loss or fever. In the majority of patients, however, backache reflects poor posture or age-related degenerative change in discs and facet joints (spondylosis).

A common complaint is of low back pain after standing for too long, or sitting in a poor position. Symptoms tend to be worse as the day progresses and better after resting or on rising in the morning. This pattern is usually due to poor posture and related ligament stresses. Sometimes contributory factors such as leg length inequality or psychosocial problems can be identified.

In contrast, insidious onset of backache and stiffness in a young adult suggests inflammatory disease such as ankylosing spondylitis. Symptoms are usually worse in the morning or after inactivity and ease with movement. Morning stiffness is more marked than in osteoarthritis, lasting 30–60 minutes. There may be other clues to the diagnosis, such as peripheral joint involvement, extra-articular features or a positive family history.

Acute onset of low back pain in a young adult, often associated with bending or lifting, is the typical presentation of acute disc protrusion (*slipped disc*). The acute episode may be superimposed on a background of preceding mild episodic backache due to disc degeneration. Activities such as coughing or straining to open the bowels exacerbate the pain. There may be symptoms of lumbar or sacral nerve root compression (*cauda equina syndrome*). If the sacral nerve roots are involved there may be loss of sphincter control and perianal sensation.

Acute back pain in the middle aged, elderly or those with preceding factors, e.g. steroid therapy, may be due to osteoporotic fracture. This is eased by lying, exacerbated by spinal flexion and is not usually associated with neurological symptoms.

An acute onset of severe progressive pain, especially if associated with systemic features such as malaise, weight loss or night sweats, may indicate pyogenic or tuberculosis infection of the lumbar spine. The patient may have a past history of diabetes mellitus, immunosuppression, e.g. steroid therapy or HIV infection, and complain of pain and great difficulty in moving. The infection may involve the intervertebral discs and adjacent vertebrae and may track into the psoas muscle sheath presenting as a painful flexed hip or a groin swelling.

In patients with unremitting spinal pain of recent onset, often disturbing sleep, consider malignant disease involving a vertebral body. Other clues are a previous history of cancer, and systemic symptoms or weight loss. Tumours rarely affect intervertebral discs.

10.19   'Red flag' features for acute low back pain
History

• Age < 20 years or > 55 years
• Recent significant trauma (fracture)
• Pain:
  – thoracic (dissecting aneurysm)
  – non-mechanical (infection/tumour/pathological fracture)
• Fever (infection)
• Difficulty in micturition
• Faecal incontinence
• Motor weakness
• Sensory changes in the perineum (saddle anaesthesia)
• Sexual dysfunction (e.g. erectile/ejaculatory failure)
• Gait change (cauda equina syndrome)
• Bilateral 'sciatica'

Past medical history
• Cancer (metastases) • Previous steroid use (osteoporotic collapse)
System review
• Weight loss/malaise without obvious cause (e.g. cancer)

> Cauda equina syndrome and spinal cord compression are neurosurgical emergencies. If you suspect them, refer the patient immediately for assessment and possible surgical decompression.

Intermittent discomfort or pain in the lumbar spine occurring over a long period of time is typical of degenerative disc disease. There is stiffness in the morning or after immo-bility. Pain and stiffness are relieved by gentle activity but recur with, or after, excessive activity. Over years there is gradual loss of lumbar spine mobility, sometimes with spontaneous improvement in pain as the facet joints become increasingly stiff.

Diffuse pain in the buttocks or thighs brought on by standing too long or walking is the presenting symptom of lumbosacral spinal stenosis. This can be difficult to distin-guish from intermittent claudication (see p. 111). Some-times the pain is accompanied by tingling and numbness and can be difficult for the patient to describe. Typically, it is relieved by rest or spinal flexion. Stooping, or holding onto a supermarket trolley may increase exercise tolerance. Narrowing of the spinal canal or neural exit foraminae is usually caused by degenerative changes in the intervertebral discs and facet joints and there is often a long preceding history of discomfort typical of degenerative joint disease.

▶ Examination sequence

Look
→ Examine the patient standing. Look for obvious deformity such as decreased/increased lordosis, obvious scoliosis, soft tissue abnormalities such as a hairy patch or lipoma that might overlie a congenital abnormality e.g. spina bifida.

Feel
→ Palpate the spinous processes and paraspinal tissues. Note the overall alignment and focal tenderness (the L4/5 interspinous space is palpable at the level of the iliac crests). After warning the patient, lightly percuss the spine with your closed fist and note any tenderness.

Move (Fig. 10.23)
→ *Flexion.* Ask the patient to try to touch his toes with his legs straight. Record how far down the legs the patient can reach; a certain amount of such movement is dependent on hip flexion. Note any abnormality of this movement. Usually the upper segments should flex before the lower ones, and this progression should be smooth.
→ *Extension.* Ask the patient to straighten up and lean back as far as possible (normal 10–20° from neutral erect posture).
→ *Lateral flexion.* Ask the patient to reach down to each side touching the outside of the leg as far down as possible while keeping the legs straight.

Special tests

Schober's test for forward flexion. Mark the skin in the midline at the level of the dimples of Venus which overlie the sacroiliac joints (Fig. 10.24; mark A). Using a tape measure, draw two marks, one 10 cm above (mark B) and one 5 cm below this (mark C). Place the end of the tape measure on the upper mark (B) and ask the patient to 'touch the toes'. The distance from mark B to mark C should increase from 15 to more than 20 cm.

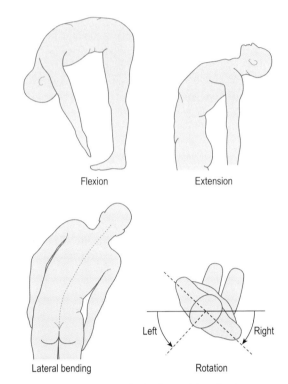

Fig. 10.23 **Movements of the lumbar and dorsal spine.**

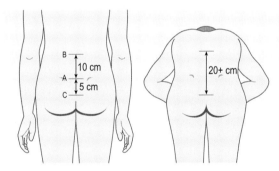

Fig. 10.24 **Schober's test.** Measuring forward flexion of the spine.

Root compression tests. Prolapse of an intervertebral disc causing pressure on a nerve root occurs most often in the lower lumbar region, causing compression of the corresponding nerve roots.

The femoral nerve lies anterior to the pubic ramus, so straight-leg raising or other forms of hip flexion do not increase its root tension. Problems with the femoral nerve roots may cause quadriceps weakness and/or diminished knee jerk on that side.

The sciatic nerve runs behind the pelvis, so manoeuvres designed to put tension on the lower nerve roots (L4 exiting the L4/5 foramen, L5 exiting the L5/S1 foramen) differ from those for the upper lumbar nerve roots (L2, L3).

Straight leg raise. This tests for L4, L5, S1 nerve root tension, e.g. in L3/4, L4/5 and L5/S1 disc prolapse (respectively). With the patient lying supine, lift the foot to flex the hip passively with the knee kept straight. Measure the angle between the couch and the flexed leg to determine any limitation (normal 80–90° hip flexion). If a limit is reached, raise the leg to just less than this level, and test for nerve root tension by dorsiflexing the foot (Fig. 10.25).

Tibial nerve stretch test. With the patient supine, flex the hip to 90°. Then extend the knee. In this position the tibial nerve 'bowstrings' across the popliteal fossa. Press over either of the hamstring tendons, and then over the nerve in the middle of the fossa. The test is positive if pain occurs when the nerve is pressed, but not the hamstring tendons (Fig. 10.25E).

Femoral nerve stretch test. With the patient lying on the front (prone) flex the knee and then extend the hip (Fig. 10.26). This stretches the femoral nerve. A positive result is when pain is felt in the back or the front of the thigh.

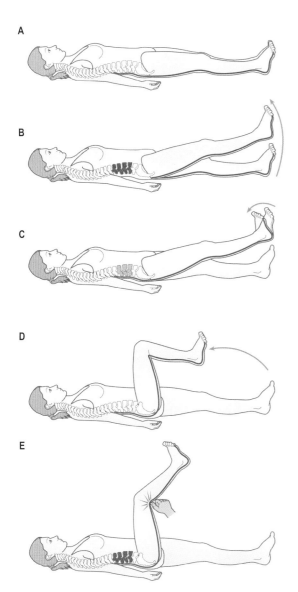

Fig. 10.25 Stretch tests – sciatic nerve roots. (A) Neutral position – nerve roots slack. (B) Straight leg raising limited by tension of root over prolapsed disc. (C) Tension increased by dorsiflexion of foot (Bragard's test). (D) Root tension relieved by flexion at the knee. (E) Pressure over centre of popliteal fossa bears on posterior tibial nerve which is 'bowstringing' across the fossa causing pain locally and radiation into the back.

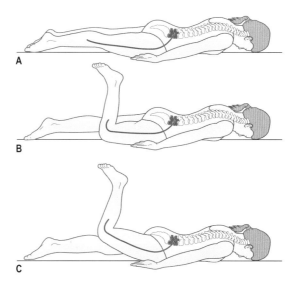

Fig. 10.26 Stretch test – femoral nerve. (A) Neutral position, nerve roots slack. The pain may be triggered by (B) knee flexion alone or (C) in combination with hip extension.

⊙ Examine this patient with acute lumbar back pain

1. With the patient standing, look for spinal deformity, e.g. decreased lordosis, scoliosis, scars, and for skin abnormality, e.g. hairy patch found in *spina bifida*.
2. Feel the spinous processes and paraspinal tissues for any focal tenderness.
3. Gently percuss the vertebral column with your closed fist, noting any tenderness.
4. Ask the patient to 'try to touch your toes with legs kept straight' and record how far down the patient can reach.
5. Ask the patient to 'straighten up and lean back as far as you can' and record amount of movement.
6. Ask the patient to 'reach down to each side, touching the outside of the leg as far as possible' and record amount of flexion.
7. Perform straight leg raising test.
8. Perform femoral stretch test.

Flip test. If a degree of functional overlay is suspected; ask the patient to sit on the end of the couch with the hips and knees flexed to 90°. Examine the knee reflexes, and then extend the knee, as if to examine the ankle jerk. The genuine sufferer will lie back ('flip'); otherwise you will have effectively demonstrated a difference between the straight leg raise test when lying and when seated (Fig. 10.27).

The sacroiliac joints. Tests for movement and pain in these joints are unreliable but compressing the pelvis or pressing down on the sacrum with the 'heel' of your hand with the subject lying prone may produce pain if these joints are inflamed.

THE UPPER LIMB

Distinguish between systemic and local conditions. Systemic conditions, e.g. rheumatoid arthritis, usually cause pathology at several sites. Local conditions cause a single-site problem but must be distinguished from referred or radicular pain. Work out whether the condition is likely to be inflammatory or non-inflammatory on the basis of the pattern of diurnal stiffness and pain.

The prime function of the upper limb is to position the hand appropriately in a volume of space. This requires a range of movements at the shoulder, elbow and wrist. The hand may function in both precision and power modes. The intrinsic muscles of the hand allow both grip and fine manipulative movements, and the forearm muscles provide the power and stability. The patient should be seated, facing you with the arms and shoulders exposed.

The shoulder

The shoulder joint consists of the glenohumeral joint and the acromioclavicular joint, but movement also occurs between the scapula and the posterior chest wall (Fig. 10.28).

Movements of the shoulder girdle, especially abduction and rotation, also produce movement at the sternoclavicular joint.

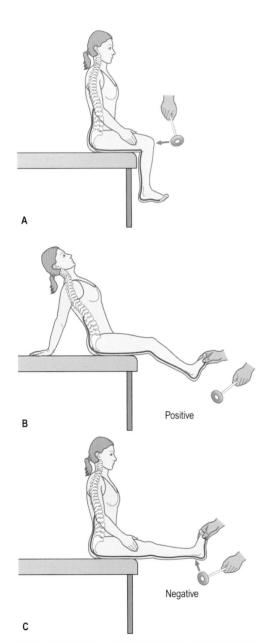

A

B

Positive

C

Negative

Fig. 10.27 Stretch test – sciatic nerve root. In the 'flip' test, when attention is diverted to the tendon reflexes the patient with actual nerve root compression cannot permit full extension of the leg.

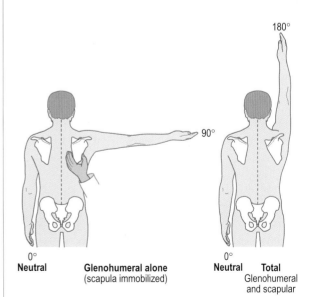

180°

90°

0°
Neutral

Glenohumeral alone
(scapula immobilized)

0°
Neutral

Total
Glenohumeral and scapular

Fig. 10.28 Movements at the shoulder joint.

10.20	Causes of shoulder girdle pain
Rotator cuff	Degeneration, tendon rupture, calcific tendonitis
Subacromial bursa	Calcific bursitis, polyarthritis
Capsule	Adhesive capsulitis
Head of humerus	Tumour, osteonecrosis, fracture/dislocation
Joints	Glenohumeral, sternoclavicular – synovitis, osteoarthritis, dislocation Acromioclavicular – osteoarthritis

10.21 Common conditions affecting the shoulder

Non-trauma

- Rotator cuff syndromes, e.g. supraspinatus, infraspinatus tendonitis
- Impingement syndromes (involving the rotator cuff and subacromial bursa)
- Adhesive capsulitis ('frozen shoulder')
- Calcific tendonitis
- Bicipital tendonitis
- Rheumatoid arthritis

Trauma

- Rotator cuff tear
- Glenohumeral dislocation
- Acromioclavicular dislocation
- Fracture of the clavicle
- Fracture of the head or neck of the humerus

Pain is a prominent feature of shoulder conditions (Tables 10.20 and 10.21) and is frequently referred to the upper arm. Glenohumeral pain may be over the anterolateral aspect of the upper arm. Pain felt at the shoulder may be referred from the cervical spine, nerve root, diaphragm and sub-diaphragmatic peritoneum via the phrenic nerve. The commonest cause of referred pain is cervical spondylosis where disc space narrowing and osteophytes cause nerve root impingement and inflammation.

Stiffness and limitation of movement around the shoulder, caused by adhesive capsulitis of the glenohumeral joint, is common after immobilization or disuse following injury or stroke. This is sometimes termed 'frozen shoulder', but movement can still occur between the scapula and chest wall.

A significant component of stability and movement (especially abduction; Fig. 10.29A) at the glenohumeral joint comes from the rotator cuff muscles and their tendinous insertions into the shoulder capsule.

The rotator muscles are: supraspinatus, subscapularis, teres minor and infraspinatus. Some rotator cuff disorders, especially impingement syndromes and tears present with a painful arc (Fig. 10.29B).

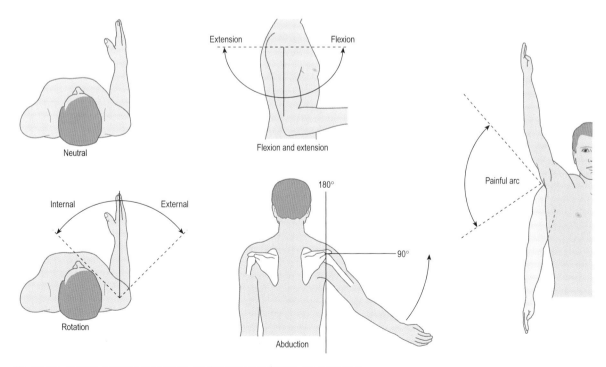

Fig. 10.29 Testing shoulder movement. (A) Shoulder movements. (B) Painful arc.

➔ Examination sequence

Look

➔ Examine the whole shoulder girdle front and back including the axilla for:

  ➔ *Deformity.* The deformities of anterior glenohumeral and complete acromioclavicular joint dislocation are usually obvious (Fig. 10.30), but the shoulder contour in posterior glenohumeral dislocation may only appear abnormal when you stand above the seated patient and look down on the shoulder.

  ➔ *Swelling.* In dislocations, proximal humeral fractures, haemarthrosis and inflammatory conditions.

  ➔ *Muscle wasting* – especially of the deltoid, supraspinatus and infraspinatus. Wasting of supraspinatus or infraspinatus usually indicates a chronic tear of their tendons.

  ➔ *The size and position of the scapula* (i.e. elevated or depressed). A small elevated scapula occurs in the rare conditions of Sprengel's shoulder and Klippel–Feil syndrome. 'Winging' of the scapula occurs with paralysis of the nerve to serratus anterior (Fig. 10.31).

Feel

➔ Start at the sternoclavicular joint and palpate along the clavicle to the acromioclavicular joint. Clavicular fractures and acromioclavicular joint injuries are accompanied by deformity and local tenderness.

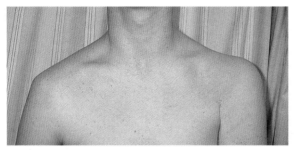

A

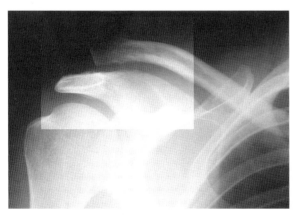

B

Fig. 10.30 Dislocations around the shoulder. (A) Right anterior glenohumeral dislocation. (B) X-ray of right acromioclavicular dislocation.

➔ Palpate the acromion and coracoid (2 cm inferior and medial to the clavicle tip) processes, the scapula spine and the biceps tendon in the bicipital groove.

➔ Palpate the supraspinatus tendon by extending the shoulder to bring supraspinatus anterior to the acromion process. Tenderness is present with ligamentous tears and calcific tendonitis.

Move

➔ *Screening tests for shoulder dysfunction.* Stand behind the patient. Ask the patient to put both hands behind the head, then to put the arms down and to reach behind the back to touch the shoulder blades. If you note pain, swelling or limitation of movement proceed to full examination.

➔ *Range of movement.* Determine the range of active and passive movement:

  ➔ Ask the patient to flex and extend the shoulder as far as possible.

  ➔ To test abduction ask the patient to lift the arm away from the side of the body. 50–70% of abduction occurs at the glenohumeral joint (the rest occurs with movement of the scapula on the chest wall), but this increases if the arm is externally rotated. To determine how much movement occurs at the glenohumeral joint, palpate the inferior pole of the scapula between your thumb and index finger to detect scapular rotation, or place your hand on the lateral clavicle and acromion. During abduction note the degree and smoothness of scapular movement. If the glenohumeral joint is excessively stiff then movement of the scapula over the chest wall will predominate. If there is any limitation or pain (painful arc) associated with abduction, test the rotator cuff.

  ➔ Measure internal and external rotation with the patient's arm by the side of the body and the elbow flexed at 90°. Internal rotation is expressed as the highest lumbar spinous process that the thumb can reach.

  ➔ Assess the ability of the deltoid to abduct against resistance – compare side with side.

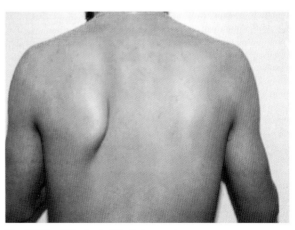

Fig. 10.31 'Winging' of the left scapula.

Special tests

Rotator cuff problems. Ask the patient to abduct the arm from the side of the body against resistance. If abduction cannot be initiated or is painful this suggests a rotator cuff problem.

Impingement:

- Test for a painful arc by passively abducting the arm fully and asking the patient to lower (adduct) it slowly. A painful arc occurs between 60° and 120° of abduction.
- If the patient cannot initiate abduction, passively abduct the patient's internally rotated arm to 30–45° while placing your hand over the scapula to confirm there is no scapular movement. Ask the patient to continue to abduct the arm. Pain on active movement, especially against resistance suggests an impingement syndrome.

Ligamentous tears and injuries. To test the component muscles of the rotator cuff, neutralize the effect of other muscles crossing the shoulder. Discrepancy between active and passive ranges suggests a tendinous tear – in particular with subscapularis where there may be an excessive range of passive internal rotation.

- *Subscapularis* and *pectoralis major* produce powerful internal rotation of the shoulder. To isolate subscapularis, test internal rotation with the patient's hand behind the back. Loss of power suggests a tear, while pain on forced internal rotation suggests tendonitis.
- *Supraspinatus.* With the arm by the side test abduction. Loss of power suggests a tear, while pain on forced abduction at 60° suggests tendonitis.
- *Infraspinatus and teres minor.* Test external rotation with the arm in the neutral position, but with 30° flexion to reduce the contribution of deltoid. Loss of power suggests a tear, while pain on forced external rotation suggests tendonitis.

Bicipital tendonitis:

- Palpate the bicipital tendon in its groove noting any tenderness.
- Ask the patient to supinate the foream, and then flex the arm against resistance. Pain is produced in bicipital tendonitis.

The elbow

The elbow joint has humero-ulnar, radio-capitellar, and superior radio-ulnar articulations. The medial and lateral epicondyles are the flexor and extensor origins for the forearm muscles respectively. These two prominences and the tip of the olecranon are easily palpated. They normally form an equilateral triangle when the elbow is flexed to 90° and lie in a straight line when the elbow is fully extended. A subcutaneous bursa overlies the olecranon and may become inflamed or infected (bursitis). Pain at the elbow may be localized or referred from the neck. Rheumatoid arthritis and epicondylitis are common causes of pain at the elbow.

➔ Examination sequence

Look
- ➔ At the overall alignment of the extended elbow. There is normally a valgus angle of 11–13° when the elbow is fully extended (the 'carrying angle').
- ➔ For swelling, bruising, and scars.
- ➔ For evidence of synovitis between the lateral epicondyle and olecranon.
- ➔ For olecranon bursitis.
- ➔ For rheumatoid nodules on the proximal extensor surface of the forearm.

Feel
- ➔ The bony contours of the lateral and medial epicondyles and olecranon tip, defining an equilateral triangle with the elbow flexed at 90°.
- ➔ Synovitis feels spongy or boggy when the elbow is fully flexed. Feel for sponginess on either side of the olecranon and ask about tenderness.
- ➔ Focal tenderness, over the lateral or medial epicondyle. When isolated to one site this may indicate 'tennis' (lateral) or 'golfer's' (medial) elbow. Tenderness at multiple sites may be part of fibromyalgia syndrome.
- ➔ For bursae – fluid-filled sacs, usually soft but if acute or infected may be firm.
- ➔ For rheumatoid nodules on the proximal extensor surface of the forearm.

Move
- ➔ Assess the extension–flexion arc. Ask the patient to touch the shoulder on that side and then straighten the elbow as far as possible. The normal range of movement is 0–145°; a range less than 30–110° will cause functional problems.
- ➔ To assess supination and pronation ask the patient to put the elbows by the side of the body and flex them to 90°. Now ask the patient to turn the hands upwards to face the ceiling (supination – normal range 0–90°) and then downwards to face the floor (pronation – normal range 0–85°).

Special tests

Tennis elbow (lateral epicondylitis). Ask the patient to flex the elbow to 90°. Pronate and flex the hand/wrist fully. Support the patient's elbow. Ask the patient to extend the wrist against your resistance. Pain is produced at the lateral epicondyle and may be referred down the extensor aspect of the arm.

Golfer's elbow (medial epicondylitis). Ask the patient to flex the elbow to 90° and supinate the hand/wrist fully. Support the patient's elbow. Ask the patient to flex the wrist against your resistance. Pain is produced at the medial epicondyle and may be referred down the flexor aspect of the arm.

The hand and wrist

The wrist joint is complex with metacarpocarpal, inter-carpal, ulnocarpal and radiocarpal components. There are a wide range of possible movements including flexion, extension, adduction (deviation towards the ulnar side), abduction (deviation towards the radial side) and circum-duction (a composite movement where the hand can move in a conical fashion on the wrist).

When examining and documenting the fingers use their *names*, to avoid confusion (Fig. 10.32).

In the hand, the proximal and distal interphalangeal (PIP and DIP) joints are hinge joints and allow only flexion and extension. The metacarpophalangeal (MCP) joints allow flexion and extension, and abduction/adduction that is greatest when the MCP joints are extended.

The patient will often localize complaints of pain, stiffness, loss of function, contractures, disfigurement and trauma. If symptoms are more vague or diffuse, then consider referred pain or a compressive neuropathy (e.g. median nerve in carpal tunnel syndrome; Fig. 10.33).

The radial, median and ulnar nerves are essential for normal hand and wrist function. The radial nerve innervates the wrist and finger extensors. The ulnar nerve innervates the adductor of the thumb and most of the small muscles of the hand (interossei and lumbricals). The median nerve supplies the opponens and abductor muscles of the thumb and most of the wrist and finger flexors.

▶ Examination sequence

Look
→ *Colour change.* Erythema suggests acute inflammation caused by soft tissue infection, septic arthritis, tendon-sheath infection or crystal-induced disease (gout and pseudogout).

→ *Swelling.* Swelling at the MCP and/or IP joints suggests synovitis (Fig. 10.34). Swelling of MCP joints produces loss of interdigital indentation on the dorsum of the hand especially when the MCP and IP joints are fully flexed (loss of normal 'hill–valley–hill–valley' aspect). Swelling at the PIP joints produces a 'spindling' appearance which is typically seen in rheumatoid arthritis and collateral ligament injuries.
→ *Deformity:*
→ The fingers are long and thin in Marfan's syndrome (arachnodactyly; see Fig. 2.28B, p. 57).
  → Phalangeal fractures may produce rotational deformity. This is best detected by flexing the fingers together (Fig. 10.35) and then in turn. Normally, with the MCP and IP joints flexed, the fingers should not cross, and should point to the scaphoid tubercle in the wrist.
  → At the IP joints (Fig. 10.36):
    → 'Mallet' finger – a flexion deformity at the DIP joint which is passively correctable. This is usually caused

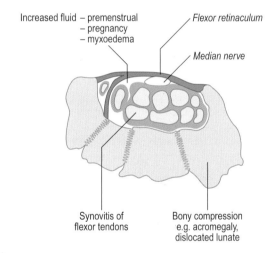

Increased fluid – premenstrual
          – pregnancy
          – myxoedema

Flexor retinaculum

Median nerve

Synovitis of flexor tendons

Bony compression e.g. acromegaly, dislocated lunate

A

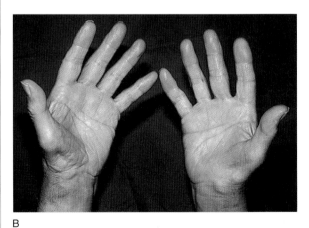

B

Fig. 10.33   Carpal tunnel syndrome. (A) Causes of median nerve compression. (B) Thenar muscle wasting.

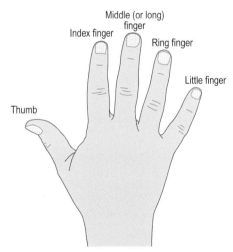

Middle (or long) finger

Index finger

Ring finger

Little finger

Thumb

by minor trauma disrupting the terminal extensor expansion at the base of the distal phalanx, either with or without bony avulsion.

→ Boutonnière (or button-hole) deformity – a flexion deformity at the PIP joint with hyperextension at the DIP joint (imagine the tip of the finger pressed firmly onto a button) and fixed flexion at the PIP joint.

→ 'Swan neck' deformity – hyperextension at the PIP joint with flexion at the DIP joint.

→ At the MCP joints:

→ Ulnar deviation of the MCP joints is typical of rheumatoid arthritis.

→ Dupuytren's contracture affects the palmar fascia, resulting in the MCP and PIP joints of the little and ring fingers becoming fixed in flexion (Fig. 10.37).

→ At the wrists: anterior (or volar) displacement – partial dislocation of the wrist may be seen in rheumatoid arthritis.

→ *Extra-articular signs* (Table 10.22):

→ Small muscle wasting, especially of the interossei in inflammatory arthritis (T1 nerve root lesion or ulnar nerve palsy).

→ Vasculitis of the fingers – most commonly detected in the nail folds (see Fig, 2.17E).

→ Palmar erythema.

→ Nail changes, e.g. pitting (psoriasis) and loosening of the nail from its bed (onycholysis) in psoriatic arthritis (see Fig. 2.17B).

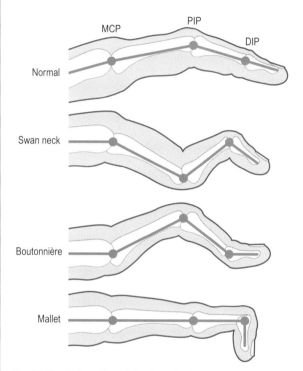

Fig. 10.36 Deformities of the finger in rheumatoid arthritis.

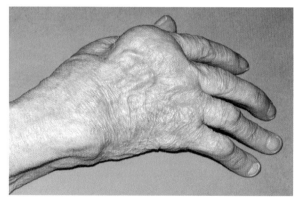

Fig. 10.34 Rheumatoid hand showing ulnar deviation of the fingers, small muscle wasting and synovial swelling at carpus, metacarpophalangeal and proximal interphalangeal joints.

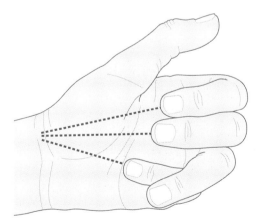

Fig. 10.35 Flexion of the fingers showing rotational deformity of the ring finger.

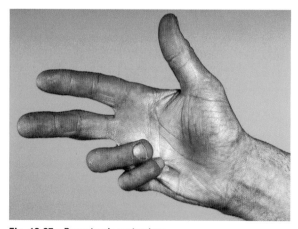

Fig. 10.37 Dupuytren's contracture.

10.22 Examples of visible abnormalities of the hands

Abnormality	Appearance and consistency	Typical site	Associated disease
Heberden's nodes	Small bony nodules	Dorsum and DIP joints	Osteoarthritis
Bouchard's nodes	Small bony nodules	Dorsum and PIP joints	Osteoarthritis
Rheumatoid nodules	Fleshy and firm	Extensor surface of knuckles	Rheumatoid arthritis
Tophi	White subcutaneous	Juxta-articular	Gout
Calcific deposits	White subcutaneous	Finger pulp	Scleroderma, dermatomyositis
Dilated capillaries	(Use magnifying glass)	Nail folds	Scleroderma, dermatomyositis, systemic lupus erythematosus

Feel

→ *Hard swellings* suggest bony outgrowths (osteophytes) characteristic of osteoarthritis, mucous cysts or rarely tumours. Heberden's and Bouchard's nodes occur at the DIP and PIP joints respectively.

→ 'Squaring' of wrist due to osteophytes at the first carpometacarpal joint.

→ *Soft swellings* suggest synovitis:
  → Test the IP joints by squeezing them from the sides with the finger and thumb of one hand and test for sponginess from top to bottom with the finger and thumb of your other hand.
  → Test the MCP joints by examining for sponginess within the interphalangeal space by pressing the metacarpal heads between your finger and thumb.
  → Detect synovitis in the PIP joints by squeezing the joint gently with your thumb and index finger while using the thumb and index finger of your other hand above and below the joint to apply pressure and detect sponginess.
  → Palpate the flexor tendon sheaths in the hand and fingers to detect local swellings or tenderness. If you detect any swelling (usually just proximal to the MCP joints) look for triggering or 'locking' during extension of the previously flexed finger.
  → To detect crepitus, place your index finger across the patient's fully extended fingers and ask the patient to open and close the fingers.
  → Swelling, tenderness and crepitus are found over the tendon sheaths of abductor pollicis longus and extensor pollicis brevis in De Quervain's tenosynovitis. Symptoms are aggravated by movements at the wrist and thumb. Crepitus at this site is often felt as a creaking sensation and may even be audible.
  → Crepitus may also occur with movement of the radiocarpal joints in osteoarthritis, most commonly secondary to old scaphoid or distal radial fractures.

Move

→ Active movements of the hand:
  → Ask the patient to make a fist, then extend (stretch out) the fingers fully. To test the power of grip, ask the patient to squeeze two of your fingers inserted from the thumb side into the palm of the patient's hand. Lack of full extension of one or more fingers may indicate tendon rupture.

→ Assess flexor tendon sheath abnormalities by passive movements of the hand to look for triggering.
→ Active movements at the wrist:
  → To assess extension, ask the patient to put the palms of the hands together and extend the wrists fully 'prayer sign' (normal is 90° of extension) (Fig. 10.38A).
  → To assess flexion, ask the patient to put the backs of the hands together and flex the wrists fully 'reverse prayer sign' (normal 90° of flexion) (Fig. 10.38B).

Examining the wrist and hand with a wound

Specifically test the tendons, nerves and circulation in a patient with wound(s) to the wrist or hand. The site of the wound and position of the hand at the time of injury indicate the structure(s) possibly damaged. There are limitations to clinical examination as normal movement may still be possible even if 90% of a tendon has been divided. Careful surgical exploration is often needed for correct diagnosis and treatment. The sensory aspects of nerve injury are covered on page 271.

Examination sequence

Muscles and tendons

→ *Flexor digitorum profundus.* This is the only flexor of the DIP joint. Ask the patient to flex the DIP joint while you hold the PIP joint in extension (Fig. 10.39A).
→ *Flexor digitorum superficialis.* This flexes the PIP joint, but to test for flexor digitorum superficialis you have to eliminate the action of flexor digitorum profundus as it can also flex the PIP joint. Do this by holding the other fingers fully extended and asking the patient to flex the PIP joint in question (Fig. 10.39B).
→ *Extensor digitorum.* With the patient's wrist in the neutral position, ask the patient to extend the fingers (Fig. 10.39C).
→ *Flexor and extensor pollicis longus.* Hold the proximal phalanx of the patient's thumb firmly and ask the patient to flex and extend the IP joint (Fig. 10.39D).
→ *Extensor pollicis longus.* Ask the patient to place the hand palm down on a flat surface and to extend the thumb like a hitch-hiker (Fig. 10.39E). If the tendon is intact, the patient will be able to do this. If pain is produced, it may indicate De Quervain's disease.

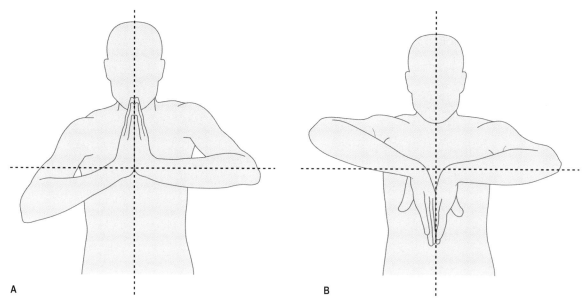

Fig. 10.38 Assessing (A) extension and (B) flexion at the wrist.

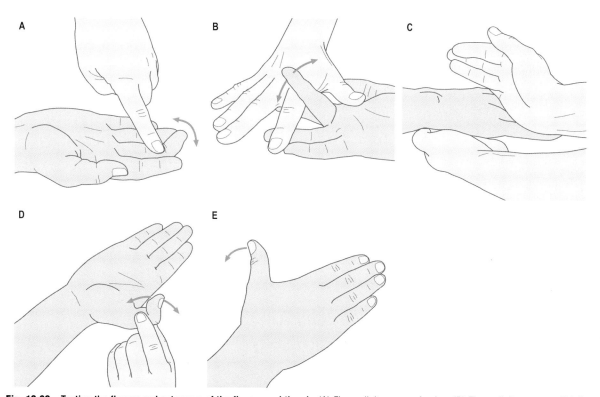

Fig. 10.39 Testing the flexors and extensors of the fingers and thumb. (A) Flexor digitorum profundus. (B) Flexor digitorum superficialis. (C) Extensor digitorum. (D) Flexor pollicis longus. (E) Extensor pollicis longus.

Nerves (motor function only)

→ The *median nerve* supplies the thenar muscles which abduct and oppose the thumb.

  → Place the patient's hand flat, palm up, on a table. Ask the patient to abduct the thumb (a vertical movement up from the palm) and to hold it in that position against resistance (Fig. 10.40A).

  → To test opposition, ask the patient to touch the tip of the little finger and keep it there against resistance (Fig. 10.40B).

→ The *ulnar nerve* supplies the interossei and adductor pollicis muscles.

  → To test the interossei ask the patient to hold a sheet of light card between the little and ring fingers (Fig. 10.40C). Note: the fingers must be fully extended.

  → Test the first dorsal interosseus muscle by asking the patient to abduct the extended index finger against resistance (Fig. 10.40D).

→ To test adductor pollicis ask the patient to grip a piece of card between the palm and the adducted thumb. If the adductor is weak, the thumb cannot be held straight and will flex at the MCP and IP joints (Froment's sign) (Fig. 10.40E).

→ The *radial nerve* supplies the extensors of the wrist and fingers.

  → Ask the patient to flex the elbow to 90° and pronate the wrist. Support the wrist with your hand and ask the patient to extend the fingers and then extend the wrist (Fig. 10.40F). When assessing finger extension watch the MCP joints as extension of the IP joints can also be produced by the interossei and lumbrical muscles supplied by the median and ulnar nerves.

  → For extensor pollicis longus ask the patient to bend the thumb and extend it against resistance.

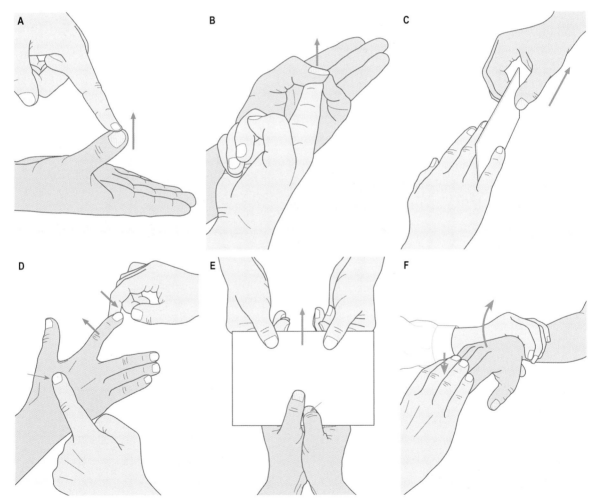

Fig. 10.40 Testing motor function of the median, ulnar and radial nerves. (A and B) The median nerve: (A) abducting the thumb; (B) testing opposition. (C–E) The ulnar nerve: (C) testing the interossei; (D) testing the first interosseus; (E) testing adductor pollicis. (F) The radial nerve: testing the extensors of the wrist and fingers.

THE LOWER LIMB

The hip

The hip is a ball and socket joint. It normally allows movements of flexion, extension, abduction, adduction, internal/external rotation and the combined movement of circumduction. With age, the commonest restrictions in movement are extension and internal rotation, followed by abduction.

Pain is the predominant hip symptom. It is usually felt in the groin, but can be referred to the anterior thigh, the knee or buttock. Hip pain from most causes is usually aggravated by activity, but certain disorders, e.g. avascular necrosis and tumours of the hip may be painful at rest and at night. Lateral hip or thigh pain, particularly aggravated when lying on the side at night, suggests trochanteric bursitis.

Distinguish pain arising from the hip from:

- lumbar nerve root irritation (see p. 324)
- spinal or arterial claudication (see p. 111)
- abdominal causes, e.g. herniae (see p. 173)
- knee pain referred to the hip.

Find out how the pain restricts patients' activities. In particular, ask about walking in terms of the time and distance they manage out of the house, and up and down stairs; whether they do their own shopping and which walking aids they use. Associated stiffness and decreased range of movement are common.

Fracture of the neck of femur is common following relatively minor trauma in postmenopausal women and those aged over 70 years. The fracture may be minimally displaced or impacted and need not have the classical appearance of a shortened, externally rotated leg (see Fig. 10.56). The patient may even be able to weight-bear.

◢ Examination sequence

→ Patients should undress to their underwear and remove socks and shoes. You should be able to see the iliac crests so you may need to pull down the top of their underpants.

Look

→ *Gait.* Assess as described above.
→ *General inspection.* With the patient standing, observe:
→ From the front, whether:
→ stance is straight
→ the shoulders are parallel to the ground and placed symmetrically over the pelvis
→ there is a pelvic tilt (which may mask a hip deformity or true shortening of one leg)
→ there are deformities of hip, knee, ankle, foot
→ there is muscle wasting (from polio or disuse secondary to arthritis)
→ From the side, whether there is a stoop or increased lumbar lordosis (both may result from a flexion contracture)
→ From behind, whether:
→ the spine is straight or curved laterally (scoliosis) – if there is scoliosis, note the relative positions of the shoulders and pelvis, and measure leg lengths
→ there is any gluteal atrophy
→ Around the hip, whether there are scars, sinuses, dressings, skin changes.

Shortening

Shortening is an important feature of hip and other lower limb conditions. *Apparent* shortening is present if the affected limb appears shortened usually because of an adduction or flexion deformity at the hip.

To measure shortening, the patient should lie face up on the couch with both legs stretched out as far as possible and in equivalent positions to eliminate the effect of any soft tissue contracture/abnormal posture. Measure with a tape.

- from umbilicus to medial malleolus – the apparent length
- from anterior superior iliac spine to medial malleolus – the 'true length' (Fig. 10.41).

Confirm any limb length discrepancy by 'block testing'. Ask the patient to stand with both feet flat on the ground. Raise the shorter leg using a series of blocks of graduated thickness until the pelvis is level as assessed by palpation of both iliac crests.

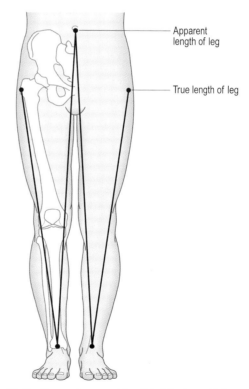

Apparent length of leg

True length of leg

Fig. 10.41 True and apparent lengths of the lower limbs.

10.23	Causes of true shortening of the lower limb
Hip	

- Fractures, e.g. neck of femur
- Following total hip arthroplasty
- Slipped upper femoral epiphysis
- Perthes' disease (juvenile osteochondritis)
- Unreduced hip dislocation
- Septic arthritis
- Loss of articular cartilage (arthritis, joint infection)
- Congenital coxa vara
- Missed congenital dislocation of the hip

Femur and tibia

- Growth disturbance secondary to:
  - poliomyelitis
  - fractures
  - osteomyelitis
  - septic arthritis
  - epiphyseal injury

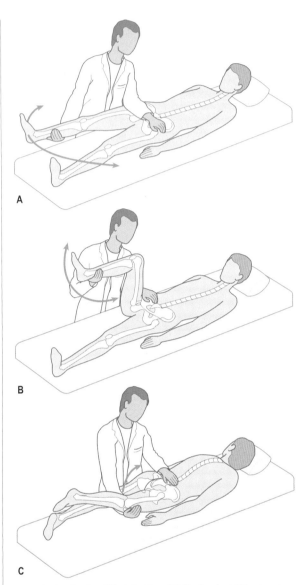

A

B

C

Fig. 10.42 Testing (A) abduction, (B) flexion and (C) extension of the hip.

Table 10.23 lists causes of true shortening of the lower limb.

➡ Examination sequence

Feel

→ Tenderness on palpation over the greater trochanter suggests trochanteric bursitis.

→ Tenderness over the lesser trochanter and ischial tuberosity is common in sporting injuries due to strains of the iliopsoas and hamstring muscle insertions respectively.

Move

→ With the patient face up on the couch, check the pelvic brim is perpendicular to the spine.

→ *Flexion.* Place your left hand under the back (to detect any masking of hip movement by movement of the pelvis and lumbar spine – see Thomas's test) and check the range of flexion of each hip in turn (normal 0–120°).

→ *Abduction and adduction.* Stabilize the pelvis by placing your left hand on the opposite iliac crest. With your right hand abduct the extended leg until you feel the pelvis start to tilt (normal 45°). Test adduction similarly by crossing one leg over the other and continuing to move it medially (normal 25°) (Fig. 10.42A).

→ *Internal and external rotation.* Test with the leg in full extension by rolling the leg on the couch and using the foot to indicate the range of rotation. Then test with the knee (and hip) flexed at 90°.

→ Move the foot medially to test external rotation and move the foot laterally to test internal rotation (normal 45° for each movement) (Fig. 10.42B).

→ *Extension.* Ask the patient to lie face down on the couch. Place your left hand on the pelvis to detect any movement. Lift each leg in turn to assess the range of extension (normal range 0–20°) (Fig. 10.42C).

Special tests

Trendelenburg's test. Stand in front of the patient and ask the patient to stand on one leg for 30 seconds and to repeat with the other leg. Normally, the iliac crest on the side with the foot off the ground should rise. The test is abnormal if the hemipelvis falls below the horizontal (Fig. 10.43). It may be caused by gluteal weakness or inhibition from hip pain, e.g. osteoarthritis, or structural abnormality of the hip joint (e.g. coxa vara or developmental hip dyplasia).

Thomas's test. Do not perform the test if the patient has a hip replacement on the non-test side, as forced flexion may cause dislocation.

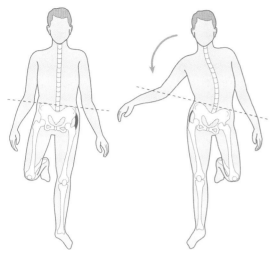

Fig. 10.43 Trendelenburg's sign. Powerful gluteal muscles maintain the position when standing on the left leg; weakness of the right gluteal muscles results in pelvic tilt when standing on the right leg.

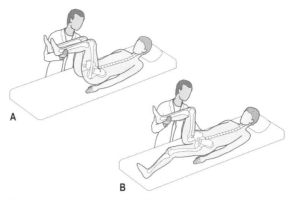

Fig. 10.44 Thomas's test examining the left hip.

The knee

The knee is a complex hinge joint with tibiofemoral and patellofemoral components. It has a synovial capsule that extends under the quadriceps (the suprapatellar pouch), reaching about 5 cm above the superior edge of the patella. The joint is largely subcutaneous, allowing easy palpation of the patella, tibial tuberosity, patellar tendon, tibial plateau margin and femoral condyles.

For stability the knee depends on its muscular and ligamentous structures (Fig. 10.45A).

Flexion is produced by the hamstring muscles. Extension requires the quadriceps muscles, quadriceps tendon, patella, patellar tendon and tibial tuberosity. Disruption of this 'extensor apparatus' at any level causes inability to straight leg-raise. Alternatively it can give rise to an extensor lag; a difference between active and passive ranges of extension.

The medial collateral ligament resists valgus stress whereas the lateral collateral ligament resists varus stress. The anterior cruciate ligament prevents anterior subluxation of the tibia on the femur, whereas the posterior cruciate ligament resists posterior translation. The medial and lateral menisci are crescentic fibrocartilagenous structures that lie between the tibial plateaux and the femoral condyles.

There are several important bursae around the knee: anteriorly the suprapatellar, prepatellar (between the patella and the overlying skin), and infrapatellar bursae (between the skin and the tibial tuberosity/patellar ligament); and posteriorly several bursae lie in the popliteal fossa (Fig. 10.45B).

Thomas's test measures fixed flexion deformity (incomplete extension). This deformity may be masked by compensatory movement at the lumbar spine or pelvis and increasing lumbar lordosis.

The test must be performed with the patient lying face up on a hard surface.

- Place your left hand palm upwards under the patient's lumbar spine.
- Passively flex both the patient's legs (hips and knees) as far as possible.
- Keep the non-test hip maximally flexed (you will feel that the lordotic curve of the lumbar spine remains eliminated).
- Now ask the patient to extend the test hip.
- Incomplete extension in this position indicates a fixed flexion deformity at the hip (Fig. 10.44).

Possible difficulties with Thomas's test are:

- If the contralateral hip is not flexed enough, lumbar lordosis will not be eliminated.
- Fixed flexion deformity of the ipsilateral knee will confuse the issue. In this case the test can be performed with the patient lying on the side.

⊙ Examine this patient with acute hip pain felt in the groin

1. Ask the patient to walk and observe gait from the front and side.
2. Perform Trendelenburg's test.
3. Measure leg lengths.
4. Examine movements at the hip in all directions (abduction/adduction, internal/external rotation, flexion).
5. Perform Thomas's test for fixed flexion deformity.

Knee symptoms

Pain. Take a detailed history of the mechanism of injury. The direction of impact, load or deformation are predictive of what structures are injured. Remember that pain in the knee may be referred from the hip.

Swelling. The presence of an effusion indicates intra-articular pathology. An effusion may be due to synovial

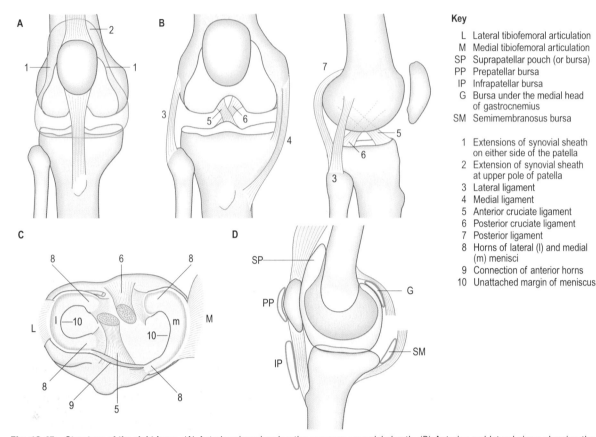

Key

L	Lateral tibiofemoral articulation
M	Medial tibiofemoral articulation
SP	Suprapatellar pouch (or bursa)
PP	Prepatellar bursa
IP	Infrapatellar bursa
G	Bursa under the medial head of gastrocnemius
SM	Semimembranosus bursa

1 Extensions of synovial sheath on either side of the patella
2 Extension of synovial sheath at upper pole of patella
3 Lateral ligament
4 Medial ligament
5 Anterior cruciate ligament
6 Posterior cruciate ligament
7 Posterior ligament
8 Horns of lateral (l) and medial (m) menisci
9 Connection of anterior horns
10 Unattached margin of meniscus

Fig. 10.45   Structure of the right knee. (A) Anterior view showing the common synovial sheath. (B) Anterior and lateral views showing the ligaments. The arrow indicates the direction of medial rotation of the femur in knee extension, during the last 10° or so of which the ligaments are twisted taut. (C) Plan view of the menisci. (D) Bursae.

fluid, blood, pus or a mixture of these fluids. The normal volume of synovial fluid is 1–2 ml and is undetectable but this increases if the synovial membrane is inflamed, e.g. trauma, rheumatoid arthritis, septic arthritis, or synovitis.

Bleeding into the knee (haemarthrosis) is caused by injury to a vascular structure within the joint, e.g. torn cruciate ligament or intra-articular fracture. Patients with a coagulation disorder, e.g. haemophilia, or on anticoagulant therapy are particularly prone to haemarthroses. The menisci are predominantly avascular, and unless torn at their periphery or in conjunction with some other internal derangement do not cause a haemarthrosis.

In acute injury the speed of onset of swelling is a clue to the diagnosis.

- Rapid (< 30 min), severe swelling suggests a haemarthrosis.
- Swelling of a lesser degree over 24 hours is more suggestive of traumatic effusion, e.g. meniscal tear.
- Septic arthritis usually develops over a few hours and is accompanied by pain, marked swelling, tenderness, redness and extreme reluctance to move the joint actively or passively. These features may be modified by concurrent oral steroid or non-steroidal anti-inflammatory drug therapy. If you suspect that swelling is due to a septic arthritis the joint should be aspirated as an emergency and an urgent Gram stain/microscopy obtained.
- Crystal-induced arthritis (gout or pseudogout) can mimic septic arthritis. Confirm the diagnosis by looking at aspirated fluid under polarized light microscopy.

Locking.   This is a block to full extension. It may be longstanding or intermittent in nature. The two predominant causes are a loose body (e.g. from osteochondritis dissecans, osteoarthritis, or synovial chondromatosis) and a meniscal tear (Fig. 10.46). Bucket-handle and anterior beak meniscal tears are especially associated with locking. Posterior horn tears commonly cause pain on extreme flexion and prevent the last few degrees of flexion. Meniscal tears also cause local joint-line tenderness. Congenital discoid meniscus may also present with locking and clunking.

Instability ('giving way').   Any of the four main ligaments may rupture from trauma or become loose with

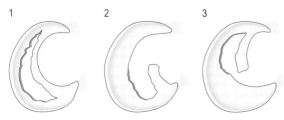

Fig. 10.46   Meniscal injury. (1) Longitudinal tear – the free edge may displace centrally as a 'bucket-handle'. (2) Anterior horn tear. (3) Posterior horn tear.

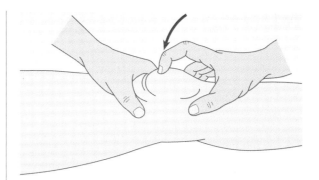

Fig. 10.47   Testing for effusion by the patellar tap.

degenerative disease. Because the normal knee has a valgus angle the patella is prone to dislocate laterally.

➋ Examination sequence

Look
→ Observe the patient walking and standing as described for gait.
→ Ask the patient to lie face up on the couch. Both legs should be fully exposed. Look for:
  → Scars, sinuses, redness or rashes.
  → Posture and common deformities, *genu valgum* (knock-knee) or *genu varum* (bow-legs).
  → Muscle wasting: quadriceps wasting is almost invariable with inflammation or chronic pain and develops within days to a fortnight. If wasting is present, measure the thigh girth in both legs at a selected distance (say 20 cm) above a defined fixed bony landmark – the tibial tuberosity.
  → Leg length discrepancy (see Fig. 10.41).
  → Flexion deformity: if the patient lies with one knee flexed this may be caused by a hip, knee or combined problem.
  → Swelling: an enlarged prepatellar bursa (housemaid's knee) and any effusion of the knee joint – a large

effusion is seen as a horseshoe-shaped swelling above the knee. Swelling extending beyond the joint margins suggests infection, major injury or rarely tumour.
→ Baker's cyst: bursa enlargement in the popliteal fossa.

Feel
→ *Warmth.* Feel the skin comparing both sides.
→ *Effusion*:
  → The patellar tap. With the knee extended, empty the suprapatellar pouch by sliding your left hand down the thigh until you reach the upper edge of the patella. Keep your hand there and with the finger tips of your right hand press down briskly and firmly over the patella (Fig. 10.47). In a moderate-sized effusion you will feel a tapping sensation as the patella strikes the femur. You may feel a fluid impulse in your left hand.
  → The 'ripple test' (Fig. 10.48). With the knee extended and the quadriceps muscles relaxed, empty the suprapatellar pouch as for the patellar tap. Then, with your fingers extended, stroke the medial side of the joint. Now stroke the lateral side of the joint and watch the medial side for a bulge or ripple as fluid reaccumulates on that side.

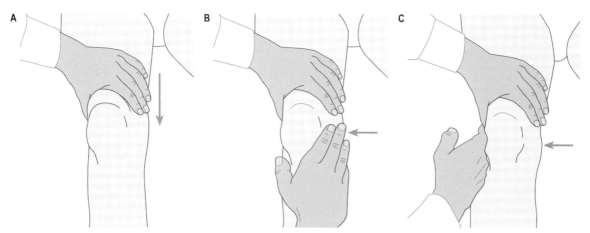

Fig. 10.48   The ripple test. (A) Empty the suprapatellar pouch as for the patella tap test. (B) Stroke the medial side of the joint to displace excess fluid to the lateral side of the joint. (C) Stroke the lateral side while watching the medial side closely for a bulge or ripple as fluid reaccumulates. This test may be negative if the effusion is tense.

→ *Synovitis*. With the knee flexed feel for sponginess by pressing posteriorly on both sides of the quadriceps tendon.

→ *Joint lines*. Feel the tibial and femoral joint lines. If there is tenderness, localize this as accurately as possible. Localized tenderness occurs over the tibial tuberosity in Osgood–Schlatter disease – a traction osteochondritis.

Move

→ *Active flexion and extension*. With the patient supine:
  → Ask the patient to flex the knee up to the chest and then extend the leg back down to lie on the couch (normal range 0–140°). Feel for crepitus between the patella and femoral condyles suggesting chondromalacia patellae (especially in younger female patients) or osteoarthritis. If there is a fixed flexion deformity of 15° and flexion is possible to 110° record this as a range of movement of 15–110°.
  → Ask the patient to lift the leg with the knee kept as straight as possible. If the patient cannot keep the knee fully extended an *extensor lag* is present, indicating quadriceps weakness or other abnormality of the extensor apparatus.

→ *Passive flexion and extension*. Normally the knee can extend so that femur and tibia are in longitudinal alignment. Record full extension as 0°. A restriction to full extension occurs with bucket-handle meniscal tears, osteoarthritis and rheumatoid arthritis. To assess hyperextension, lift both legs by the feet. Hyperextension (*genu recurvatum*) is present if the knee extends beyond the neutral position. Up to 10° is normal.

Ligament testing

Tests of stability

Collateral ligament stability. With the knee fully extended, there should be no abduction or adduction possible. If the ligament is lax or ruptured, movement can occur. If the ligament is strained (partially torn) but intact, pain will be produced but the joint will not open.

- With the patient's knee fully extended hold the ankle between your elbow and side. Use both hands to apply a valgus and then varus force to the knee. Use your thumbs to feel the joint line and assess the degree to which the joint space opens. Major opening of the joint indicates collateral and cruciate injury (Fig. 10.49A).
- If the knee is stable, repeat the process with the knee flexed to 30° to assess minor collateral laxity. In this position the cruciate ligaments are not taut.

Cruciate ligament stability.

- Flex the patient's knee to 90° and maintain this position by sitting with your thigh trapping the patient's foot.
- Check that the hamstring muscles are relaxed and look for posterior sag (posterior subluxation of the tibia on the femur). This is an important cause of a false-positive anterior drawer sign which should not be interpreted as anterior collateral ligament laxity.
  - *The anterior drawer sign*. With your hands behind the upper tibia and both thumbs over the tibial tuberosity, pull the tibia anteriorly (Fig. 10.49B). If there is significant movement (compare with the opposite knee) the anterior cruciate ligament is lax, and movement of > 1.5 cm suggests anterior collateral ligament rupture. There is often an associated medial ligament injury.
  - *The posterior drawer sign*. Now push backwards on the tibia. Posterior movement of the tibia suggests posterior cruciate ligament laxity.

Patellar stability.

The patellar apprehension test. With the knee fully extended push the patella laterally and flex the knee slowly.

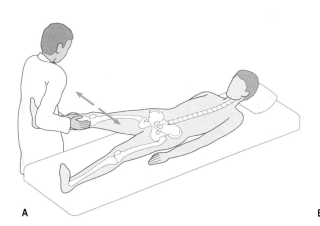

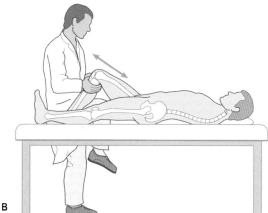

A   B

Fig. 10.49 Testing the ligaments of the knee. (A) Collateral ligaments. (B) Cruciate ligaments.

If the patient actively resists flexion, this suggests previous patellar dislocation or instability.

Special tests

Tests for meniscal tears. Meniscal tears in younger sporting patients are often the result of a specific injury, most commonly a twisting injury to the flexed weight-bearing leg. In middle-aged patients degenerative horizontal cleavage of the menisci is common and there may be no history of trauma. Associated well-localized joint-line tenderness is common. Meniscal injuries are commonly associated with small effusions especially on weight-bearing or after exercise. There may be localized joint-line tenderness.

Meniscal provocation test. With the patient face up on the couch, test the medial and lateral menisci in turn:

- *Medial meniscus.* Passively flex the knee fully, externally rotate the foot and abduct the upper leg at the hip keeping the foot towards the midline (i.e. creating a varus stress at the knee). Then extend the knee smoothly. In medial meniscus tears a click or clunk may be felt or heard accompanied by discomfort.
- *Lateral meniscus.* Passively flex the knee fully, internally rotate the foot and adduct the leg at the hip (i.e. creating a valgus stress at the knee). Then extend the knee smoothly. In tears of the lateral meniscus a click or clunk may be felt or heard accompanied by discomfort.

Squat test. Ask the patient to squat, keeping the feet and heels flat on the ground. If the patient cannot do this it indicates incomplete knee flexion on the affected side. This may be caused by a tear of the posterior horn of the menisci. The extreme range of knee flexion may also be tested with the patient face down on the couch, which makes for easy comparison with the contralateral side.

⊙ Examine this patient who complains of pain in the knee aggravated by walking

1. Ask the patient to walk and observe gait and movement of the knee from the front and side.
2. Ask the patient to lie on the couch and expose both legs.
3. Look at the lower limbs for redness, scars, muscle wasting, deformity, swollen bursae, etc.
4. Feel both knees with the back of your hand for temperature difference – warm in *septic arthritis* and *haemarthrosis*.
5. Palpate for knee effusion – found in *septic arthritis*, *trauma*, *haemarthrosis*.
6. Feel for tenderness over joint lines and soft tissues.
7. Assess active and passive movements at both knees – note crepitus.
8. Examine collateral and cruciate ligament stability.

The ankle and foot

The ankle is a hinge joint. The talus articulates with a three-sided mortise made up of the tibial plafond and the medial and lateral malleoli. This allows dorsiflexion and plantar flexion, although some axial rotation can occur at the ankle if it is plantar-flexed. During dorsiflexion the trochlea of the talus rocks posteriorly in the mortise and the malleoli are forced apart because the superior articular surface of the talus is wider anteriorly than posteriorly. The bony mortise is the major factor contributing to stability but the lateral, medial (deltoid) and inferior tibiofibular ligaments are also important (Fig. 10.50).

Foot movements are inversion and eversion and principally occur at the midtarsal (talonavicular/calcaneocuboid) and subtalar (talocalcaneal) joints. Toe movements are dorsiflexion and plantar flexion. In adults, problems involving the ankle and foot can be divided into those with a history of trauma and those without.

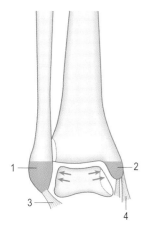
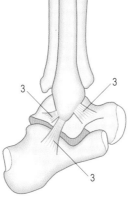
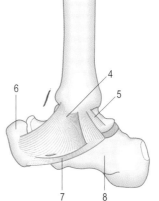

Key
1 Lateral malleolus
2 Medial malleolus
3 Lateral (external) ligament
4 Medial ligament
5 Deep fibres of medial ligament
6 Navicular
7 Spring ligament
8 Calcaneus

Fig. 10.50 The ankle ligaments.

Traumatic conditions

- A 'twisted' ankle is very common, usually related to a sporting injury or stepping off a kerb or stair awkwardly. Establish the exact mechanism of injury and the precise site of pain. Frequently there has been a forced inversion injury with involvement of the lateral ligament. A *sprain* occurs when some fibres are torn but the ligament remains structurally intact. A complete ligament tear allows excessive talar movement in the ankle mortise with instability.
- Achilles tendon rupture (Fig. 10.51) is associated with attempted sudden plantar flexion at the ankle. It is common in middle-aged patients doing unaccustomed activity, e.g. badminton, squash or the fathers' race at sports day, and some drug therapy, e.g. steroids, fluoroquinolones. Sudden pain occurs above the heel and there is often a sensation or noise of a crack. Patients may feel as if they have been kicked or even shot!
- Forefoot pain, often localized to the second metatarsal, after excessive activity such as trekking, marching or dancing suggests a stress fracture (Fig. 10.52). Symptoms are relieved by rest and aggravated by weight-bearing. X-rays in the first week may be normal.

Non-traumatic conditions

- Anterior metatarsalgia with forefoot pain is common, especially in middle-aged women. Acute joint pain with swelling suggests an inflammatory arthropathy such as rheumatoid arthritis or gout. The forefoot is commonly affected in rheumatoid arthritis, and in severe cases the

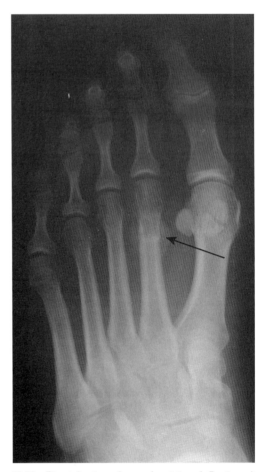

Fig. 10.52   Stress fracture of second metatarsal. Fracture site and callus are arrowed.

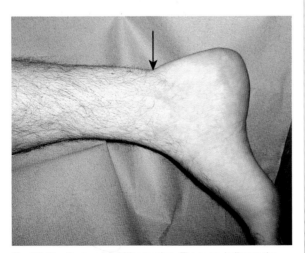

Fig. 10.51   Ruptured Achilles tendon. The arrow indicates the site of a palpable defect in the Achilles tendon.

metatarsal heads become so prominent that the patient may report a sensation of 'walking on pebbles or broken glass'.
- Plantar surface heel pain that is worse on the heel-strike phase of walking may be due to plantar fasciitis and tends to affect middle-aged patients.
- Posterior heel pain may be caused by Achilles tendonitis, an enthesopathy which may be associated with seronegative spondyloarthritis.
- Spontaneous lancinate pain in the forefoot radiating to contiguous sides of adjacent toes occurs with Morton's neuroma. A common site is in the interdigital cleft between the third and fourth toes. This occurs predominantly in women aged 25–45 years and is aggravated by wearing tight shoes.

☑ Examination sequence

→ Ask patients to remove their socks and shoes.

Look

→ Examine the soles of the shoes for any abnormal patterns of wear.

→ *Gait.* Observe as described previously. In particular, look for:
  → Increased height of step indicating 'foot-drop'
  → Ankle movement (dorsi-/plantar flexion)
  → Position of the foot as it strikes the ground (supinated/pronated)
  → Hallux rigidus.

→ With the patient standing observe:
  → From behind: how the heel is aligned (valgus/varus)
  → From the side: the position of the midfoot, looking particularly at the longitudinal medial arch. This may be flattened (*pes planus* – flat foot) or exaggerated (*pes cavus*). If the arch is flattened, ask the patient to stand on tip-toe, which will restore the arch in a mobile deformity, but not in one with a structural basis.

→ A splay-foot is one in which there is widening of the foot at the level of the metatarsal heads often associated with MTP joint synovitis.

→ Examine the ankle and foot for scars, sinuses, swelling, bruising, callosities (an area of thickened skin at a site of repeated pressure), nail changes, oedema, deformity and position (e.g. fixed plantar flexion or foot-drop).

→ *The toes.* Look for deformities of the great and other toes (Fig. 10.53).
  → Hallux valgus is very common, has a familial pattern and may be aggravated by footwear and activities such as ballet dancing (Fig. 10.53B). A bunion (a soft tissue bursal swelling) may develop over the protuberant first metatarsal head and become inflamed or infected. As the condition progresses, rotation of the hallux and overriding onto the second toe may occur.
  → Gout affecting the first MTP joint causes marked redness and soft tissue swelling. This is followed by desquamation (peeling) of the superficial skin and pain on movement or touch.
  → Swelling of the entire digit 'sausage toe' (*dactylitis*) is characteristic of psoriatic arthropathy.

→ Claw toes result from dorsiflexion (hyperextension) at MTP joints and plantar flexion at PIP and DIP joints.
→ Hammer toes are due to dorsiflexion at MTP and DIP joints and plantar flexion at PIP joints.
→ Mallet toes describes plantar flexion at DIP joints.

Feel

→ Feel the ankle and foot for focal tenderness and heat. In an acute ankle injury it is particularly important to palpate the proximal fibula, both malleoli, the lateral ligament and base of the fifth metatarsal.

→ Gently compress the forefoot. Tenderness on metatarsal compression suggests Morton's neuroma or, if associated with sponginess, synovitis due to rheumatoid arthritis. If there is toe deformity (see Fig. 10.53 and above) assess whether there is impingement on the other toes, e.g. overriding hallux valgus. Pain and stiffness at the first MTP joint suggests hallux rigidus.

Move

→ *Active.* Assess the range of plantar and dorsiflexion at the ankle and inversion/eversion of the forefoot by asking the patient to perform these movements.

→ *Passive:*
  → Ankle dorsiflexion/plantar flexion. Grip the heel with the cup of your left hand from below, with the thumb and index finger on the malleoli. Put the foot through its arc of movement (normal range 15° dorsiflexion to 45° plantar flexion). If dorsiflexion is restricted, assess the contribution of gastrocnemius (which functions across both knee and ankle joints) by measuring ankle dorsiflexion with the knee extended and flexed. If more dorsiflexion is possible with the knee flexed, this suggests a gastrocnemius contracture.
  → Foot inversion/eversion. The subtalar joint may be examined in isolation by placing the foot into dorsiflexion to stabilize the talus in the ankle mortice, then moving the heel into inversion (normal 20°) and eversion (normal 10°). This can also be performed with the patient lying face down with the knee flexed. The combined midtarsal joints are then examined by fixing the heel with your left hand and moving the forefoot with your right hand into dorsiflexion, plantar flexion, adduction, abduction, supination and pronation.

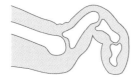 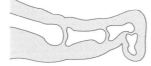 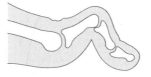 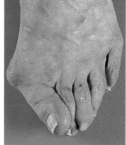

A   B

Fig. 10.53 Toe deformities. (A) Claw toe, mallet toe and hammer toe. (B) Hallux valgus overriding the second toe.

Special tests

Achilles tendon. Ask the patient to kneel with both knees on a chair. Palpate the gastrocnemius and Achilles tendon for focal tenderness and soft tissue swelling. Achilles tendon rupture is often palpable as a discrete gap in the tendon about 5 cm above the calcaneal insertion.

Thomson's (Simmond's) test. Squeeze the calf just distal to the level of maximum circumference. If the Achilles tendon is intact, plantar flexion of the foot will occur (Fig. 10.54).

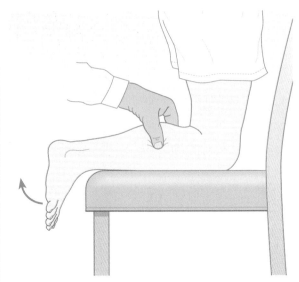

Fig. 10.54 Thomson's test. Failure of the foot to plantar flex when the calf is squeezed is pathognomonic of an acute rupture of the Achilles tendon.

FRACTURES, DISLOCATIONS AND TRAUMA-RELATED PRESENTATIONS

A *fracture* is a breach in the structural integrity of a bone. This may arise in:

- normal bone from excessive force
- normal bone from repetitive (load-bearing) activity (*stress* fracture)
- bone of abnormal structure (*pathological* fracture) (Table 10.24) with minimal or even no trauma.

The epidemiology of fractures varies widely with geographical location. In the developed world, there is an epidemic of osteoporotic fractures because of the increasing elderly population. Fractures resulting from road traffic accidents and falls from a height are decreasing because of legislative and other preventive measures such as seat belts, air bags and improved road engineering.

Osteoporosis is a systemic skeletal condition caused by loss of bone mineral density with associated micro-architectural deterioration. It is the commonest cause of abnormal bone structure and its incidence increases with age, particularly in women after the menopause (Table 10.25). In the absence of complications osteoporosis is asymptomatic. Although any osteoporotic bone can fracture, the common sites are the distal radius (Colles' fracture; Fig. 10.55), neck of femur (Fig. 10.56), proximal humerus and the spinal vertebrae. Caucasian women in Europe have a lifetime risk for a hip fracture of 11–18%.

10.24	Bone conditions associated with pathological fracture
• Osteoporosis	
• Osteomalacia	
• Primary or secondary tumour	
• Paget's disease	
• Osteogenesis imperfecta	
• Renal osteodystrophy	
• Parathyroid bone disease	

10.25	Risk factors for osteoporosis	
Age	
Sex	Female (female : male is 3 : 1)
Menstrual history	Decreased menstrual cycling, i.e. late menarche, early menopause, amenorrhoea
Past history	Hypogonadism (anorexia nervosa/excessive exercise/hyperprolactinaemia) Previous fragility fracture
Drug history	Previous or current steroid therapy
Family history	First-degree relative risk increased × 2
Social history	Immobilization, smoking, alcohol, low calcium/Vitamin D diet

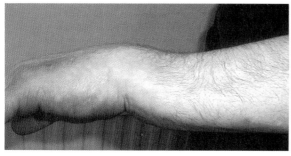

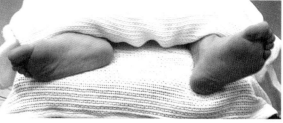

A

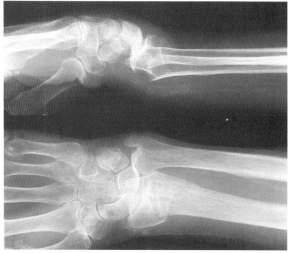

B

Fig. 10.55   Colles' fracture. (A) Clinical appearance of dinner fork deformity. (B) X-ray appearance.

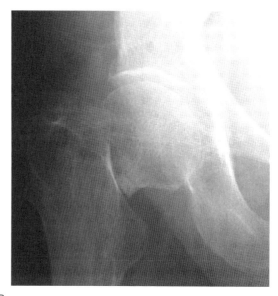

A

B

Fig. 10.56   Fracture of neck of right femur. (A) Showing shortening and external rotation of leg. (B) X-ray showing translation and angulation.

Clinical features

A fracture may occur in the context of severe trauma. If so, examine the patient according to the system in Chapter 12.

History

Establish the mechanism of injury. For instance, a patient who has fallen from a height onto his heels may have an obvious fractures of the calcaneal bones in his ankles but is also at risk of fractures of the proximal femur, pelvis and vertebral column.

Examination

Use the Look/Feel/Move approach.

Observe patients closely to see if they move the affected part and are able to weight-bear.

Look to see if the skin is intact. If there is a breach in the skin, and the wound communicates with the fracture, the fracture is open or *compound* (otherwise it is closed).

Also look for associated bruising, deformity, swelling, or wound infection.

Feel (gently) for local tenderness, and distal to the suspected fracture to establish if sensation and pulses are present.

Move. Try to establish whether the patient can move joints distal and proximal to the fracture. Do *not* move the fracture site to see if crepitus is present. This only causes additional pain and bleeding.

Investigation

For each suspected fracture, radiographs are needed, showing (at least) two views (at perpendicular planes) of the affected bone, and including the joints above and below.

Describing a fracture (Figs 10.57, 10.58 and 10.59)

- What bone(s) is/are involved?
- Is the fracture open (*compound*) or closed?

345

Anatomical divisions
E Epiphysis
EP Epiphyseal plate
M Metaphysis
D Diaphysis or shaft

Fractures
A Fracture of the
tibial diaphysis
B Fracture of the
femoral neck
C Fracture of the
greater trochanter
F Supracondylar
fracture of the femur

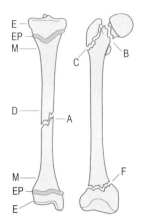

Fig. 10.57 Describing a fracture. The site of the fracture.

- Is the fracture complete or incomplete?
- Where is the bone fractured (intra-articular/epiphysis/physis/metaphysis/diaphysis)?
- What is the fracture's configuration (transverse/oblique/spiral/comminuted/butterfly fragment)?
- What deformity is present?
  - *Translation.* This is the shift of the distal fragment in relation to the proximal bone. The direction is defined by the movement of the distal fragment, e.g. dorsal or volar and is measured as a percentage.
  - *Angulation.* This is defined by the movement of the distal fragment, measured in degrees.
  - *Rotation.* This is measured in degrees along the longitudinal axis of the bone, e.g. for spiral fracture of the tibia or phalanges.

  - *Shortening.* Proximal migration of the distal fragment can cause shortening in an oblique fracture. Shortening may also occur if there has been impaction at the fracture site (e.g. in a Colles' fracture of the distal radius).
- Is there distal nerve or vascular deficit?
- What is the state of the tissues associated with fracture – soft tissues and joints (e.g. fracture blisters, dislocation).

Complications of fractures are summarized in Table 10.26.

10.26 Complications of fractures		
	Early (first 48 hours)	**Late (weeks, months, years)**
Systemic	Hypovolaemia and shock Fat embolism Adult respiratory distress syndrome	Chest infection Urinary tract infection
Bone	Osteomyelitis	Delayed union Non-union Malunion Necrosis
Joint		Stiffness Osteoarthritis Instability
Soft tissues	Compartment syndrome Muscular/tendon injury Neural injury	Reflex sympathetic dystrophy Peripheral and cord injury Ischaemic contracture
	Vascular injury Adjacent structural damage	Pneumothorax

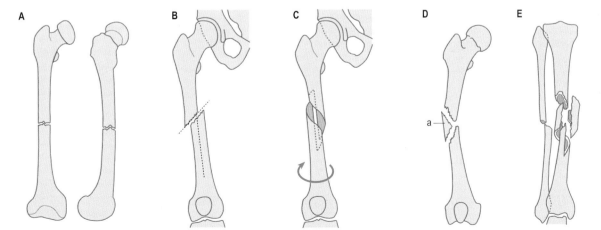

Fig. 10.58 The nature of the fracture. (A) If there is no deformity (no movement of the bone ends relative to one another), the fracture is in anatomical position. (B) Oblique fracture: the fracture runs at an oblique angle of 30° or more. (C) Spiral fracture: simple spiral fractures result from twisting (torsional) forces. (D) Multifragmentary (comminuted) fracture: there are more than two fragments. The fragment (a) is often called a butterfly fragment because of its shape. (E) Multifragmentary complex fracture: there is no contact between the main fragments after reduction.

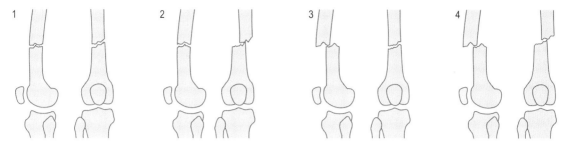

Fig. 10.59 The deformity of the fracture. Translation is present if the bone ends have moved relative to one another. The direction of translation is described in terms of movement of the distal fragment, e.g. in these fractures of the femoral shaft, there is (1) no translation, (2) lateral translation, (3) posterior translation, (4) lateral and posterior translation.

COMMON MUSCULOSKELETAL INVESTIGATIONS

10.27 Common musculoskeletal investigations	
Test	**Diagnosis**
Bedside	
Schirmer tear test	Keratoconjunctivitis sicca (dry eyes)
Urinalysis – protein	Secondary amyloid in rheumatoid arthritis and other chronic arthropathies Drug adverse effects, e.g. myocrisin, penicillamine
– blood	Glomerular disease, e.g. systemic lupus erythematosus
Microscopy for red cells and casts	Glomerular disease e.g. systemic lupus erythematosus
Haematological	
Erythrocyte sedimentation rate	Non-specific indicator of inflammation or sepsis
Full blood count	Anaemia in inflammatory arthritis, blood loss after trauma Neutrophilia in sepsis and very acute inflammation, e.g. acute gout Neutropenia in systemic lupus erythematosus, Felty's syndrome and adverse effects of antirheumatic drug therapy
Biochemical	
C-reactive protein	↑ in sepsis and inflammatory arthritis, e.g. rheumatoid arthritis
Urea and creatinine	↑ in renal impairment, e.g. secondary amyloid in rheumatoid arthritis or adverse drug effect
Uric acid	May be ↑ in gout, but levels may be normal during an acute attack
Angiotensin-converting enzyme	↑ in sarcoidosis
Calcium	↓ in osteomalacia; normal in osteoporosis
Alkaline phosphatase	↑ in Paget's disease, osteomalacia, and immediately after fractures
Serological	
IgM rheumatoid factor	↑ titres in 80% of cases of rheumatoid arthritis, occasionally low titres found in other connective diseases
Antinuclear factors	↑ titres in most cases of systemic lupus erythematosus, low titres in other connective tissue diseases and rheumatoid arthritis
Anti-Ro, Anti La	Sjögren's syndrome

Continued

10.27 Musculoskeletal investigations (*cont'd*)	
Test	**Diagnosis**
Serological	
Anti-Sm	Systemic lupus erythematosus
Anti-RNP	Mixed connective tissue disease
Antineutrophil cytoplasmic antibodies	Wegener's granulomatosis, polyarteritis nodosa
Joint aspiration	
Polarized light microscopy	+ly birefringent rhomboidal crystals – calcium pyrophosphate –ly birefringent needle-shaped crystals – monosodium urate monohydrate
Bacteriology	Raised white cell count in infection Organism may be isolated
Biopsy and histology Plain radiography (X-rays)	Synovitis – rheumatoid arthritis and other inflammatory arthritis Fractures, erosions in rheumatoid arthritis and psoriatic arthritis, osteophytes and joint space loss in osteoarthritis, bone changes in Paget's disease, pseudofractures (Looser's zones) in osteomalacia
Ultrasonography	Popliteal cysts in inflammatory knee arthritis, bursae, joint effusions
Isotope bone scan	Increased uptake in Paget's disease, bone tumour
CT scan	Atlanto-axial subluxation in rheumatoid arthritis
MR Imaging	Sacroileitis, soft tissue injury
Dual energy X-ray abnormality	Osteoporosis when assessed at lumbar spine and hip

◆ Key points

- Rest pain or pain at night suggests serious pathology.
- Bone pain with fever is osteomyelitis until proven otherwise.
- Ask about sphincter disturbance and assess perianal sensation and anal tone in every patient with back pain.
- Remember retroperitoneal causes of back pain.
- A septic joint is characteristically immobile and painful, but this may be masked in patients taking steroids or non-steroidal anti-inflammatory drugs.
- Pain out of proportion to an injury suggests compartment syndrome.
- Distal pulses may be preserved in compartment syndrome.
- Always consider the hip as a source for knee pain and vice versa.

- In aches and pains with headache or jaw pain on chewing think of temporal arteritis.
- Joint erythema implies an acute arthritis such as crystal-induced arthritis or sepsis.
- Look at the hands for diagnostic extra-articular features, e.g. small muscle wasting in rheumatoid arthritis, digital infarcts in rheumatoid vasculitis, nail pitting and onycholysis in psoriatic arthritis.
- Varus and valgus deformities at the knee are best detected with the patient standing.
- Loss of extension at the elbow is an early feature of arthritis.
- Abnormal patterns of wear on the soles of the shoes often indicate underlying foot deformity.

Section 3
SPECIAL SITUATIONS

Babies and children

IAN A. LAING • SINEAID BRADSHAW • JAMES PATON

NEONATES AND INFANTS

A neonate is a baby in the first few weeks of life. The term infant is sometimes used instead, but includes babies up to the age of one year.

Neonatal and infant assessment differs from that of older children and adults in that you need to be an opportunist and not expect to carry out your examination systematically. Defer any examination that you cannot complete and keep uncomfortable procedures to the end so that you do not disturb a contented baby. Remember the basic principles discussed in Chapter 1 and apply them to both the parents and baby.

Assessing a newborn infant serves the several functions listed in Table 11.1.

Preparation and setting

Gather your equipment together and use a well-lit warm room that is draught free. You need a stethoscope, an ophthalmoscope, an auriscope, a tape measure and some scales. Use a firm comfortable surface. Do not examine the baby immediately before or after a feed.

Introductions

Introduce yourself and find out who is going to be present and their names. Establish what their relationship is with each other and the infant. Examine the neonate in front of both parents. This is an ideal opportunity for you to identify and address any uncertainties they have. Some parents have never handled an infant before, and some will be highly experienced. Do not be judgemental about them nor intimidated yourself.

Listening. Encourage parents to share their fears and anxieties so that you can answer these. They may have ideas and expectations about the baby, and you need to clarify these. Although 9% of infants have abnormalities, mainly orthopaedic problems, many congenital abnormalities cannot be identified during this first examination.

Inform parents about the purpose of newborn examination and emphasize that not all problems are evident at birth. Record this in writing.

Information gathering

Establish the essential background (Table 11.2).

EXAMINATION

Observation is the key to diagnosis since physical signs are usually less obvious than in adults. Become familiar with the range of normal in order to be confident about what is abnormal. Experienced paediatricians often have their own individual system of examination. With time, you may develop your own, which should be based on Table 11.3. Where possible, examine the supine infant from the right side. This will allow you to be consistent in your clinical approach.

General inspection

Observe the demeanour and posture of the infant before asking a parent to undress the infant completely and remove the nappy. A normal term infant will be flexed and symmetrical, but a preterm infant, or one who is profoundly

---

11.2 Essential background information

• The infant's:
  – gender
  – name (if already given)
• The previous maternal:
  – medical history
  – obstetric history
• History of the:
  – current pregnancy
  – delivery
  – events since the infant's delivery
• Parental concerns

11.1 Functions of assessing a newborn infant

• To reassure parent and doctor that the baby:
  – appears to be normal
  – is feeding acceptably
  – has passed urine and meconium
• To identify:
  – any congenital abnormalities
  – any illnesses or infection
• To measure and record baseline data:
  – weight
  – head circumference
  – length

11.3 Sequence of examination
• General inspection • Inspection of skin and related tissues • Head, neck, ears, nose and mouth • Cardiovascular examination • Respiratory examination • Abdominal examination • Neurological examination • Final inspection

11.4 Normal ranges or values for physiological variables in the newborn		
Sign	**Preterm neonate**	**Term neonate**
Heart rate (beats per minute)	120–160	100–140
Respiratory rate (breaths per minute)	40–60	30–50

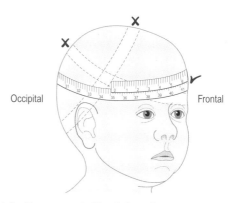

Fig. 11.2 Measurement of head circumference.

hypotonic, may adopt a more extended position. Assess whether the baby looks well and is an appropriate size for the gestation. Look for any visible congenital abnormalities like a rash or skin tag. Check that the respiratory rate is normal (Table 11.4) and whether the baby is resting or irritable. If the baby is crying, note whether the pitch and volume are normal.

Look at the limbs and count the digits noting any oligodactyly (decreased number of digits), polydactyly (increased number of digits) or syndactyly (joined digits). Open the baby's fingers and look for the palmar creases in both hands. A small percentage of the normal population have single palmar creases but it may be associated with Down's syndrome and many other chromosomal abnormalities including trisomies 13, 16 and 18.

Measure the weight, crown–heel length and occipitofrontal circumference on a centile chart appropriate to that population. Ideally weigh the baby fully undressed using electronic scales accurate to within 5 g. Measure the crown–heel length using a neonatal stadiometer (Fig. 11.1). Ask a parent or assistant to hold the baby's head still while you stretch out the legs and ensure the infant is supine and fully extended. This is the least reproducible of the three measurements.

Use a non-extendible paper tape to measure the occipitofrontal circumference round the forehead and occiput at the largest part (Fig. 11.2). Use the tape to measure three times and note the largest measurement to the nearest millimetre. Record weight, length and occipitofrontal circumference on a centile chart.

11.5 Skin characteristics
Colour
• Jaundice • Pallor • Plethora
Rash
• Distribution • Size • Colour • Macules or papules • Pus • Bleeding • Exudation

Skin

Look at the skin characteristics (Table 11.5).

The 'stork's beak mark' (Fig. 11.3A) occurs in 30–50% of newborns and is a pink discoloration at the nape of the neck, the eyelids and on the glabella. Pallor may be due to anaemia or peripheral vasoconstriction. Note any blue colour of the lips and mucous membranes of the mouth. This is central cyanosis and indicates hypoxia. *Acrocyanosis* is common in the early minutes and hours of life. The infant has blue peripheries but is centrally pink. *Plethora* is a general red colour and occurs in vasodilatation, polycythaemia and vascular overload. Jaundice is always an abnormal finding in the first 24 hours of life and needs investigation.

The texture of the skin may be normal, dry, wrinkled or vernix-covered. Describe any blisters or bullae seen. A 'collodion baby' has a varnished appearance of the skin and may be postmature.

Count and measure any pigmented naevi. A Mongolian blue spot (Fig. 11.3B) is usually over the buttocks, back and thighs. It is often large with a bluish tinge, and usually

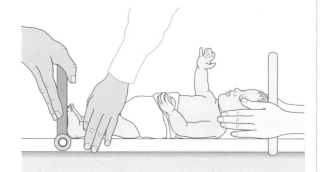

Fig. 11.1 Measuring length accurately in infants.

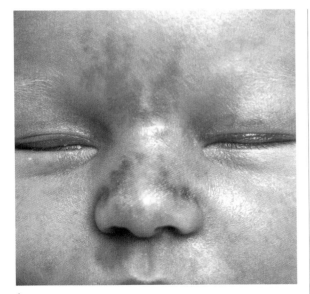

A

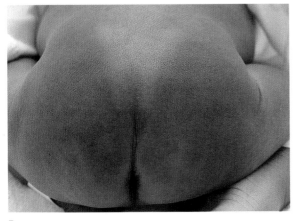

B

Fig. 11.3 (A) Stork's beak mark and (B) Mongolian blue spot.

11.6 Neonatal head shapes	
Head shape	**Description**
Microcephalic (small-headed)	Small cranial vault
Megalencephalic (large-headed)	Large cranial vault
Hydrocephalic (water-headed)	Large cranial vault due to enlarged ventricles
Brachycephalic (short-headed)	
Dolicocephalic (long-headed)	
Plagiocephalic (oblique-headed)	Asymmetrical skull

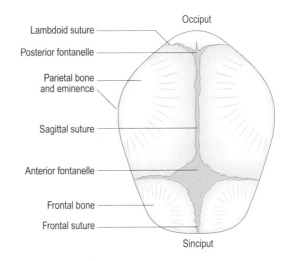

Fig. 11.4   The fetal skull from above.

fades in the first year of life. Other common skin changes are *milia* due to sebaceous gland hyperplasia, acne neonatorum, erythema toxicum, nappy dermatitis and dermatitis due to *Candida* infection.

Look for evidence of trauma. Document any scalp cuts and bruises from forceps or cardiotocography leads. Subcutaneous fat necrosis occurs as hard plaques under the skin where there has been local trauma, e.g. as a result of compression by forceps.

Head

Moulding of the head is common in the first 24 hours of life. Note the baby's head shape (Table 11.6) and any swellings. The anterior fontanelle is usually open. Feel to see if the skin is sunken, flat or bulging. Palpate all the sutures (Fig. 11.4). They may be overriding (feels like a shallow step), split apart (e.g. by raised intracranial pressure) or fused together (*synostosis*).

Eyes

Look at the eyebrows and eyelashes, eyelids and lacrimal system. Note any congenital abnormality, and asymmetry.

Pull the lower lid down gently and look for yellow sclerae. In pigmented races this is the best sign of neonatal jaundice. Note any discharge of pus from the eyes and any surrounding erythema. What size are the eyes? Small eyes (*microphthalmia*) may suggest multiple congenital abnormalities. If the eyeball appears large, gently palpate it through the baby's closed lid, using the tip of both your index fingers. If it is firm on palpation this suggests glaucoma (*buphthalmos*).

Look at the cornea. Observe any clouding and note its colour and position. A *hyphema* is a red fluid level over the iris, caused by bleeding, which varies with the child's position.

Ophthalmoscopy

Keep the instrument as close as possible to your eye, shining the light into the baby's eye with your head at the same level as that of the baby. Start about 20 cm away and look through the lens to identify the baby's pupil. Normally you should see a red or pale pink glow from the pupil – the *red reflex*, which is reflected light from the retina. If you cannot see this, there may be a cataract. Black spots in front of the retina may be small lens opacities (*cataracts*) and you should obtain a formal ophthalmological opinion. If the eyes are very puffy from oedema in the first 2 days of life you will not be able to examine them. Arrange to do so later in the first week of life.

Congenital cataract occurs in 2–3 per 10 000 births in the UK and is a cause of preventable blindness. Of babies with congenital cataract, only 35% are identified at birth.

Nose

Check that the nostrils are both patent. Block each nostril in turn with your finger and see if the infant continues to breathe through the other nostril.

Mouth

Note whether the jaw is small (*hypomandibularism* or *micrognathia*). Examining the inside of the mouth is easy in the crying infant and also in the sleeping baby if you are patient. Open the baby's mouth gently, using your finger tips to depress the lower jaw. Use the index finger and thumb of your other hand to retract the angles of the mouth. Shine a narrow-beamed torch on the palate, and feel with your little finger the pad turned towards the palate. Tongue elevators and depressors may cause local trauma so do not use them.

Tongue. A large tongue protruding from the mouth is true *macroglossia*. In Down's syndrome the baby has a normal-sized or small tongue which protrudes through a small mouth (*glossoptosis*). Look for the lingual frenulum in the midline, joining the tongue to the floor of the mouth. True tongue tie is uncommon.

Palate. Describe any cleft lip or palate. Is the cleft lip midline, unilateral or bilateral and does it involve the alveolus (gum)? Is it associated with cleft of the hard palate?

Gums. You may see eruption cysts before the neonatal teeth erupt.

Mucosa. White discoloration may be due to curdled milk from the last feed, or from thrush (*Candida albicans*). Scrape the discoloration gently using a tongue depressor.

Milk comes off easily, but thrush adheres and produces a little local bleeding when removed. A mucous cyst on the floor of the mouth is known as a *ranula*: it is related to the sublingual or submandibular salivary ducts.

Ear

Look at the size shape and position of the ears and for any auricular skin tags, usually anterior to the pinna. The helix may be temporarily folded due to local pressure in utero. Low-set ears occur if the helix joins the cranium below an imaginary line through the inner *canthi* (the inner corner of the eye where the lids meet) of the eyes.

The external auditory meatus and tympanic membrane can be inspected using an auriscope. Choose the smallest earpiece available. If the child is deeply asleep then the procedure may be carried out without any further precautions, but if the child is awake, seek help in restraining the baby (see p. 379). Hold the auriscope with the handle upwards as if you were holding a pen. Gently retract the pinna posteriorly and downwards. The external auditory meatus passes up and forwards in the neonate and you need to straighten it to visualize the tympanic membrane. Insert the earpiece into the external auditory meatus only to a depth of 0.5 cm and then move the tip gently until you see the tympanic membrane.

Neck

Asymmetry of the neck is often due to fetal posture and usually soon resolves. A lump in the sternocleidomastoid muscle is often caused by a fibrosed haematoma. This may result in *torticollis* (a wry neck) which causes the baby to rotate the neck to gaze in the contralateral direction.

Transilluminate any swellings to see if they are cystic (see Fig. 11.11). Cystic swellings glow as the light is transmitted through but solid or blood-filled swellings do not.

Palpable lymph nodes are normally present in one-third of normal newborn infants, not only in the cervical regions but also in the inguinal and axillary areas.

Cardiovascular examination

Cardiovascular problems often present with respiratory abnormalities, so count the respiratory rate for 15 seconds and multiply by four to give the rate per minute. The normal respiratory rate in a sleeping baby varies between 20–40 breaths per minute, but if the baby is hungry, crying or cold it may be above 60 breaths per minute.

Look for respiratory distress. The baby who has heart failure may be tachypnoeic but rarely uses accessory muscles of respiration. Look for the apex beat which should be visible and prominent. The apex beat of the newborn is normally positioned in the 4th or 5th intercostal space, on or within the midclavicular line. Palpate the apex beat using the palm of your hand. Note its position relative to the midclavicular line. If it is displaced lateral to the midclavicular line this may indicate cardiomegaly, or it may mean that the heart has been displaced to the left, e.g. by left lung atelectasis, right-sided pneumothorax or a right-sided pleural effusion. If the force of the heartbeat moves your hand up and down, this is a parasternal heave and if you can feel a vibration it is called a thrill.

Record the heart rate by feeling the right radial or brachial pulse. Count the number of beats in 15 seconds and multiply by four. A rate as low as 80 beats per minute or as high as 160 beats per minute can be normal depending on the state of arousal of the baby.

Feel the femoral pulses by placing your thumbs gently on either femoral triangle while moderately abducting the hips (Fig. 11.5). Good-volume femoral pulses normally indicate that there is no severe narrowing of the outflow tract from the left ventricle and no significant *coarctation* of the aorta at the time of the examination. In older children and adults you can palpate the right radial and femoral pulses together in order to identify a delayed femoral pulse compared with the radial. In neonates with a heart rate of 140 per minute it may be impossible to detect true radiofemoral delay, and only a comparison of pulse volumes is possible. Compare the femoral pulse with the brachial pulse by palpating the right femoral pulse with your right thumb and the infant's right brachial pulse with your left thumb. A neonate with low-volume femoral pulses should be referred to a paediatric cardiologist to exclude coarctation of the aorta. In neonates, you may feel the femoral pulses even when coarctation of the aorta is present, because the ductus arteriosus is open in the early hours or days and the right ventricular outflow may contribute to arterial pulsation in the lower aorta distal to the coarctation.

Palpate the abdomen and measure the size of the liver, using a tape measure in a cephalocaudal direction from the lowest rib anteriorly, in the midclavicular line.

Listen using the bell of the stethoscope, which is best for low-pitched sounds. Start using this at the apex. The diaphragm is better for high-pitched sounds and murmurs and should be used in all positions. One scheme of examination is shown in Figure 11.6.

A murmur is heard in up to 2% of neonates, but congenital heart disease occurs in only 0.6% of live-born infants. Routine examination only detects 45% of these babies with congenital heart disease because many murmurs are transient or benign.

Because the heart rate of the newborn is faster than that of an older child or adult, it is difficult to hear some sounds. However, you should still describe the rate, the quality of the first and second heart sounds, splitting of the second heart sound, additional heart sounds and the presence or absence of murmurs (see Ch. 3).

A patent ductus arteriosus may cause a murmur restricted to systole in the early days of life. This is because the pulmonary and systemic blood pressures are initially similar and left-to-right shunting of blood through the ductus is limited. The typical continuous murmur with a diastolic component is heard after a few weeks or months.

Do not measure blood pressure routinely in the newborn. It is very difficult to measure non-invasively. The baby who is well perfused and has readily palpable brachial pulses

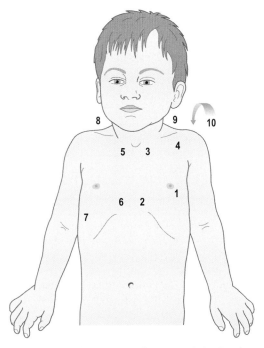

Fig. 11.6 Auscultation positions. Recommended order of auscultation: 1, apex; 2, left lower sternal edge; 3, left upper sternal edge; 4, left infraclavicular; 5, right upper sternal edge; 6, right lower sternal edge; 7, right midaxillary line; 8, right side of neck; 9, left side of neck; 10, posteriorly.

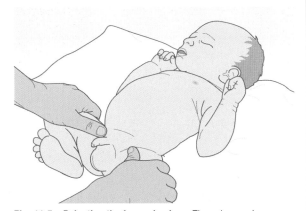

Fig. 11.5 Palpating the femoral pulses. The pulse can be difficult to feel at first; use a point halfway between the pubic tubercle and the anterior superior iliac spine as a guide.

is unlikely to be hypotensive. If you do measure BP, use a cuff width of a size two-thirds of the distance from the baby's elbow to shoulder tip. Repeat the measurement with a different cuff if the BP is unexpectedly high. In the intensive care unit, blood pressure is measured accurately by monitoring intra-arterial pressure using a cannula and a meticulously zeroed and calibrated instrument.

Respiratory examination

Note any extra breathing sounds before you handle the infant. Stridor is a sound made in the upper respiratory tract and is predominantly inspiratory.

Look for any abnormality of the shape of the chest wall after noting signs of respiratory distress. Respiratory distress shows itself in the newborn as tachypnoea, suprasternal, intercostal and subcostal recession. Remember that these signs can be caused by cardiac or respiratory tract problems. Stridor and indrawing in an otherwise well baby beginning on the second or third day of life and getting worse may be due to *laryngomalacia* (softness of the larynx). Consider the possibility of infection if there is any sign of respiratory distress.

Percussion of the newborn's chest is not helpful. It makes the baby cry, so that further respiratory examination is difficult.

Auscultate using the diaphragm symmetrically, starting anteriorly then laterally and finally posteriorly. Compare both sides and note any crackles and wheeze.

Abdominal examination

Look at the abdomen after removing the nappy. Mild abdominal distension is common because of gastric distension after a recent feed or swallowed air during crying. Because the anterior abdominal wall has poorly developed musculature in the neonate you may see the outline of the intestines. Clearly defined laddering of the intestines occurs with intestinal obstruction.

Inspect the umbilicus for any lump. The cord stump should age and drop off on the fourth or fifth day. An umbilical hernia is common and is covered with skin and subcutaneous tissue. It usually closes spontaneously. An *omphalocele* (or *exomphalos*; Fig. 11.7) is an eventration through the umbilicus containing protruding intestines covered by a thin layer of peritoneum. *Gastroschisis* is a defect in the anterior abdominal wall with herniation of intestines through the defect. By contrast to exomphalos, in gastroschisis the intestines are not covered with a membrane. The most common site of herniation is above and to the right of the umbilicus. A *granuloma* appears later as a pink fleshy lump in the umbilicus when the cord remnant has separated. A small amount of bleeding from the umbilicus is common in the neonate, but check that the infant has received vitamin K supplementation. A halo of

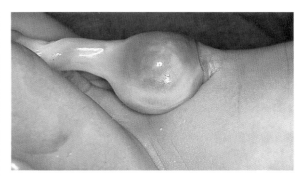

Fig. 11.7 Small exomphalos with loops of bowel in the umbilicus.

erythema round the umbilicus suggests infection causing omphalitis which may require urgent treatment.

Look at both groins for swellings. Hydroceles are the most common scrotal swelling and contain only fluid, while inguinal hernias contain bowel. These are best differentiated by palpation. Transillumination (see Fig. 11.11) may help but can be misleading since both a hydrocele and a hernia of thin-walled bowel may transilluminate. Hydroceles usually resolve spontaneously in the early months of life.

Indirect inguinal hernias are common in the newborn, especially in boys and preterm infants with chronic lung disease (Fig. 11.8). Check that any hernia can be readily reduced. Gently push the hernia contents upwards from the scrotum towards the inguinal canal and abdomen. An irreducible hernia may become incarcerated and requires urgent surgical repair.

To palpate the abdomen make sure your hands are warm, and be gentle. Stand on the supine infant's right side. Use the flat of your hand rather than probing with your finger tips. Always start with superficial palpation before

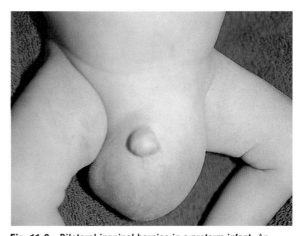

Fig. 11.8 Bilateral inguinal hernias in a preterm infant. An inguinal hernia is primarily a groin swelling; only when it is large does it extend into the scrotum.

feeling deeper structures. In the neonate the kidneys are often palpable, especially if ballotted. The neonate's spleen enlarges down the left flank rather than towards the right iliac fossa. Gently palpate the suprapubic region to establish bladder fullness; the baby may respond by passing urine.

The neonatal perineum

Female

Look at a girl's genitalia with the baby on her back. Hold her thighs gently and wait for her to relax. Gently abduct the legs and use your thumbs to separate the labia. You will often see a milky substance in the vagina; this is normal, not due to an infection. Later in the first week of life you may see a little vaginal bleeding (*pseudomenses*) as the neonatal uterus withdraws from the influence of maternal hormones. Gently retract the labia majora. You may see a mucosal tag attached to the wall of the vagina; this needs no treatment. In preterm infants the labia minora appear prominent because the labia majora are positioned laterally. This may give a masculinized appearance, but it will resolve spontaneously over the next few weeks.

Male

Look at a boy's genitalia for any abnormality in the shape or size of the penis. The outlet of the urethra should be at the tip of the penis. It may be malpositioned on the ventral aspect of the glans, along the ventral shaft of the penis or rarely in the scrotum or further posteriorly in the perineum. This phenomenon, which occurs in 1 in 400 boys, is *hypospadias* (Fig. 11.9). If you are in any doubt about the position of the meatus ask the mother to watch the baby urinating (Fig. 11.10A).

Do not attempt to retract the child's foreskin. The meatus may occasionally be seen on the dorsum of the penis: an abnormality known as *epispadias*. *Chordee* is a tethering of the foreskin and often causes the glans to be curved ventrally (Fig. 11.10B).

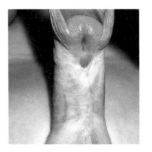
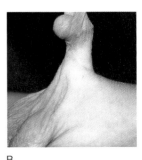

A   B

Fig. 11.10 Hypospadias and chordee. (A) Penile shaft hypospadias with dorsal hooded foreskin. (B) In lateral view, the ventral curvature of the penis (chordee) can be seen.

Look at the scrotum and the testicles. Palpate both testes with warm hands. The right testis usually descends from the abdomen into the scrotum later than the left testis, and ends up higher in the scrotum. If the testes are larger than usual the commonest cause is a hydrocele. Confirm this by transillumination (Fig. 11.11).

If you cannot identify the testes in the scrotum, exclude undescended or retractile testes. Using your right hand, start above the inguinal region on that side. Feel for any smooth lumps, moving your fingers down towards the scrotum, and then check the other side with your left hand. The testis is smooth, soft and about 0.7 × 1 cm across. You may feel a retractile testis just below the inguinal canal. Try gently milking it along the line of the inguinal canal to see if you can bring it down into the scrotum. Note any cryptorchidism or maldescent of one or both testes. It may be difficult to palpate the testes if there is a large pad of suprapubic fat. If there is any doubt about the position of the testes arrange for the infant to be examined at 6 weeks.

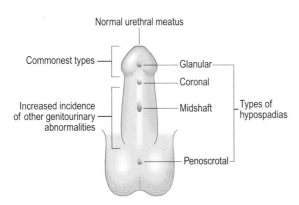

Normal urethral meatus

Commonest types

Glanular

Coronal

Increased incidence of other genitourinary abnormalities

Midshaft — Types of hypospadias

Penoscrotal

Fig. 11.9 Varieties of hypospadias.

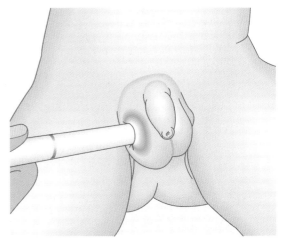

Fig. 11.11 How to transilluminate a scrotal swelling.

Neurological examination

This consists principally of assessing tone, posture, movement and primitive reflexes. Sensory examination is more limited.

Look at the baby and note any asymmetry in posture and movement. Erb's palsy post-delivery affects the upper brachial plexus roots (C5, C6) producing reduced movement of the arm, medial rotation of the forearm and failure to extend the wrist (Fig. 11.12).

The rarer Klumpke's palsy may be seen after breech delivery and is due to damage to nerve roots C8, T1, with weakness of the forearm and hand.

Facial nerve palsy causes reduced movement of the affected cheek muscles, and that side of the mouth does not turn down when the baby cries. Note any muscle wasting present in, e.g. *talipes equinovarus* (primary club foot).

Check sensation by seeing if the baby withdraws from stimuli, e.g. stroking the child's feet. Do not inflict painful stimuli or use a pin or needle. The eyesight of newborn infants can be checked crudely if they are alert, by carrying them to a dark corner where they may open their eyes wide. Then take them to a brightly lit area such as a window in daylight, and they will screw up their eyes to the bright light. If there is any doubt about vision refer to a neonatal ophthalmologist.

Test hearing by noting the startle response to a loud sound. In the UK there are plans to introduce electronic audiological screening for all infants.

Tone is the resistance to passive movement across a joint. It is a subjective judgement and requires experience before you can judge it reliably. A normal infant's tone changes so the baby may feel 'floppy' after a large feed. Hypotonic infants may have a frog-like posture with abducted hips and extended elbows. Causes of hypotonia include Down's syndrome.

Increased tone may cause back and neck arching, limb extension and the baby to feel stiff when picked up. Causes include meningitis, asphyxia or an intracranial haemorrhage. Neonates are often tremulous but this also occurs in subarachnoid haemorrhage or drug withdrawal if the mother has been abusing opiates in pregnancy. Infrequent jerks in light sleep are common and normal but regular clonic or tonic jerks are abnormal.

Power is difficult to assess and depends on the arousal of the infant. Look for strong symmetrical limb and trunk movements.

Assess the primitive reflexes in the following order:

- grasp response of feet
- grasp response of hands
- pull to sit
- ventral suspension
- pelvic response to back stimulation
- vestibular responses
- place and step reflexes
- Moro reflex
- root and suck responses
- tonic neck reflex.

Grasp responses. Stroke the sole of the foot, and the toes will flex and curl round your examining finger. Stimulate the palm of the baby's hands and observe the reflex grasping of your finger. Make sure the response is not inhibited by inadvertently stimulating the dorsal aspects of feet and hands.

Pull to sit. Hold the baby's hands and gently pull to sit (Fig. 11.13). Watch the sternocleidomastoid muscles which should bilaterally anticipate the pull to sit; the head flexes for a moment before head lag occurs.

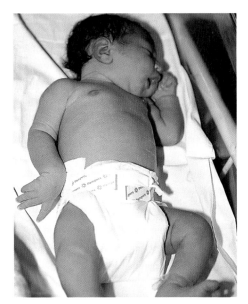

Fig. 11.12   Erb's palsy. The right arm is medially rotated and the wrist is flexed.

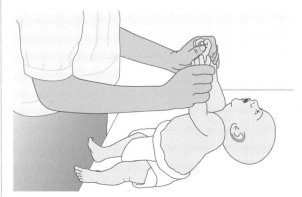

Fig. 11.13   Pulling to sit.

Ventral suspension/pelvic response to back stimulation. Turn the baby prone and look for good neck extension. Observe the extensor response to firmly stroking the skin over the vertebral column. Pelvic response to stimulation of the back and flanks should be symmetrical.

Vestibular responses. Demonstrate vestibular responses by holding the baby upright at your eye level, and then rotating the baby in an arc around your body. The baby's eyes should gaze in the direction of travel. Once the baby is a few days old it is normal to see *optokinetic nystagmus*, a horizontal jerking movement of the eyes in response to the arc rotation movement.

Place and step reflexes. The place response is elicited by holding the child vertical and stimulating the dorsum of the foot on the edge of the examination table. This results in the infant flexing the knee and hip and placing the sole of the foot on the table (Fig. 11.14).

Hold the baby under the arms facing towards you and lower the baby down towards the surface of the table or couch. When the feet touch the surface a walking movement occurs. Both these responses depend on arousal of the baby.

Moro reflex. The Moro response should always be elicited with the infant safely on the examining couch. Support the trunk and head at an angle of 70° to the couch.

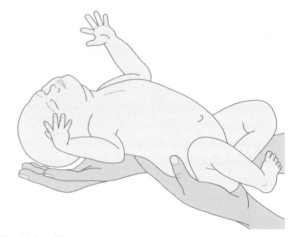

Fig. 11.15 The Moro response.

With your right hand supporting the head, allow it to drop 1 cm on to your right hand. The normal baby throws out both arms quickly with symmetrical abduction and spreads the fingers (Fig. 11.15). This is often followed by jerky adduction of the arms as though the hands were reaching for an unseen security.

An asymmetrical Moro response may be due to a previously unsuspected fracture of the clavicle or Erb's palsy.

If primitive reflexes persist into later infancy this may be the first indication of neurodevelopmental abnormality.

Root and suck responses. Efficient infant feeding depends on rooting, sucking, swallowing and defending the airway. Test the first two by gently stroking the baby's cheek. The hungry baby immediately turns to that side and opens his mouth as though for a nipple. This is called rooting. If the baby sucks on your finger it is often very vigorous.

Tonic neck reflex. This is the most difficult of all the primitive reflexes to demonstrate. In theory, if you turn the recumbent infant's head to the left, then the left arm and leg extend and the right arm and leg will flex (Fig. 11.16).

The tonic neck reflex appears at 37 weeks' gestation but is most prominent at 1 month.

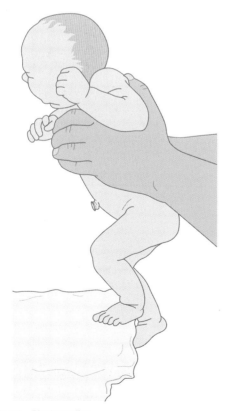

Fig. 11.14 Placing reflex.

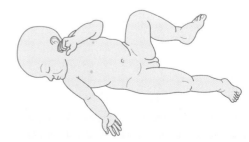

Fig. 11.16 Tonic neck reflex.

Final inspection

The final inspection ensures that you do not omit anything and allows the parents a further opportunity to ask questions and clarify points.

Begin at the top of the scalp and progress down to the feet. Look at the scalp again and feel for any abnormalities. Re-inspect all aspects of the head and neck.

Re-inspect the chest and abdomen. Breast engorgement is benign and resolves spontaneously.

Turn the baby over and feel along the length of the vertebral column starting at the neck. Particularly note and record that the sacrum and coccyx are present if the mother is diabetic; sacral agenesis is associated with maternal diabetes. A hairy or pigmented patch over the lower spine may indicate spina bifida occulta. If you find a sacrococcygeal pit visualize the bottom of it by separating the surrounding skin in good light. It is usually possible to see that the pit is lined with dry skin, which excludes pathological communication with the spinal cord.

Look at the anus to confirm it is present. Check the margins for any signs of a fissure, which can be demonstrated as a local split in the protecting epidermis of the anal ring. The position of the anus may be abnormal, either too anterior or too posterior. See if it is patent; confirm this by checking that the baby has passed meconium. If the anus pouts, gently stimulate the sphincter by touching it with your finger and seeing that the muscle reacts by contracting. Do not routinely carry out a digital rectal examination; it can cause an anal fissure. There are few indications for digital rectal examination in a neonate. They include suspected rectal atresia or stenosis and delayed passage of meconium. If there is mucus or bleeding per rectum it is more valuable to visualize the rectal mucosa using an auriscope and a well-lubricated earpiece. Perform a rectal examination by putting on gloves and using lubrication on your fifth finger. Gently press your finger tip against the anus until you feel the muscle resistance relax and insert your finger up to your distal interphalangeal (DIP) joint only.

Look at the baby's legs for any malformations. Hold the lower half of each leg in your hands and gently flex and extend them to gain an impression of the infant's tone. Count the toes and note whether any override each other. In talipes equinovarus the foot is plantar flexed and rotated so that the sole is directed medially. Check that you can gently manipulate the foot and ankle into the correct position. Normal findings include forefoot adduction and tibial bowing caused by the fetal position in utero.

Finally examine for dislocation of the hip, now called 'developmental dysplasia of the hip' because there is evidence that some dysplasias identified at 1 year are not evident in the first few weeks. The incidence of developmental dysplasia of the hip detected depends on the experience of the examiner and is around 1 in 1000 in the UK.

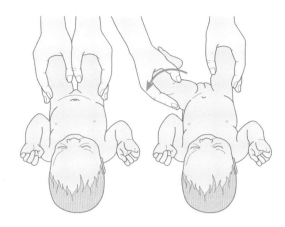

Fig. 11.17 Examination for developmental dysplasia of the hip. (A) The hip is dislocated posteriorly out of the acetabulum (Barlow manoeuvre). (B) The dislocated hip is relocated back into the acetabulum (Ortolani manoeuvre).

Lay the baby supine on a firm but comfortable surface. Look at the thighs for symmetry of the thigh creases.

Examine each hip separately. Hold the thigh with the knee flexed and your thumb on the medial aspect of the thigh. Move the proximal end of the thigh laterally and then push down towards the examining table (*Barlow manoeuvre*) (Fig. 11.17A). A clunk implies dislocatability of the hip. Then abduct the thigh. If you feel a clunk this indicates that the head of the femur has been dislocated and has been returned into the acetabulum (*Ortolani manoeuvre*) (Fig. 11.17B). Diagnose dislocated hips if the femoral head is very lax and you feel a clunk without doing the lateral and downward movement, i.e. the Ortolani manoeuvre without requiring the Barlow manoeuvre.

You can often feel minor clicks produced at the hip or knee by tendon movements. If you are in any doubt refer the infant for a senior opinion, preferably an orthopaedic surgeon with expertise in paediatrics. An ultrasound screening program is available in some centres.

◆ Key points

- ◆ The neonatal clinical examination can only identify those abnormalities present at the time of the examination. It does not guarantee the identification of all congenital abnormalities.
- ◆ Even after a normal neonatal examination you cannot be certain that the baby is free of congenital abnormalities.
- ◆ Always listen to the parents' concerns and address these. If a parent thinks that the baby has a problem you must take this seriously.
- ◆ Parents appreciate it if you are enthusiastic about their new baby: remember to congratulate them.

- Be opportunistic and do not expect to carry out your examination systematically.
- Defer any examination that you cannot complete.
- Keep uncomfortable procedures to the end so that you do not disturb a contented baby.
- You need experience to appreciate the normal range of neonates and infants. Seek advice from a senior colleague if you are in doubt.

- If you identify any abnormalities give parents a clear written plan of treatment and follow-up.
- Give parents information about other appropriate sources of advice about their infant's care in the coming days and weeks.

CHILDREN

Introduction

Children are not miniature adults. Illness and abnormality in children differ from those in adults because they occur within an individual who is constantly growing and developing. While many clinical methods used in adults are directly relevant in children, skills frequently need to be adapted for examining children.

GENERAL PRINCIPLES

Setting the scene

Your environment

Before you meet any family, think carefully about your environment. Is it likely to lead to a successful consultation? Have you enough chairs? Are they arranged in a way that minimizes barriers between you and the family? Make sure that the floor and surfaces are uncluttered and safe for an inquisitive toddler to roam around. A small table and chairs with colourful books and toys suitable for a range of ages makes entering a strange space more welcoming for a child. If you are likely to be discussing something that should be confidential make sure that the space is private.

Think about the way you are dressed – is it appropriate? Paediatricians generally adopt informal styles of dress but remember that children are often rather conservative. They frequently have clear views about how staff should dress; one study found that children viewed doctors dressed in casual clothes as caring but not competent, while doctors in white coats were competent but not caring.

If you wear dangling jewellery, children will be quite happy to pull it. If parents are worrying about whether their child will injure you, they cannot concentrate on what you are trying to say.

Infectious illnesses are common in children and are often transmitted via contaminated hands. Dirty hands and finger-nails are never attractive and may be positively dangerous. Scrupulous hand washing is therefore particularly important. Most staff working with children wear short sleeves to make frequent hand washing easier.

Equipment

Before you start, make sure you have everything you need for the examination; Table 11.7 provides a list of things that are commonly used.

Talking with parents

One important way in which a paediatric history differs from an adult one is that the paediatric history is nearly always given by a third party, usually a parent. However, all the principles in Chapter 1 still apply. At the outset, introduce yourself, and clarify the relationship between the person giving the history and the child, for instance is it mother, grandmother or childminder? Introduce other doctors or students and ask permission for them to remain.

The most valuable account almost always comes from the person who spends most time with the child. Always listen carefully to and acknowledge the ideas, concerns and expectations of the parents (or main carer where others have parental responsibility). They are experts in their child, and only by exploring their ideas and anxieties will you be able to fully address their problems.

11.7 The equipment
• Auriscope with a properly functioning bright light and range of clean earpieces
• Disposable spatulas for examining the throat
• Ophthalmoscope
• Paediatric stethoscope
• Equipment for measuring blood pressure with a selection of cuffs of different sizes
• Accurate measuring equipment for height (stadiometer) and weight (scales)
• Prader orchidometer
• Disposable paper tape measure
• Centile charts for plotting measurements
• A selection of toys for children to play with
• For a developmental assessment:
– 8 × 1 inch bricks
– pencils and paper
– a selection of picture and reading books

One common difficulty in medical history taking from a third party is that you receive an interpretation of events rather than a first-hand account of the symptoms and signs as experienced by the patient. Attempt to clarify exactly what was witnessed. Certain terms can be ambiguous, e.g. fit, constipation, wheeze. Listen carefully and clarify by summarizing your understanding of the situation and relating it back to the parents. This helps to reassure parents that you are listening to what they are saying.

Careful use of non-verbal communication through eye contact, attentive concentration, active listening and encouraging sounds will facilitate the story. Try to let the story flow without interruption. Remember that most people only talk for a few minutes before stopping.

Communicating with children

Always remember to talk to children and explain what you are doing. If possible ask them to describe the nature of the problem, e.g. the site of a pain, and encourage them to tell you about it. When it comes to examining children be gentle and be prepared to compromise, e.g. they may be more comfortable letting you palpate their abdomen with their own hand underneath.

Children vary in the rate of their language and cognitive development. Therefore, you have to think carefully about how much the child will be able to understand and communicate. Before they can communicate, children have to develop linguistic and cognitive skills. By 12–18 months, a child normally uses single words. By 3–4 years, an average child has a vocabulary of 850–1500 words and will be using three-word sentences. Children's understanding of illness also changes as they get older. Preschool children tend to attribute illness to coincidence or magic. In primary school, the idea of contagion develops and contracting disease is associated with contamination from other people or objects. Older children perceive that they fall ill through ingestion or inhalation of a 'germ'. Only in adolescence can young people conceive of psychological explanations for illness.

The importance of play

Part of the art of examining children is in engaging the child's cooperation. At the start, it is usually best to pause rather than diving in; much useful information can be obtained from watching a child play while you chat to the parents. Playing games with any equipment you are going to use can make the actual examination less frightening. All doctors develop their own tricks and games for working with children:

- Get down to the child's eye level.
- Compliment children about their clothes, hair adornments, etc.

- Refer to popular characters, e.g. Bob the Builder.
- Tailor your language appropriately.
- Talk playfully.
- Play games with equipment, e.g. listening to dolly, blowing out the light of the auriscope.
- Give 'I've been brave at the doctor's' stickers.

What is normal?

Most doctors come to paediatrics with knowledge of normal adults – you will have an idea of the range of heights, weights and behaviours that can be expected in adults. Children grow and develop, so everything changes as they get older. This makes it much more difficult to recognize deviations from normal. Parents often have similar difficulties, and many referrals and consultations are from parents who want reassurance that their child is not abnormal.

Unfortunately, there are no short cuts to differentiating normal from abnormal. Practice certainly helps. However, even experienced paediatricians use specific tools such as growth charts (Fig. 11.18) to allow them to distinguish normal from abnormal.

Information gathering

The important attributes for success in gathering information are:

- an observant eye
- an attentive ear
- a practised hand
- an open mind.

Structuring your clinical history and examination

In children, most information comes from careful observation. Observation includes formal inspection but is much more. From the time you first encounter children, you should be looking carefully at them and their interaction with people and their environment. This can provide important clues about the severity of their illness, their growth and nutrition, about their development, and about their relationships with their parents.

You should structure your approach to the examination by having a series of logical questions in your mind.

Is the child ill? The most important initial question is whether a child is acutely unwell and needs resuscitation or urgent treatment. Figure 11.19 provides a list of key observations for assessing illness severity in children.

Is there any obvious abnormality? Look for obvious abnormalities as the child approaches you – is there any abnormality of posture or gait? Are there any obvious dysmorphic features such as low-set ears, slanting eyes or a large tongue? Check whether the child's features are similar to those of the parents or siblings.

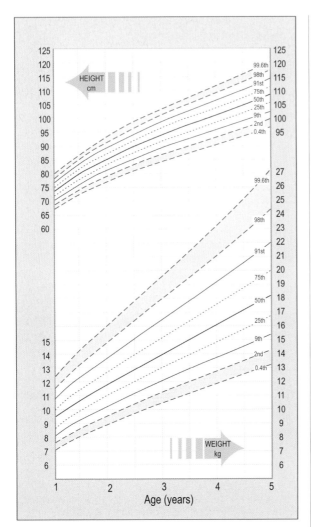

Fig. 11.18 Growth chart.

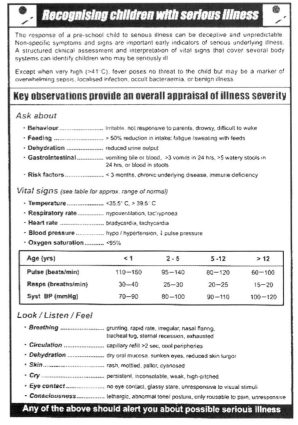

Fig. 11.19 Rapid cardiopulmonary evaluation.

You cannot expect to remember every unusual syndrome. However, you should be able to describe, record and, if necessary, measure what you see.

Is the child well grown and cared for? Healthy children grow normally and so growth provides a valuable indication of a child's overall well-being. Every child should have a growth chart within their medical records documenting measurements of height and weight, and head circumference in infants (see Fig. 11.18).

Measuring height. Height is measured using a *stadiometer*, a vertical scale with a rigid armpiece under which the patient stands barefoot and erect (Fig. 11.20). There are standard procedures for making accurate and reproducible measurements of height and length (detailed on the back of most growth charts) which need to be followed.

Scales and weighing. Toddlers and children should be weighed in their underwear. Infants are weighed naked without nappies. Scales need to be accurately calibrated and standard procedure followed if accurate measurements are to be made.

Previous measurements are often available from a child's personal health record, so serial growth over time can be plotted. In older children, you may need to evaluate the child's progress through puberty (Fig. 11.21).

If a child is unusually tall or short, measure the parents' heights and calculate the mid-parental height centile so that you can make allowances for the child's genetic background. A prediction of final adult height can be calculated using the parental heights, which are added together and the total halved to produce the mean. To correct this for gender, add 7 cm in the case of a boy and subtract 7 cm for a girl. This is the mid-parental height which should be plotted at the farthest end of the age scale, 18 years. The range 10 cm above and below that figure is the target centile range for the child, creating a 'normal' distribution curve skewed for this particular family spanning 2 standard deviations.

The child's appearance, demeanour, behaviour and interactions with carers are also important indicators of well-being. Doctors working with children always need to be vigilant for signs of neglect or abuse. Any suspicious or

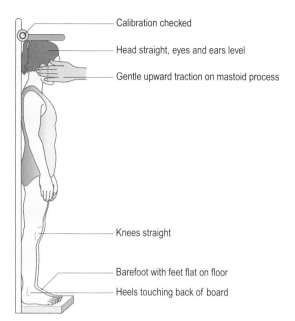

Fig. 11.20 **Stadiometer for measuring height accurately in children.**

- Calibration checked
- Head straight, eyes and ears level
- Gentle upward traction on mastoid process
- Knees straight
- Barefoot with feet flat on floor
- Heels touching back of board

unusual bruises or injuries must be carefully detailed. It is important to ask how any injury occurred, to decide whether the injuries are consistent with the explanation given and to note if there has been any delay before presentation.

Is the child developing normally?

Careful observation can also give important clues about a child's developmental progress.

What is the problem?

Traditionally, medical students have been taught to obtain a detailed history and to complete a full examination which should lead to a differential diagnosis. This list of diagnoses is then confirmed or refuted. In paediatrics, this is not always necessary or possible. Instead, a logical problem-based approach helps focus on the relevant facets of the history and examination.

How and why did the problem develop?

Start with the child's name, age and sex. Not only can you address children by their correct name but knowing the age and sex rapidly limits the range of diagnostic possibilities.

Ask the parents to describe the problem and how it developed. The way an illness develops and how it varies over time may be important clues to the diagnosis.

Check what the parent thinks about the problem and its cause and find out why the child has been brought to the doctor at this time.

Has this problem or others happened before?

Enquire about any significant previous episodes of ill health particularly any that led to hospital referral or admission; document their investigation, treatment and outcome. Note any operations, accidents or injuries, and what they were. Find out if previous problems resolved satisfactorily.

Find out what medications are currently being used. Remember to record the dose, route and frequency of administration, and to ask about drugs bought over the counter and complementary remedies. Ask about any adverse reactions such as rashes, diarrhoea or anaphylaxis that may have been caused by medication.

Has the problem been present from birth?

Enquire about the pregnancy and delivery:

- Was the pregnancy uneventful?
- Did labour start spontaneously?
- Was the baby preterm?
- What were the gestation and birth weight?
- Were there any complications at delivery?
- Did the baby require resuscitation, special or intensive care?
- Were there any other neonatal problems?
- Were any medications used during pregnancy?

Have there been any problems with the child's growth or nutrition?

Ask about this particularly in children with poor appetite, faltering growth (Table 11.8), constipation, diarrhoea and

11.8 **Some causes of short stature in children**
Intrinsic shortness
• Familial (genetic) short stature • Turner's syndrome
Delayed growth
• Constitutional delay in growth (adult height often normal) • Subtle undernutrition • Physical and/or psychological abuse/child neglect • Underlying systemic diseases of mild to moderate severity
Attenuated growth
• Chronic renal failure • Metabolic acidosis • Malignancy (including effects of chemotherapy and radiotherapy) • Glucocorticoid excess • Pulmonary disease (e.g. cystic fibrosis and severe asthma) • Congenital heart disease • Gastrointestinal disease (e.g. coeliac disease and Crohn's disease) – patients often underweight as well as short • Hypothyroidism • Advanced HIV infection • Severe protein and calorie malnutrition

A Female breast changes

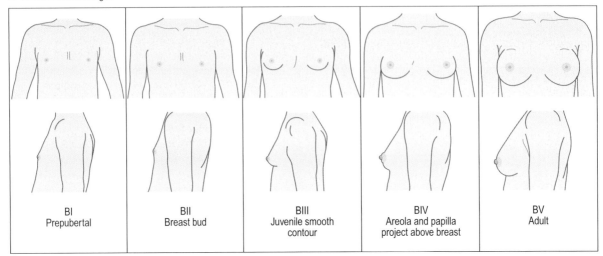

| BI Prepubertal | BII Breast bud | BIII Juvenile smooth contour | BIV Areola and papilla project above breast | BV Adult |

B Pubic hair changes–female and male

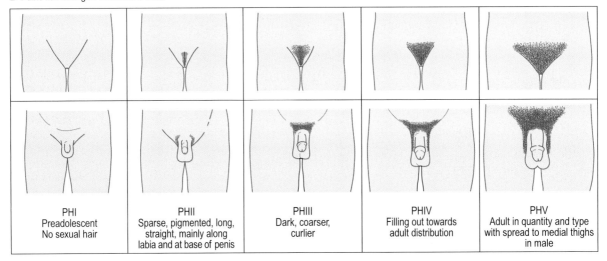

| PHI Preadolescent No sexual hair | PHII Sparse, pigmented, long, straight, mainly along labia and at base of penis | PHIII Dark, coarser, curlier | PHIV Filling out towards adult distribution | PHV Adult in quantity and type with spread to medial thighs in male |

C Male genital stages

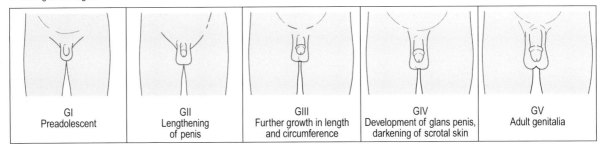

| GI Preadolescent | GII Lengthening of penis | GIII Further growth in length and circumference | GIV Development of glans penis, darkening of scrotal skin | GV Adult genitalia |

Fig. 11.21A–C Stages of puberty in males and females. Pubertal changes are shown according to the Tanner stages of puberty.

D Timing of puberty

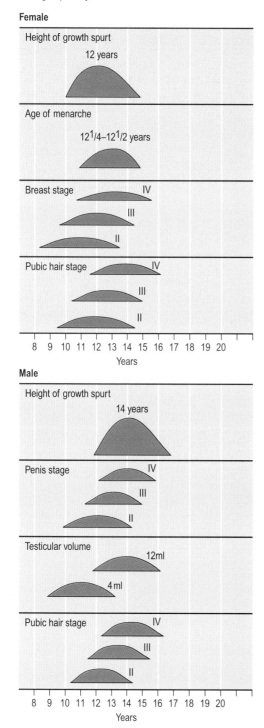

Fig. 11.21 D Timing of puberty in males and females.

vomiting, possible food allergies or if there are parental concerns. Check that parents understand and follow instructions on preparing artificial feeds. If they are not preparing bottle milk appropriately, it may explain why the child is unwell.

- Is/was the child bottle- or breastfed?
  - If breastfed, what was the duration of exclusive breastfeeding?
  - If bottle-fed, what was/is the volume and frequency of feeds and how are they prepared? (useful rules of thumb for appropriate feeding are 30 ml = 1 oz with 5 oz (150 ml) formula/kg/day)
- At what age was unmodified cow's milk introduced into the diet?
- What was the age of weaning and which foods were given?
  - How were they administered, e.g. by bottle, or spoon or as finger food?
- Can the child chew, suck and swallow without difficulty, e.g. choking?
- What makes the parents think the child is allergic?

Have there been any problems with the child's development?

The progressive acquisition of movement and motor skills and intellectual and cognitive development is one of the key tasks of childhood. It is closely related to maturation of the nervous system. Ask about this when there is parental concern regarding delay in development, epilepsy, an unusual (dysmorphic) appearance or a recognized syndrome, an abnormal shape or size of the skull.

If children have reached their milestones satisfactorily it makes many other conditions less likely. In young children check the age when they first sat, walked, and talked. In school-age children check whether they are attending normal school and making good progress.

What are the child and family's social circumstances?

It is always important to locate the presenting illness in the context of the child's life. Try to understand the family dynamics and relationships.

Family

- Are the child's mother and father living together? If not, what contact does the patient have with the absent parent?
- Who else is in the household? What are their occupations?
- How many siblings are there and are they all healthy? Note their ages and sex.
- What are the child care arrangements?
- Are the family restricted because of the child's illness?

Housing and household

- Are there any problems with housing, e.g. damp?
- Are there enough bedrooms and bathrooms, adequate facilities for cooking and room for safe play?
- Are there any smokers in the house?
- Does the family have pets?

School

- What has the child's school attendance been like?
- How is the child performing?
- Document the name of the school and teacher.
- Has there been bullying or behaviour problems?
- What is the impact of the symptom/s at and after school?
- Does the illness interfere with the child's day-to-day activities, e.g. playing, sports, activities of daily living, and ability to keep pace with peers?

Does the problem run in the family?

Ask about this if the child's appearance is dysmorphic or if a genetic disease or inborn error of metabolism is suspected. Establish if the parents are related, because for some illnesses consanguinity is a key finding. If the problem seems to occur within the family then it may be useful to draw up a detailed family tree (see p. 15).

Might the problem be infectious?

Think of this in a child with acute onset fever, rash, respiratory symptoms such as stridor, lymphadenopathy, diarrhoea and vomiting.

- Is the child up to date with all relevant immunizations?
- For certain groups check if there have been any additional immunizations such as:
  - BCG in certain ethnic minorities
  - hepatitis B in parental infection/intravenous drug use.
- If the child is not immunized, find out why not:
  - are there parental concerns about certain vaccinations such as MMR?
  - has there been a previous adverse reaction?
- Has there been:
  - any infectious contact?
  - any recent foreign travel?
  - any adverse reaction to antibiotics, particularly a rash or anaphylaxis?

Do you sense a psychological or psychiatric component?

Problems with emotions, behaviour or relationships ('troubles and muddles') are common and can present with sleeping difficulties, temper tantrums, faddy eating and school refusal. Some physical disorders such as abdominal pain or headache can have a psychological basis and some psychiatric problems, e.g. depression or school refusal, can complicate genuine physical illnesses.

The aim of the psychiatric history is to elucidate the symptoms, explore their impact and look at the child's risk factors for mental health problems and strengths or protective factors (sirs) (Fig. 11.22). If you directly question children about their behaviour and emotions it can be intimidating. Usually it is more illuminating to sensitively observe children's facial expression, body language, play, drawing and interactions as you talk with them. Once you have grasped the presenting symptoms, ask about specific symptoms of mood disorder such as appetite and sleep disturbance, physical symptoms, attention and concentration and separation anxiety. Enquire about any significant events in the child's life, e.g. starting school, moving home, the death of a family member or parental divorce. How does the child respond? Empathetic, open-ended questions to the child such as 'That sounds difficult. How did it make you feel?' can be useful.

It is important to understand why the child has become a focus for concern. Sometimes problems arise because of a disturbance in the mental health and coping skills of the parents. Use the family tree to document family functioning by enquiring about relationships between parents and siblings.

EXAMINATION

Careful observation throughout the consultation is nearly always the key when examining children. Observation means more than simply looking at the child, it means taking note of the child's appearance, demeanour and interaction with you and the family. More direct methods of examination such as palpation and auscultation are usually less informative because specific localized signs in children are uncommon. You do not need to examine every system in all children. If you combine detailed observation and a careful history you should be clear about which system to target.

When examining children, always look first, before touching them. Capturing their interest, be it by playing with a toy or talking about a television programme, can provide a way to carry out a great deal of examination without the child realizing it. Leave any unpleasant parts of the examination, such as examining the throat, to the end.

General inspection

Initial observations can tell you a lot about a child (see Fig. 11.19):

- Does the child appear ill or well?
- Is the child cyanosed, or dehydrated?
- Is there any obvious abnormality, e.g. unusual dysmorphic features that suggest a particular syndrome?
- Is the child appropriately grown and nourished?
- Is the child behaving appropriately for age and size?

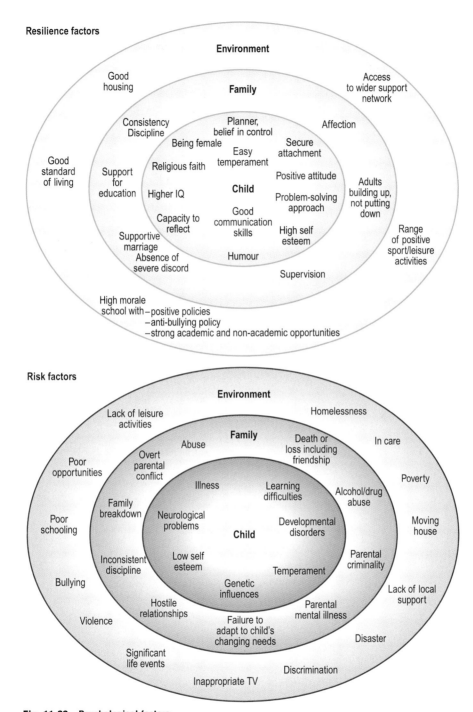

Fig. 11.22 Psychological factors.

Skin, hair, and nails

Examine these in detail if there is any evidence or history of a rash.

Making a drawing or diagram of any rash can be helpful in making your observations more accurate and systematic.

Special diagrammatic charts with outline drawings of body shapes are available. Take a photograph, especially if accurate recordings are necessary, e.g. medicolegal documentation of bruising due to suspected child abuse.

Rashes are discussed in more detail in Chapter 2.

What to look for

- Colour
- Distribution
- Size and nature of individual lesions making up the rash
- Whether the lesions are separate or run together
- Whether the rash is itchy or not.

What to feel for

- Is the rash raised?
- Do the individual lesions contain fluid?
- What type of fluid?

Lymph nodes

Parents may see or feel an enlarged lymph node, particularly in the child's neck or groin. Often, such glands are normal. Such 'normal glands' are not tender, may be multiple and tend to be small ('shotty'). Parents may have unspoken anxiety about leukaemia or cancer, but fortunately, malignant conditions are rare in children (Table 11.9). Children with skin conditions such as eczema may have enlarged lymph nodes draining the affected area. Check for any abnormality in the surrounding region of skin.

What to look for

- Are any swollen lymph glands visible?

What to feel for

- Carefully palpate the affected area and note carefully:
  - size
  - number
  - consistency
  - temperature
  - tenderness

11.9   Causes of lymph node enlargement
Cervical lymphadenopathy
• Tonsillitis, pharyngitis, sinusitis • Chronic gingivostomatitis • 'Glandular fever' (infectious mononucleosis/cytomegalovirus) • Tuberculosis (uncommon in developed world)
Generalized lymphadenopathy
• Acute exanthemata • 'Glandular fever' • Systemic juvenile chronic arthritis (Still's disease) • Acute lymphatic leukaemia • Drug reaction • Mucocutaneous lymph node syndrome (Kawasaki syndrome)

- whether they are mobile or attached to skin or deeper structures?
- Check all the other regional lymph node areas.
- Check for liver and spleen enlargement.

Respiratory system

Examine this in any child with a cough, difficulty breathing, wheezing, poor feeding or fever.

What to look for

Watching the child's breathing carefully, count the respiratory rate over 30–60 seconds. Fast breathing (tachypnoea) is a sensitive marker for acute respiratory infection (Table 11.10).

Look for cyanosis or alteration in the child's colour. Ideally use a pulse oximeter to measure oxygen saturation (SaO_2); the normal saturation in children is 95% or above. Cyanosis only becomes clinically apparent when there is sufficient deoxyhaemoglobin circulating in the blood and usually occurs when SaO_2 is 85% or less. You can miss mild but significant desaturation by relying only on observation.

Look for signs of difficulty breathing such as subcostal, intercostal or supraclavicular retraction. In more severe respiratory distress there may be an indrawing of the trachea in the suprasternal notch during inspiration (*tracheal tug*) and flaring of the nostrils. Is the chest hyperinflated or is there asymmetry of chest wall movement? In children, chest expansion is best checked by watching carefully from the end of the bed. In asthma with hyperinflation, the chronic pull from a displaced diaphragm leads to fixed indrawing of the lower ribs with flaring of the diaphragm (*Harrison's sulcus*). Observe the pattern of breathing. In obstructive airway diseases such as asthma, there is a more prolonged expiratory phase compared with inspiration.

If the child has a prominent cough, note if it sounds moist and productive or dry. A persistent, productive cough is uncommon in children and is not a feature of asthma.

Look at any sputum produced and its colour. The colour of sputum usually correlates with the presence of infection because neutrophilic inflammation produces myeloperoxidase, which colours the sputum green.

11.10 Respiratory rate in children (breaths/min)		
Age	**Normal**	**Tachypnoea**
Neonate	30–50	> 60
Infants	20–30	> 50
Young children	20–30	> 40
Older children	15–20	> 30

Look for finger clubbing which occurs most commonly in children with cystic fibrosis and cyanotic congenital heart disease and not with asthma.

What to feel for

Feel the position of the trachea. Percussion is occasionally helpful if you suspect consolidation or effusion from the quality of the breath sounds. Restrictive disorders are rare in children so chest expansion is only very rarely of value.

What to listen for

Note any respiratory noise such as an expiratory grunt, inspiratory stridor or an audible wheeze. Respiratory noises are often audible without a stethoscope. Some noises may even be palpable. If there is a noise, establish whether it originates in the chest or throat or both.

Use your stethoscope and listen for crackles and wheeze. The respiratory sounds heard on auscultation are usually high pitched so use the diaphragm. Note the type of sound and whether this is symmetrical or focal. Localized differences point to focal lung lesions. Wheezing is an important pointer towards a diagnosis of asthma. Record if it is present and whether or not it is heard all over the chest.

Cardiovascular system

Examine this in any child with shortness of breath, syncope, cyanosis, feeding difficulties or in the presence of a murmur.

What to look for

Look for central cyanosis and check the SaO_2 using a pulse oximeter. Count the respiratory rate and look for any sweating, finger clubbing, oedema and any abnormality of the precordial area such as a precordial bulge.

What to feel for

Feel if the child is warm and well perfused and record the time for capillary return.

Check the femoral and brachial pulses; note the rate, strength and whether the pulses on the two sides are symmetrical. The normal pulse rate varies with the child's age as well as with fever, excitement or distress and exercise (Table 11.11). It can be surprisingly difficult to feel normal femoral pulses in small chubby children. Note whether the pulse is of small, normal or full volume. Small-volume pulses are difficult to feel and distal pulses may be more difficult than proximal pulses. Full-volume pulses are bounding, and if this is the case you should feel the more peripheral pulses easily.

Feel the apex beat and the chest for a heave or thrill. The apex beat is normally in the fourth–fifth intercostal space. A thrill is a palpable murmur and is always significant. Check the suprasternal notch with your index finger as thrills from aortic stenosis may only be palpable there.

Auscultation

Listen for the heart sounds, identify the first and second sounds. Note particularly the quality and intensity of the second sound and whether it is single or split. If there are any murmurs note where they are loudest, whether they are systolic and/or diastolic and where they are conducted to. Murmurs associated with a thrill (grades 4–6) are always pathological, but innocent murmurs (Table 11.12) are common in children. If you find a suspicious murmur, refer the child to the paediatric cardiologist. Listening to the heart is conventionally left to last but if children are cooperative or asleep use the opportunity to listen while they are quiet (Ch. 3).

Blood pressure

Automatic Doppler, oscillometric or ultrasonic machines have made measuring the blood pressure much simpler. Like other vital signs in children, blood pressure varies with age. Measure the blood pressure with a cuff that is two-thirds of the distance from the elbow to the shoulder tip and have the child seated or standing. Note the size of cuff and whether the child was seated or standing. Keep the child's heart, arm and sphygmomanometer at the same level and explain what you are going to do before you start. A single elevated reading should be repeated with a larger cuff if necessary.

11.11	Normal resting pulse rate in children	
Age	**Beats/min**	
< 1 year	110–160	
2–5 years	95–140	Increased with stress, exercise, fever, arrhythmia
5–12 years	80–120	
> 12 years	60–100	

11.12 Characteristics of innocent murmurs
• Soft – grades 1–3 intensity and often midsystolic
• Localized
• Poorly conducted
• Not usually conducted posteriorly
• Variable with position and with respiration

Gastrointestinal system

Carry out a detailed abdominal examination if the child has any of the following symptoms: vomiting, diarrhoea, constipation, abdominal swellings or abdominal pain.

What to look for

Check for jaundice, anaemia or finger clubbing. Look for abdominal distension. In normal toddlers and children the abdomen is often protuberant because of an exaggerated lumbar lordosis. Abdominal movement with respiration is normal up to school age. Look for fullness in the flanks which may occur if there is ascites. If there is any swelling note its size and if it is local or generalized. The site of the swelling may suggest the cause. Fat, fluid, faeces and flatus all cause generalized swelling. Localized swellings may be due to a hernia, distended bowel loops, masses or enlarged organs. Umbilical and inguinal hernias are common and with gross ascites the umbilicus may be everted. Visible peristalsis occurs in pyloric stenosis or intestinal obstruction.

What to feel for

Make sure that the child is as relaxed as possible because the abdominal muscles need to be relaxed for you to perform an adequate examination, and achieving this often takes skill and patience. Ideally, the child should lie on his back. Always ask children whether their abdomen is sore before you start. In younger children, watch their face carefully during palpation for any sign of discomfort. Palpate methodically round the abdomen, feeling for the size and position of the abdominal organs and for any masses or fluid.

The liver can normally be felt 1–2 cm below the costal margin in the midclavicular line. Start palpating in the left iliac fossa so that you do not miss a very large liver. Define the upper edge by percussion, then measure the distance in centimetres between the top and bottom edge in the midclavicular line. Record the liver breadth in centimetres and note whether the edge is soft or firm. A very hyper-inflated chest as occurs in severe bronchiolitis can flatten the diaphragm and push the liver down, so measuring the liver span helps differentiate a large liver from one that is palpable and of normal size but pushed down.

Palpate for the spleen, which may occasionally be felt in normal children. Start in the right iliac fossa and work towards the left costal margin.

Palpate for the kidneys, keeping your left hand underneath the child and using your right hand on top for both sides. The kidneys are not easy to feel in young children except in a hypotonic neonate, so if you do feel them, they are probably enlarged. You may feel a full bladder and sometimes see it arising from the pelvis in infants and young children. Note if there are any abdominal masses, the commonest cause in children being faeces. If you suspect there is ascites, you will need to check for shifting dullness. Finally, always check the groins to make sure there are no swellings or lumps that might indicate a hernia.

Auscultation

Bowel sounds are accentuated in intestinal obstruction and absent in peritonitis or paralytic ileus.

Examining the anus and rectum

Remember to look at the anus when you examine the abdomen. A rectal examination is not routine in a child. However, it may provide valuable information in some circumstances, e.g. 'redcurrant jelly stool' in a suspected intussusception. If it is required, explain clearly what you are going to do. Use your little finger in infants and small children and lots of lubricant jelly. Feel carefully for any masses, or local tenderness, and check for blood or other material on your examining finger (see Ch. 7).

Genitourinary system

Abnormalities of the genitalia are common especially in little boys. If you are examining the genitals make sure you have a chaperone or a parent with you and record this in the notes. If there is any hint of sexual child abuse from the history or from your assessment of the situation, then refer the child for a more detailed assessment.

In boys

What to look for. Look at the size of the penis and the position of the urethral opening, which should be at the tip. Check that the scrotum is of normal size and rugosity and that both testes are present within it. Transilluminate any swellings by placing a pen-torch against the skin over the swelling and see if the light is transmitted across the swelling. This indicates a fluid-filled swelling, most commonly a hydrocele (see p. 358).

What to feel for. Palpate the scrotum with the boy standing. If you are trying to decide if a testis is truly undescended or just retractile, ask the child to squat. This abolishes the cremasteric reflex and allows you to feel a retractile testis. Testicular volume is measured using a Prader orchidometer (Fig. 11.23).

In girls

What to look for. With the child lying on her back look for enlargement of the clitoris, labial adhesions, the position of the vagina and the presence and the nature of any vaginal discharge. In older children, you can stage progress through

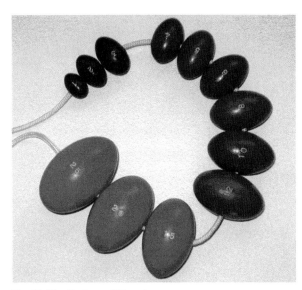

Fig. 11.23 Prader orchidometer.

puberty using charts of pubertal staging. The charts use the extent of pubic hair growth, breast development (in girls) or penile and testicular development (in boys) to assign a pubertal stage (see Fig. 11.21).

Musculoskeletal system

Common presenting complaints are joint, bone or limb pain. Parents may be concerned about unusual postures such as bow legs or knock knees. The musculoskeletal system is one area where specific descriptive labels, usually derived from Greek (e.g. *phocomelia* – a seal-like limb) or Latin (*talipes* – club foot) are common. Do not worry if you do not know the name but always describe exactly what you see.

What to look for

Watch how the child moves around. For infants, note if they crawl or bottom-shuffle, for older children see if they can hop, skip and jump and look for a waddle or a limp. See if there is any bony deformity or joint swelling or redness. Note any limb abnormalities. Some findings will only become obvious when a child is undressed. There may be extra toes or fingers. Check for evidence of muscle wasting or alternatively hypertrophied muscle groups.

What to feel for

Always try to avoid causing the child any pain. Ask children's permission before you touch them and watch the child's face carefully throughout your examination. Work out which joints are involved and feel for signs of inflammation. The pattern of affected joints is important

as it helps in making the diagnosis. Note if small or large joints, or both, are affected and whether affected joints are proximal or distal.

Always check active movements before attempting passive ones.

Nervous system

Carry out a detailed neurological examination in a child with a history of seizures, headaches, an abnormal or unsteady gait, any weakness and any increase or decrease in tone.

A quick assessment

In virtually all children your initial observations and a few simple points of history allow a brief but detailed assessment of a child's neurological system.

Motor function. In an infant who is not yet mobile, a good assessment of gross motor function is the 180-degree test:

- With the baby supine, pull him by the hands to a sitting position and look for head lag.
- Does the baby sit unsupported?
- Put your hands under the axillae and raise the baby up, noting his tone.
- Bring the feet down to touch the table, note if the baby takes his weight.
- Turn the baby quickly face down; note if the baby supports his head.
- Watch for the protective parachute reflex, seen from 6–9 months, as you lay the baby down. The baby suddenly extends the arms as if to protect himself.
- Note if the baby pushes his chest up off the floor by extending his arms.
- Does the baby roll from front to back and from back to front?

A child usually starts walking between 12–18 months. From then on, observe children running, walking, jumping and hopping. Check fine motor skills by watching them play with toys, and draw, copy or write if they are old enough. This should allow you to assess whether there are any problems with the child's vision.

Special senses and social skills. Carefully observe how children interact with their parents, whether they talk and respond to commands and how they behave. Watch to see whether they fix and follow your face. If you offer an object, do they take it from you?

Full examination

General points. In an older child, detailed neurological examination is carried out as in an adult. In younger children, the nervous system is developing and their comprehension and cooperation are much less. Therefore, in the younger the child the examination of development and the nervous system are intertwined.

Head

What to look for. Look at the shape, size and the fontanelles. Note if the head shape is normal. Some head shapes are associated with particular syndromes (see p. 354).

Palpation. Measure the occipitofrontal circumference using a disposable paper tape. Place the tape around the head at the level of the occiput and forehead. Make sure this is at the largest circumference and then measure at least three times, noting the largest measurement, to the nearest millimetre (see Fig. 11.2). Plot the measurement on centile charts (see p. 364). Feel the fontanelles and the cranial sutures and note if they are open or closed. The posterior fontanelle closes soon after birth, and the anterior at 15–18 months. Delay in closure suggests increased intracranial pressure, bone disease such as rickets or other abnormalities of the skull bones.

Neck stiffness

More than 80% of cases of meningitis occur in children. Neck stiffness is an important sign but can be unreliable in infants and young children. Children who are very ill with meningitis may have none but tonsillitis may give neck stiffness.

What to look for. Look for signs of passive resistance. Do children lie rigid or can they turn their head from side to side? Ask them to flex their chin onto to their chest. If meningeal irritation is severe, the child may lie with head extended.

What to feel for. Gently flex the neck while supporting the occiput by putting both your hands behind the child's head. Feel for resistance and watch for a change in the child's facial expression. In older children, ask them to kiss their knees. If meningism is present, the child will not be able to do this without discomfort.

Head jolt may be a more sensitive test of meningeal irritation. Standing to the right of the child and facing the child's head, place your hands on either side of the head. Turn it from side to side fairly rapidly and note any resistance.

Central nervous system: cranial nerves

In older children test the cranial nerves as you do in adults. In preschool children and infants you require skill and ingenuity. Observe common activities such as the child following a face, smiling, crying, chewing or drinking. Asking the child to open his mouth and stick out his tongue can give a lot of information. Parents will often give a very

accurate assessment of whether they think there are any problems with the child's hearing and vision.

What to look for

- Facial expression, movements and feeding
- Eyes:
  - visual fixation and following
  - corneal light reflection
  - red reflex
- Ears
  - responds to loud sudden sounds
- Posture.

What to feel for

- Tone
- 180-degree test (see p. 373)
- Reflexes
- Withdraws from tickling.

Checking special senses. Always ask the parents or carers if they think the child hears and sees all right. If not, clarify exactly what they think is the problem.

Vision. Watch to see if the child fixes and follows; if so the child can see. Remember that children follow faces not torchlight. Look for a squint (see Ch. 8). Observe if the light reflection is in the same position on the cornea in both eyes. By 6 weeks, both eyes should move together.

Check whether a red reflex is present using your ophthalmoscope (see p. 355). This will be obscured if there is a cataract, corneal clouding or a retinal tumour. Test vision and manipulation together by seeing whether a child can pick up small objects such as raisins.

Fundoscopy takes practise and patience in children and testing visual acuity in young children is a specialist skill.

Hearing. Detecting deafness is important but surprisingly difficult. Because of this, in the UK, universal hearing screening is being introduced in the neonatal period. If this is not available, then hearing is usually checked at around 8 months using distraction testing. This test is hard to do and requires properly trained staff. For the non-specialist, check with the parents about the child's hearing behaviours (Table 11.13) and refer for specialist assessment if there are any concerns.

Peripheral nervous system

Motor function.

What to look for. Check for any abnormal postures such as scissoring of the legs which may indicate that the underlying tone is increased (Fig. 11.24).

In infants, primitive reflexes, e.g. sucking and palmar grasping, are present (see p. 359). As the child matures, these primitive reflexes must be lost before new, more advanced skills can be acquired. If they persist, there may be underlying neurological abnormality.

11.13	Hearing checklist for parents
Shortly after birth	Startles and blinks at a sudden noise, e.g. slamming of door
By 1 month	Notices sudden prolonged sounds, e.g. a vacuum cleaner, and pauses and listens when they begin
By 4 months	Quietens or smiles to the sound of your voice even when he cannot see you. He may also turn his head or eyes towards you if you come up from behind and speak to him from the side
By 7 months	Turns immediately to your voice across the room or to very quiet noises made on each side, so long as he is not too occupied with other things
By 9 months	Listens attentively to familiar everyday sounds and searches for very quiet sounds made out of sight. Should also show pleasure in babbling loudly and tunefully
By 12 months	Shows some response to his own name and to other familiar words. May respond when you say 'no' and 'bye-bye' even when he cannot see any accompanying gesture

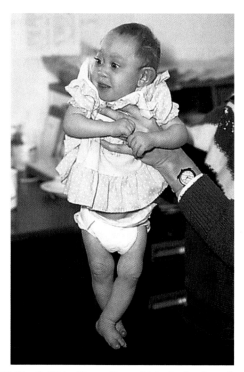

Fig. 11.24 A child with spastic quadriplegia showing scissoring of the legs from excessive adduction of the hips, pronated forearms and 'fisted' hands.

In older cooperative children, power can be tested as in adults. In younger children, watch for movements against gravity and behaviours such as sitting, crawling and walking.

What to feel for. Pick infants up and feel their tone. If they are excessively floppy they may slip through your fingers when you hold them upright; increased tone may make them feel stiff so they seem to move as if in one piece. Pull them to sit and look for evidence of head lag.

In an older child, check tone by gently testing passive movements of a limb around a single large joint.

Test the tendon reflexes in the same way as in an adult. Increased reflexes are easier to assess than decreased ones. If the reflexes are pathologically increased or decreased, you should find other evidence that the underlying tone is altered. An upgoing plantar response provides additional evidence of upper motor neurone dysfunction (see Ch. 8).

Sensation. Detailed testing of sensation requires co-operation and is carried out as for adults. A useful screening test in younger children is to check whether they withdraw from tickling.

Development

Development is usually considered under four main headings:

- movement and posture
- vision and manipulation
- hearing and speech
- social behaviour.

There is a wide range in the ages of attainment of each milestone and it is not unusual to be slow in reaching one, and advanced in another. When you are assessing children make allowances if they are tired, hungry or just uncooperative. If a child does not achieve certain milestones at a single examination it does not necessarily indicate a problem. A list of warning signs that should lead to a more detailed developmental examination is given in Table 11.14.

Delay in development may be global, where it encompasses all categories of development, or specific, affecting one category in particular, e.g. motor delay in cerebral palsy or social impairment and language delay in autism. Several standardized tools facilitate developmental examination, e.g. Griffiths Score, Denver Scale, Schedule of Growing Skills and the Woodside System (Fig. 11.25). One simple approach used in the community is illustrated.

Inspection

Careful observation can reveal a great deal of information about developmental progress.

Movement and posture. In a non-mobile infant, use the 180-degree test (see p. 373). An infant's first steps usually occur between 12–18 months, although babies who bottom-shuffle may not walk until the age of 2 years.

11.14	Warning signs in developmental milestones

The supine infant – around 6 weeks

- Marked head lag (in cerebral palsy, excessive extensor tone can mimic advanced motor development)
- Asymmetry of movements
- Absence of visual fixation and following
- Excessive placidity or hyper-excitability
- Difficulty with sucking and swallowing

The sitting infant – 7–10 months

- Inability to sit unsupported
- Inability to raise head and chest when prone
- Hand preference (right or left *dominance* should not be present until age 2 – before this it suggests a problem with the neglected hand)
- Absence of hand transfer, inability to handle two objects
- Absence of visually directed reach
- Poor vocalization
- Inability to chew or swallow

The mobile toddler – around 2 years

- Unsteady gait
- Unable to climb stairs
- Mouthing or casting objects
- Unable to build a tower of cubes
- Lack of intelligible speech
- No meaningful three-word combinations; subject–verb–object
- Unable to name pictures

The talking child – 3–4 years

- Unable to stand on one foot
- Unable to peddle a tricycle
- Unable to copy a circle
- Solitary or obsessional play
- Inability to use sentences of at least six words
- Inability to separate from mother

Vision and manipulation. Check at 6 weeks for congenital cataract and squint. If in doubt refer to a specialist ophthalmologist.

At 3 months assess palmar grasp by seeing if the baby holds on to a 1-inch wooden cube. The essential pincer grip should emerge at 8–10 months. Test this along with vision by presenting a small object such as a raisin which the baby will rake with the pointer finger before successfully opposing the thumb to pinch it and pick it up. Quickly take it away before the baby puts it in his mouth!

Hearing and language. Always take parental concerns about their child's hearing very seriously at any age and arrange formal audiometry. Hearing-impaired infants fail to startle at a loud noise only if severely deaf. They will still cry and vocalize. At 8 months the infant should babble in a sing-song fashion, while the vocalizations of a child with impaired hearing will be monotonous and not tuneful.

Test hearing at 8 months using the distraction test.

Distraction test. This requires three testers and ideally should take place in a sound-proofed room. The baby sits on the mother's knee and is distracted by a tester sitting opposite so that the baby faces forward. The second tester is stationed behind the baby and makes a series of sounds which should be measurable. In practice, a high-frequency rattle, a whisper and a low-pitched coo, emitted from left and right are used. The test is passed if the baby turns toward the sound.

Non-verbal communication of needs through gestures such as pointing, gaze and facial expression, and behaviours such as crying or squealing precede word formation. At 2 years you can assess language development using a naming pictures book, when the child should name three to five objects. Vocabulary expands rapidly and at 3 years children should be able to recount their experiences to a parent. Phonetic immaturities such as substituting 'th' for 's' are common and gradually diminish over time. Reassure parents that speech will naturally develop into adult pronunciation over time, usually without intervention from speech therapy. The combination of slow language development and abnormal communication with lack of eye contact and facial expression for social interaction should raise suspicion of autism.

Social behaviour and play. The eagerly awaited first smile is the first milestone of social development and occurs by 6 weeks. From then, there is a developing response to human contact, maturing feeding behaviour, evolving awareness and control of bodily functions, self-care and imaginative and interactive play.

Feeding ties in with language development in that the ability to chew at 8 months is an important marker of intraoral coordination.

The skill of finding a toy under a cup at 1 year suggests the child has developed the concept of object permanence, such that the object no longer ceases to exist when out of sight.

As far as toilet training is concerned, children are often out of daytime nappies by age 2, but more challenging is the change from night nappies. Half of 3-year-olds are dry by night, but 10% of 5-year-olds and 5% of 10-year-olds continue to wet the bed (enuresis).

Ears, nose and throat

Common symptoms that should lead you to carry out a detailed examination of the ears and throat include earache or discharge, a runny or blocked nose, sore throat, and fever.

Ears

What to look for. Is the external ear normal in shape and position? Normal ears have approximately one-third of the pinna above an imaginary coronal plane between the inner canthi. Ears which are low-set have less than one-third of the pinna above this line. Low-set ears are found in syndromes such as Down's syndrome.

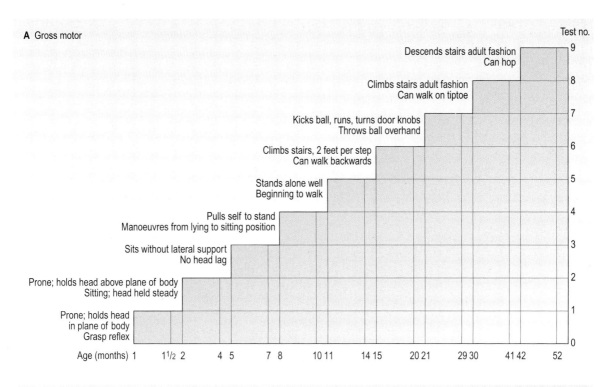

A Gross motor

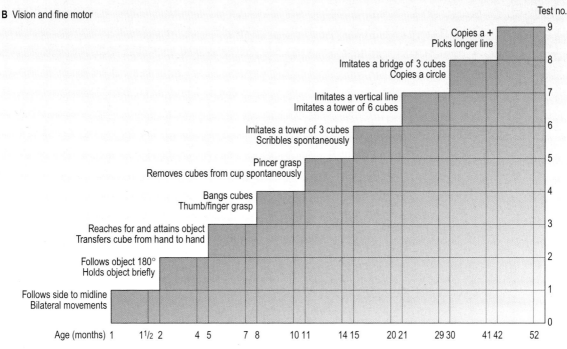

B Vision and fine motor

Fig. 11.25A–B Woodside System of developmental assessment.

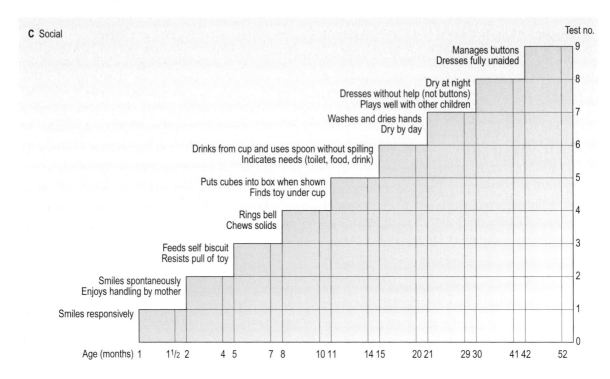

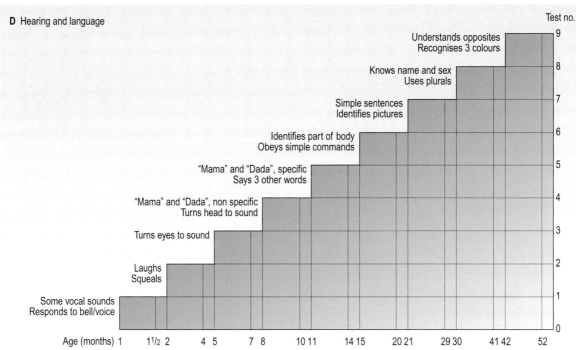

Fig. 11.25C–D Woodside System of developmental assessment.

Young children are often reluctant to allow their ears to be examined. You need the child to be properly held (Fig. 11.26), the largest speculum that fits in the external auditory meatus and a bright light from your auriscope. If the child is not held properly and struggles, the examination will be painful leading to more struggling.

In the infant pull the pinna down because the canal is directed upwards. In an older child pull the pinna back and up. Look at the tympanic membranes for anatomical landmarks, swelling, perforation, redness, dullness and fluid (see Ch. 10).

Nose

What to look for. Does the nose look normal? Note if the child is breathing through the nose and whether there is a nasal discharge. If so, is it clear, pus or blood? You may see a small crease in the skin near the tip of the nose. This is caused by a child with allergic rhinitis persistently rubbing his nose upwards – the 'allergic salute'.

In a cooperative older child, use an auriscope with a large speculum to check the nasal mucosa. Note whether the mucosa is inflamed or swollen and whether any pus is present.

Mouth and throat

Examine these in a child with sore throat, unexplained fever or mouth ulcer (Fig. 11.27).

What to look for. Young children usually object to having their mouth and throat examined. Leave these and the ears to the end. A bright light and a firmly held child are important but you still may only get a brief look, so practise. Try asking young children to do an alligator's yawn or to show you what they had for breakfast by opening their mouth even wider. If they are uncooperative, slip a tongue depressor along the side of the mouth between the lips and teeth to touch the back of the throat. When the child gags you will get a glimpse of the throat. Use this only when it is important to visualize the throat but never in a child with stridor.

Look at the tongue and jaw size. A protruding tongue is a seen in a number of conditions such as Down's syndrome. Look for redness, exudates or secretions on the oropharynx, or palatal petechiae which are seen in glandular fever. In thrush, there is a white exudate that is difficult to scrape away.

Check the tonsils for ulceration or exudates. Tonsillar size does not matter but note if they are huge and touching in the middle. The size is only significant if they produce symptoms of airway obstruction during sleep.

Look at the palate for any cleft of the soft or hard palate. It is surprisingly easy to miss a cleft palate. If you cannot get a good view, use a spatula to inspect this part clearly.

If the child has a sore throat, and is toxic, febrile and drooling, beware. The child may have epiglottitis. Check if the child has had *Haemophilus influenzae* b (Hib)

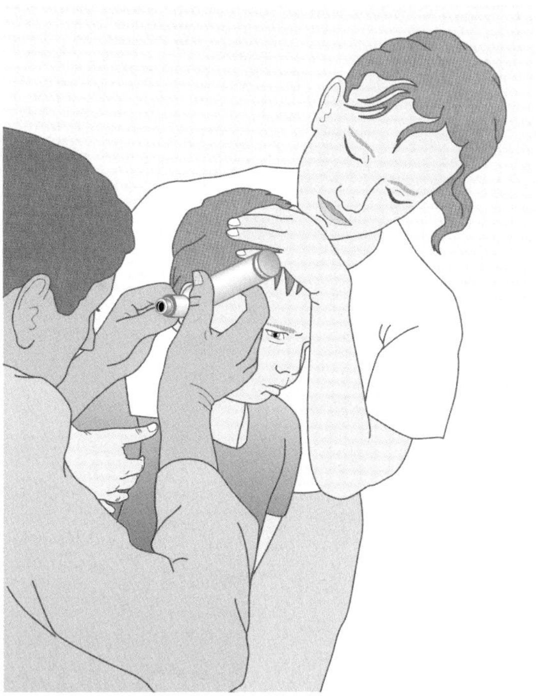

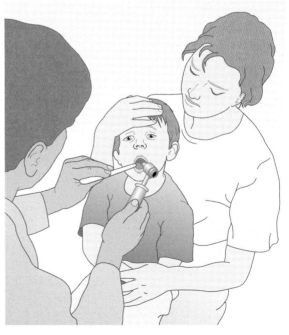

Fig. 11.26   How to hold a child to examine the ear.

Fig. 11.27   How to hold a child to examine the mouth and throat.

immunization and *do not* examine the throat because you may precipitate complete airway obstruction.

Teeth

Check the teeth for dental caries and the gums for any abnormalities. Suggest that the child sees a dentist for full assessment if necessary.

PUTTING IT ALL ALTOGETHER – WHAT IS THE PROBLEM?

Having looked, listened and examined (the 'observant eye', the 'attentive ear' and the 'practised hand'), you should usually be able to arrive at a differential diagnosis. In children, the list of possibilities is often quite short. From these you can start to work on a plan of investigation and treatment.

By the end of the consultation, everyone should have an agreed view of what is the expected outcome and plan.

It is important that parents know what to look out for and how to respond if things do not develop as expected. You should tell them signs that might suggest deterioration or the development of a more dangerous problem, along with a plan of how to respond. This is called 'safety-netting'. In some conditions such as asthma, this is often formalized into a written asthma action plan.

Communication: sharing information

Parents often feel they receive insufficient information about their children's health. They are looking for explanations and detailed advice to help them manage their sick child confidently. An important role of the children's doctor is to educate the parents and to provide them with the information they want.

Developments such as parent-held records and sending parents copies of clinic letters help to promote partnership between parents and clinicians.

◆ Key points

- ♦ Listen carefully to the parents' concerns about their child. If they think there is a problem you must take this seriously. They will usually be telling you the diagnosis.
- ♦ Observation is the key to paediatric examination; closely watch children from the first moment you see them.
- ♦ Children often do not cooperate to allow a full, formal examination, so examine what you can, when you can and return another time to complete it.
- ♦ Always measure and chart growth and check on the child's development.
- ♦ You need experience to appreciate the range of normal. Check with more experienced colleagues if in doubt.
- ♦ Parents want explanations and detailed advice.
- ♦ By the end of the consultation, everyone should have an agreed view of the expected outcome and plan.
- ♦ Leave uncomfortable procedures to the end.

The critically ill patient

ALASDAIR GRAY • COLIN ROBERTSON

EXAMINATION OF THE CRITICALLY ILL PATIENT

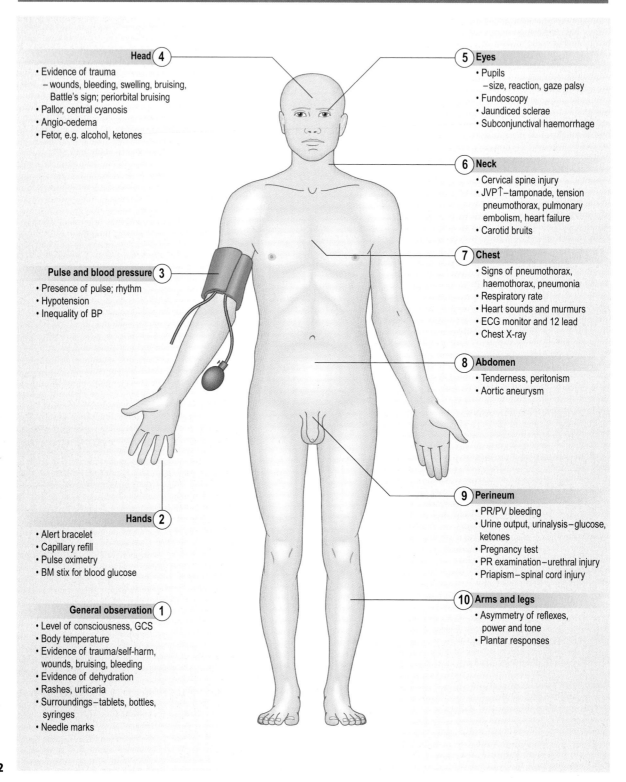

Head (4)
- Evidence of trauma
  – wounds, bleeding, swelling, bruising,
    Battle's sign; periorbital bruising
- Pallor, central cyanosis
- Angio-oedema
- Fetor, e.g. alcohol, ketones

(5) **Eyes**
- Pupils
  –size, reaction, gaze palsy
- Fundoscopy
- Jaundiced sclerae
- Subconjunctival haemorrhage

(6) **Neck**
- Cervical spine injury
- JVP↑–tamponade, tension
  pneumothorax, pulmonary
  embolism, heart failure
- Carotid bruits

(7) **Chest**
- Signs of pneumothorax,
  haemothorax, pneumonia
- Respiratory rate
- Heart sounds and murmurs
- ECG monitor and 12 lead
- Chest X-ray

Pulse and blood pressure (3)
- Presence of pulse; rhythm
- Hypotension
- Inequality of BP

(8) **Abdomen**
- Tenderness, peritonism
- Aortic aneurysm

(9) **Perineum**
- PR/PV bleeding
- Urine output, urinalysis–glucose,
  ketones
- Pregnancy test
- PR examination–urethral injury
- Priapism–spinal cord injury

Hands (2)
- Alert bracelet
- Capillary refill
- Pulse oximetry
- BM stix for blood glucose

General observation (1)
- Level of consciousness, GCS
- Body temperature
- Evidence of trauma/self-harm,
  wounds, bruising, bleeding
- Evidence of dehydration
- Rashes, urticaria
- Surroundings–tablets, bottles,
  syringes
- Needle marks

(10) **Arms and legs**
- Asymmetry of reflexes,
  power and tone
- Plantar responses

INTRODUCTION

The general and systematic approach to examination described earlier is inappropriate for critically ill patients because you may need to intervene immediately to save the patient's life, e.g. in cardiac arrest or tension pneumothorax, or to halt or stabilize processes which, untreated, would lead to death, e.g. hypovolaemic shock. Therefore, for a critically ill patient, examination and interventions are often performed simultaneously. This is a temporary phase, which must always be followed by a full history and clinical examination when the patient is 'stable'.

IDENTIFYING THE CRITICALLY ILL PATIENT

The clinical features of critically ill patients are listed in Table 12.1. Although using these criteria may lead to a relative over-triage, up to 20% of patients will require admission to the high dependency or intensive care unit.

Critical illness is a condition which, if unrecognized or untreated within the next few minutes or hours, may lead to death or serious disability. Paradoxically, the nature of the disease process may not necessarily determine whether a patient is critically ill or not. It is the time course of the disease process that is more relevant, and initially you may not be able to make a definitive diagnosis. Your aim is to stabilize the patient's condition temporarily to allow full diagnosis, specialist investigations and definitive therapy.

Preventing patients from becoming critically ill is as important as treating them later. Emergency departments, intensive care and high dependency units need adequate staff and facilities to detect early signs of deterioration and institute corrective procedures. In hospital if your patient has any of the features in Table 12.1, immediately call senior experienced medical and nursing personnel and the medical emergency team. Out of hospital, urgently call the ambulance or emergency services.

The clinical manifestations of critical illness

Critical illness usually presents in one of three ways:

- altered conscious state (Table 12.2)
- acute respiratory compromise (Table 12.3)
- acute cardiovascular compromise (Table 12.4).

In cardiac arrest, where immediate recognition and intervention are vital, all three of these are present. Others more often present with a single manifestation, but if untreated, the remaining two may develop. For example a patient with a pneumothorax developing tension initially has respiratory symptoms. As increasing tension occurs, cardiovascular compromise develops and leads to loss of consciousness and ultimately death.

What do you do?

When you see a patient for the first time, you may not know the preceding events or time frame concerned. If you concentrate on the system which appears to be most likely to have caused the problem this may be misleading, time-wasting and further compromise the patient. An ABC

12.1 Clinical features of the critically ill patient
Airway and breathing
<ul><li>Respiratory arrest</li><li>Obstructed or compromised airway</li><li>Respiratory rate < 8 or > 35/min</li><li>Respiratory distress: stridor, inability to speak in complete sentences, use of accessory muscles, intercostal indrawing</li></ul>
Circulation
<ul><li>Cardiac arrest</li><li>Pulse rate < 40 or > 140/min</li><li>Systolic BP < 100 mmHg</li><li>Features of shock: altered conscious level, peripheral perfusion, urine output < 0.5 ml/kg/h</li></ul>
Neurological
<ul><li>Failure to obey commands</li><li>Glasgow Coma Scale < 10, or sudden fall in GCS 2 points</li><li>Frequent or prolonged seizures</li></ul>
Other
<ul><li>Any patients you are seriously concerned about even if they do not have any of the above criteria</li></ul>

12.2 Common causes of altered conscious state
Non-CNS causes
<ul><li>Hypoxia</li><li>Hypovolaemia</li><li>Hypoglycaemia</li><li>Drugs and poisons, e.g. opioids, alcohol, carbon monoxide, benzodiazepines, tricyclic antidepressants</li><li>Metabolic: – type II respiratory failure ($\uparrow PaCO_2$), hepatic or renal failure – thyrotoxicosis/myxoedema/Addisonian crisis, non-ketotic hyperosmolar states</li><li>Hypo- or hyperthermia</li></ul>
CNS causes
<ul><li>Intracranial haemorrhage, e.g. subarachnoid haemorrhage</li><li>Ischaemia: thrombosis, embolism</li><li>Trauma: concussion, white matter shearing (diffuse axonal shearing), haemorrhage (extradural, subdural and/or intracerebral)</li><li>Infections: meningitis, encephalitis, cerebral malaria</li><li>Seizures</li><li>Primary or secondary tumour</li><li>Hypertensive encephalopathy</li></ul>

12.3 Common causes of acute respiratory compromise
Airway obstruction
<ul><li>Altered conscious state (see Table 12.2)</li><li>Upper airway trauma</li><li>Maxillofacial injury</li><li>Tracheolaryngeal injury</li><li>Foreign body</li><li>Infections (e.g. epiglottitis, quinsy)</li><li>Angio-oedema</li><li>Tumours</li></ul>
Pulmonary conditions
<ul><li>Pneumothorax (especially if tension is present or bilateral)</li><li>Chest injury<ul><li>blunt: rib fractures, flail segment, lung contusion</li><li>penetrating: pneumothorax, open chest wound, major vessel injury with haemothorax</li></ul></li><li>Acute severe asthma</li><li>Pulmonary embolism</li><li>Pneumonia</li><li>Acute pulmonary oedema<ul><li>cardiogenic: acute left heart failure</li><li>non-cardiogenic: smoke, toxic fume inhalation</li></ul></li><li>Adult respiratory distress syndrome</li><li>Exacerbation of chronic obstructive pulmonary disease</li><li>Massive pleural effusion</li></ul>
Non-pulmonary conditions
<ul><li>Metabolic acidosis<ul><li>diabetic ketoacidosis</li><li>severe renal or hepatic failure</li><li>lactic acidosis</li><li>overdose – methanol, ethylene glycol, (late) salicylate</li></ul></li><li>Severe anaemia</li><li>Pyschogenic hyperventilation</li></ul>

12.4 Common causes of acute cardiovascular compromise
Cardiac
<ul><li>Cardiac arrest</li><li>Acute myocardial infarction or ischaemia</li><li>Acute valve dysfunction, e.g. endocarditis, mechanical valve failure or obstruction</li><li>Arrhythmia</li><li>Pericardial tamponade:<ul><li>trauma</li><li>malignancy</li></ul></li><li>Cardiomyopathy: viral, alcohol related, postpartum</li></ul>
Vascular
<ul><li>Dissection, or rupture, of abdominal or thoracic aortic aneurysm</li><li>Mesenteric infarction</li></ul>
Massive pulmonary embolus
Blood loss
<ul><li>Gastrointestinal:<ul><li>upper: varices, peptic ulcer, tumour, Mallory–Weiss tear, non-steroidal anti-inflammatory drugs</li><li>lower: diverticular disease. angiodysplasia, ischaemic bowel, Meckel's diverticulum, tumour</li></ul></li><li>Trauma:<ul><li>overt: wounds especially to scalp, face long bone or pelvic fractures</li><li>concealed: chest – haemothorax abdomen – splenic and/or hepatic injury, retroperitoneal</li></ul></li><li>Obstetric/gynaecological:<ul><li>placenta praevia</li><li>miscarriage</li><li>ectopic pregnancy</li><li>trauma</li><li>tumour</li></ul></li><li>Anticoagulant use or bleeding diathesis</li></ul>
Miscellaneous
<ul><li>Anaphylaxis</li><li>Hypothermia</li><li>Hyperthermia</li><li>Electric shock/lightning injury</li><li>Envenomation (bites or stings from snakes, insects, jellyfish)</li></ul>

approach is the simplest and safest approach. This may seem overly simplistic, but many patients die suddenly or unexpectedly from simply treatable conditions. In the heat of the moment, the ABC approach allows you to address and correct conditions using a logical framework. It can be used by either a single inexperienced clinician or a full specialist team.

THE ABC APPROACH

The ABC approach has (up to) four interlinked phases:

1. Preparation before you see the patient (where possible)
2. The primary survey
3. The secondary survey
4. Definitive care or intervention.

Alone, you cannot manage a critically ill patient adequately. Get senior, experienced help as soon as possible. If you have to work alone, only proceed to the next item once the preceding one has been dealt with adequately. If you are part of a team the separate elements can be dealt with simultaneously, but the team leader must ensure that all components are covered and, if a patient's condition deteriorates, must immediately review the ABC sequence.

Preparation

Often you will be unable to take a history from patients because of their condition. If so, use all other possible sources of information for your preliminary data (Table

12.5	**Preliminary key data**
A	Allergies
M	Medication
P	Past medical history
L	Last meal
E	Events leading up to presentation and environment

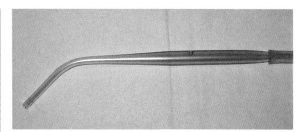

Fig. 12.1 Yankauer catheter.

12.5). Include previous general practice or hospital records, relatives, friends or bystanders, emergency or ambulance service personnel. Look in the patient's pockets, wallet, purse for diabetic/steroid/anticoagulant cards and medications. Look for Alert bracelets and necklaces (see Fig. 2.1). If possible, contact the patient's general practitioner who is often a key source of current and background information.

THE PRIMARY SURVEY

The primary survey, investigations and interventions should take only 5–10 minutes unless a life-saving intervention such as tracheal intubation needs to be undertaken. Use a stepwise approach for all these stages.

A: Airway

Approach patients so that they can see you if conscious and able to open their eyes. This is particularly important for patients who are supine and immobile because of splintage, pain or paralysis. Speak slowly and clearly. If the patient talks back to you normally, the airway is clear and the patient can protect it. There is currently circulation of blood to the brain and, if the speech is lucid, cerebral function is adequate. Give the patient a high inspired concentration of oxygen by mask, and move on to B (Breathing).

If there is no response, usually because the patient has altered consciousness, perform a more detailed assessment of the airway. Use simple, basic techniques first. Look, listen and feel. Open the mouth and remove any significant secretions, blood, vomit or foreign material by gentle suction with a Yankauer catheter (Fig. 12.1) under direct vision. Leave well-fitting dentures or dental plates in place as they help maintain the normal airway anatomy, but if they are loose or poorly fitting, remove them. Listen for upper airway noises (Table 12.6). Gurgling, snoring or stridor, suggest partial airway obstruction. Absence of any breath sounds indicates either complete airway obstruction and/or absence of breathing.

Open the airway by tilting the head and lifting the chin (Fig. 12.2). In patients with suspected neck injury, control the head and neck by manual in-line control and open the airway using the jaw-lift technique (Fig. 12.3). Do not move the neck. Appropriately sized airway adjuncts, such as nasopharyngeal or oropharyngeal (Guedel) airways,

12.6	**Airway noises**
No noise (the 'silent airway')	Implies complete airway obstruction and/or absence of, or minimal, respiratory effort
Snoring	Caused by partial upper airway obstruction from soft tissues of the mouth and oropharynx
Gurgling	Caused by fluids (secretions, blood or vomit) in the oropharynx
Hoarseness	Caused by partial laryngeal obstruction associated with oedema
Wheeze	A 'musical' noise, best heard on chest auscultation. When heard loudest in expiration relates to obstruction in the small bronchi and bronchioles, most often in asthma and chronic obstructive pulmonary disease
Stridor	A harsh noise caused by partial obstruction around the larynx or main bronchi. It is usually loudest in inspiration. In a febrile patient, consider epiglottitis or retropharyngeal abscess. Otherwise, foreign bodies, laryngeal trauma, burns or tumours are possible

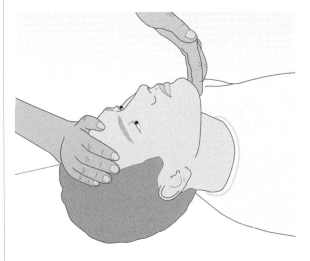

Fig. 12.2 Opening the airway by tilting the head and lifting the chin.

A

B

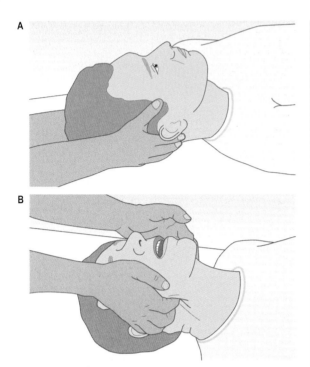

Fig. 12.3 In patients with suspected neck injury (A) control the head and neck manually and (B) open the airway using the jaw-thrust technique.

may help to maintain the airway in patients with altered consciousness (Fig. 12.4). Do not use a nasopharyngeal airway if you suspect a skull-base fracture or if epistaxis, nasal trauma or deformity is present or the patient is taking anticoagulant therapy. Maintain the patient's airway as described until senior experienced help arrives. Tracheal intubation may then be undertaken if the patient cannot maintain a patent airway, but should only be performed by an experienced clinician (Table 12.7).

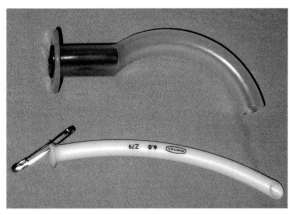

Fig. 12.4 Guedel airway (top); nasopharyngeal airway (bottom).

12.7	Principal indications for emergency advanced airway and ventilation techniques

- Apnoea
- Inability to maintain a patent airway by simple airway manoeuvres and adjuncts (Fig. 12.4)
- Inability to protect the airway, e.g. facial trauma, uncontrolled vomiting/bleeding
- Glasgow Coma Scale < 9
- Inability to maintain adequate oxygenation and ventilation
- Requirement for controlled ventilation, e.g. because of raised intracranial pressure
- Potential for subsequent clinical deterioration, e.g. orofacial or respiratory burns
- Patients at potential risk due to environment, e.g. CT/MR scanning or ambulance transfer

B: Breathing

Give the patient oxygen. Hypoxia hastens and causes death. Give the highest possible concentration of oxygen initially. Use a tight-fitting anaesthetic mask, or an oxygen mask with a reservoir bag and an oxygen flow rate of 15 l/min (Fig. 12.5). The *only* exception to this initial treatment is where you know the patient has chronic obstructive pulmonary disease with CO_2 retention (type II respiratory failure). These patients lose the hypoxic stimulus to breathe if given high concentrations of oxygen. They then develop progressive hypoventilation, hypercapnoea and CO_2 narcosis.

Recognize and treat open pneumothorax or a pneumothorax under tension at this stage. Expose the patient's chest and abdomen and look for wounds (usually gunshot or stab) producing an open defect in the chest wall (Fig. 12.6). Remember to examine the back and axillae. An open chest wound equalizes pressure between the pleural space and atmosphere by direct communication and the affected lung is unable to expand or contract normally with respiration.

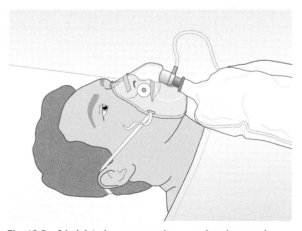

Fig. 12.5 Administering oxygen using a mask and reservoir bag.

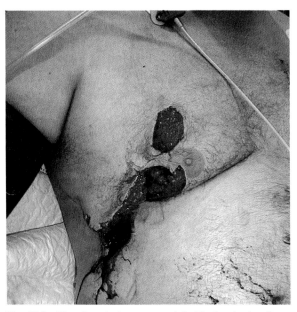

Fig. 12.6 **Wound producing an open defect in the chest wall.**

During inspiration and expiration, you can often hear air movement and see a spray of blood at the wound site. Cover the wound with a sterile occlusive dressing (in extremis use a small sheet of polythene) and secure it on *three* sides only. This allows air to escape from the pleural space during expiration and impedes air entry during inspiration. A formal tube thoracostomy with underwater seal drainage is then needed.

Tension pneumothorax occurs when lung injury produces a one-way valve effect (Fig. 12.7). With each inspiration air escapes from the lung and accumulates in the pleural space where it is unable to escape. As the pleural pressure increases, the ipsilateral lung progressively collapses and the mediastinum is shifted to the opposite side. This, and the increased intrathoracic pressure, reduces venous return to the heart and eventually causes cardiac arrest.

Suspect tension pneumothorax in any patient who develops severe respiratory and cardiovascular distress over a period of minutes. It occurs most commonly in penetrating or closed chest injury, patients having positive-pressure ventilation or those with underlying lung disease (especially when ventilated). The diagnosis is a clinical one. The patient appears acutely breathless, agitated, has a rapid pulse and may be cyanosed. Hypotension, bradycardia and altered consciousness are preterminal features. Quickly examine for jugular venous distension, tachycardia, and absent breath sounds on the affected side. Tracheal deviation to the contra-lateral side may be present. Do not delay resuscitation to perform a chest X-ray. Immediately insert a large-bore (16 or 18 FG) intravenous cannula through the second intercostal space in the midclavicular line on the affected side. Remove the needle. A hiss of air escaping from the cannula confirms the diagnosis and should be followed by rapid improvement in the patient's clinical state. Formal tube thoracostomy with underwater seal drainage can then be performed.

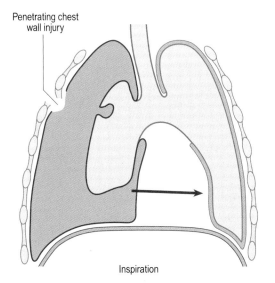
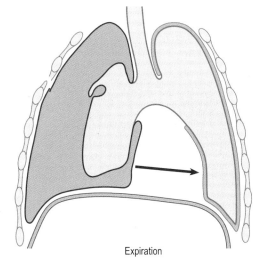

Penetrating chest wall injury

Inspiration

Expiration

Fig. 12.7 **Tension pneumothorax.** Right pneumothorax under tension; air enters the pleural cavity via the punctured lung during inspiration. The lung defect acts as a one-way valve and air cannot escape from the pleural cavity during expiration. The injured right lung progressively collapses. The increased pleural pressure shifts the mediastinal structures to the left.

For the subsequent assessment of B (Breathing) follow the format of Chapter 2. Note, however, that the patient may be unable to sit up, necessitating a supine examination. If the oxygen mask is 'misting' on exhalation the patient has (some) respiratory effort. Look for movements of the chest (including the accessory muscles) and the abdomen. Paradoxical respiration, movement of the abdomen exactly out of phase with that of the chest, is a sign of respiratory compromise. It is most often due to fatigue of the muscle of the diaphragm and/or upper or lower airway obstruction. Look for abnormal breathing patterns (Table 12.8). Signs of injury (bruising, pattern imprinting, wounds) and of flail segment may be seen in trauma patients. In a 'flail' segment the affected area moves paradoxically with respiration, i.e. it moves outwards with respect to the rest of the chest wall during expiration and inwards during inspiration. To detect a flail segment kneel at the patient's side and look tangentially across the chest wall. The area is often well localized and clearly seen. Identification is important as it implies that at least three ribs are broken in at least two places (Fig. 12.8), and underlying lung injury is common.

Feel in the suprasternal notch to assess the position of the trachea. In trauma patients, systematically palpate the chest gently to identify any areas of injury. Rib and sternal fractures are associated with localized discomfort. Subcutaneous emphysema feels like 'crackling' under your fingers. Examine for consolidation, pneumothorax, pleural effusion or haemothorax.

Auscultate for breath sounds and added sounds, such as wheezes, crackles and pleural or pericardial rubs. Critically ill patients may not have the signs you expect. For example,

12.8	**Respiratory patterns**
	Common causes
Tachypnoea	Anxiety, pain, asthma, metabolic acidosis, chest injury, pneumothorax, pulmonary embolus, brain stem stroke
Bradypnoea/apnoea	Cardiac arrest, opioids, central neurological causes (stroke, head injury)
Cheyne–Stokes respiration	Left ventricular failure, central neurological causes (stroke, head injury), overdose (barbiturates, γ-hydroxybutyrate, opioids)
Küssmaul respiration	Metabolic acidosis – diabetic ketoacidosis, uraemia, hepatic failure, shock (lactic acidosis), overdose (methanol, ethylene glycol, salicylate)
Paradoxical respiration	Respiratory failure, Guillain–Barré syndrome, high spinal cord lesions

a patient with life-threatening asthma may have little or no wheeze (a silent chest) because airflow into the lungs is so poor.

Central cyanosis is a late and unreliable sign of hypoxia. Even in states of critical hypoxia, cyanosis may be completely absent because of severe anaemia or massive blood loss.

Pulse oximetry is a useful adjunct to clinical examination. It is a simple, non-invasive and relatively inexpensive method to assess peripheral oxygenation. Attach a probe to a finger tip (Fig. 4.24) or ear lobe. An SaO_2 of < 92% indicates hypoxia.

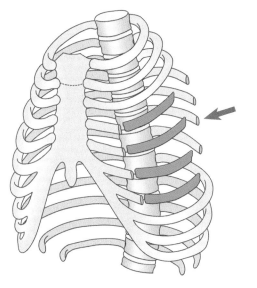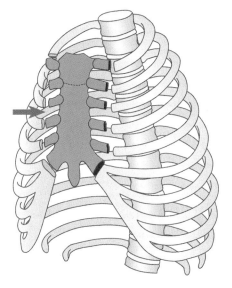

Fig. 12.8 Flail chest. (A) A direct blow (arrowed) that fractures several ribs at two points will result in a flail segment. (B) A severe blow to the sternum (arrowed) may cause multiple bilateral costochondral fractures, resulting in a flail chest.

In the following situations pulse oximetry may either not be possible or give misleading values:

- shock
- hypotension
- poor peripheral perfusion
- hypothermia
- excessive movement
- nail varnish, false fingernails
- severe anaemia
- abnormal haemoglobins, e.g. met- or sulphhaemoglobin
- carbon monoxide poisoning
- skin pigmentation or excessively dirty fingers.

C: Circulation

If the patient is not responding, feel for a central (carotid or femoral) pulse for 10 seconds. If you cannot feel a pulse *and* the patient is unresponsive, treat as for cardiac arrest (Figs 12.9 and 12.10). In responsive patients, you can feel for a peripheral (most commonly radial or brachial) pulse but if you cannot palpate a peripheral pulse this suggests that the patient is significantly hypotensive. Note the pulse rate, rhythm, volume and character. Assess peripheral perfusion by pressing on the finger tip pulp for a few seconds, removing your finger and estimating the capillary refill time (normal < 2 s). Attach the patient to an ECG monitor and note the ventricular rate and the rhythm.

Control external blood losses from wounds or open fractures by direct firm pressure with a sterile dressing placed over the site. Minimize blood loss from long bone fractures (femur, tibia/fibula, humerus and forearm) by splintage.

Insert a large-bore (16 FG, 1.7 mm internal diameter or bigger) IV cannula and ensure that it is securely taped to the skin. In trauma patients, and those in whom you suspect

12.9 Initial venous blood samples
All patients
<ul><li>Stix test for blood glucose and formal blood glucose</li><li>Blood grouping and save serum</li><li>Full blood count</li><li>Urea, creatinine and electrolytes</li></ul>
Selected patients
<ul><li>Amylase</li><li>Cross-matching</li><li>Toxicology screen</li><li>Coagulation screen</li><li>Liver function tests</li><li>Blood cultures</li></ul>

hypovolaemia, insert and secure two large-bore cannulae. Take initial blood samples (Table 12.9) from the cannula and then attach an IV fluid-giving set. Commence volume replacement, if needed, with warmed 0.9% saline or Ringer's solution.

Examine the neck to determine the jugular venous pressure (JVP). In a sitting or semirecumbent patient, elevation of the JVP in the presence of shock suggests a major problem with the heart's pumping ability, e.g. acute left heart failure, cardiac tamponade, massive pulmonary embolus, tension pneumothorax, or an acute valvular problem.

Check the patient's blood pressure.

Examine the precordium and heart as described in Chapter 3, in particular identifying the presence of added heart sounds or murmurs.

Insert a urinary catheter (unless there is evidence of urethral or prostatic injury – blood at the urethral meatus and/or a high-riding, 'boggy' prostate on rectal examination), to monitor urine output.

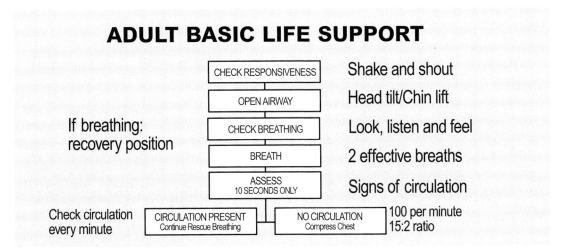

Fig. 12.9 Adult basic life-support algorithm.

12.10 Clinical features of shock
• Altered consciousness, confusion, irritability
• Pallor, cool skin, sweating
• Heart rate > 100/min
• Hypotension (systolic BP < 100 mmHg): *NB. hypotension is a late sign*
• Respiratory rate > 30/min
• Oliguria (urine output < 0.5–1 ml/kg/h)

At a cellular level the term 'shock' implies that the oxygen and blood supply to an organ or tissue is inadequate for its metabolic requirements. Clinically, shock is recognized by a combination of features (Table 12.10). The extent to which each feature is present depends upon the cause of the underlying shock process (Table 12.11) and the time course. In certain groups of patients signs of shock may be delayed or obscured by their condition. These include athletes, pregnant women, those on vasoactive drugs (beta-blockers, calcium-channel blockers, angiotensin-converting enzyme inhibitors), those with pacemakers and the very young and old.

Tachycardia (pulse rate > 100/min) and hypotension (systolic blood pressure < 100 mmHg) are not necessarily required to diagnose shock. The heart rate may be normal, or even low, in hypoxic shocked patients or those on drugs such as beta-blockers. Blood pressure may be temporarily maintained by excess sympathetic activity and peripheral vasoconstriction. In critically ill patients non-invasive cuff blood pressure measurements are often inaccurate. Do not concentrate on absolute figures of systolic or diastolic blood pressure. Readings of 90/50 mmHg are normal in many healthy young women, while 120/70 mmHg indicates significant hypotension in a patient whose pressures are usually 195/115 mmHg. Trends in pulse and BP give far more information than initial or isolated readings. If a patient who you think has hypovolaemia has a rising pulse rate with a falling blood pressure and reduced urine output, this strongly implies continuing volume loss and inadequate replacement.

In a trauma patient the most likely cause of shock is blood loss leading to hypovolaemia. External blood loss from wounds and compound fractures is usually apparent, but haemorrhage into abdomen, chest and from closed long bone or pelvic fractures will be less obvious. Examine these areas as part of the primary survey.

D: Disability

Rapidly assess the patient's Glasgow Coma Score. Record the three components: eye opening, verbal response and motor response (see Table 8.7, p. 237). Examine the limbs for localizing signs or paraplegia. Check the pupils for size, reactivity and equality of reaction to light. In coma patients the presence or absence of a pupillary light reflex helps differentiate structural (intracranial haemorrhage, infarction) from metabolic (poisoning, hypoglycaemia, sepsis) causes. In structural causes of coma the light reflex is usually absent; in metabolic causes it is usually present. Difference between the pupil sizes (anisocaria) may help: a difference in pupillary diameters > 1 mm suggests a structural cause.

Hypoglycaemia

Check every patient's blood glucose using a Stix test (Fig. 12.11). Hypoglycaemia usually causes a global neurological deficit with reduced consciousness, but may present with irritability, erratic or violent behaviour (sometimes mistaken for alcohol or drug intoxication), seizures or focal neurological deficits, e.g. hemiplegia.

If the Stix test reading is < 3 mmol/l take a venous sample for formal blood glucose measurement, *but do not wait for this result before giving treatment*. Give 25–50 ml of 50% dextrose IV followed by a flush of saline to reduce the development of thrombophlebitis (the dextrose solution is very hypertonic). If you cannot obtain venous access rapidly, give 1 mg glucagon by subcutaneous or intramuscular injection. If hypoglycaemia is the cause of the altered mental state the patient's conscious level should start to improve in 10–20 minutes. Repeat the Stix test to confirm correction of hypoglycaemia. Persistent altered consciousness in a patient whose hypoglycaemia has been adequately corrected implies coexistent pathology, e.g. stroke, or the development of cerebral oedema from prolonged neuroglycopenia. In patients with hypoglycaemia where you suspect chronic alcohol use or withdrawal, or malnutrition, give 100 mg IV thiamine to prevent and treat Wernicke's syndrome.

12.11 Classification of shock	
Hypovolaemic	
Blood loss	Trauma, GI or obstetric haemorrhage, abdominal aortic aneurysm rupture
Fluid loss	Burns, GI loss (diarrhoea, vomiting), severe dehydration, diabetic ketoacidosis, 'third space' losses, e.g. sepsis, pancreatitis, ischaemic bowel
Cardiogenic	Arrhythmia, myocardial infarction, myocarditis, acute valve failure, overdose of negatively inotropic drugs, e.g. calcium-channel or β-blocker
Obstructive	Major pulmonary embolism, tension pneumothorax, cardiac tamponade, acute valve obstruction
Neurogenic	Major cerebral or spinal injury
Others	
Toxic causes	Carbon monoxide, cyanide, hydrogen sulphide, poisons causing methaemoglobinaemia
Anaphylaxis	

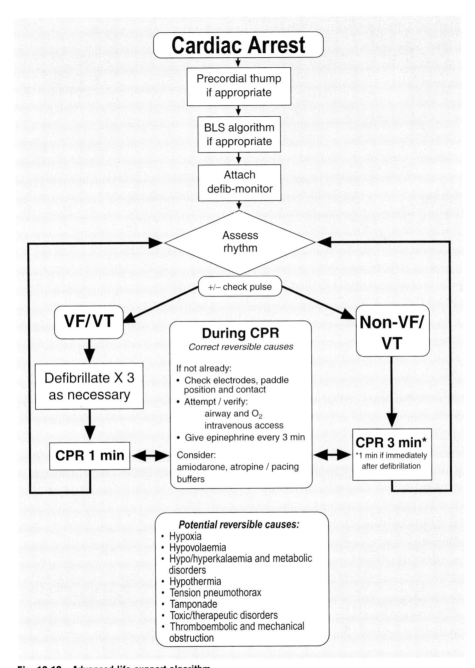

Fig. 12.10 Advanced life-support algorithm.

Overdose

If you cannot clearly identify a cause for the patient's altered conscious state consider drug overdose. The commonest drugs to threaten life acutely are opioids. Cardinal features of opioid overdose are altered consciousness, respiratory depression (reduced respiratory rate and volume) and small pupils. Naloxone is a specific opioid antagonist with no agonist activity. Give 0.8–2 mg IV naloxone as a diagnostic aid and definitive treatment to *any* patient in whom you have not identified a clear cause for altered consciousness. If the patient's altered consciousness is due solely, or in part, to opioid intoxication, a response is seen within 30–60 seconds of IV administration. If IV access is difficult, naloxone can be given by subcutaneous or intramuscular routes. If the patient responds, further doses will probably be needed.

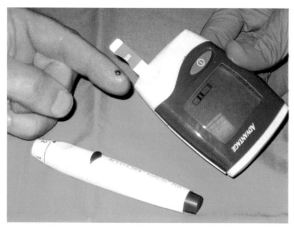

Fig. 12.11 Monitoring blood glucose with a testing strip and meter.

Naloxone has a short duration (minutes), while the half-life of most opioids and their active metabolites is hours/days.

Seizures (fits)

Give immediate treatment to stop active focal or generalized seizures. First-line therapy is a benzodiazepine such as lorazepam (0.5–1 mg/min up to 4 mg) or diazepam (1–2 mg/min up to 10–20 mg) given IV in aliquots. If seizures continue despite this you may require other agents such as phenytoin.

Manage a seizure in a pregnant woman using the ABC approach but consider the fetus as well. Get senior obstetric and neonatal support immediately. In women > 20 weeks' gestation, position the patient in the left lateral position (most easily achieved by placing one or two pillows under the right hip). This prevents the gravid uterus obstructing venous return to the heart with consequent hypotension. Eclampsia may be the underlying cause of seizure(s) in pregnant and postpartum patients. Eclamptic seizures are associated with hypertension (diastolic BP > 100 mmHg), oedema (usually generalized and often affecting hands and face) and proteinuria. IV magnesium sulphate is a first-line treatment for eclampsia.

E: Exposure and environment

If patients are not fully undressed, remove (cut off if necessary) the remainder of their clothes. Cover them with a gown and warm blankets to prevent hypothermia and maintain their dignity. Critically ill patients lose heat rapidly and cannot maintain normal body temperature. Trauma patients may arrive on a rigid spinal board with neck immobilization. Remove them from the board to make them more comfortable, reduce the chance of pressure sores and facilitate radiological examination. If patients are conscious tell

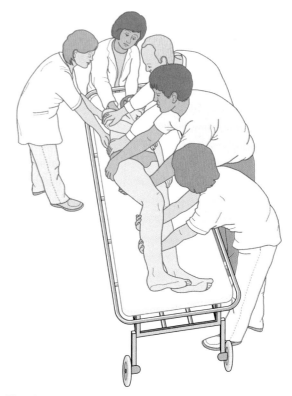

Fig. 12.12 Deployment of personnel and hand positions used when log-rolling a patient from the supine to the lateral position.

them what you are going to do before they are 'log-rolled' and lifted (Fig. 12.12). The process needs five people: one holds the head/neck and directs the procedure; one removes the spinal board and other debris including clothes and glass and quickly examines the back and spine; and the remaining three roll and hold the patient. While the patient is rolled perform a rectal examination, assess anal tone and perianal sensation and check the core temperature.

Examine the patient's skin surface rapidly, but comprehensively. Look for signs of injury including bruises and wounds. In particular, examine the scalp, perineum and axillae. Note open fractures and rashes, e.g. the non-blanching purpuric rash of meningococcal septicaemia, and hyperpigmentation (hypoadrenalism).

The stages of the primary survey are summarized in Table 12.12.

THE SECONDARY SURVEY

The secondary survey reassesses the patient after the initial examination and emergency interventions of the primary survey are complete. This is a careful, systematic and detailed top-to-toe examination to fully document additional signs and identify injuries in the trauma patient. Only start

12.12	The primary survey: investigations and interventions
A	Administer high-flow oxygen
B	Measure respiratory rate and SaO_2
C	Monitor the ECG continuously and measure BP (by cuff) every 5 min Insert and secure large-bore IV cannula(e) and take venous blood samples 'Stix' test for blood glucose
D	Record the Glasgow Coma score Record pupil size and reactivity
E	Measure core (rectal or tympanic membrane) temperature
Others	Arterial blood gas measurement 12-lead ECG Chest X-ray (+ pelvic and cervical spine views in multiply injured) Urinary catheter[a] (and measure urine output hourly) Urinalysis (Stix test) for blood, protein, glucose, ketones, nitrite, bilirubin and urobilinogen Urine pregnancy test in females Nasogastric tube[b]

[a] Contraindicated if urethral injury suspected
[b] Contraindicated if skull-base fracture suspected

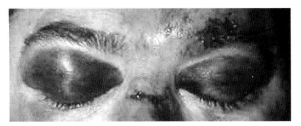

Fig. 12.13 Periorbital bruising ('racoon' or 'panda' eyes).

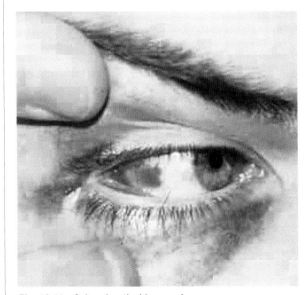

Fig. 12.14 Subconjunctival haemorrhage.

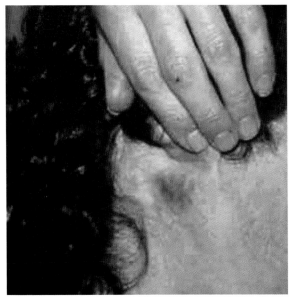

Fig. 12.15 Battle's sign.

the secondary survey once you are confident that there is no immediate need for further resuscitation and if the patient does not need immediate transfer for definitive care, e.g. to theatre for a patient with a ruptured abdominal aortic aneurysm.

Make sure that the patient is not in pain. Adequate analgesia is needed for *all* patients in pain. There is no 'standard' dose. In critically ill patients the optimal approach is to slowly titrate an opioid drug, e.g. morphine, IV in 1–2 mg aliquots to achieve the desired effect. The amount needed varies with the patient and any adverse effects produced by the opioid. An antiemetic, e.g. cyclizine is often required.

Examine the entire body surface including the scalp, eyes, ears, mouth and face. Carry out a more detailed examination of all relevant systems. Organize further investigations and treatment after this to confirm the cause of the patient's condition. Continually re-evaluate patients to see that they are responding to treatment. If they deteriorate, or you are unsure about their clinical status, return to the primary survey.

Start by examining the head. In the trauma patient palpate the scalp for areas of swelling and look for wounds which may be hidden in thick or tangled hair. Look for signs of skull-base fracture. These include periorbital bruising ('racoon' or 'panda' eyes) (Fig. 12.13), subconjunctival haemorrhage (usually without a posterior margin) (Fig. 12.14), oto- or rhinorrhoea, and bleeding from the ear or behind the tympanic membrane (haemotympanum). Battle's sign (bruising over the mastoid process) (Fig. 12.15) may be seen but usually takes 1–3 days to develop. Examine the eyes for foreign bodies including retained contact lenses (remove them at this stage) and signs of chronic disease such as jaundice or anaemia. If corneal abrasions are suspected, stain the eye with fluorescein to identify them. Assess the pupils for size, shape, and reactivity to light and accommodation. Then examine the eye movements, visual acuity and the optic fundi. Refer urgently to a specialist ophthalmologist any patient with penetrating injury, disruption of the globe or loss of vision.

Look in the mouth for injury to the palate, tongue and teeth. Check the ears and throat for potential sources of infection. Smell the patient's breath. The sweet odour of ketones in diabetic ketoacidosis is unmistakable, but not everyone can detect it. Severe uraemia has a 'fishy' quality to the smell and the fetor hepaticus of hepatic failure a 'mousy' one due to methyl mercaptan. Note if a patient smells of alcohol but *never* attribute altered conscious level to alcohol alone. Blood or breath alcohol level measurements are unnecessary in an emergency since neither correlate usefully with conscious state.

Assume that the spine and/or spinal cord is injured in all trauma patients especially those with altered consciousness. Conscious patients may complain of localized neck or back pain, but may be distracted by pain from other sites of injury. Maintain spinal immobilization until you can exclude underlying injury. This is rarely possible in the initial assessment period, and in many cases you will need imaging by plain X-ray, CT or MR scan to exclude cord or bony injury (Fig. 12.16).

If there is no history of trauma, ask the patient to flex the neck to touch the chin on the chest. If this causes discomfort, *gently* flex the neck passively. Meningeal irritation causes spasm of the paraspinal neck muscles with neck stiffness. Meningitis and subarachnoid haemorrhage are common causes and may be associated with photophobia and a positive Kernig's sign (see p. 240). Neck stiffness may, however, be absent in early presentations of these conditions or if the patient has altered consciousness.

Re-examine the chest and precordium in detail as outlined in Chapter 3. The back of the chest should be examined during the log-roll process. A 12-lead ECG and chest X-ray are needed in all critically ill or injured patients. In these circumstances an anteroposterior chest X-ray is usually taken with the patient supine. This produces apparent enlargement of the heart and mediastinum. Small or moderate-sized pneumothoraces, pleural effusion and haemothoraces are often difficult to identify.

Examine the abdomen with the pelvis and perineum. Perform a rectal and vaginal examination if necessary. A

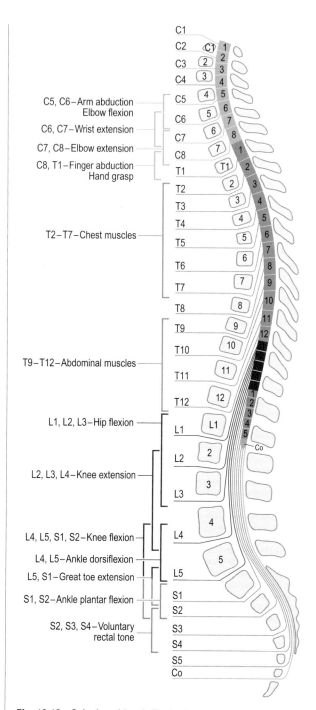

Fig. 12.16 Spinal cord level. The level can be delineated by physical examination, including a detailed neurological examination.

rectal examination, to help identify gastrointestinal bleeding, is mandatory in patients presenting with signs of hypovolaemia. In trauma patients examine the perineum, rectum and urethral orifice before inserting a urinary catheter. In male patients urethral disruption (a contraindication to urethral catheterization) is usually associated with blood at the urethral meatus, and a 'boggy' high-riding prostate.

Check perianal sensation and rectal sphincter tone to assess potential spinal cord injury. Perform a urinary pregnancy test in all women of child-bearing age and consider retained tampon as a cause of septic shock in all menstruating females. Clinical assessment of the pelvis is often misleading. A pelvic X-ray is required in patients with significant injury, as major blood loss can occur from the pelvis. Do not 'spring' the pelvis to assess stability as this may precipitate further bleeding.

Examine each limb in turn. Include a musculoskeletal examination in injured patients. Look for wounds, swelling and bruising; palpate all bones and joints for tenderness and crepitus and assess passive and active joint movements. Always examine the neurovascular integrity of the limb distal to any injury.

Now perform a full neurological examination. This is particularly important in patients with altered conscious level or possible spinal injury. The neurological examination gives a good opportunity to examine the entire skin surface. Do not omit examination of the genital area and perineum.

Certain skin colours may give clues as to the underlying diagnosis including, pallor (blood loss or anaemia), jaundice (hepatic failure), vitiligo or pigmentation in sun-exposed areas, recent scars and skin creases (Addison's disease). Look for rashes (in particular, the non-blanching purpuric rash of meningococcal disease) (Fig. 12.17), foci of infection (cellulitis, abscesses, erysipelas), bruising and

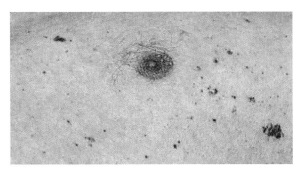

Fig. 12.17 Meningococcal rash.

wounds. Examine joints for swelling suggesting septic or reactive arthritis.

Remember to ensure tetanus prophylaxis for all trauma patients who are non-immune. Antibiotic therapy is mandatory at this stage for patients with presumed meningococcal disease, septic shock and those with open fractures but otherwise the timing and agent(s) used should be determined by further investigation and response.

Accurately document all investigations, therapy and response to treatment. Do not wait for a complete assessment or for results of investigations before getting senior help. Stop the assessment process if you identify the need for immediate definitive care or investigation. Let the receiving team know the exact stage of the assessment process you have reached when you hand over care of the patient.

DEFINITIVE TREATMENT

Once stable, the patient will need to be moved to a critical care area, theatre, scanning room or another hospital. This is a high-risk process and you need to ensure you are sufficiently trained to accompany the patient. The critically ill patient needs to be adequately monitored and as 'stable' as possible. All relevant documentation and investigation results should go with the patient and there should be clear lines of communication between clinicians.

You may discover during the primary or secondary surveys that the patient is terminally ill and that this crisis is not unexpected. It may not be appropriate for the patient to be given aggressive or 'heroic' treatment. Recognizing and preparing for a patient's death is difficult but essential. Whenever possible, communicate with the patient, the family, the GP and the senior clinician involved in the patient's prior care. The patient must be cared for in a dignified manner, with especial emphasis on analgesia, relief of distressing symptoms and the highest quality of nursing care.

◆ Key points

- Get senior experienced help now.
- Simple things save lives. Follow the ABC approach.
- 'Classical' signs of shock are often unreliable and late.
- A patient in pain needs appropriate and adequate analgesia.
- Trends in parameters (heart rate, BP, respiratory rate, SaO_2) are more important than isolated values.
- If the patient deteriorates, re-evaluate from the beginning of the ABC sequence.

Index